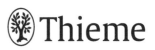

Stuttering and Related Disorders of Fluency

Fourth Edition

Patricia M. Zebrowski, PhD, CCC-SLP
Professor Emerita
Department of Communication Sciences and Disorders
University of Iowa
Iowa City, Iowa, USA

Julie D. Anderson, PhD, CCC-SLP
Associate Professor
Department of Speech, Language and Hearing Sciences
Indiana University
Bloomington, Indiana, USA

Edward G. Conture, PhD, CCC-SLP
Professor Emeritus
Department of Hearing and Speech Sciences
Vanderbilt University
Nashville, Tennessee, USA

78 illustrations

Thieme
New York • Stuttgart • Delhi • Rio de Janeiro

Library of Congress Cataloging-in-Publication Data is available from the publisher.

Important note: Medicine is an ever-changing science undergoing continual development. Research and clinical experience are continually expanding our knowledge, in particular our knowledge of proper treatment and drug therapy. Insofar as this book mentions any dosage or application, readers may rest assured that the authors, editors, and publishers have made every effort to ensure that such references are in accordance with **the state of knowledge at the time of production of the book**.

Nevertheless, this does not involve, imply, or express any guarantee or responsibility on the part of the publishers in respect to any dosage instructions and forms of applications stated in the book. **Every user is requested to examine carefully** the manufacturers' leaflets accompanying each drug and to check, if necessary in consultation with a physician or specialist, whether the dosage schedules mentioned therein or the contraindications stated by the manufacturers differ from the statements made in the present book. Such examination is particularly important with drugs that are either rarely used or have been newly released on the market. Every dosage schedule or every form of application used is entirely at the user's own risk and responsibility. The authors and publishers request every user to report to the publishers any discrepancies or inaccuracies noticed. If errors in this work are found after publication, errata will be posted at www.thieme.com on the product description page.

Some of the product names, patents, and registered designs referred to in this book are in fact registered trademarks or proprietary names even though specific reference to this fact is not always made in the text. Therefore, the appearance of a name without designation as proprietary is not to be construed as a representation by the publisher that it is in the public domain.

Thieme addresses people of all gender identities equally. We encourage our authors to use gender-neutral or gender-equal expressions wherever the context allows.

Thieme Medical Publishers, Inc.
333 Seventh Avenue,
New York, NY 10001, USA
+1 800 782 3488,
customerservice@thieme.com

Cover design: © Thieme
Related Fluency Disorders icon:
© AlexBlogoodf/stock.adobe.com

Typesetting by TNQ Technologies, India

Printed in Germany by Beltz Grafische Betriebe   5 4 3 2 1

ISBN: 978-1-68420-253-9

Also available as an e-book:
eISBN (PDF): 978-1-68420-254-6
eISBN (epub): 978-1-63853-707-6

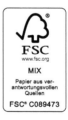

For Ray—my steadfast partner then, now, and everywhere in between. I love you. And for the mentors, students, colleagues, and the people who stutter and have shared themselves with me. You have been my greatest teachers, and I am forever grateful for what I learned from you.

Patricia M. Zebrowski

To my family who have always been there for me, my students who have challenged me to be a better professor, and my cats who kept me company as I wrote (even though they sometimes made it difficult to type or sat on the keyboard).

Julie D. Anderson

To the many family members, friends, mentors, professors, students, and teachers who helped me take the road, in the words of Robert Frost, "...less traveled by, and that has made all the difference."

Edward G. Conture

Contents

Section I: Some Characteristics and Theories

Section II: Processes Associated with Stuttering

Contents

Section IV: Treatment of Stuttering

Section V: Additional Treatment Considerations

15   Pharmacological Considerations 236

Lisa LaSalle, Angharad Ames, and Gerald Maguire

Section VI: Related Fluency Disorders

16   Cluttering: Etiology, Symptomatology, Identification, and Treatment...................... 259

Kathleen Scaler Scott, Hilda Sønsterud, and Isabella Reichel

Contents

17 Acquired Stuttering: Etiology, Symptomatology, Identification, and Treatment 271
Catherine Theys and Luc F. De Nil

Videos

Video 17.1: This video provides supporting information for the case study in the chapter. The selected video clip shows B. while having a spontaneous conversation with a reporter for a TV interview. This interview was recorded 1 month before B.'s first stroke and provides evidence of her prestroke fluent speech.

Video 17.2: This video provides supporting information for the case study in the chapter. The selected video clip shows B. while having a spontaneous conversation with the speech language pathologist during the first assessment session. It shows the occurrence of poststroke stuttering disfluencies.

Video 17.3: This video provides supporting information for the case study in the chapter. The selected video clip shows B. while using the paced speech approach toward the end of the first treatment block. It shows the increase in fluency while using this technique.

Foreword

When I received an invitation from Patricia M. Zebrowski, Julie D. Anderson, and Edward G. Conture to write this foreword for their book, it provided me with an extraordinary and unexpected opportunity to consider the current evidence in the field, especially as it relates to our clients and families. I have sat at the feet of these authors (literally, on one occasion, as there were no empty seats in the auditorium at ASHA!). I am in awe of their astonishing intellect, their phenomenal clinical skills, and their vast experience in the world of stuttering and I know that anything they teach is worth learning, anything they say is worth listening to, and anything they write is worth reading.

Throughout this text, one can hear the authors' voices—their personal styles shine through in a very engaging way. Their depth of knowledge and enthusiasm for their area of expertise jump out from their chapters. They bring therapy to life in the case examples they describe. I am fortunate to know most of these contributors and you will too by the time you have finished reading their chapters. And if you are wise, you will open other journals and books and attend conferences and courses and webinars, where you will encounter them and other talented colleagues who share this quest to understand more about stuttering to be the best researcher, teacher, and therapist you can be.

It is my honor to follow in the footsteps of—and currently head up—a team of phenomenally talented therapists at the Michael Palin Centre. As a specialist center for stammering, as we Brits call it, it is our responsibility to maintain the highest possible level of knowledge and expertise to support our clients—children, teenagers, parents, adults—as well as our therapy colleagues. Some questions from clients and families truly stretch us, necessitating some research before we can give an informed response. We hold a responsibility to impart knowledge and advice and to deliver therapy services which are based on sound and contemporary theoretical evidence and learning from our expert colleagues in other settings. To that end, this text is an extraordinary synthesis of a vast array of academic, research, and clinical expertise. The editors have invited contributions from the key authorities in the world of stuttering and related fluency disorders. Readers will acquire a comprehensive understanding of the wide range and depth of research and practical methodology.

In sections I and II, various authors who are at the heart of the current explosion in our knowledge base take us through the common characteristics and the theories of stuttering, going into depth on the genetic, speech, language, and cognitive, neural and physiological, and the temperamental and emotional processes associated with stuttering. An in-depth and yet concise summary of the research and our theoretical understanding about stuttering are presented by those who have undertaken the studies and made the learning accessible so that it can be translated into our clinical practice. These chapters are a wonderful resource as we seek to understand stuttering so that we can, in turn, explain it to our students, our therapist colleagues, the children, young people, parents, and adults who seek our help, as well as wider society. These six chapters will equip us for this task as well as point us to more sources of research to encourage us to keep learning and deepening our understanding.

In section III, a range of expert therapists in pre-school, school-age, adolescent, and adult stuttering provide us with detailed and highly practical descriptions of the assessment and diagnosis of stuttering. A therapist who is not sure what to do with a child or adult who is referred for evaluation can simply follow the content of these chapters. In doing so, they will cover all the important aspects which will equip them and their clients to make sound decisions about next steps.

Section IV takes the reader through the many therapy options across the age ranges, with contributions from highly experienced therapists, covering a wide range of approaches. Importantly, the theoretical framework and rationales are presented, enabling readers to consider how different approaches might suit different children and clients. Further reading and training will help the therapists to develop their knowledge and skills with these different approaches, and this comprehensive summary will help steer that ongoing process.

In section V, we are provided with an invaluable understanding of language, phonological, bilingual, and multicultural considerations in assessment and treatment, followed by a summary of the research on pharmacology. The authors are leaders in these fields, and in these chapters, the reader will find answers to many questions we are asked by families and colleagues, as well as pointers to further research to give depth to our knowledge. Finally, section VI covers cluttering and acquired stuttering. It may be that these are conditions that therapists encounter less frequently and about which they consequently feel less knowledgeable, skillful, and confident. The two chapters in this section present an up-to-date and concise summary of the relevant research and therapy approaches, again from researchers and therapists who are expert in these areas, equipping us all to expand our own spheres of understanding, confidence, and expertise.

I have had the privilege of working in the field of stuttering and cluttering for many years than I care to admit. How come I have not diversified, become bored with this area, branched out into something shiny and new? The simple answer is because I have never stopped learning, being challenged, being inspired. I am where I am because I have learned so much from my colleagues across the globe. There is always something shiny and new to learn about, to challenge my preconceptions, to stretch my thinking, to try out and evaluate. We are all a work in progress and this book is an invaluable tool in our ongoing development.

Elaine Kelman
Consultant Speech and Language Therapist
Head of the Michael Palin Centre for Stammering
London, United Kingdom

Preface

"Life is divided into three terms—that which was, which is, and which will be. Let us learn from the past to profit by the present and from the present live better in the future."

William Wordsworth (b. 1770, d. 1850)

Inspired by Mr. Wordsworth's philosophy, our goal for the revised edition of this book is to provide students with an understanding of how the past informs our present understanding of stuttering. Our hope is that by honoring both, we will create a bright future of promise for people who stutter and the clinicians and researchers who are their allies.

Initially developed over 30 years ago, the first three editions of this book bore the same title; the first two were edited by the late Dr. Richard F. Curlee and the last was co-edited by Dr. Curlee and Dr. Edward G. Conture. Dr. Curlee was a broad-minded clinician and scholar, whose wide and deep knowledge of stuttering was the catalyst for bringing together a diverse set of contributors in those earlier editions of this book. Walking in the footsteps of Dr. Curlee, we believe and hope that this fourth edition is true to the notion, as Wordsworth proposed, that the discoveries of the past are the bedrock of the present and the inspiration for our future explorations into the nature and treatment of stuttering. Beginning with basic facts and theories, the chapter contents transition to describe the key factors that likely contribute to the emergence and development of stuttering. This content sets the stage for subsequent chapters on the comprehensive evaluation and treatment of stuttering and related fluency disorders across the lifespan.

We received contributions from among the best and brightest academicians, clinicians, and researchers in the field of stuttering and related disorders. Their names and reputations speak for themselves, but it is the collective wisdom and experience of each one of these authors that makes the whole of the book greater than the sum of its parts. Each chapter has been thoroughly edited and reviewed by the co-editors to ensure that the material is as accessible as possible to both students and instructors alike. Some of the areas covered in this book may be on the frontiers of some readers' knowledge, but rest assured all represent active, current, and important topics that need to be included in any modern-day, comprehensive discussion of the nature and treatment of stuttering.

Last, but not least, we acknowledge our friends and loved ones who often had to share our attention and time "with the book." Their advice, suggestions, and support along the way have been invaluable. That said, whatever flaws that remain are totally the editors' doing. We remain humbled by the enormity of the landscape our chapter authors have helped us traverse, while at the same time remain excited by the positive impact this work will have on the future of people who stutter and their families.

As Daniel Goleman, of emotional intelligence fame, has suggested, "Nothing important gets done alone." Nothing more truly describes the combined efforts of chapter authors, book co-editors, and Thieme staff in the development of this book!

Patricia M. Zebrowski, PhD, CCC-SLP
Julie D. Anderson, PhD, CCC-SLP
Edward G. Conture, PhD, CCC-SLP

Contributors

Angharad Ames, MD, MA
Chief Resident
Department of Psychiatry and Neuroscience
Riverside School of Medicine
University of California
Riverside, California, USA

Julie D. Anderson, PhD, CCC-SLP
Associate Professor
Department of Speech, Language and Hearing Sciences
Indiana University
Bloomington, Indiana, USA

Hayley S. Arnold, PhD
Associate Professor
Speech Pathology and Audiology Program
School of Health Sciences
Kent State University
Kent, Ohio, USA

Deryk Beal, PhD
Senior Scientist
Bloorview Research Institute
Holland Bloorview Kids Rehabilitation Hospital
Toronto, Ontario, Canada

Janet Beilby, BS, MS, PhD, FSPA, MPSPA, MASLHA
Associate Professor
Dementia Program Lead Curtin enAble Institute
Faculty of Health Sciences
Curtin School of Allied Health
Perth, Australia

Jennifer E. Below, PhD
Associate Professor
Department of Medicine
Division of Genetic Medicine
Vanderbilt University Medical Center
Vanderbilt Genetics Institute
Nashville, Tennessee, USA

Courtney Byrd, PhD, CCC-SLP
Professor
Department of Speech, Language, and Hearing Sciences
Arthur M. Blank Center for Stuttering
    Education and Research
University of Texas at Austin
Austin, Texas, USA

Dahye Choi, PhD
Associate Professor
Department of Speech Pathology and Audiology
University of South Alabama
Mobile, Alabama, USA

Craig Coleman, MA, CCC-SLP, BCS-F, ASHA-F
Assistant Professor and Department Chairperson
Department of Communication Sciences and Disorders
Edinboro University
Pennsylvania Western University
Edinboro, Pennsylvania, USA

Edward G. Conture, PhD, CCC-SLP
Professor Emeritus
Department of Hearing and Speech Sciences
Vanderbilt University
Nashville, Tennessee, USA

Anthony DiLollo, PhD
Professor and Director
Davies School of Communication Sciences and Disorders
Texas Christian University
Fort Worth, Texas, USA

Kurt Eggers, BA, MA, PhD
Professor
Department of Rehabilitation Sciences
Ghent University
Ghent, Belgium;
Department of Speech-Language Pathology
Thomas More University of Applied Sciences
Antwerp, Belgium;
Department of Psychology and Speech-Language
    Pathology
University of Turku
Turku, Finland

Julie Fortier-Blanc, PhD
Associate Professor Emerita
Ecole d'Orthophonie et d'Audiologie
University of Montreal
Montreal, Quebec, Canada

Marie-Christine Franken, PhD
Fluency Expert and Speech and Language Research Lead
Department of Otorhinolaryngology, Speech and
   Hearing Center
Sophia Children's Hospital
Erasmus University Medical Center
Rotterdam, The Netherlands

Julianne Garbarino, PhD
Research Affiliate
Department of Hearing and Speech Sciences
University of Maryland
College Park, Maryland, USA

Hope Gerlach-Houck, PhD, CCC-SLP
Assistant Professor
Department of Speech, Language, and Hearing Sciences
Western Michigan University
Kalamazoo, Michigan, USA

Corrin I. Gillis, PhD, CCC-SLP
Associate Professor
Department of Communication Disorders and
   Special Education
Old Dominion University
Norfolk, Virginia, USA

Nancy E. Hall, PhD, CCC-SLP
Professor
Department of Communication Sciences and Disorders
University of Maine
Orono, Maine, USA

Anna Hearne, PhD
Speech Language Therapist
Massey University
Albany, New Zealand

Caryn Herring, MS, CCC-SLP
Doctoral Candidate
Communicative Sciences and Disorders
Michigan State University
East Lansing, Michigan, USA

Eric S. Jackson, PhD, CCC-SLP
Assistant Professor
Department of Communicative Sciences and Disorders
New York University
New York, New York, USA

Kia Noelle Johnson, PhD, CCC-SLP
Associate Professor
Department of Speech, Language, and Hearing Sciences
Arthur M. Blank Center for Stuttering
   Education and Research
University of Texas at Austin
Atlanta, Georgia, USA

Robin Jones, BS, MA, PhD
Assistant Professor
Department of Hearing and Speech Sciences
Vanderbilt Bill Wilkerson Center
Vanderbilt University Medical Center
Nashville, Tennessee, USA

Ellen M. Kelly, PhD, CCC-SLP, BCS-F
Director of Educational Innovation
Arthur M. Blank Center for Stuttering Education and
   Research
Moody College of Communication
University of Texas at Austin
Franklin, Texas, USA

Shelly Jo Kraft, PhD, CCC-SLP
Associate Professor
Department of Communication Sciences and Disorders
Wayne State University
Detroit, Michigan, USA

Lisa LaSalle, PhD, CCC-SLP
Professor
Department of Communication Sciences and Disorders
University of Redlands
Redlands, California, USA

Kenneth J. Logan, PhD, CCC-SLP
Associate Professor
Department of Speech, Language, and Hearing Sciences
University of Florida
Gainesville, Florida, USA

Gerald Maguire, MD
Professor
Department of Psychiatry
California University of Science and Medicine
Colton, California, USA

Sharon Millard, PhD
Research Lead
The Michael Palin Centre for Stammering
Whittington Hospital NHS Trust
London, United Kingdom

Luc F. De Nil, PhD
Professor
Department of Speech-Language Pathology
University of Toronto
Toronto, Ontario, Canada

Katerina Ntourou, BA, MA, PhD
Assistant Professor
Department of Communication Sciences and Disorders
Health Sciences Center
University of Oklahoma
Oklahoma City, Oklahoma, USA

Nan Bernstein Ratner, EdD
Professor
Department of Hearing and Speech Sciences
University of Maryland
College Park, Maryland, USA

Isabella Reichel, EdD
Professor
Graduate Program in Speech and Language Pathology
Touro University
Brooklyn, New York, USA

Naomi Rodgers, PhD, CCC-SLP
Assistant Professor
Department of Special Education & Communication
    Disorders
University of Nebraska-Lincoln
Lincoln, Nebraska, USA

Kathleen Scaler Scott, PhD, CCC-SLP
Associate Professor
Department of Speech-Language Pathology
Monmouth University
West Long Branch, New Jersey, USA

Cara M. Singer, PhD, CCC-SLP
Assistant Professor
Department of Communication Sciences and Disorders
Grand Valley State University
Grand Rapids, Michigan, USA

Hilda Sønsterud, PhD
Senior Advisor and Associate Professor
Department of Speech and Language Disorders
Faculty of Education and Arts
Statped, Nord University
Oslo, Norway

Anna Tendera, PhD
Department of Communication Sciences and Disorders
Faculty of Rehabilitation Medicine
University of Alberta
Edmonton, Canada

Catherine Theys, PhD
Senior Lecturer
School of Psychology, Speech, and Hearing
University of Canterbury
Christchurch, New Zealand

Victoria Tumanova, PhD
Associate Professor
Communication Sciences and Disorders
Syracuse University
Syracuse, New York, USA

Evan Usler, PhD
Assistant Professor
Department of Communication Sciences and Disorders
University of Delaware
Newark, Delaware, USA

Stacy Wagovich, PhD
Associate Dean for Research & Scholarship
College of Health Sciences
University of Texas at El Paso
El Paso, Texas, USA

J. Scott Yaruss, PhD, CCC-SLP, BCS-F, F-ASHA
Professor
Communicative Sciences and Disorders
Michigan State University
East Lansing, Michigan, USA

Patricia M. Zebrowski, PhD, CCC-SLP
Professor Emerita
Department of Communication Sciences and Disorders
University of Iowa
Iowa City, Iowa, USA

Hatun Zengin-Bolatkale, BS, MA, PhD
Assistant Professor
Communicative Sciences and Deaf Studies
California State University
Fresno, California, USA

Section I

Some Characteristics and Theories

1 Common Characteristics

Edward G. Conture, Victoria Tumanova, and Dahye Choi

Abstract

The purpose of this chapter is to describe and discuss some of the more *common characteristics* of stuttering, particularly in children. The chapter begins with a definition of stuttering, incidence and prevalence, the types of speech disfluencies most apt to be judged as stuttering, measures of stuttering and associated variables as well as nonspeech behaviors associated with stuttering. Following that, the chapter describes basic facts about stuttering, for example, variability, an important hallmark of stuttering. Finally, the chapter discusses some of the more common behaviors (e.g., singing) and conditions (e.g., delayed auditory feedback) associated with decreases in stuttering. Underlying the above information is the fact that stuttering begins in early childhood, with more children exhibiting mild than severe stuttering, and that more children recover (70–80%) from stuttering than persist (20–30%). Although the precise mechanism that causes stuttering to emerge in young children remains unclear, multifactorial perspectives suggest that causation involves interactions among a finite number of variables. Available information further suggests that stuttering does not randomly occur within an utterance; rather it appears to be associated with speech-language aspects of the utterance (e.g., adjectives, adverbs, nouns, and verbs). Some of these speech-language aspects associated with instances of stuttering may be *unique* to the individual who stutters (e.g., stuttering on words that begin with "f"), while others are more *common* for many people who stutter (e.g., stuttering on words in the beginning of the utterance).

Keywords: stuttering, common characteristics, basic facts, children

1.1 Purpose

The purpose of this chapter is to describe the most common and well-documented characteristics of stuttering. Although no single chapter can include all such characteristics, our description should provide readers with a broad perspective regarding stuttering behaviors and associated phenomena. With such a perspective, the reader will better appreciate the information presented in subsequent chapters discussing constitutional and environmental processes associated with stuttering as well as assessment and treatment of stuttering.

1.2 Common Characteristics: Definitions of Stuttering, Speech Disfluency Types and Stuttered and Nonstuttered Disfluencies

1.2.1 Definition

Stuttering is a speech disorder that typically emerges in early childhood (i.e., for most children, stuttering onset occurs between 2.5 and 4 years of age). Stuttering is typically characterized by frequent repetitions of sounds (e.g., "S-s-see the dog") and monosyllabic words (e.g., "I-I-I am going"), sound prolongations, and interruptions in the forward flow of speech, often accompanied by physical muscle tension and struggle. The disorder has a lifetime incidence of approximately 5 to 8%, with prevalence of approximately 1% at any one point in time.[1,2] Stuttering can significantly impact children's academic, emotional, and social abilities as well as their later vocational potential and achievements.[3,4] As is true with many disorders, early detection followed by appropriate intervention has been shown to increase the odds of a successful outcome.

Stuttering can also occur, although less commonly, in older individuals experiencing neurodegenerative disease, stroke, traumatic brain injury, tumors, emotional trauma, and psychiatric disorders. For the purpose of this chapter, we will focus on developmental stuttering, which typically begins in early childhood. Adult-onset stuttering is discussed in detail in ► Chapter 17 of this book.

1.2.2 Speech Disfluency Types

Speech disfluency refers to any interruption in the rhythm and forward flow of speech. For example, when saying the sentence, "Bobby look at this," someone may say the word "Bobby" as "B-B-Bobby," repeating the first sound of the word multiple times. This type of speech disfluency is described as a "sound/syllable repetition" (i.e., "part-word repetition"). If in the same sentence someone repeats the first word multiple times, "Bobby-Bobby look at this," then this speech disfluency would be described as a multisyllabic whole-word repetition.

1.2.3 Stuttered and Nonstuttered Disfluencies

Naïve listeners as well as expert clinicians and researchers most frequently judge the following types of speech disfluencies to be "stuttered": sound/syllable repetitions, audible and inaudible sound prolongations (the latter, in particular, often referred to as "blocks"), monosyllabic whole-word repetitions, and within-word pauses. Listeners are apt to notice these speech disfluencies in someone's speech and perceive them as different, atypical, or abnormal. People who stutter often report that these "stuttered" disfluencies are associated with a feeling of loss of control and tension. On the other hand, listeners more typically perceive phrase repetitions, revisions of words, phrases, and sentences, interjections (e.g., "uh," "um"), and repetitions of multisyllabic words to be normal, "not stuttered," or typical. Often, listeners do not notice these speech disfluencies in their own or someone else's speech. Further, speakers do not usually associate these more typical speech disfluencies as being connected with any specific feeling, such as loss of control or tension.

To assess someone's speech fluency, clinicians and researchers count both types of speech disfluency: stuttered (e.g., "I-I-I will go") and nonstuttered (e.g., "I will-I will go"). The typical way to do this is to obtain a speech sample, usually during a conversation, and an oral reading sample for those children and adults who can read. Based on these samples and associated counts of stuttered and nonstuttered disfluencies, the examiner can determine the frequency of stuttered and nonstuttered disfluencies, important measures of any comprehensive assessment of stuttering. We will provide a bit more detail regarding these measures in the following sections.

Of these two categories of stuttered and nonstuttered disfluencies, it is the stuttered disfluency that is of primary focus during an assessment for stuttering. Typically, the examiner focuses on stuttered disfluencies because he or she is trying to determine whether someone stutters as well as determine the severity of their stuttering. Measures of stuttering frequency and severity are clinically important because they contribute to the diagnosis of stuttering and inform the decisions about the need for therapeutic intervention.

It should be noted, however, that although stuttering frequency and severity are related to one another, they are not identical measures (more about each measure later). As suggested earlier, these two measures—stuttering frequency and stuttering severity—are usually considered together to achieve a comprehensive index of stuttering. Although we described "stuttered" and "nonstuttered" as two different types of disfluencies earlier, it should be noted that some stuttered disfluencies (e.g., brief sound prolongations) are not always perceived as stuttering. Likewise, some nonstuttered disfluencies may be perceived as stuttered (e.g., multiple repetitions of an interjection). Despite these challenges to measurement accuracy, ▸ Table 1.1 provides examples of the different types of speech disfluencies and whether they are most apt to be judged by listeners as stuttered or nonstuttered (i.e., typical).

1.3 Common Characteristics: Measures of Stuttering and Associated Variables

1.3.1 Stuttering Frequency

As mentioned earlier, stuttering frequency and severity are the two most common measures of stuttering. Again, the first

measure, stuttering frequency, involves a count of the number of stuttered disfluencies per X number of syllables or words spoken (often expressed as "percent syllables stuttered" or "percent words stuttered"). Although counting *syllables* versus *words* when measuring stuttering frequency is the source of some debate among clinicians and researchers, both measures allow the examiner to come reasonably close to the same conclusion in terms of the frequency of stuttering.

1.3.2 Stuttering Severity

The second measure of stuttering is stuttering severity. In general, stuttering severity is a description of the degree to which stuttering interferes with typical speaking/communication. The degree of severity ranges from not very serious (i.e., mild) to quite serious (i.e., severe). Specifically, stuttering severity is often indexed by an overall or composite score that may be based on several measures. For example, the Stuttering Severity Instrument, fourth edition (SSI-4)[5] determines stuttering severity by considering the following measures: (1) *frequency* of instances of stuttering (stuttered disfluencies), (2) the average *duration* of the three longest instances of stuttering, and (3) the *quantity* and *quality* of associated nonspeech behaviors (see the explanation later). The SSI-4 is one of the norm-referenced assessments of stuttering severity although other assessments can also be employed to assess stuttering severity (e.g., Test of Childhood Stuttering [TOCS]).[6]

1.3.3 Associated (Non) Speech Behaviors

The speech and nonspeech behaviors associated with stuttering—also referred to in the literature as *accessory* or *secondary* behaviors as well as *physical concomitants*—can run the gamut from minimally to very apparent.[2,7] Indeed, as experienced clinicians can attest, parents may have little concern about their child's repetition of whole words (e.g., "I-I-I want a cookie"). However, if the child also tightly closes his or her eyelids and/or sharply turns his or her head to the side while saying "I-I-I- want a cookie," the parents are much more likely to be concerned and seek professional advice, whether from a speech-language pathologist or a pediatrician.

The quantity and quality of these associated behaviors are quite varied across people who stutter. However, in young

Table 1.1 Speech disfluencies most apt to be associated with listener judgments of stuttering and not stuttering

Instances of stuttering	Instances of not stuttering
*Speech disfluencies with **high** probability to be judged by listener as **stuttered***	*Speech disfluencies with **high** probability to be judged by listener as **not stuttered***
Sound or syllable repetitions (e.g., "I l-l-l- like vanilla ice-cream")	Sound or syllable repetitions seldom judged as not stuttered
Several iterations of single-syllable word repetition (e.g., "**I-I-I-I-** like vanilla ice cream")	One iteration single-syllable word repetitions (e.g., "**I-I** like vanilla ice-cream")
Audible sound prolongation **longer** than 0.500 seconds (e.g., "**Mmmmmm**ore cake please")	Audible sound prolongations **shorter** than 0.500 seconds (e.g., "**Mm**ore cake please")
Inaudible sound prolongation (block) **longer** than .500 seconds (e.g., "T-[0.750 seconds silence while person holds articulatory posture for 't']-oday is Monday")	Inaudible sound prolongations **shorter** than 0.500 seconds (e.g. "T-[0.250-second silence while person holds articulatory posture for 't']-oday is Monday")
Interjections (**repeated multiple times**); e.g., "I will, **ah, ah, ah, ah,** be late"	Interjections (**repeated once**); e.g., "I will, **ah,** be late"
Revisions seldom judged as stuttered	Revisions utterance (e.g., "She is—**she was** here")
Phrase repetitions seldom judged as stuttered	Phrase repetitions (e.g., "**I was—I was** here")

children who stutter, these behaviors can include eyeball movements (e.g., looking to one side or the other), eyelids opening and closing (or sometimes even fluttering), turning of the head to one side or the other, lip pressing, or pitch rises (these behaviors are just examples; such behaviors may occur with some but not every instance of stuttering). Movements of the arms and torso as well as alterations in breathing may also accompany instances of stuttering, but such "larger muscle" movements are more apt to be observed in older children, teens, and adults who stutter than in younger children.

Speaker's associated nonspeech behaviors may "…reflect a variety of cognitive, emotional, linguistic and physical events associated with childhood stuttering".[7] The following describes but a few examples of what these nonspeech behaviors may reflect:

- *Overflow behavior:* Facial or bodily acts and movements that one might see, for example, when a person is having trouble opening a jar.
- *Reduction in aversive listener feedback or reaction:* A child closing his or her eyelids, for example, during an instance of stuttering to minimize viewing a listener's startled or concerned expression or reaction.
- *Ongoing cognitive or emotional activity:* A person's attempt to avoid or not stutter, for example, by consciously selecting words believed to be less likely to be stuttered and/or an (un)conscious emotional reactions to an instance of stuttering.

Despite the apparent "uniqueness" of these associated (non) speech behaviors, most clinicians focus on modifying the child's speech disfluencies and/or any concomitant speech-language processes (e.g., difficulties with speech sound articulation[8]) that seems to contribute to these speech disfluencies. Nevertheless, the relation between the nonspeech behaviors associated with instances of stuttering remains a very intriguing window of observation through which to view the possible mechanisms associated with and/or underlying instances of stuttering.

1.3.4 Speaking Rate and Speech Naturalness

Speaking rate and speech naturalness are two additional measures (besides stuttering frequency and severity) that can be considered when determining the degree to which stuttering interferes with verbal communication.

Speaking rate is important to consider because instances of stuttering consume a portion of a person's speaking time. Thus, the more instances of stuttering a speaker produces, the more speaking time is consumed. This, in turn, impacts the number of overall words spoken for any time period, which can interfere with successful and efficient communication. There are two ways that speaking rate can be measured. One way is to measure how many words or syllables a person says during their utterances. This measure includes pauses that speakers normally have in their utterances. The resulting measure is called the *overall speaking rate.* It is relatively easy to calculate and only requires a stopwatch. Another way to measure speaking rate is by *only* considering *fluent* sounds and words produced by a speaker. This measure is called the *articulatory rate.* Articulatory rate is computed by calculating the number of fluent sounds or syllables produced per unit of time, with all

disfluencies and pauses longer than 250 milliseconds removed from the total length of the speaking sample. The resulting articulatory rate reflects the speaker's rate of producing fluent speech. Articulatory rate calculation requires the use of acoustic analysis software and is more time-consuming than the calculation of the overall speaking rate, which may be the reason why it is mostly used in research. Further, articulatory rate does not distinguish children who do from those who do not stutter, but overall speaking rate does. That is, higher frequency and longer duration of speech disfluencies produced by children who stutter yield them a significantly slower overall speaking rate when compared to their nonstuttering peers.

Speech naturalness is another measure of how much stuttering interferes with typical communication. This measure includes clinical judgments about how typical and natural someone's speech sounds and its degree of intelligibility. Although some clinical tests for stuttering assessment (e.g., SSI-4) include a Likert-type scale (e.g., 0 = very mild to 7 = very severe), judgments of speech naturalness are less often similarly scaled. In general, factors mentioned earlier (i.e., frequency and severity of stuttering, presence of associated [non]speech behaviors, speaking rate) affect listener's judgments of speech naturalness. Nevertheless, since different listeners may have unique criteria for how "natural" speech should sound, ratings of speech naturalness remain somewhat subjective. Regardless, for people who stutter, speech naturalness remains an important consideration for the diagnosis and treatment of stuttering, especially given that few treatments of stuttering are designed to result in unusual or unnatural sounding speech.

In sum, although all of the measures reviewed earlier can augment one's description of stuttering, the primary measures used to index a change in stuttering, especially change associated with therapeutic intervention, are measures of stuttering frequency and overall stuttering severity.

1.4 Common Characteristics: Variability (General Aspects)

1.4.1 Variability

One of the more common characteristics of instances of stuttering is that they change, fluctuate, or vary in frequency of occurrence. To understand stuttering is to understand that it *varies.* Although there is variability in stuttering *between* people who stutter (not all people stutter in the same way), in the following we will focus on the variability that can occur *within* a person who stutters. Simply put, a person who stutter's stuttering may change if there are changes in the speaking environment (e.g., home vs. clinic), listeners (e.g., parent vs. clinician or friends vs. strangers), nature of the speaking task (e.g., conversation vs. reading), time of day (e.g., morning vs. afternoon), fatigue level (e.g., after a restful night's sleep vs. after a day of intense cognitive and physical activity), presence of positive emotion (e.g., child speaking at their birthday party),[9] and so on.[10]

People who stutter and their family are usually aware of and perplexed by such day-to-day or moment-to-moment changes in stuttering frequency and are unlikely to know how to interpret such variability. One helpful thing to keep in mind is that the knowledge regarding stuttering variability can (and should) temper one's concern after observing a day's worth of frequent stuttering. With such knowledge, an observer may be better able to see that *over*-concern about a day of highly frequent stuttering is no wiser than *under*-concern about a day's worth of totally fluent speech! This inherent quality of stuttering—its variability—also has important implications for clinicians who treat and researchers who study stuttering. For example, to capture the true nature of stuttering during assessment, a clinician may need to obtain several samples of speaking at beginning, middle, and end of assessment as well as across days or weeks and then calculate the person's central tendency (i.e., average) as well as minimum and maximum frequency of stuttering across such time spans. Alternatively, a clinician could ask the child's parent or caregiver (or the person who stutters) how representative the speech sample was of the child's stuttering in everyday life (e.g., did the child [you] stutter more, less, or about the same as they [you] usually do?).

Such variability is one reason why some clinicians will ask the child's caregivers—particularly when the type or frequency of the child's speech disfluencies is on the cusp between normal and stuttered—to record a speech sample from home or to bring the child back in 3 months or so for a second evaluation and/or before formal therapy begins. In this way, the child's performance at the first evaluation and the second evaluation can be compared and contrasted. Similar multisampling advice may

be applied to tracking treatment progress over time. To illustrate this point, ▶ Fig. 1.1 graphically illustrates *stuttering variability* exhibited by a young child who stutters across several weekly therapy sessions (as measured by their clinician). Experienced clinicians will continue to sample and record stuttering frequency at consecutive therapy sessions to thoroughly document ongoing changes in the child's speech fluency.

In sum, it is important to understand that for an individual who stutters their stuttering frequency of today may differ from their stuttering frequency of tomorrow. Such fluctuations, while a common characteristic of stuttering, are important to note for both the diagnosis and treatment of stuttering.

1.4.2 Non-normally Distributed

Students and clinicians alike may wonder when they see the header "non-normal distribution" why a "statistical" issue is presented in a more clinically oriented text. The reason is simple: stuttering frequency (at least in children) is not normally distributed. That is, rather than the usual bell curve that represents the so-called normal distribution, the curve of stuttering in children is skewed to the right.[11,12] This means that for the population of children who stutter, there are more children whose stuttering frequency is relatively low (▶ Fig. 1.2). In essence, more children cluster at the low (less often) end of the

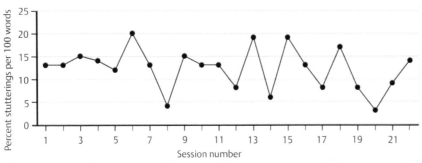

Fig. 1.1 Example of a child's variability of stuttering across treatment sessions. Fluctuations in or variability of a young child's instances of stuttering during speech-language therapy. Specifically, the figure displays the percent stuttering (i.e., sound-syllable repetitions + sound prolongations + monosyllabic whole-word repetitions) per 100 spoken words for each therapy session (1 = initial therapy session, 22 = final therapy session).

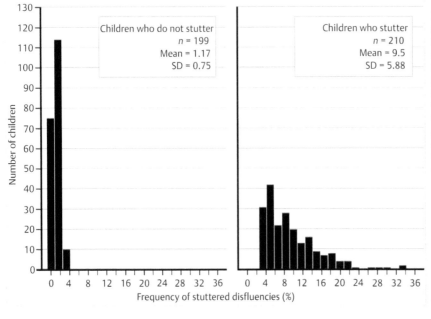

Fig. 1.2 Non-normal distribution of stuttered disfluencies in preschool-age children who do stutter ($n = 210$) and who do not stutter (typically fluent; $n = 199$). These graphs display these two groups of preschool-age children's percent stuttered disfluencies per total words spoken during conversational speech. (Adapted from Tumanova et al.[12]) The number of children for each vertical bar of stuttering are represented on the ordinate or vertical axis for each talker group. Although 10 children who did not stutter had 2.6% stuttered disfluencies in their speech, the graphical software used to make this figure rounded that value to 3.

stuttering frequency distribution than the high (more often) end of the stuttering frequency distribution. Why should students and clinicians care?

People who diagnose, treat, and study stuttering should care because the non-normal distribution of stuttering means that student-clinicians, practicing clinicians, and researchers are more apt to encounter children with lesser than greater amounts or frequencies of stuttering. Below we provide an illustration of variability of stuttered disfluencies across a relatively large sample of children who stutter.[12] It is important to know that children with relatively low stuttering frequency (and likely less severe stuttering) are truly children who stutter, not merely some relatively fluent normally fluent children. And yes, normally fluent children produce speech disfluencies, just not as frequently and far less of the kind that children who stutter more frequently produce (i.e., sound/syllable repetitions and sound prolongations). Indeed, it is this fact—greater numbers of children with low rather than high frequency of stuttering—that may cause some children with bona fide but relatively low stuttering frequency to fall through the cracks and not receive needed treatment. This fact also suggests that many reported studies of stuttering, particularly in children, may include more children with low (compared to high) frequency of stuttering. Forearmed is forewarned.

1.5 Common Characteristics: Variability (Specific Aspects)

In the earlier section, we discussed variability of stuttering in *general*. We should note, however, that there are *specific* conditions in which stuttering varies in a relatively predictable way. In the following section, we discuss these conditions and their implications for clinical practice.

1.5.1 Adaptation Effect

One of the earliest studied aspects of stuttering variability was "adaptation" or, as it is commonly referred to, the "adaptation effect." The adaptation effect was initially observed in adults when they read aloud the same passage several times in a row.[13] This initial study was published over 80 years ago and was followed by numerous empirical studies of stuttering adaptation in

children and adults. Indeed, adaptation of stuttering was one of the more frequently studied basic characteristics of stuttering; however, more recently, there have been fewer published investigations of the phenomenon.

In brief, adaptation of stuttering (or the "adaptation effect") refers to *decreases* in stuttering frequency during successive oral readings or speaking of the same material (as shown in ▶ Fig. 1.3 for one individual who stutters). This decrease, averaged across people who stutter, is about 50%. In other words, there is a 50% decrease in stuttering from the first to the fifth oral reading of the same text.[13,14] Thus, adaptation, as described here, is a specific condition in which stuttering varies in a relatively predictable way.

The adaptation effect can be mitigated (i.e., the reduction in stuttering would be smaller during successive oral readings) in several ways, including (1) increasing the time interval in between successive readings, (2) increasing the number of listeners with each successive oral reading, and (3) changing the material that is read or spoken in each of the successive readings. Thus, when discussing stuttering variability associated with adaptation, it is important to specify the nature of the material being read, the type and number of listeners, the nature of the situation in which the person reads, and so forth.

As with the non-normal distribution of stuttering frequency, some might wonder why adaptation is of relevance to clinical practice. Frankly, to date some findings regarding stuttering adaptation are more theoretical than clinical in significance. However, the fact remains that many (but not all) people who stutter decrease stuttering during repeated oral readings if the material, listener, time interval between readings, and listener remain the same. For the clinician, therefore, this observation suggests the possibility that some of the changes that occur during treatment, with the same clinician, room, and speaking/reading material, may be associated with adaptation (and not merely the influence of the treatment regimen). Clinicians who understand this will then be sure to account for it by varying therapy contexts (i.e., location, timing of breaks, where the client and clinician sit, etc.) and activities within and between sessions. Certainly, these simple, matter-of-fact changes make the treatment setting a bit less constant. However, such changes also make the therapy setting more closely reflective of the continual change the person who stutters experiences outside of the clinical setting. Indeed, a client's ability to generalize

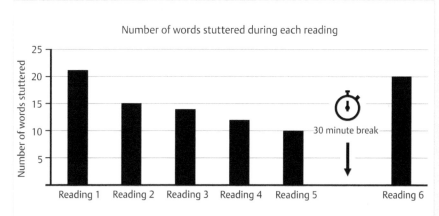

Number of words stuttered during each reading

30 minute break

Fig. 1.3 Example of adaptation of stuttering and temporary effects of stuttering. Adaptation effect: The steady decrease in the number of stuttered words (i.e., decrease in stuttering frequency) from 21 to 10—from Reading 1 to 5—across five successive readings of a 133-word passage by a young adult who stutters. This individual read this passage five times in a row, with no stopping or resting between each of the five readings. Temporary effect of adaptation: After the fifth reading, the same individual had a pause of no reading or speaking for 30 minutes, and then read the passage a sixth time, with their stuttering frequency on the sixth reading returning to the same frequency they exhibited during Reading 1.

change in stuttering from a nonchanging (clinical) to an ever-changing (everyday) environment may be quite challenging for some clients.

1.5.2 After the Effects of Adaptation Have Dissipated

Given the fluency-inducing effect of adaptation, one might think that an individual's stuttering could be solved merely by having them read or speak the same material over and over. However, this is not the case. For as we will see immediately below, the effect of adaptation is temporary. If a person who stutters takes a break after repeatedly reading or speaking the same material, their stuttering frequency tends to return to about the same level as they exhibited on the first oral reading.[15,16,17] For example, let us say a person stutters on 8% of the words read (or 8 stuttered disfluencies per 100 words read) in the first oral reading of a passage. By virtue of adaptation, they then stutter on 4% of the words by the fifth reading of the same passage. If, however, following that fifth reading, the person takes a 30-minute break and then reads the same passage for the sixth time, their stuttering returned to 7% (or 7 stuttered disfluencies per 100 words read). The person's 7% stuttering on the sixth reading is nearly the same frequency of stuttering they exhibited in the first reading. This temporary effect of adaptation is relatively common.[16,17,18] Again, as with most such effects, some people exhibit total return to their typical stuttering frequency, some less so, and some very little. Although the reasons for the adaptation-related decreases and increases in stuttering have long been of interest to both clinicians and researchers, there remains no agreed-upon explanation for why such changes in stuttering frequency occur. At the risk of redundancy, we note that the one constant about stuttering is that it changes!

1.5.3 Consistency Effect

Similar to the adaptation effect, the consistency effect was also first described over 80 years ago in a study that asked adults to repeatedly read the same passage aloud.[13] The consistency of stuttering (▶ Table 1.2) refers to the fact that people who stutter tend to stutter on the same words when they repeatedly read the same text aloud.[13,19] Although the consistency effect was primarily studied with adults, it also applies to children who stutter.[20,21] This suggests something quite important to an understanding of stuttering: some features or stimuli within the reading material appear to either "set the occasion for" or elicit an instance of stuttering. In other words, stuttering is not produced in a random or haphazard fashion; rather there is

consistency in the places within an utterance where stuttering is produced. The frequency of stuttering at certain places in utterances is significantly higher than chance, although not totally predictable within and between individuals who stutter. The percentage of words that are consistently stuttered across multiple oral readings of the same material has been reported to range from about 50 to 100% with an average of 77%.[20,22,23] In general, the cues (e.g., position of word within sentence, grammatical function of the word, etc.) associated with consistency seem to be related to a mix of factors (1) *unique* to each individual who stutters and (2) *common* to the group of individuals who stutter. These cues or stimuli have been described as the "loci of stuttering" (with "loci" the plural of "locus").

1.5.4 Loci of Stuttering

About the time that adaptation and consistency of stuttering were being studied, so too were the loci of stuttering. The loci of stuttering refer to the *characteristics* (e.g., sounds, syllables, and words) of those places that are consistently stuttered. Specifically, the loci of stuttering are often associated with longer words, words at the beginning of the sentence, and the like.[24,25] As with the consistency effect, the loci of stuttering highlights the fact that instances of stuttering are (1) not random and (2) associated with specific linguistic qualities of a word, phrase, utterance, or sentence.

Initially, the loci or characteristics of consistently stuttered words were thought to involve (1) longer words (five or more letters); (2) words that begin with a consonant; (3) words that are in the first three positions of a sentence; and (4) words that were nouns, adjectives, verbs, or adverbs.[26] This observation was mainly based on adults who stutter; however, when researchers began to study the loci of stuttering in the *conversational* speech of children, the picture changed somewhat. That is, young children appeared to stutter mainly near the beginning of sentences and on *function words* (e.g., conjunctions, prepositions, and pronouns). This finding is in contrast to adults who stuttered on *content* words (i.e., nouns, verbs, adverbs, adjectives). These tendencies appeared to apply not only to English but also to other languages, such as Spanish, German, and Portuguese. Recently, however, loci of stuttering have been examined in children who speak Korean, a language where function words are less likely to occur in the sentence-initial position compared to English.[27] Findings indicated that unlike English-speaking children who stutter, Korean-speaking children who stutter stuttered more on content words than function words. These findings support the contention that it is not the function or content words that are associated with stuttering, but rather their position within an utterance.[24]

Table 1.2 Example of consistency of stuttering

Reading 1: "**You** wish to know all about my **grandfather**. Well, he is **nearly ninety**-three **years** old."
Reading 2: "**You** wish to know all about my **grandfather**. Well, he is **nearly ninety**-three **years** old."
Reading 3: "You wish to know all about my **grandfather**. Well, he is nearly ninety-three years old."
Reading 4: "You wish to know all about my **grandfather**. Well, he is nearly ninety-three years old."
Reading 5: "You wish to know all about my **grandfather**. Well, he is nearly ninety-three years old."

Note: ▶ Table 1.1 depicts an individual who stutters reading the same sentence five times in a row, with each sentence read immediately after one another. The words read for each of the five sentences that were stuttered during each of the five readings are highlighted in **bold** font. From this table, it can be seen that the word "grandfather" is consistently stuttered across all five readings and the words "ninety-three" across two of the five readings.

Although theoretical accounts of the factors associated with loci go beyond the scope of this chapter, research has consistently pointed to the *nonrandom* nature of stuttering loci. For example, a child may not always stutter on every utterance-initial word, but when the child does stutter many of his instances of stuttering will be on utterance-initial words. This stuttering characteristic has encouraged researchers to study such factors as speech *production* (i.e., speech motor control) and speech-language *planning* (e.g., expressive vocabulary, sentence construction) in people who stutter in attempts to determine whether they have clinical or subclinical difficulties with these processes. Indeed, the association between these processes and stuttering will become clearer in the later chapters of this book. Likewise, in subsequent chapters, authors will discuss the translational or applied implications of stuttering loci for the diagnosis and treatment of stuttering.

1.6 Other Common Characteristics: Age at Onset, Gender, Persistence, and Recovery from Stuttering

1.6.1 Age at Onset

Within the above definition of stuttering is the phrase "…first emerges in early childhood." Thus, it should not be surprising to find that stuttering typically begins in early childhood, with onset ranging in age from 2 to 5 years of age with a mean age of 33 months.[28] Can stuttering begin outside of this age range? Certainly. It is quite possible for stuttering to begin in older children, teens, and adults. Although possible, it is much less probable.

Why would stuttering begin for most children during early childhood? What might be occurring during that time period that contributes to stuttering? At present, we lack precise answers to such questions. However, in the chapters ahead, this book presents several credible possibilities, for example, subtle but important differences in speech/language planning, neurological processes, speech motor control, and emotional reactivity and regulation. The notion that "multiple factors" contribute to early-childhood onset of stuttering has led to the development of what are called "multifactorial" theories.[29,30,31]

A detailed description of the multifactorial theory is beyond the scope of the present chapter; however, the basic tenet of such a theory is that there is no single factor that, in and of itself, causes stuttering. Rather, there are a finite number of clusters, constellations, or groupings of factors that contribute to the onset of stuttering. For example, for one grouping of children, all factors—speech/language, neurological, speech motor, and emotion—may play a role, with challenges to speech motor processes weighting more heavily than the other factors. For another grouping of children, on the other hand, the same factors might be involved, but weigh more heavily toward language and emotional factors. Again, further discussion of factors that may contribute to stuttering onset and development is beyond the scope of this chapter, but it will be discussed in the chapters that follow.

At present, it does appear that ascribing the reason that stuttering begins in early childhood to one single factor is less than appropriate given available information.

1.6.2 Gender

In general, boys (who have XY chromosomes) are more likely to exhibit a full range of developmental disorders (such as language-learning and reading problems) than girls (who have XX chromosomes). However, gender disparities are the rule rather than the exception for many disorders, which raises the possibility that stuttering is associated with sex-linked, genetic processes.[32] Therefore, it should not be particularly startling to learn that stuttering is more apt to be exhibited by boys than girls. (One exception to this rule is that boys and girls, near the onset of stuttering, are roughly equally represented.) Why such a gender disparity? We could certainly ask the same question regarding gender disparities for other disorders, for example, attention deficit/hyperactivity disorder, obsessive compulsive disorder, etc. Be that as it may, why do more boys than girls (and, ultimately, men than women) develop stuttering in early childhood?

Like the former question regarding stuttering and age of onset, we lack a precise answer as to why stuttering is more apt to emerge in boys than in girls. Still, the sex discrepancy for stuttering remains a fact. And such facts typically, like iron filings to a magnet, attract a variety of explanations. For example, some have suggested that in general, when compared to girls, boys' speech and language matures later and/or is more apt to be disordered. Others have suggested that genetic influences for at least some other nonspeech and language disorders are more prevalent for boys than for girls. Still others have suggested that environmental influences, for example, differences in parental attitudes and child-rearing practices, account for stuttering to be more prevalent in boys than in girls. Or epigenetic processes (i.e., environmental and learning influences on gene expression that do not involve changes in the deoxyribonucleic acid [DNA] sequence) might be at play differently for boys than for girls. Perhaps the truth lies in the possibility that both genetic and environmental factors contribute to the unequal sex ratio, possibilities that will be explored in greater depth in the following section, in ▶ Chapter 3 discussing the association between genetic factors and stuttering.

In contrast, one can still find mutually exclusive accounts for why more boys than girls stutter, for example, mainly genetic versus mainly environment. These explanations lie counter to the fact—as discussed earlier—that many that treat and research stuttering have increasingly embraced more multifactorial accounts of its etiology. Hence, it is possible that a multifactorial approach may be—in the long run—a more productive account for the sex ratio of stuttering than more unifactorial accounts. This is consistent with other developmental and behavioral disorders in that a *single* factor is neither necessary nor sufficient to account for the emergence of such disorders. Indeed, a multifactorial perspective seems reasonable given the fact that one-factor perspectives have not led to particularly resounding clarity regarding the cause of stuttering as well as the fact that more males than females stutter.

1.6.3 Stuttering Persistence and Recovery

It has long been known that some children recover from stuttering without intervention, while others persist in stuttering. In recent years, however, the exact percentage of persistence and recovery has become more apparent.[33] Indeed, the percentage of children who exhibit unassisted recovery (roughly 70–80%) is greater than for those whose stuttering persists (roughly 20–30%). Specifically, children for whom stuttering *persists* (relative to those who recover) have been shown to exhibit lower receptive and expressive vocabulary,[34] more variable speech articulation,[34,35] stronger and more frequent negative emotions (such as fear) per parent report,[34] differences in neurological function,[36] and greater psychophysiological reactivity (i.e., skin conductance) to stress at initial assessment.[37]

Therefore, measurable, though sometimes subtle, differences in speech, language, and emotional processes seem to be associated with the persistence of stuttering. Nevertheless, it is important to mention that while children who stutter (CWS) may differ from children who do not stutter (CWNS) on these various measures (1) CWS's abilities generally remain within normal limits and (2) there is no evidence, to date, that any one deficit is necessary or sufficient to cause stuttering.

Although we are far from knowing all there is to know about the factors associated with the persistence of stuttering, a broad theory characterized by the interaction of multiple factors is beginning to emerge, one that will be elaborated upon in the chapters to follow, from both basic and applied perspectives. Of course, establishing an association between two variables should not be taken to suggest that one causes the other. Indeed, the exact mechanisms by which any of these speech, language, and emotional processes "cause" stuttering to persist, if any of them do, will only be uncovered by future research.

1.7 Common Characteristics: Behaviors and Conditions that Decrease Stuttering

Several *behaviors*, on the part of the person who stutters, and *conditions*, when experienced by the person who stutters, are known to be associated with a *decrease* in stuttering frequency. Usually, however, once the behavior is stopped or the condition changed, the frequency of stuttering returns to its previous level (this is a bit like the increase of stuttering once the adaptation paradigm is completed). The section provides a brief description of the more common behaviors and conditions associated with decreases in stuttering frequency.

1.7.1 Behaviors Associated with Decreases in Stuttering

Behaviors associated with decreases in stuttering (i.e., fluency-inducing behaviors and conditions) are fairly common events (e.g., singing). Indeed, these behaviors can lead to a dramatic reduction in the frequency of stuttering for people who stutter. Most speaking-related behaviors described below are associated with decreases in stuttering in most, but not necessarily

all, people who stutter. Because of their temporary impact on stuttering (i.e., they are only associated with decreases in stuttering when they are employed), modern-day clinicians generally do not include these behaviors as a part of their stuttering therapy program.

Furthermore, these behaviors may not seem appropriate or desirable for typical communication (e.g., a person who stutters is unlikely to choose to sing instead of speaking when ordering food at a drive-through). Suffice it to say, at present, the underlying mechanisms or reasons why these various behaviors impact stuttering are not fully understood. Some have suggested that the fluency-inducing effects, specifically paced speech, and singing may be related to more effective coupling of auditory and motor systems (e.g., efficient self-monitoring).[38] Others have noted that different brain activation patterns (e.g., increased right hemisphere activation of speech-related regions) in people who stutter have also been reported during these times.

Singing

Singing is commonly associated with decreases in stuttering.[38,39] Of course, as suggested earlier, we do not precisely know why singing decreases stuttering but we will provide some educated guesses. First, most singing differs from typical conversational speech and language in that songs are generally memorized. Singing a song, in whole or in part, generally involves little changing or improvising the words to the song. Conversely, most conversational speech is not memorized; rather, it involves spontaneous, on-the-fly responses. Such responses may occur, for example, when the speaker shifts from one thought to the next. Or when the listener asks the speaker questions or the speaker or listener creates shifts in the topic(s) of conversation, shifts that require the speaker to respond on the fly. Second, singing is often accompanied by music—either played by the singer or other external sources—which has a melody and a rhythm. Conversational speech, on the other hand, is seldom associated with external cadences, melodies, or rhythm. Third, when someone sings, they are seldom interrupted. That is, once someone begins to sing a song, unless they are rehearsing for a play or recording the song, the "singer" is seldom corrected or interrupted in mid-song. In contrast, corrections, disagreements, questions, and other interruptions are an integral part of everyday conversational speech.

In short, as mentioned earlier, we lack a definitive answer regarding why singing decreases stuttering. However, we do know that singing represents a significant departure from natural, everyday speech and language planning and production. As a result, singing—as a means for everyday conversational speech—is not apt to be tolerated or used by most individuals who speak, whether they stutter or not, as their go-to means for communication. So, although many of us enjoy listening to music and singing, few would select singing to conduct their daily conversational communication, which begs the question: Why would we ever expect a person who stutters to tolerate such a "cure"?

Whispering

In contrast to singing, during whispering, the vocal folds are typically held apart (i.e., moved and held away from midline of the speaker's glottis), which minimizes the speaker's ability to *vocalize* (i.e., when a speaker whispers, their vocal folds are minimally if at all vibrating).[40,41,42] Conversely, during typical conversational speech, vocal folds rapidly shift between vibration and no vibration. Such shifting in vocalization during speaking—between voiced and voiceless sounds—is required to produce vowels and voiced consonants, whereas voicing is not required to produce voiceless consonants. Thus, quite different behaviors—one where voicing is absent (i.e., whispering) and the other where voicing is very present (i.e., singing)—seem to decrease instances of stuttering.

The diametrically opposed nature of these two behaviors—whispering and singing—may be telling us that merely adjusting vocal fold activity does not completely explain why these behaviors impact stuttering. Importantly, just as with singing, continually whispering when we speak is less than a desirable means for everyday communication (if not impossible when there is loud ambient or background noise). Therefore, requiring a person who stutters to whisper more or less constantly when they speak would appear to be a "cure" that is likely to be more unsatisfactory than the concern, embarrassment, inconvenience, and less-than-typical communication associated with stuttering itself!

Speaking While Performing in a Play

It has often been observed that people who stutter may decrease their stuttering while performing in a play.[43] To the authors' knowledge, there is no definitive explanation for this observation. Again, it should be mentioned that there is one major difference between the lines spoken by someone in a play and the words, phrases, sentences, and thoughts expressed during everyday conversation. The former—performing in a play—is generally well rehearsed and memorized, while the latter—everyday conversational speech—is typically not (as mentioned earlier). Further, a stage or performance speaking style typically involves using a slower rate, increased volume, and overarticulation—all resulting from using the speech production system differently than the way we use it for everyday talking.

As with singing, when we act in a play, we are seldom questioned or interrupted by our listeners. Indeed, most if not all interruptions by actors are a priori scripted, often rehearsed, and thus fairly quite predictable to the actor. In contrast, and as mentioned earlier, a speaker's natural conversation often constitutes on-the-fly changes. These frequent, if not sudden, stops and starts for the speaker in a conversation are often related to the speaker's listener(s) interrupting, questioning, and talking over the speaker's conversational utterances. Thus, our *natural*, conversational speech and language planning and production cannot, and should not, be *memorized* to achieve fluent speech. Such memorization, of course, is appropriate for acting in a play, giving a speech, or performing a religious ritual. However, for naturally occurring conversational speech? Not so much.

Speaking in a Slow, Prolonged Manner

Speaking in a slow, prolonged manner (i.e., prolonged speech) also has been shown to lead to decreases in stuttering frequency.[44,45] When employing prolonged speech, people who

stutter are typically instructed to significantly (1) decrease their rate of speech (by 50%),[46] (2) elongate their syllables and words, and (3) maintain continuous voicing across words and syllables. The fluency-inducing effect of slow, prolonged speech has been attributed to increased vowel and syllable durations.[47,48] Unlike singing and whispering, speaking in a slow, prolonged manner has been included in some stuttering therapy approaches.[49,50] Depending on how slow the person needs to speak to achieve the fluency-inducing effect, people who stutter may find that routinely employing slow, prolonged speech sounds feels unnatural, both to themselves and their listeners, and for that reason is less than an ideal means for maintaining natural everyday communication.

1.7.2 Conditions Associated with Decreases in Stuttering

Conditions associated with decreases in stuttering include, but are not limited to, the following: (1) delayed auditory feedback (DAF), (2) loud noise, and (3) external rhythmic stimulus. Digital technology allows these conditions to be readily manufactured, which has led to continuing discussion about their clinical applicability as a central or peripheral part of a stuttering therapy program. Several questions remain regarding the appropriateness and usefulness of these conditions for people who stutter. Nevertheless, for the sake of completeness, we provide below some brief description and discussion of these conditions.

Delayed Auditory Feedback

DAF, in essence, "takes" the speaker's air-conducted or airborne auditory sidetone while speaking and delays the arrival of this sidetone to the speaker's ears (i.e., auditory system) by fractions of a second.[51,52] When a speaker, whether they stutter or not, speaks in the presence of DAF, they typically change their speech in response. In the case of a person who stutters, this "change" can involve decreases in stuttering, at least during certain speaking conditions (e.g., reading aloud). In other words, "changes" (e.g., slowing down their speech rate) in natural conversational speech—similar to whispering or singing—may be induced by DAF. This slowing of speaking rate may be one reason why DAF decreases stuttering, along with possible increased attention paid to kinesthetic and proprioceptive cues. Another possible contributor, suggested by some,[53] is that DAF somehow compensates for a deficit that people who stutter have in their auditory feedback for speech. Commercially available DAF units, similar in size to modern-day hearing aids, appear to be of help for some adults who stutter, especially those who stutter more severely and/or did not have success with other available treatments.

Rhythmic Stimulation

Rhythmic stimulation (i.e., metronome effect) as a means to ameliorate stuttering has a long history.[54,55] When people who stutter speak to the beat of a metronome (or the metronome's "tick-tock-tick-tock, etc." sound), they typically are more fluent. Similar to DAF, rhythmic stimulation changes the naturalness of one's speaking. This is because synchronizing or timing one's speech to the beat of a metronome typically results in a slower, less typical sounding speaking pattern. With rhythmic stimulation, the speaker's speech sounds singsong, staccato, or rhythmical. Although such rhythmic stimulation is associated with an appreciable reduction in stuttering, the speaker's speech both feels and sounds far less than natural. Given this less-than-natural quality of speech-language production, many people who stutter are likely to prefer to speak and stutter than speak to the beat of a metronome. In short, what most people who stutter want—similar to most people who do not stutter—is typical sounding speech. They do not seem to be seeking to replace one less than typical sounding speech (e.g., "th-th-th-this is different") with a second less than typical sounding speech (i.e., "th-is-dif-fer-ent").

Loud Noise

Loud noise (e.g., white noise effect), whether naturally present in the environment or deliberately introduced while a person who stutters is speaking, can be associated with a decrease in stuttering.[54,56,57,58] When people speak in the presence of masking noise, regardless of whether they stutter or not, they tend to increase the loudness of their own speech (for the interested reader, this is called the "Lombard effect").[59] Although speaking louder appears to decrease stuttering, at least to some degree, the loud noise also presents a threat to the speaker's hearing system (i.e., has potential to contribute to at least a temporary noise-induced hearing loss; this is why construction workers using jackhammers wear ear protectors). Further, it is hard to imagine successful communication when someone not only has to raise their voice level or loudness but also has to listen to a loud noise in their headphones while trying to engage in conversational speech! Therefore, routinely speaking in a loud voice, with or without ambient loud noise, is not a particularly desirable means for ameliorating stuttering.

Summary of Behaviors and Conditions Associated with Decreases in Stuttering

Before we end our discussion regarding behaviors and conditions associated with decreases in stuttering, we would like to make some general comments regarding both. First, we are unable to cover all such behaviors and conditions in this space, just some of those most commonly noted (see Bloodstein's seminal overviews[43,60,61]). Second, whether whispering or speaking to the beat of a metronome, these behaviors and conditions are associated with not only changes in stuttering but also changes in the naturalness of conversational speaking. Thus, most behaviors and conditions that induce fluency do so—at least in part—by creating a significant departure from speaking naturalness. This departure from natural conversational speech makes us question the routine use of most such behaviors and conditions with people who stutter. Third, some of these behaviors and conditions involve memorized, noninterrupted speaking events. Such memorization is simply not feasible for speakers to employ, whether they stutter or not, in everyday conversation. Nor, for that matter, can speakers, whether they stutter or not, expect to engage in conversational speech that is noninterrupted. Fourth, some of these behaviors and conditions, DAF, for example, represent "speaker-passive" rather than "speaker-active" means for changing stuttering. Rendering a speaker more or less passive in the generation of his or her own speech fluency can be problematic, especially if the behavior or condition does not appreciably ameliorate stuttering (keeping in mind that few things work for everyone, in all circumstances).

Nevertheless, these various behaviors and conditions (► Fig. 1.4) may be telling us something about the variables associated with increased fluency for people who stutter. ► Fig. 1.4 presents a summary for the common features of some fluency-inducing behaviors and conditions. For example, some of these behaviors and conditions seem to induce a more regulated, less changeable, more predictable, and slower form of "speaking." Importantly, these changes in speech planning and production concurrently induce a significant departure from the ever-changing tempo of natural conversational speaking. The fluency gained with these behaviors and conditions comes, however, at the cost of significantly altering the naturalness (and sometimes speaking rate) of speaking. We would like to suggest that such alterations in speech-language planning and production—especially speech naturalness—is a price that most

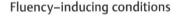

Fluency–inducing conditions

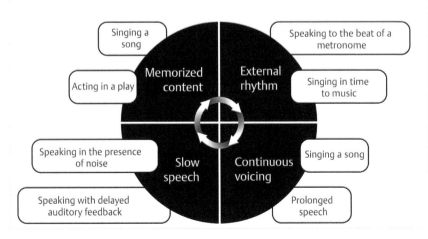

Fig. 1.4 Common characteristics of some fluency-inducing (i.e., decreases in stuttering) behaviors and conditions. Note: Some of these fluency-inducing behaviors/conditions, as ► Fig. 1.4 suggests, can be associated with two or more characteristics. For example, the condition of singing can be associated with the following characteristics: it is often memorized, it involves nearly continuous voicing, it is often produced slower than conversational speech, and it can occur with external rhythm.

speakers, whether they stutter or not, are generally not willing to pay. Indeed, as we shall see in later chapters covering the treatment of stuttering, changing stuttering is best, and with most long-term benefits, accomplished in a "nonhomogenized" environment of ever-changing, natural speech and language. Or, by way of analogy, a ship in harbor is safe, but that is not what ships are built for.

1.8 Future Directions

Future investigations of stuttering will undoubtedly study the various contributors to stuttering, for example, constitutional, developmental, and environmental factors in stuttering development. Such study will include investigations of genetic underpinnings of stuttering, developmental processes related to speech, language and temperament, and contributions of environmental factors such as caregiver interaction style, among others. Of course, some of these directions will be shaped by developments in methodology, for example, neuroimaging, as well as theoretical models suggesting new, fruitful avenues of investigation, for example, cortical/neurological antecedents to the development of anxiety. Likewise, the development of more advanced means of measurement will lead to more fine-grained understanding of the perceptual as well as behavioral aspects of instances of stuttering. All such informational, methodological as well as theoretical advances—from behavior to neurological processes—will further our understanding of stuttering as well as improve our basic study of and clinical diagnosis/treatment of stuttering. This enhanced general knowledge of stuttering may be augmented by specific study of possible subgroups of people who stutter. Results from such specific studies, it is thought, should contribute to our ability to more narrowcast the treatment of stuttering to the individual needs of people who stutter.

1.9 Conclusion

Stuttering is a speech disorder that typically begins in early childhood. In its early stages, stuttering is equally distributed between boys and girls, with more boys than girls developing chronic stuttering. The disorder is characterized by relatively frequent production of sound/syllable repetitions, (in)audible sound prolongations, and repetitions of monosyllabic words, with more young children exhibiting mild rather than severe stuttering. Stuttering frequency is quite variable within and between people who stutter, but, importantly, the loci of stuttering within an utterance are not random. For example, stuttering most often occurs in the beginning of an utterance.

Various nonspeech behaviors may be associated with stuttering, for example, eyelid opening and closing, and turning of the head away from the listener. However, the precise reason(s) for the occurrence of these behaviors is unclear. More children recover from stuttering without therapy than develop chronic stuttering. However, for those children who persist, stuttering can significantly impact their academic, emotional, and social abilities as well as their later vocational potential and achievements.

Given that the loci of stuttering are not random, stuttering appears to be a relatively *predictable* reaction to specific stimuli, some of which are seemingly *unique* to the individual who

stutters (e.g., words that begin with "f"), while others are more *common* to the problem of stuttering itself (e.g., words at the beginning of the utterance). Often, as will be discussed in greater detail in later chapters, instances of stuttering are associated with the linguistic content of the speaker's message. For example, longer, more grammatically complex utterances will be more apt to contain instances of stuttering than shorter, less grammatically complex utterances. Is this apparent difficulty with more complex linguistic content due to the (1) linguistic abilities of the person who stutters, (2) the inherent challenges of longer, more complex utterances, or (3) a combination of both? At present, the answer to this question is not clear.

What is clear, as subsequent chapters will describe, is that both clinicians and researchers alike are continuing to develop a more comprehensive, data-based understanding of such issues, a fact that following chapters will strongly affirm. Therefore, if Hobbes (1668) is correct, that knowledge is power, the future, for both people who stutter and those who treat them, should be full of bright promise.

1.10 Definitions

Adaptation (of stuttering): The *decrease* in stuttering frequency that occurs during successive oral readings or speaking of the same material. This is sometimes called the *adaptation effect*.

Associated (non) speech behaviors: Any speech (e.g., overly loud production of a word) or nonspeech (e.g., tight closure of eyelids) behavior associated with an instance of stuttering. These behavioral events are also referred to as *accessory*, *concomitant*, or *secondary* behaviors.

Consistency (of stuttering): The tendency of people who stutter to stutter on the same words when they repeatedly read the same text aloud. This is sometimes called the *consistency effect*.

Delayed auditory feedback (DAF): This procedure enables a speaker to listen to his or her own speech a fraction of a second later.

Fluency-inducing behavior and conditions: Any behavior (e.g., whispering) or condition (e.g., speaking to the beat of a metronome) that is associated with a noticeable decrease in stuttering (hence an increase in speech fluency).

Lifetime incidence: The percent of people who have stuttered sometime in their life.

Loci (of stuttering): The *characteristics* (e.g., sounds, syllables, and words) of those places within an utterance that are consistently stuttered, for example, longer words, words at the beginning of the sentence, etc.

Non-normal distribution (of children's stuttering): For the population of children who stutter, there are *more* children whose stuttering frequency is relatively low (i.e., they cluster at the low end of the distribution) rather than high (fewer children are at the middle or upper end of the distribution).

Monosyllabic repetition: Repetition of one- or single-syllable words (e.g. "I-I-I am going").

Multifactorial perspectives: The idea, hypothesis, notion, or theory that stuttering is caused, develops, or is maintained by several different factors or variables (e.g., emotion, linguistic, and motor), with some of these factors contributing more than others and whose relative contributions to stuttering differ among people who stutter.

Prevalence: The percent of people who stutter at any one point in time (e.g., presently).

Rhythmic stimulation: A fluency-inducing condition whereby a person who stutters speaks to the beat of a metronome and decreases their stuttering. This is sometimes called the *metronome effect.*

Sound prolongation: Increased or lengthened duration of a speech sound (e.g., "Sssssso I am going").

Sound/syllable repetitions: Reiteration of sounds and syllables (e.g., "S-s-see the dog").

Speech naturalness: A listener's judgment of how typical or natural someone's speech sounds and its degree of intelligibility.

Speaking rate: The speed at which sounds, syllables, or words are spoken for any time period, for example, 180 words per minute.

Speech disfluency: Any interruption in the rhythm and forward flow of speech (e.g., "B-b-b-bobby").

Stuttering: A speech disorder typically characterized by frequent repetitions of sounds (e.g., "S-s-see the dog"), monosyllabic words ("I-I-I am going"), sound prolongations, and interruptions in the forward flow of speech. These disruptions in the forward flow of speech are often accompanied by physical muscle tension and struggle (see associated speech/nonspeech behaviors above).

Stuttering frequency: A count or tabulation of the number of stuttered speech disfluencies per number of syllables or words spoken (often expressed a "percent syllables/words spoken").

Stuttering persistence and recovery: The tendency for some children who stutter to continue to stutter, while other children who stutter experience unassisted/spontaneous recovery.

Stuttering severity: A listener's judgment/description of the degree to which stuttering interferes with typical speaking communication, with the degree of severity ranging from not very serious (i.e., mild) to quite serious (i.e., severe).

Variability (of stuttering): Any change—either increase or decrease—in stuttering frequency that occurs within or between speaking situations.

References

[1] Craig A, Hancock K, Tran Y, Craig M, Peters K. Epidemiology of stuttering in the community across the entire life span. J Speech Lang Hear Res. 2002; 45 (6):1097–1105

[2] Guitar B. Stuttering: An Integrated Approach to Its Nature and Treatment. 5th ed. Philadelphia, PA: Wolters Kluwer; 2019

[3] Erickson S, Block S. The social and communication impact of stuttering on adolescents and their families. J Fluency Disord. 2013; 38(4):311–324

[4] Klein JF, Hood SB. The impact of stuttering on employment opportunities and job performance. J Fluency Disord. 2004; 29(4):255–273

[5] Riley G. SSI-4: Stuttering Severity Instrument. 4th ed. Austin, TX: Pro-Ed; 2009

[6] Gillam RB, Logan KJ, Pearson NA. TOCS: Test of Childhood Stuttering. Austin, TX: Pro-Ed; 2009

[7] Conture EG, Kelly EM. Young stutterers' nonspeech behaviors during stuttering. J Speech Hear Res. 1991; 34(5):1041–1056

[8] Conture EG, Louko LJ, Edwards ML. Simultaneously treating stuttering and disordered phonology in children: experimental treatment, preliminary findings. Am J Speech Lang Pathol. 1993; 2(3):72–81

[9] Adams MR. Childhood stuttering under "positive" conditions. Am J Speech Lang Pathol. 1992; 1(3):5–6

[10] Johnson KN, Karrass J, Conture EG, Walden T. Influence of stuttering variation on talker group classification in preschool children: preliminary findings. J Commun Disord. 2009; 42(3):195–210

[11] Jones M, Onslow M, Packman A, Gebski V. Guidelines for statistical analysis of percentage of syllables stuttered data. J Speech Lang Hear Res. 2006; 49(4): 867–878

[12] Tumanova V, Conture EG, Lambert EW, Walden TA. Speech disfluencies of preschool-age children who do and do not stutter. J Commun Disord. 2014; 49:25–41

[13] Johnson W, Knott JR. Studies in the psychology of stuttering: I. The distribution of moments of stuttering in successive readings of the same material. J Speech Disord. 1937; 2(1):17–19

[14] Frank A, Bloodstein O. Frequency of stuttering following repeated unison readings. J Speech Hear Res. 1971; 14(3):519–524

[15] Jones EL. Explorations of experimental extinction and spontaneous recovery in stuttering. In: Johnson W, ed. Stuttering in Children and Adults. Minneapolis, MN: University of Minnesota Press; 1955:226–231

[16] Leutenegger RR. Adaptation and recovery in the oral reading of stutterers. J Speech Hear Disord. 1957; 22(2):276–287

[17] Newman PW. A study of adaptation and recovery of the stuttering response in self-formulated speech. J Speech Hear Disord. 1954; 19(4): 450–458

[18] Jamison Do. Spontaneous recovery of the stuttering response as a function of the time following adaptation. In: Johnson W, ed. Stuttering in Children and Adults: Thirty Years of Research at the University of Iowa. Minneapolis, MN: University of Minnesota Press; 1955:245–248

[19] Williams DE, Silverman FH, Kools JA. Disfluency behavior of elementary-school stutterers and nonstutterers: the consistency effect. J Speech Hear Res. 1969; 12(2):301–307

[20] Bloodstein O. The development of stuttering. I. Changes in nine basic features. J Speech Hear Disord. 1960; 25:219–237

[21] Neelley JN, Timmons RJ. Adaptation and consistency in the disfluent speech behavior of young stutterers and nonstutterers. J Speech Hear Res. 1967; 10 (2):250–256

[22] Yairi E, Seery CH. Stuttering: Foundations and Clinical Applications. Upper Saddle River, NJ: Pearson; 2015

[23] Johnson W, Inness M. Studies in the psychology of stuttering, XIII: a statistical analysis of the adaptation and consistency effects in relation to stuttering. J Speech Disord. 1939; 4(1):79–86

[24] Buhr A, Zebrowski P. Sentence position and syntactic complexity of stuttering in early childhood: a longitudinal study. J Fluency Disord. 2009; 34(3):155–172

[25] Zackheim CT, Conture EG. Childhood stuttering and speech disfluencies in relation to children's mean length of utterance: a preliminary study. J Fluency Disord. 2003; 28(2):115–141, quiz 141–142

[26] Brown SF. The loci of stutterings in the speech sequence. J Speech Disord. 1945; 10(3):181–192

[27] Choi D, Sim H, Park H, Clark CE, Kim H. Loci of stuttering of English- and Korean-speaking children who stutter: preliminary findings. J Fluency Disord. 2020; 64:105762

[28] Yairi E, Ambrose NG. Early Childhood Stuttering for Clinicians by Clinicians. Austin, TX: Pro-Ed; 2005

[29] Smith A. Stuttering: a unified approach to a multifactorial, dynamic disorder. In: Ratner N, Healey C, eds. Stuttering Research and Practice: Bridging the Gap. Mahwah, NJ: Lawrence Erlbaum Associates, Inc.; 1999

[30] Smith A, Kelly E. Stuttering: a dynamic, multifactorial model. In: Curlee R, Siegel G, eds. Nature and Treatment of Stuttering: New Directions. 2nd ed. Boston, MA: Allyn & Bacon; 1997

[31] Smith A, Weber C. How stuttering develops: the multifactorial dynamic pathways theory. J Speech Lang Hear Res. 2017; 60(9):2483–2505

[32] Suresh R, Ambrose N, Roe C, et al. New complexities in the genetics of stuttering: significant sex-specific linkage signals. Am J Hum Genet. 2006; 78 (4):554–563

[33] Månsson H. Childhood stuttering: Incidence and development. J Fluency Disord. 2000; 25(1):47–57

[34] Ambrose NG, Yairi E, Loucks TM, Seery CH, Throneburg R. Relation of motor, linguistic and temperament factors in epidemiologic subtypes of persistent and recovered stuttering: initial findings. J Fluency Disord. 2015; 45:12–26

[35] Usler E, Smith A, Weber C. A lag in speech motor coordination during sentence production is associated with stuttering persistence in young children. J Speech Lang Hear Res. 2017; 60(1):51–61

[36] Usler E, Weber-Fox C. Neurodevelopment for syntactic processing distinguishes childhood stuttering recovery versus persistence. J Neurodev Disord. 2015; 7(1):4

[37] Zengin-Bolatkale H, Conture EG, Walden TA, Jones RM. Sympathetic arousal as a marker of chronicity in childhood stuttering. Dev Neuropsychol. 2018; 43(2):135–151

[38] Stager SV, Jeffries KJ, Braun AR. Common features of fluency-evoking conditions studied in stuttering subjects and controls: an H(2)15O PET study. J Fluency Disord. 2003; 28(4):319–335, quiz 336

[39] Andrews G, Howie PM, Dozsa M, Guitar BE. Stuttering: speech pattern characteristics under fluency-inducing conditions. J Speech Hear Res. 1982; 25(2):208–216

[40] Zimmermann G. Stuttering: a disorder of movement. J Speech Hear Res. 1980; 23(1):122–136

[41] Ingham RJ, Bothe AK, Jang E, Yates L, Cotton J, Seybold I. Measurement of speech effort during fluency-inducing conditions in adults who do and do not stutter. J Speech Lang Hear Res. 2009; 52(5):1286–1301

[42] Rami MK, Kalinowski J, Rastatter MP, Holbert D, Allen M. Choral reading with filtered speech: effect on stuttering. Percept Mot Skills. 2005; 100(2):421–431

[43] Bloodstein O. Conditions under which stuttering is reduced or absent; a review of literature. J Speech Disord. 1949; 14(4):295–302

[44] Cordes AK. Current status of the stuttering treatment literature. In: Cordes A, Ingham R, eds. Treatment Efficacy for Stuttering: A Search for Empirical Bases. San Diego, CA: Singular Publishing Group; 1998:117–144

[45] Finn P. Evidence-based treatment of stuttering: II. Clinical significance of behavioral stuttering treatments. J Fluency Disord. 2003; 28(3):209–217, quiz 217–218

[46] Ingham RJ, Martin RR, Kuhl P. Modification and control of rate of speaking by stutterers. J Speech Hear Res. 1974; 17(3):489–496

[47] Packman A, Onslow M, van Doorn J. Prolonged speech and modification of stuttering: perceptual, acoustic, and electroglottographic data. J Speech Hear Res. 1994; 37(4):724–737

[48] Webster RL, Morgan BT, Cannon MW. Voice onset abruptness in stutterers before and after therapy. In: Peters H, Hulstijn W, eds. Speech Motor Dynamics in Stuttering. New York, NY: Springer; 1987:295–305

[49] Ingham RJ, Andrews G. Stuttering: the quality of fluency after treatment. J Commun Disord. 1971; 4(4):279–288

[50] Packman A, Onslow M, Menzies R. Novel speech patterns and the treatment of stuttering. Disabil Rehabil. 2000; 22(1)(−)(2):65–79

[51] Foundas AL, Mock JR, Corey DM, Golob EJ, Conture EG. The SpeechEasy device in stuttering and nonstuttering adults: fluency effects while speaking and reading. Brain Lang. 2013; 126(2):141–150

[52] Kalinowski J, Stuart A, Sark S, Armson J. Stuttering amelioration at various auditory feedback delays and speech rates. Eur J Disord Commun. 1996; 31(3):259–269

[53] Foundas AL, Bollich AM, Feldman J, et al. Aberrant auditory processing and atypical planum temporale in developmental stuttering. Neurology. 2004; 63(9):1640–1646

[54] Brayton ER, Conture EG. Effects of noise and rhythmic stimulation on the speech of stutterers. J Speech Hear Res. 1978; 21(2):285–294

[55] Martin RR, Johnson LJ, Siegel GM, Haroldson SK. Auditory stimulation, rhythm, and stuttering. J Speech Hear Res. 1985; 28(4):487–495

[56] Adams MR, Hutchinson J. The effects of three levels of auditory masking on selected vocal characteristics and the frequency of disfluency of adult stutterers. J Speech Hear Res. 1974; 17(4):682–688

[57] Stager SV, Denman DW, Ludlow CL. Modifications in aerodynamic variables by persons who stutter under fluency-evoking conditions. J Speech Lang Hear Res. 1997; 40(4):832–847

[58] Conture EG. Some effects of noise on the speaking behavior of stutterers. J Speech Hear Res. 1974; 17(4):714–723

[59] Brumm H, Zollinger SA. The evolution of the Lombard effect: 100 years of psychoacoustic research. Behaviour. 2011; 148(11–13):1173–1198

[60] Bloodstein O. Hypothetical conditions under which stuttering is reduced or absent. J Speech Disord. 1950; 15(2):142–153

[61] Bloodstein O. A rating scale study of conditions under which stuttering is reduced or absent. J Speech Hear Disord. 1950; 15(1):29–36

Further Readings

Andrews G, Howie PM, Dozsa M, Guitar BE. Stuttering: speech pattern characteristics under fluency-inducing conditions. J Speech Hear Res. 1982; 25(2):208–216

Choi D, Conture EG, Tumanova V, Clark CE, Walden TA, Jones RM. Young children's family history of stuttering and their articulation, language and attentional abilities: an exploratory study. J Commun Disord. 2018; 71:22–36

Foundas AL, Mock JR, Corey DM, Golob EJ, Conture EG. The SpeechEasy device in stuttering and nonstuttering adults: fluency effects while speaking and reading. Brain Lang. 2013; 126(2):141–150

Smith A, Weber C. How stuttering develops: the multifactorial dynamic pathways theory. J Speech Lang Hear Res. 2017; 60(9):2483–2505

Tumanova V, Conture EG, Lambert EW, Walden TA. Speech disfluencies of preschool-age children who do and do not stutter. J Commun Disord. 2014; 49:25–41

Williams DE, Silverman FH, Kools JA. Disfluency behavior of elementary-school stutterers and nonstutterers: the consistency effect. J Speech Hear Res. 1969; 12(2):301–307

2 Some 20th- and 21st-Century Theories of Stuttering: A Brief Overview

Edward G. Conture, Julie D. Anderson, and Patricia M. Zebrowski

Abstract

This chapter begins with a brief description of both theories and speculations about stuttering prior to the age of enlightenment or reason (i.e., from about biblical time to about the time of Francis Bacon [mid to late 1600s]). Subsequently, from about the beginning of the age of enlightenment and the scientific method that it engendered, the chapter provides a succinct overview of theories of stuttering from the 1700s through the early 1900s. Following that, the chapter provides a bit more expansive overview of theories of stuttering from the mid-20th to early 21st century. The chapter ends with a discussion of these theoretical foundations, followed by some conclusions. It should be noted that not ***all*** theories of stuttering are described in this chapter, nor are those selected comprehensively discussed. Rather, we chose theories that are (1) the most prominent and/or cited, (2) better reasoned and possibly testable, and/or (3) associated with data that either support or refute the theory's premises. Such theories range from broad to narrow focus on variables thought to contribute to the onset, development, and maintenance of stuttering. Knowledge of these theories should help readers better appreciate subsequent chapters that cover the knowledge base, diagnostic, and treatment protocols for stuttering across the lifespan.

Keywords: stuttering, fluency disorder, theories, models, etiology, cause

2.1 Introduction

"If I have seen further it is by standing on the shoulders of Giants."

Sir Isaac Newton (b. 1642, d. 1727)

The past, it is said, is prologue. Certainly, that is the case with theory. Theories of yesterday inform, to greater or lesser degrees, those of today. Thus, this overview of past and present theories of stuttering begins by providing some historical context.

Readers are briefly introduced to the medical/scientific world that *predates* modern-day approaches to science, medicine, human health, etc. The pre-modern-day approaches are mainly focused on the opinions and writings of a select number of authorities, whereas the modern-day approaches are more focused on hypothesis generation, testing, and evaluation. Such early (prescientific method) conceptualizations of stuttering, theory, and therapy were often based on a very different model of human health and its disorders: the humoral system. As suggested earlier, the "humoral" perspective was highly influenced by the ideas, theories, and writings of past authorities. Such influence meant, for investigators and practitioners alike, that there was little to no attempt or incentive to make new, exact observations and/or systematically collect data. Our brief exploration of pre-modern-day approaches to human health and disorders should help provide background and context for our later coverage of modern-day theoretical accounts of stuttering.

"The body of man has in itself blood, phlegm, yellow bile and black bile; these make up the nature of this body, and through these he feels pain and enjoys health."

Hippocrates (b. circa 460 BC, d. circa 375 BC)

2.2 Humoral System of Medicine

Up until the late 1600s through the early 1800s, the humoral system of medicine influenced much of the theory and therapy regarding human disorders, including stuttering. Suffice it to say, this early system of medical practice is quite foreign and/or unknown to early 21st-century readers of this chapter. Yet its influence carried on long after its demise, even impacting some of our modern-day terminology. To provide such historical perspective, the following brief overview discusses some of the seemingly more salient early antecedents to as well as prominent mid-1990s to early 2000s theories of stuttering. Similar discussion is available elsewhere, for example, Duffy's[1] discussion of older to modern health care, in general; Rieber and Wollock's[2] discussion of ancient to mid-1990s approaches to stuttering; and Van Riper's[3] discussion of 1800s to 1900s stuttering therapies.

In brief, the ancient, humoral view of human health and its disorders held that our universe has four basic *qualities*: cold, dryness, heat, and moisture. Combining these qualities in pair-like fashion, four *elements* are created: cold and dryness (*earth*), cold and moisture (*water*), heat and dryness (*fire*), and heat and moisture (*air*). Based on this conceptualization, ancient physicians and scholars considered humans to be a miniature or microcosmic version of this universe. These early practitioners and scholars appeared to believe that the human equivalent of these four elements was the four *humors* (bodily fluids): yellow bile, blood, black bile, and phlegm. Everyone was believed to have their own unique balance of humors, which was referred to as their *natural temperament*.[2]

According to this belief, there were four broad categories of natural temperaments that determined mental and physical health. If someone had too much *yellow bile*, then they were *choleric* (hot and dry). This was taken to mean that they were easily angered, aggressive, and smart. Someone who was *sanguine* (hot and moist), on the other hand, had an abundance of *blood* in their body. As a consequence of such abundance, the individual was assumed to be "fleshy," yet physically vigorous and optimistic. In present-day terms, we might say that an individual has a "fiery disposition" (i.e., choleric) or another person has a "happy-go-lucky" disposition (e.g., sanguine). In contrast, a *melancholic* (cold and dry) individual was believed to have an excessive amount of *black bile*, which resulted in an anxious, fearful, and brooding temperament. Finally, if *phlegm* was the dominant humor, then the person had a *phlegmatic* temperament, which gave them the unfortunate distinction of being fat, "soft," dull, and cowardly.[2] Nowadays, hearing the phrase "She is in good humor today" is a verbal remnant of the ancient humoral system! Whatever the case, these humors and their associated temperaments were the basic building blocks upon which ancient/early physicians and scholars approached human health, including stuttering.

Perhaps most curious for readers living in the early part of the 21st century is that ancient health care providers considered their client's "temperaments" as important to treat as the symptoms of the disorder itself.[2] For these early practitioners, the various temperaments were thought to contribute to the client's problem, symptoms, and treatment, in that the "disease" was not, for example, stuttering but an imbalance in the humors that impacted the whole person. This also meant that people with the same disease could have different etiologies; for example, stuttering in a person with a choleric temperament would have a very different cause than someone with a phlegmatic temperament. In a way, such possible differences among people are reflected in the present-day notion of "individual differences" in abilities, sensitivities to drugs, reactions to stress, etc. Regardless of the presumed etiology, however, bringing the client's humors back into balance was viewed as crucial to bringing the client's physical and mental health back to normal.

So, what does the above have to do with theories of stuttering? A good deal, or at least the way the ancients thought about stuttering. For example, a person with a melancholic temperament was theorized to have rapid motion(s) of the imagination (today we might say cognition/language formulation). This was a problem because the tongue of the melancholic person could not easily "keep up with" the mental concepts they were processing. Stated in more modern terms, Rieber and Wollock[2] suggested that early scholar-physicians believed that "stuttering… (is) a failure of synchronization between the processes of thinking and speaking." Whether valid or not, this "desynchronization" idea comes close to being one of the first of what we might consider to be a theory or at least hypothesis regarding stuttering. However, the only thing constant is change. So, as we will see, the age of enlightenment or reason would put the humoral system firmly in its rearview mirror.

To obtain some insight into the role that the humoral system played in ancient/early medical practice, it is instructive to consider the circumstances surrounding the death of the U.S. President George Washington. In the early morning hours of December 14, 1799, Washington woke his wife Martha complaining that he felt quite sick and that he was having trouble breathing and talking. Shortly thereafter, Washington asked his estate overseer to bleed him. At that time, bloodletting was a practice based on the humoral system of medicine and, in this case, used to treat George Washington.

His doctors arrived a bit later that day, assessed George's condition, and drained even more blood from Washington. His throat was swapped with a salve as well as a preparation made from insects, and other treatments were used in apparent attempts to address Washington's serious illness. Although it is difficult to be precise based on written notes made over

200 years ago, modern-day estimates suggest that, in total, the bloodlettings removed 40% of Washington's blood from his body. Likewise, present-day examination of the records suggests that the former president most likely died from a serious infection of the epiglottis at around 10 or 11 p.m. on December 14, 1799; however, it seems safe to say that the loss of so much blood probably did little to improve an already very serious situation.

For further details, see DM Morens' article titled "Death of a president."[4]

"Half of science is putting forth the right questions."

Francis Bacon (b. 1561, d. 1626)

2.3 The Beginnings: Shifting from Humoral to Scientific Approaches

In its earliest days, Francis Bacon was a major contributor to what we now call the scientific method or scientific investigation. People such as Bacon and Isaac Newton were not satisfied with repeating the words and thoughts of the authorities before them. Rather, enamored as they were with scientific investigation and observation, they advocated for the idea that one must test those words and thoughts. Despite this philosophical change in the zeitgeist, however, the past humoral system was not far behind. And this makes sense, for like the pendulum of a clock that swings from one side to the other, it too must pass through the middle. Or in Bacon's writings:

"Divers, we see, doe stut. The Cause, may bee, (in most,) the Refrigeration of the Tongue; Whereby it is lesse apt to move. And, therefore wee see that Naturalls doe generally Stut. And wee see that in those who stut, if they drinke Wine moderately, they Stut less, because it heateth…."[2]

Bacon's quote points out, once again, the earlier theory based on the humoral system that the tongue of (most) people who stutter is weak or cold. With that as the basic assumption, it was suggested that heat, like that provided by the alcohol in wine, rectifies the "refrigerated condition" of the tongue of people who stutter. So, it would seem, such early "treatment" was consistent with early theory. Of course, to subscribe to such theory requires one to ignore other possible explanations casting doubt on Bacon's basic premise that alcohol "heats" a "cold" tongue and thus leads to increased fluency.[2] For example, perhaps the person habitually inhibits the smooth, fluent flow of their speaking by overly self-correcting, editing, and revising their speech-language planning and production. Thus, drinking alcohol may disinhibit the person's habitual and frequent inhibiting tendency. And by so doing, the person exhibits an increase in fluent speech!

Be that as it may, it is not our intent to use the advances in knowledge and procedures of the 21st century to critique Bacon's 17th-century notion of stuttering. Rather, it is to show that Bacon and his predecessors held theories about the cause and treatment of stuttering that were influenced, at least in part, by the tenets of the humoral system. Even so, Bacon and his fellow travelers of that time were unique in that they were some of the first to suggest that merely relying on the word of authority about x, y, or z phenomena was inadequate to obtain a true understanding of such phenomena. Bacon and those who followed him, such as Voltaire, Darwin, and Pasteur, would instead push for exact, rigorous observation (and, if possible, testing) of events, stimuli, and phenomena. Truly this, called the "scientific method," laid down the blueprints that much of our current research continues to follow and refine.

"But by far the greatest obstacle to the progress of science and to the understanding of new tasks…is found in this—that men despair and think things impossible."

Francis Bacon (b. 1561, d. 1626)

2.4 The 18th and 19th Centuries: Establishment of the Scientific Method

Beginning in the late 17th century with the work of Bacon/Newton and continuing through the early 19th century, the age of enlightenment or reason held sway throughout much of Europe. This period was noted for many things, but for our purposes we will focus on its rejection (without criticism) of the words and thoughts of authority and emphasis on the scientific method. Indeed, much of our modern-day scientific method saw its beginning during this time.

Of relevance is this period's emphasis on the process of acquiring and/or developing knowledge, to test hunches, hypotheses, ideas, and theory. This method then insisted on (and still does now) careful/exact observation, applying objectivity/skepticism toward that which is observed, and from these observations, developing, testing, and refining or rejecting hypotheses. As more and more investigators followed these principles of the scientific method, more and more objective information about and understanding of stuttering was developed and reported.

Ideas die hard, however, and many were not overly impressed with the scientific method, relying instead on the thoughts and words of authorities through much of the 19th century. This is particularly true when it comes to theories of stuttering during the 19th century (i.e., the 1800s). This was the age of *nosology* (i.e., classification of diseases), which lead to the classification of speech and hearing disorders. Some of these classification schemes were focused on symptomatology, whereas others also included etiologies, anatomy, and therapy procedures for each disorder. Of these elements of classification, we turn to etiology for that is, in essence, theory.

"There is no short cut to truth, no way to gain a knowledge of the universe except through the gateway of scientific method."

Karl Pearson (b. 1857, d. 1936)

Of the various classification schemes, Erasmus Darwin's[2] non-humoral system account bears special mention. This is because of his strong interest in normal as well as disordered speech and language. In general, his theory of stuttering appears based on the law of association or contiguity: two objects become linked with one another when they are perceived or thought of simultaneously or in close association. (This is a bit like the American behavioral psychologist Edwin Guthrie's principle of contiguity learning, i.e., a combination of stimuli that accompany a movement will, on its recurrence, be followed by that movement. Or, the modern-day neuroscience principle, "those things that fire together wire together.") Specifically, Darwin theorized that when the person who stutters is considerably focused on an idea, the associated fear of failure is so strong that muscular motions and/or articulations become impaired.

What is important here is that Darwin's theory specifically implicated simultaneously occurring psychology and physiological processes in stuttering and did so in a way that comes close to being testable and possibly falsifiable (falsifiability refers to the ability of a theory or hypothesis to be contradicted and is one important cornerstone of the scientific method). His theory clearly breaks with earlier humoral system accounts and points to increasing use of the scientific method to better understand stuttering.

"Observation, reason, and experiment make up what we call the scientific method."

Richard P. Feynman (b. 1918, d. 1988)

2.5 The 19th and 20th Century: Physiological and Psychological Theories

Although the scientific method was, at least at its outset, more amenable to the study of observable anatomical and physiological structure and functioning, during the 1800s psychological processes were increasingly considered. Quite naturally, this orientation has carried into therapeutic and theoretical accounts of stuttering. It should be noted that during this period, physiology was thought to have considerable impact on psychology. Indeed, many appeared to believe that the brain, either in general or specifically, determined an individual's psychological assets and liabilities.

At this time, we find theorists suggesting that psychological processes, emotions, and the like may contribute to stuttering. One such theorist—Edward Warren[2]—suggested in the mid-1800s that stuttering is a nervous system disorder and that when this "weakness" is associated with or exacerbated by fear, true stuttering occurs. Warren appears to be one of the first to suggest that the cause of stuttering was both mental and physical in nature. Interestingly, Warren also suggested that people who stutter often exhibit a "nervous temperament." Indeed, considerable discussion during the 1800s regarding temperament and stuttering, as well as refinement in the nature and variety of temperaments occurred, presaging a return to this area of study in the first two decades of the 21st century.

"The deepest sin against the human mind is to believe things without evidence. Science is simply common sense at its best— that is, rigidly accurate in observation, and merciless to fallacy in logic."

Thomas H. Huxley (b. 1825, d. 1895)

In 1914, John M. Fletcher published a paper (really more like a monograph)—An Experimental Study of Stuttering[5]—that reported the findings of a series of empirical studies of stuttering.

Although smaller studies before and larger studies after were published, Fletcher's study is notable for its systematic application of the scientific method, not to mention its emphasis on the "psychology" of stuttering. Heretofore, most theories of stuttering, with some exceptions, focused on possible anatomical, physiological, and neurological contributions to stuttering. Indeed, as we cover more modern-day theories, it will be become apparent that some are primarily based on a "nature" (i.e., genetic, congenital, biological) perspective, some primarily a "nurture" (i.e., environmental, learned, psychosocial) perspective, and others an "interactive" nature plus nurture (e.g., slow-to-develop speech-language abilities interacting with emotional sensitivity) perspective.

As mentioned earlier, for further detail pertaining to stuttering therapies and the theories behind them during the 1800s through mid-1900s, see Van Riper.[3] His extensive coverage, especially those based on translations of non-English publications, provides a good breadth and depth description of various approaches to stuttering. Further, Van Riper's writing gives the sense that many aspects of stuttering therapy/theory believed to be "novel" actually have a considerable history of application and reported results. Of course, these earlier studies do not always meet the 21st-century standards of scientific study, but applying the 21st-century standards to 19th-century research is less than reasonable. What does seem reasonable, however, is to admire these earlier investigators increased willingness to experiment and test hunches, hypotheses, and ideas about stuttering instead of merely accepting and following authoritative but nontested opinions and pronouncements about stuttering.

Before we begin our discussion of some of the more prominent theories of the 20th and 21st centuries, it is worth noting that at their heart lies the notion of causality—that is, "what causes stuttering?" The search for "cause" is, of course, a challenging but not insurmountable task, as modern-day theories meet up with ever-more refined, sophisticated methodology.

Technically, for A to *cause* B, three conditions must be met: (1) A (cause) must happen before B (effect); (2) A (cause) and B (effect) must covary (e.g., if more of A more of B); and (3) no plausible alternative "causal" variable should be readily apparent. Unfortunately, these causality conditions have not always been applied to modern-day theories of stuttering, especially those that are more formal and testable using the scientific method.

Just importantly, however, such lack of application does not render theories meaningless, particularly if they lead to further scientific exploration that reveals more truths about stuttering that were not previously known. However, that few such theories have met these formal "causality" conditions should create a degree of humbleness for both theorists and therapists alike. In the latter part of this chapter, we will return to the issue of causality, the criteria for establishing it, and challenges to meeting those conditions when empirically examining stuttering.

"In the real world there is no nature vs. nurture argument, only an infinitely complex and moment-by-moment interaction between genetic and environmental effects."

Gabor Maté (b. 1944)

2.6 The Early to Mid-20th Century: Physiological and Psychosocial Theories

2.6.1 Nature Perspectives

The brain, of course, is fundamental to what we do and say. It should, therefore, come as no surprise that one of the first prominent 20th century theories of stuttering involved the brain and its processes. Indeed, empirical studies of one aspect of this theory—namely, the notion that people who stutter have insufficient cerebral dominance—continue to this day. As we shall see later in the chapter, some of the more rigorously pursued modern-day approaches toward identifying causal contributors to stuttering involve cortical and subcortical processes.

Cerebral Dominance Theory

One of the more notable theories of this period, the cerebral dominance theory of stuttering,[6,7,8,9] posited that people who stutter have ambiguous or uncertain laterality of cortical dominance, particularly for the speech-language centers of the brain. The underlying assumption of the cerebral dominance theory was that during normal speech there was synchronization in timing between the two cerebral hemispheres for control of the left and right halves of the speech musculature. This synchronization was believed to be possible because one hemisphere, usually the left, was dominant over the other. This theory suggested, however, that people who stutter did not have this normal pattern of cerebral dominance and this led to poor synchronization of the speech musculature and, in turn, stuttering.

Research Findings

Technology and research methods available in the late 1920s and some decades thereafter made it decidedly difficult to *directly* test the notion of "laterality of cortical dominance." However, handedness (i.e., being right-handed, left-handed, or ambidextrous), which can be related to cerebral dominance, has been thoroughly studied during the first and second halves of the 1900s. During this time, a multiyear exploration of the relation between handedness and stuttering was therefore, initiated to test, albeit indirectly, whether uncertain cerebral laterality was associated with stuttering.

To begin with, some of the earlier studies appeared to support a lack of cerebral dominance in people who stutter, but a series of studies, employing larger numbers of participants, did not. More recently, Geschwind and Behan[10] reported that in relatively large samples of "highly" righted-handed and "highly" left-handed individuals, self-reports indicated that 4.5% of the left-handed stuttered and 0.9% of the right-handed stuttered. Following, a robust meta-analysis[11] of cortical activity, mainly involving adults, indicated that people who stutter are more apt to exhibit right (or anomalous) lateralization.

There were no differences, however, in cerebral lateralization between either older[12] or younger[9] children who do and do not stutter. These differences in findings between children and adults who stutter have led some[13] to suggest that anomalous lateralization in adults who stutter results from "neoplastic adaptation." In other words, adults who have stuttered since childhood change, shift, or switch their "cortical resources" for speech production from the left to the right hemisphere following a lifetime of *adapting* to or dealing with stuttering. Whatever the case, the cerebral dominance theory of stuttering presages early 21st-century scientific studies. These more recent theories of the brain and stuttering have employed various modern, sophisticated neuroimaging and related methodology. Although perhaps obvious, these more modern procedures for studying brain function and structure were not available in the 1920s to 1940s when the cerebral dominance theory was first proposed and tested. We will return to these more recent cortically oriented theories later in this chapter.

2.6.2 Nurture Perspective

It is difficult to categorically dismiss the notion that environmental factors/variables contribute to human development and health. Indeed, it is highly likely that similar to other developmental disorders, environmental factors significantly contribute to the onset, development, and maintenance of stuttering. Like the brain, however, saying that environmental processes may contribute to stuttering is about like saying that oxygen contributes to our well-being. Such is a foregone conclusion; what is unknown, however, are the *specifics* of these contributions, be they cortical (nature) or environmental (nurture). The following sections, along with the preceding coverage of theory, attempt to "fill in" some of the specifics.

Diagnosogenic Theory

If the cerebral dominance theory of stuttering was largely "nature," Johnson's[14,15,16] diagnosogenic theory of stuttering was largely "nurture." Specifically, according to the diagnosogenic theory, the speech (dis)fluencies of children who stutter, at least those occurring near the onset of stuttering, were assumed to be similar to those of children who do not stutter. What differed, according to this theory, was that some parents "diagnosed" stuttering in their children on the basis of brief, "effortless" repetitions of sound, syllables, words, and phrases. For example, the theory suggested that when a child produces a "normal" disfluency, the parents may perceive it as stuttering, and react to it with concern, worry or upset. If the parent reacted that way, according to the theory, the child might try harder *not* to produce the parent-reacted-to disfluency to avoid disapproval from the parents. Consequently, the theory suggests, the child's ensuing struggle would transform his or her normal disfluency into a stuttered disfluency and, after repeated occurrences, the child would go on to develop stuttering. On the other hand, if the child's normal disfluency was perceived as just that—a normal disfluency—then the child would develop typically fluent speech. Thus, the diagnosogenic theory states that a child's stuttering starts after, not before, being diagnosed by an adult, typically one or both parents. In general, the model is often summarized by saying, "stuttering begins in the ear of the parent rather than the mouth of the child."

Research Findings

If one is to stay true to the scientific method, handed down and refined by our predecessors, then one should probably use Johnson's theory to develop testable hypotheses, empirically test the same, report the findings, and discuss whether findings support or refute the hypotheses. That is all well and good, but if the problem begins with the parent's diagnosis, how might a researcher study that event? Our answer: not very easily. So, although the diagnosogenic theory appears somewhat reasonable and tantalizing, it is in essence incapable of being readily falsifiable. In short, the theory cannot be tested, at least not easily. This lack of testability is important if one is going to rest their beliefs and understanding on facts and data, and not on seemingly logical but untestable speculation of authority. Further, more recent genetic findings, for example,[17] strongly suggest that inheritance or *nature* plays an important role in the onset and development of stuttering. This does not render the diagnosogenic theory completely invalid, but it does, once again, suggest caution, humbleness, and thoughtfulness when promoting pure or solely *nurture* or environmental accounts of stuttering.

Approach-Avoidance Conflict Theory

In his approach-avoidance conflict theory, Sheehan[18,19] proposed that stuttering resulted from opposing drives or tendencies to both speak and refrain from speaking. This notable theory was probably the first to heavily rely on theory and research findings from psychology. According to this theory, for a person who stutters, *speaking* has two "tendencies": one positive (e.g., I can say what I want) and one negative (e.g., I do not want to stutter). Furthermore, this theory suggests that the person will *approach* the positive and *avoid* the negative.

Consequently, if the positive tendency outweighs (i.e., is stronger than) the negative, the person who stutters will approach talking and speak fluently. Conversely, if the negative tendency outweighs the positive, the person who stutters will avoid and not talk. However, when the two tendencies are roughly comparable in strength, they intersect and the ensuing conflict (i.e., "do I approach or avoid?") results in an instance of stuttering. A similar situation occurs when the person who stutters considers not speaking; there is a positive tendency (I will not stutter) and a negative tendency (I will not say what I want to say). The conflict between the desire to both approach and avoid not talking (i.e., silence) is, in a sense, the mirror image of the conflict that occurs between approaching and avoiding speaking (hence this theory is often referred to as double-approach-avoidance conflict for speaking and not speaking).

Research Findings

Of the three early to mid-20th-century theories we have examined thus far, the approach-avoidance conflict theory is perhaps the most formal and logical. Formal and logical, however, does not always translate into testable. Others[20] have said much the same, "A theory may be poor not because it is untrue, but because it is logically incapable of verification as stated." Certainly, avoidance of speaking, especially in older children, teens, and adults who stutter can and does occur; however, whether the mechanism that Sheehan suggests accounts for such avoidance remains unclear. What seems clearer, however, is that there is a lack of data, facts, and/or findings that either support or refute the fundamental tenets of the approach-avoidance conflict theory of stuttering. This lack of factual support is no doubt related to the challenges of empirically testing such a theory.

"Whenever a theory appears to you as the only possible one, take this as a sign that you have neither understood the theory nor the problem which it was intended to solve."

Karl Popper (b. 1902, d. 1944)

2.7 The Late 20th Century: Learning and Multifactorial Theories

2.7.1 Nurture Perspectives

Related to environmental contributions to stuttering is the notion that *learning* underlies some, if not much of, stuttering. As with many human disorders, stuttering is likely to be somehow related to processes of learning. These processes involve a myriad of events, for example, developing behavior, knowledge, insights, and understanding through experience. Furthermore, these learning processes can be conscious, unconscious, or some combination of both. The following two theories of stuttering, two-factor theory and operant conditioning theory, go beyond the general in attempts to account for the specific nature of learning and its contributions to stuttering and associated behavior.

Two-Factor Theory

In general, the two-factor theory of stuttering[21,22] and other learning-based models (e.g., operant conditioning) shifted focus away from nature (e.g., in-born or innate abilities, attributes, traits) to a more nurture (e.g., experiential, environmental factors) account of stuttering. Specifically, the "two-factor model" proposed that instances of stuttering (e.g., sound-syllable repetitions) were developed through classical conditioning. It also proposed that associated, concomitant or secondary behaviors (e.g., head jerks, eyelids closing, eyeballs turning to the side, etc.[23]) were developed through operant conditioning. Accordingly, instances of stuttered speech were thought to result from emotional arousal that became associated with speech through classical conditioning. For example, during one occasion a child might experience negative emotion (e.g., fear) when speaking to a teacher. If such occasions are repeatedly experienced, the child's negative emotion (and related increases in anxiety, stress, or tension) may become more generally associated with the act of speaking with the teacher. These repeated "pairings," in this example negative emotion plus speaking with a specific individual (in this case the teacher), are posited, by this theory, to result in disruptions in fluent speech production.

Again, after repeatedly experiencing such encounters, the child will begin to more frequently produce stuttered speech whenever he speaks to his teacher, thus marking the beginnings of stuttering. On the other hand, associated behaviors, such as lowering eyelids or moving eyeballs to the side when talking, were thought to be acquired or learned through operant

conditioning, largely through escape and avoidance. For example, a child might "accidentally" escape a moment of stuttering by closing their eyes as he attempts to get a particular word out. According to the two-factor theory, the momentary relieve or reprieve the child experienced from escaping an instance of stuttering would serve as reinforcement, increasing the likelihood that the behavior (i.e., closing the eyes) will occur again.

As with the approach-avoidance conflict model, clinicians have employed therapeutic approaches that are based on the theoretical underpinnings of the two-factor theory. This theory-to-therapy connection seemingly rests on two points.

The *first point* relates to the model's assumption that instances of stuttering resulted from disruptions of speech by "fear reactions" that have been classically conditioned. Thus, therapies attempting to treat these "fear reactions" have employed "systematic desensitization." That is, the person who stutters is helped, by the clinician, to reach a state of deep relaxation. While in that state, the client is asked to imagine feared speaking situations, beginning with those that are less feared. Once the client indicates that the imagined situation no longer evokes fear or distress for them, the procedure is then repeated, gradually increasing, over time, the degree of fearfulness of the imagined situations. The relaxation is thought to inhibit or minimize the various cognitive, emotional, and physical events associated with fearfulness, as the two states of being (i.e., relaxed, nonfearful vs. nonrelaxed, fearful) presumably cannot occur simultaneously.[24]

The *second point* relates to the model's assumption that associated, concomitant, or secondary behaviors (e.g., head jerks) were developed through operant/instrumental conditioning and as such could not be mitigated by systematic desensitization. Instead, these operantly conditioned behaviors were thought to be changed through the process of reactive inhibition.[25] With this therapy, a person who stutters would engage in mass (i.e., repetitive) practice of these concomitant behaviors. These repeated productions of associated behaviors (e.g., looking away from the listener) were thought to build up fatigue (i.e., reactive inhibition)[20] and, therefore, diminish or inhibit the reinforcement that supposedly developed these behaviors in the first place.

Research Findings

Although the theory and logic behind the two-factor theory appear reasonable, there have been relatively few published reports of empirical testing that either support or refute its tenets. Those that have been reported[26,27] indicate that, in general, various forms of "punishment" have no appreciable impact on stuttering. In fact, in one single-participant study,[28] punishment was reported to actually increase the frequency of prolongations. Others,[29] however, have reported that making a loud auditory stimulus contingent on sound prolongations and repetitions reduced these speech disfluencies. If, as the two-factor account suggests, instances of stuttering are not instrumentally or operantly learned, then stuttering should not decrease because of punishment; however, in at least one study it did.

Currently, therapy procedures based on the two-factor model are not widely used. Still, some individuals with a long history of stuttering may find it helpful to learn how to cognitively, emotionally, and physically relax when speaking. This is particularly true for those who have developed fears and worries about both talking and stuttering. In hindsight, perhaps the biggest contribution of the two-factor theory was to shift the emphasis from cortical/physiological accounts of stuttering to learning and environmental contributions. This shift in emphasis helped the field better understand the challenge of employing relatively *invariable* (nature) accounts as the sole means for explaining *variable* behavior such as stuttering (a point we will return to at the end of this chapter). Immediately below, we shall see at least one more prominent theory of stuttering—operant conditioning theory—that also shifted the frame of reference concerning the etiology of stuttering.

Operant Conditioning Theory

The operant conditioning account of stuttering (e.g., Flanagan et al,[30] Shames and Sherrick,[31] Ingham and Andrews,[32] and Ingham[33]) was based on Skinner's[34] theory of learning. According to this account, instances of stuttering are "operants" or behaviors that "operate" on the environment that can be modified by their consequences.[34] As such, these operant behaviors can be learned or established through response-contingent reinforcement.

Relating operant conditioning to stuttering, instances of stuttering are thought to be developed, established, or learned according to the principles of operant conditioning. Specifically, there may be something positive in the environment that reinforces the behavior (i.e., stuttering). For example, say that a child produces a repetition, and this has the effect of getting the parent's attention. The increased parental attention being paid to the child may serve as a positive reinforcer, making it more likely that the child will produce a repetition in the future, when he desires the parent's attention. (Of course, parental attention, in this example, is assumed to be desired by the child, something the child would do nothing to avoid and if not desired, parental attention may not be reinforcing.)

Although positive reinforcement is an important aspect of operant conditioning, so too is negative reinforcement (and negative reinforcement is not the same as punishment). Negative reinforcement may occur if there is cessation or removal of a non-positive environmental event contingent upon a behavior or the consequence thereof. For example, removal or cessation of parental frowning can be "negatively" reinforcing if contingent on or the consequence of a child's attending rather than ignoring the parent. In other words, the parent ceases to frown when the child attends. If applied consistently each time the child attends, at least in theory, cessation of parental frowning should increase the frequency of the child's attentiveness. Be that as it may, for the purpose of this overview of theories of stuttering, we will limit our discussion of the operant theory of stuttering to "positive" reinforcers or reinforcement.

The elegant simplicity of this theory was attractive to both theorists and clinicians alike. This was because, at least in part, the theory was based on measurable, observable behaviors or events that could be counted and compared across settings and/or over the course of treatment. Indeed, the "observable" aspect of this model is completely in line with the position taken by Francis Bacon; he would only theorize and discuss that which was observable.

In keeping with Skinner's ideas, researchers and clinicians who viewed stuttering as an operant behavior would count instances of stuttering as an index of "learning." Again, the beauty of this approach was its steadfast adherence to identifying learning through measurable, observable behavior by using means readily available to other researchers and clinicians. In other words, such measurable, observable behaviors could be readily replicated from one observer to the next. Accordingly, any aspect of stuttering that *changed* due to response-contingent reinforcement (or punishment) was considered, by definition, to be an operant. These operant behaviors are fundamentally different from classically conditioned behaviors, which involve stimulus substitution (e.g., a light stimulus substituting for a loud, annoying alarm bell) as the mechanism for learning. Further, this theory, because of its reliance on measuring only that which is observable, eschews more abstract constructs such as feeling, thinking, etc.—unless, of course, one would assume, they could be clearly connected to or considered observable behavior.

Research Findings

Research has shown that overt stuttering can either decrease or increase in response to environmental events. These findings lend support to the hypothesis that various aspects of stuttering behavior are operant in nature. One of the nontrivial inconsistencies with the operant model of stuttering, however, is that there have been reported instances of stuttering *increasing* with punishment.[35] If a behavior is truly an operant, according to the theory, it should *decrease* with punishment or negative consequences/contingencies. Indeed, clinically oriented studies of young children who stutter, for example,[36,37] have reported that apparently neutral to benign verbal corrections, reprimands, or punishment for stuttering *decrease* stuttering (putting aside, for the sake of argument, the decrease in stuttering that at least 70% of children who stutter will eventually experience *without* formal therapeutic intervention).

These differences in the behavioral responses between children and adults to response-contingent reinforcement, have led to at least two observations: (1) we cannot readily extrapolate backward from the behavior of adults who stutter to that of children who stutter, and (2) we cannot readily extrapolate forward from the behavior of children who stutter to that of adults who stutter. Thus, there remains some uncertainty regarding the influence of chronological age and/or experience on operant-oriented treatments for stuttering. There is less uncertainty that early enthusiasm for theoretical consideration of stuttering as an operant behavior has not seemingly been maintained in recent years. Nevertheless, despite waning of theoretical interest in operant theories of stuttering, there remains enthusiasm, by some clinicians, for operant-informed treatments of stuttering. Specifically, clinical approaches, based solely or in part, on operant theory/method, especially for young children who stutter, continue to be employed in the form of "verbal contingencies" for both fluent and stuttered productions.[36] Such clinical approaches have reportedly resulted in significant improvement in stuttering for these children.[37]

2.7.2 Nature and Nurture Interaction Perspectives

Demands and Capacities Model

The demands and capacities model (DCM) of stuttering is straightforward in suggesting that stuttering occurs when the "demands" (social or otherwise) that are being placed on a child for fluent speech *exceed* the child's "capacities" (social-emotional maturity, language formulation, cognitive skills, and/or speech motor) for producing fluency.[38,39,40] If the demands continue to exceed the child's capacity, the child will struggle more during speaking, particularly during instances of disfluency, leading to the development of stuttering. The DCM was a truly interactive model in that environmental pressure, requirements, or stimuli were thought to interact with the child's inherent or innate capabilities. Although the model attempts to account for stuttering in people who stutter as a group, it has the potential to account for individual cases as well. That is, the DCM allows for many permutations of demands exceeding capacities involving one or more constructs (i.e., linguistic, motor, etc.). Interestingly, the converse—capacity exceeding demand—does not seem to be, according to the DCM model, a potential pathway to producing stuttering. In other words, the interaction between demand and capacity seems uni- rather than bidirectional in nature.

Research Findings

It is worth noting that in 2000 an entire issue of the *Journal of Fluency Disorders*[41] was devoted to a critical appraisal of the DCM's theoretical and clinical implications. In the absence of testable hypotheses and empirical data, it is difficult to adequately assess the validity of this volume other than saying that the DCM engendered a robust pros and cons debate. A bit closer to testing the DCM, or at least some of its basic assumptions, it would seem, are the findings of a series of studies by a German researcher, Bosshardt.[42] Although these studies involved adults rather than children who stutter, some of the findings are relevant to the DCM. In essence, Bosshardt's studies examined the effect of changes in "processing load" (one form of demand, it may be argued), using a dual-task paradigm (think about driving a car while talking on a telephone), on the frequency of stuttering. The adults who stutter were reported to exhibit increased disfluency and/or lower linguistic productivity, suggesting that the "heightened demands" of the task exceeded their capacity for fluent speech and/or language formulation. Whether these findings are directly related to the DCM, the implications of these results for hypotheses and theory are exactly the type of knowledge generation/theory testing that the founders of the enlightenment like Bacon, Newton, and Voltaire had in mind.

2.8 Late 20th to Early 21st Century: Prominent Contemporary Theories

As the 20th century turned the corner into the 21st century, theories of stuttering became increasingly influenced by advances in a variety of related disciplines (e.g., psycholinguistics,

speech motor control, etc.). The application of these advances moved from the general (e.g., demands and capacity model) to much more specific processes (e.g., the covert repair hypothesis [CRH], execution and planning [EXPLAN] model, etc.). Indeed, the past 20 to 25 years of theory relating to the causation of stuttering have increasingly relied on understanding of findings and speculation from outside the area of speech-language pathology. These theories are noted not only for this reliance but also for their formality and ability to generate hypotheses that are both testable and capable of being falsifiable. The speech-language formulation and computational/ neurocomputational models discussed in this section are based on a nature perspective, whereas the multifactorial theories are clearly interactive—that is, they adopt both a nature and nurture orientation.

2.8.1 Speech-Language Planning Theories

Covert Repair Hypothesis

Arising from a psycholinguistic perspective regarding (a)typical speech-language planning and production, Dutch researchers Postma and Kolk formulated and reported on the CRH.[43,44] The CRH provides a decidedly different approach to understanding stuttering. In brief, the model takes a psycholinguistic perspective that focuses on the interactions between linguistic and psychological factors. As such, psycholinguists study the psychological and neurological underpinnings of human language comprehension and production.

Beginning with their landmark theoretical-position paper,[43] Postma and Kolk's CRH was created to explain both typical and atypical speech disfluencies. The model rests on the reasonable assumption that all speakers occasionally produce errors during language processing. For example, when prompted to name a picture of a cat, a speaker might inadvertently select the wrong phoneme (/r/), saying "rat" instead of "cat." Most theories of language production propose that the accuracy of speech can be monitored before production and if an error is detected, it can be corrected. To repair the error, speech is interrupted, with the by-product of this repair being a normal or stuttered disfluency—that is, the very aspects of speech output that characterize instances of stuttering.

The CRH appears rooted in the idea that unlike normally disfluent individuals, people who stutter are presumed to have difficulty with phonological processing (see ▶ Chapter 4). As a result of these assumed phonological processing difficulties, individuals who stutter have many more opportunities to correct their (more frequent) errors, and thus, create, as a by-product, more disfluency. The model was quite unique and generated a great deal of attention from researchers and clinicians alike, resulting in a fair amount of empirical testing. It is also one of the only models that have attempted to explain the production of different types of disfluencies (e.g., why a speaker might sometimes produce a sound repetition and at other times a sound prolongation).

Research Findings

In general, some research findings support the basic notion(s) of the CRH and some do not. Regardless, such testing is a step forward to the truth of the matter and for that, the CRH has moved our understanding of stuttering forward. For an example, it has been reported that slips of the tongue (e.g., saying "coffee cot" for "coffee pot") are related to instances of stuttering produced by children who stutter.[45] Likewise, articulatory accuracy is lower for children whose stuttering persists compared to those who recover.[46] Studies of syntactic (i.e., grammatical formulation level)[47] and lexical (i.e., word-selection level) processing[48] have further indicated that these aspects of speech-language planning and production differ between children who do and do not stutter. Interestingly, at the phonological level (i.e., sound-selection level), there appears to be no difference in performance between children who do and do not stutter. However, children who stutter, unlike their normally disfluent peers, exhibit a significant correlation between their articulation test scores and their overall reaction times to name age-appropriate pictures.[49]

Finally, one study of phonological processing[50] inspired by the CRH investigated whether children who stutter, when compared to their typically fluent counterparts, exhibit less mature (i.e., holistic) than mature (i.e., incremental) forms of phonological encoding. Holistic processing involves processing of speech at the syllable level, whereas incremental processing involves processing of speech at the individual sound level. Overall, findings from this study were taken to suggest that young children who stutter were delayed in shifting from holistic to incremental forms of processing. This developmental challenge may impact their abilities to begin and maintain fluency as they encounter increasingly more complex verbal expression as they age, findings and speculation consistent with the CRH.

The above findings provide mixed support for the basic tenets of the CRH. However, findings appear sufficiently robust to warrant empirically investigating this model with different, more fine-grained means of measurement. For example, employing precise measures of speech reaction time (e.g., measuring electrical activity in the brain using electroencephalography) may provide more definitive evidence to either support or refute the CRH.

Execution and Planning Model

The EXPLAN model[51,52,53] is similar to the CRH in that both are psycholinguistic in orientation. According to the EXPLAN model, which was developed by the British researcher Howell, speech disfluencies are related to a dyssynchrony (i.e., a timing or temporal mismatch) between language planning and motor execution. Specifically, speech disfluencies are thought to occur when the processes involved with language planning (i.e., PLAN) are delayed or slower than the rate of execution (i.e., EX) of speech.

In essence, there are two interrelated phases to EXPLAN. Given that the formulation of a language plan occurs *before* motor execution, the first phase consists of a delay in language planning resulting in no speech (available) to execute. In the second phase, when faced with no speech available to execute, the speaker adopts one of two processes to "gain" or "buy" time for further processing. Typically or normally fluent speakers (i.e., nonstutterers) do this by means of a "stalling process." This "stalling process" involves repeating the previously produced word or inserting a filled (e.g., ummmm, errrrr) or unfilled

(e.g., silent) pause until the language plan becomes available for execution. In contrast to the "stalling process" employed by typically fluent speakers, this model posits that people who stutter employ an "advancing process" whereby they repeat portions of the word that is presently being processed. This "advancing process" is thought to result in sound/syllable repetitions (e.g., "m-m-m-more"), blocks (e.g., "muh [long silent pause] ore"), or sound prolongations (e.g., "mmmmmore").

Research Findings

There is an intuitive feel to EXPLAN. That is, the model, although much more sophisticated and technical in nature than models of the early to mid-20th century, shares some of the same assumptions. For example, in 1826, Combe[2] suggested that stuttering relates to "the ineffectual struggle of a small organ of language to keep pace with the workings of larger organs of intellect." In essence, these early-day scholars were proposing "a lack of synchronization between language and thought."[2] Of course, 19th-century notions of "language" and "thought" do not readily map onto current, more data-based terms, like "execution" and "planning," but the key similarity is the notion of less-than-appropriate synchronization between related but different processes. And given that instances of stuttering seem to disrupt the "temporal flow" of speech, as mentioned earlier, there is intuitive appeal for a model like EXPLAN in which disturbances in timing are thought to be central to stuttering.

Of course, just because something seems intuitive (rather than evidence based) does not necessarily mean it is wrong. Indeed, many well documented theories start out from intuitions, hunches, and observations made during the process of clinical practice. Whether intuitive or not, Howell[52] proposes that EXPLAN's account of stuttering involves an "autonomous theory"—that is, a theory that assumes that the production system works independent of perception. As such, Howell argues, "…many features of stuttering can be explained in an autonomous production model in which the problem arises at the point where linguistic and motor processes interact." Here again, there is intuitive appeal to EXPLAN in that stuttering is quite often associated with the first word of an utterance, a word spoken that is not apparently reliant on perception of one's own overt speech.

Interestingly, the "autonomous" nature of EXPLAN contrasts with other models (e.g., Kolk and Postma[44]) that assume a link between perception and production. Which approach best fits actuality or data—that is, perception linking with production versus perception autonomous from production—will not be solved in these pages. However, both CRH and the EXPLAN model have benefitted greatly from the confluence of modern-day psychological and linguistic constructs in research. In short, both models have expanded the parameters as well as framework within which to view the possible means by which instances of stuttering are generated and, hence, elevated and furthered our understanding of stuttering.

2.8.2 Multifactorial Theories

Dual-Diathesis Stressor Model

The dual-diathesis stressor (DD-S)[54,55,56] model of stuttering builds on the earlier Monroe and Simons' diathesis stress model[57] in the field of psychology. As applied to stuttering, the DD-S model rests on several assumptions. Below are brief descriptions of the diathesis stressor model in general as well as specific assumptions made when applying the model to stuttering.

The word "diathesis" comes from the Greek term for predisposition or sensibility. A diathesis (thought to be an inherited or innate vulnerability/weakness) can take many forms, for example, biological, genetic, or psychological. Stress or stressors are typically considered to be related to environmental or life challenges, events, or experiences. Taken together, this model, typically considers the diathesis to be a biological or genetic trait (but other forms are possible, e.g., the early life experience of loss or death of a parent) and stress to be an environmental event or experience. Central to the diathesis-stress model is the notion that a diathesis, predisposition, or vulnerability *interacts* with stress (stressors) associated with environmental factors. The model assumes that when the combination or interaction of the diathesis-stress exceeds a threshold, the individual may be at risk of developing a disorder, especially if this combination is experienced repeatedly or routinely. If this model sounds like one that assumes that nature (diathesis) interacts with nurture (stressors), that is because it is such a model! Furthermore, the model assumes that diatheses vary across individuals. Thus, if two individuals, with different diatheses, are exposed to similar life experiences, their responses or outcomes are likely to differ, according to this model.

Briefly, the DD-S model's application of diathesis-stress theory to stuttering, involves specific assumptions. First, the DD-S model assumes two different diatheses, one emotional and the other speech-language, with some people who stutter having one or the other or both. Second, the DD-S model assumes that neither diatheses nor stressors need be pathological or markedly disparate from the norm to activate underlying predispositional vulnerabilities. Rather, the model assumes that there merely needs to be a confluence of the two—the diathesis and stressor—that exceeds some threshold for an instance of stuttering to occur and/or a problem with stutter to develop or exist. Third, the DD-S model of stuttering assumes that processes thought to contribute to stuttering—such as cognitive, emotional, linguistic, and motoric processes—concurrently interact with one another and that these processes are likely sources of diatheses. Fourth, and perhaps obvious, the DD-S model assumes that people who stutter may have a biological or genetic diathesis (i.e., a vulnerability) that can be activated by domain-specific stress. Domain-specific stress is specific to each diathesis, for example, planning or formulating speech-language at a rate of speech (the stressor) that well exceeds one's motoric abilities to produce speech fluently (the diathesis). Fifth, and finally, the DD-S model assumes that these diatheses—again, frequently thought to be biological and/or inherited in nature—represent "open" genetic variables. This means that they are "open to" or permit considerable environmental interaction and influence (i.e., epigenetic).

In general, the DD-S model of stuttering posits that one or both diatheses (i.e., emotions and speech-language) contribute to stuttering, each with its own domain-specific stressors (as mentioned earlier). Specifically, the DD-S model hypothesizes that a diathesis (e.g., high emotional reactivity and/or low emotional regulation) that is *intermittently but predictably activated* by environmental events or experiences increases the likelihood of instances of disfluency occurring and/or a stuttering problem developing or existing. The confluence or combinations of diatheses-stress (be they emotional, speech-language, or both) intermittently challenge the speaker's ability to plan and produce on-the-fly speech and language fluently and quickly. These two "combinations" can occur concurrently or singularly. Most importantly, the notion of "intermittently activated" is consistent with the model's basic assumption that the cause of stuttering is neither static nor invariant, thus accounting for variability in stuttering itself (with *variability* being a hallmark of stuttering).

Research Findings

To date, the DD-S model of stuttering has been tested at least three times.[55,56,58] The first empirical test,[55] with young children who do and do not stutter, indicated that emotion and language diatheses in preschool children are associated with not only stuttering but also coping strategies and situational emotional stressors. For example, children who exhibited more negative emotions and lesser abilities to regulate their emotional reactivity produced more stuttering, whereas those with more negative emotions and greater regulation produced fewer stuttering (see ▸ Chapter 6). Findings from a second study[56] with young children demonstrated that increases in stuttering were associated with higher levels of both positive and negative emotions—that is, the more emotionally aroused a child was, the more likely they were to stutter, regardless of whether the emotions were positive or negative. Findings from a third study[58] of older children who stutter appear to support the basic diathesis-stress tenet of the DD-S model. The authors of this third study[58] interpret their findings as supporting the notion that a child's temperament may be, for example, an "intrinsic sensitivity" (diathesis) that is "triggered and boosted by external agents" (stressors) "to influence the emergence of disfluencies" (p.10).

However, given that these three studies involved young and older children, it remains unclear if their findings also apply to teens and adults who stutter. Further, as findings suggest,[58] there may be temperamental differences between younger and older children who stutter (differences confounded by the fact that younger children, when compared to older children, who stutter are more likely to recover from their stuttering without formal treatment). Whatever the case, at least for pre-school and school-age children who stutter, emotional processes would appear to warrant inclusion as one variable related to stuttering, the diagnosis as well as stuttering, the behavior (see ▸ Chapter 7 for further discussion of the assessment of emotional contributions to the assessment of stuttering in preschoolers).

Multifactorial Dynamic Pathways Theory

As an outgrowth of a long-standing program of empirical study of stuttering, Smith et al[59,60] developed the multifactorial dynamic pathways (MDP) theory of stuttering. This theory would appear to provide, a "grand amalgam" of many factors operating in concert to contribute to stuttering. At the heart of this "multifactorial" model is a disruption in motor speech production that is impacted by cognitive, linguistic, and emotional variables. The centrality of motor disruption is consistent with the near universal nature of instances of stuttering, such as sound/syllable repetitions and prolongations. In essence, a single "source of disruption" is hypothesized to create homogeneity in the symptoms of stuttering. This hypothesis is somewhat at odds with the observation that stuttering is heterogeneous in terms of the variables that impact its frequency and severity. That is, for some people who stutter, emotional factors seem to predominate, whereas for others, linguistic factors are most salient. And yet for still others, a combination of variables seems to be of greatest import. To account for such heterogeneity, the MDP theory proposes that cognitive, emotional, etc., variables interact with as well as condition the underlying motor disruptions, making them more or less capable of creating a disruption in speech fluency. In other words, the theory appears to be suggesting that a select number and nature of motor disruptions are the reason the "symptoms" of stuttering are essentially universal across people who stutter, whereas individual differences in cognitive, emotional, and linguistic factors are viewed to be the reason for variation in at least the frequency of overt expression of these symptoms.

According to the model, this interaction among variables that contribute to stuttering is dynamic in nature. The word "dynamic" implies that the contribution of the variables themselves and their interactions differ with time, circumstances, and/or context. For example, a child with strong reaction to a new or unfamiliar situation, change, and difference may experience cognitive or emotional stress. Such stress leads to a scanning of the situation for "threat," creating the potential for impacting the child's cognitive, linguistic, and motor systems in a manner that disrupts, at least to a degree, the child's speech fluency. In other situations, emotion and cognitive variables may be of less salience, for example, a person describing all the features of a new bicycle over the phone to someone (who cannot see the bicycle). In this example, of greater salience is the fact that such description requires the use of new words and phraseology that can increase linguistic demand on an already vulnerable motor system, resulting in speech disfluencies.

In short, the multifactorial model describes a reasonably select number of variables that may contribute to stuttering. Further, it suggests that such variables may combine in various permutations to undermine a person's speech fluency. These various possible permutations would appear to increase theoretical as well as clinical flexibility and thoughtfulness when accounting for group and individual differences across various investigations.

Research Findings

There appears to be developing empirical support for the multifactorial model.[61,62] For example, the notion that one variable can create the conditions for another variable to emerge can be seen by findings[61] that longer, more complex sentences may be associated with more variable speech motor production for children and adults who stutter, one convergence of events that may undermine speech fluency. The question remains, however: why doesn't this impact all speakers?

Perhaps it does, but the impact is thought to be slight compared to the person who stutters with a vulnerable motor system, prone to disruption by certain variables or combinations of variables. The stress, at least for some people who stutter, could be as straight forward as thought-processes that render an automatic act like speaking into one that is far more deliberate

(i.e., thinking more about how they speak than the thoughts they want to express). Whatever the case, the multifactorial model covers many of the variables reasonably thought to contribute to stuttering. Furthermore, its manifold possible accounts of stuttering open, to a degree, various pathways for research and clinical exploration. If it is true that standing for most anything leads to falling for most anything, the long-term influence of this theory is unknown, but for the present its comprehensive approach to stuttering is refreshing and quite empirically testable.

2.8.3 Computational/ Neurocomputational Models

SimpleDIVA and Related Models

The last theory discussed in this chapter is the SimpleDIVA (Directions into Velocities of Articulators)[63] model. This model was "streamlined" from its predecessor models to better characterize individuals with speech disorders. As mentioned, SimpleDIVA was derived from its "parent" models developed by Guenther and colleagues: the DIVA model[64,65] and its subsequent version, Gradient Order DIVA (GODIVA).[66,67,68] These earlier, more comprehensive models provide a robust and testable neurocomputational account of speech motor control and sound sequencing. Although the DIVA family of models are not models of stuttering per se, some elements of these (DIVA and GODIVA) models have been applied to stuttering.[69,70] Detailed, further explanation of the first two models—DIVA and GODIVA—goes well beyond the purpose and scope of the present, brief overview chapter. Instead, we will briefly cover the essentials of SimpleDIVA, the most recent model in the DIVA family of models. Again, whereas DIVA and its offshoots are not models of stuttering per se, they have been applied to the empirical study of stuttering and will undoubtedly receive further study employing computer simulations as well as other experimental methodologies.

In short, SimpleDIVA addresses three fundamental components of the DIVA model:[64,65] (1) auditory feedback, (2) somatosensory feedback, and (3) feedforward control processes. Feedforward control refers to a mechanism in a system that monitors performance *inputs* rather than *outputs* and reacts so as to maintain a specified state by correcting errors or problems *before* they occur. So, in a sense, feedback "looks back" to what *has happened* and feedforward "looks forward" to what *may or is about to happen.*

These three components of SimpleDIVA and their interactions are perhaps best viewed through the lens of a sensorimotor adaptation experiment. In such an experiment, the speaker's acoustic signal is disrupted or shifted over some period of time (i.e., their auditory feedback is perturbed/shifted). Consequently, the speaker changes their speech production (which alters their somatosensory feedback) in opposition to the shift, in order to make their perception better match what they intended to say (which engages their feedforward control processes). The processes the speaker uses to make such adjustments involve a complex combination of feedback and feedforward controls, processes that are very much involved with normal speech and language production.

The SimpleDIVA publication[63] used real data from an existing dataset in computer simulations to test the model's fit. To the present authors' knowledge, SimpleDIVA has not been specifically applied to stuttering. If applied, differences between individuals who do and do not stutter in their relative use of auditory feedback, somatosensory feedback, and feedforward control processes during speech production may provide some insight into the underlying mechanisms associated with speech motor control in stuttering. At the very least, the perturbations to the auditory/motoric processes associated with instances of stuttering would seem fertile ground for SimpleDIVA application. Furthermore, SimpleDIVA's relatively clear, straightforward framework and predictions make it an accessible entrance point for the interested reader, clinician, or researcher interested in the DIVA/GODIVA model.

Research Findings

Results of recent studies of stuttering, which were either generated or interpreted by the DIVA/GODIVA models, can be found in Daliri et al[69] and Garnett et al.[70] For example, findings from this latter study indicated that children whose stuttering persisted exhibited reduced thickness in their left motor and lateral premotor cortices, a morphological difference that may be associated with impaired neural processing. These differences may make it difficult for the basal ganglia motor loop to identify/provide the proper sensorimotor context for initiating the next gesture in a speech sequence, resulting in stuttering. Specifically, the authors interpreted their findings from two possible perspectives regarding directionality of effect: (1) impaired ventral motor/premotor cortex processing makes it difficult for the basal ganglia to initiate the next gesture in a speech sequence, creating instances of stuttering; or (2) impaired basal ganglia neural processing leads to less effective motor programs in the ventral motor/ventral premotor cortices, creating instances of stuttering. Chang and Guenther's[71] recent review of such research provides, within the neurocomputational framework of DIVA, a general takeaway applicable to stuttering. Specifically, this review suggests that stuttering behaviors may be associated with impairment within the basal ganglia; impairment of axonal projections between cerebral cortex, basal ganglia, and thalamus; and impairment in cortical processing. Certainly, these are intriguing, thought-provoking possibilities. However, such possibilities must await results of future research for refinement, refutation, or confirmation.

Whichever perspective on the directionality of effect is eventually best supported by objective results, these DIVA-/GODIVA-interpreted findings are an excellent example of the power of producing data to examine testable hypotheses generated by a model (a "test-your-theory" process that was previously discussed and championed by Newton, Pasteur, Voltaire, and others in the development of and support for the "scientific method"). Whether hypotheses generated by SimpleDIVA will be empirically tested regarding the cause and/or origins of instances of stuttering remains an open question, but the future shines bright for the DIVA family to further illuminate our understanding of stuttering.

"The greatest tragedy of science—the slaying of a beautiful hypothesis by an ugly fact."

Thomas H. Huxley (b. 1825, d. 1895)

2.9 Further Considerations

The previous section represents a brief coverage of some of the more prominent theories of stuttering and related phenomena from the early-mid 20th to early 21st centuries. As mentioned at the outset, this description was not intended to represent *all* theories of stuttering nor was it meant to be comprehensive in describing those selected. It was, however, representative of theories that were mainly nurture, mainly nature, or amalgams of both. Furthermore, although some theories have been directly tested by empirical studies, others have not been tested due to the challenges that such study would entail. Still, other theories have either gained or lost support due to studies that indirectly tested its assumptions; for example, the theory that stuttering is mainly learned was less than able to readily account for findings from genetic studies indicating heritable aspects of the disorder.

Thus, theories may rise or fall, in whole or part, due to the emergence of new data, facts, or information. Such theoretical comings and goings are not easily charted by a straight line. However, science, as may be apparent by now, does not proceed in a straight line but often along a crooked one. Certainly, science is not a full-contact sport, but neither is it for the faint of heart. Likening science to ships, it is said that ships are safe in the harbor. But ships were not built for the harbor.

Whatever the case, there are general considerations regarding theories of stuttering that deserve mention as well as some thought. The following are among the more germane considerations, provided neither to critique nor support the above theories as much as to provide perspective. And, like the present authors' coverage of the theories themselves, these considerations are not intended to be nor will be comprehensive of *all* such matters.

2.9.1 Theories of Stuttering Etiology

Most theories of stuttering attempt, more or less, to put forth or describe the causes of stuttering. At the least, these theories try to provide a conceptual framework with which to understand and view the cause or etiology of instances of stuttering. Putting forth both—description of cause and conceptual framework—is helpful and needed. It provides the natural rationale for accounting for known facts and theory development. Nevertheless, it is critical for us to think about what we mean when we say that X *causes* Y. Doing so, the authors believe, gives us pause about how far along the various theories of stuttering have progressed towards formulation of cause.

Indeed, and as briefly discussed earlier, individuals in the philosophy of science have suggested that to *conclusively* indicate that X causes Y, the following **three** conditions must be met:
- X (cause) must happen *before* Y (effect), that is, there must be "temporal precedence."
- X (cause) and Y (effect) must *covary* (i.e., a relation must be established), so that the following occurs:
  - If X, then Y.
  - If not X, then not Y.
    OR
  - If more of X, then more of Y.
    OR
  - If less of X, then less of Y.
- There should be *no plausible alternative* explanation.

Although some theories of stuttering meet some of these criteria, more than a few meet none or perhaps only one of the requisites to establish cause–effect. Certainly, the preceding criteria set a high bar to hurdle. However, one might welcome more explicit attempts to meet such criteria. By so doing, we might better move forward in our quest to establish the cause of stuttering. Of course, stuttering is not unique in this regard, for across the array of speech-language disorders, few theories can meet these criteria for establishing cause–effect. Indeed, some of these conditions are difficult to meet regarding stuttering. For example, consider whether the relative thinness of cortical tissue "causes" persistent childhood stuttering (something the authors of the previously mentioned study[70] *did not* suggest). The following question could be asked: Was the cortical morphologic difference present before the child began to stutter or did it appear after the child began to stutter? Given our present lack of precursor indicators *prior to* the onset of stuttering in young children, this question is difficult, if not impossible, to answer.

The bottom line is that understanding the criteria for determining causation, and our challenges in meeting such criteria, should make us careful about our statements of cause. Achieving such humbleness, uncertainty of thought and expression, should not stifle our attempts to advance our understanding/knowledge of cause(s) of stuttering. Neither, however, should it suggest that we know (let alone have answered) all the questions surrounding what causes stuttering.

"I am an agnostic; I do not pretend to know what many ignorant men are sure of."

Clarence Darrow (b. 1857, d. 1938)

2.9.2 Antecedents to versus Consequences of Stuttering

We are often puzzled when we observe and study the behaviors, events, processes, and experiences associated with stuttering, either those that are antecedents (occur before) or consequences (occur after) of the disorder. Arguably, if we could go back in time to the period before the person began to stutter, we might have a better understanding of this puzzle. However, even if time travel were possible, we would still have problems because our ability to predict stuttering from infancy remains an inexact science (keeping in mind that most stuttering begins between 2.5 and 4.0 years of age, not during infancy). That said, at present it remains challenging to precisely discern whether a phenomenon associated with stuttering is an antecedent or a consequence. Some may express knowledge about what preceded what, but certainty about the uncertainty does not make the latter disappear. It merely puts it out of sight, and often out of mind. And to paraphrase Aldous Huxley, facts, in this case uncertainty regarding antecedents and consequences, do not cease to exist (simply) because they are ignored.

The conundrum of what is antecedent and what is consequent becomes even more problematic when one assumes consequence and in addition to that assumption, assigns a causal chain of events. For example, nonspeech associates of stuttering (e.g., eye blinking) can have many possible originating sources[18] that have little or nothing to do with learned avoidance or escape, one of the more common explanations for the occurrences of nonspeech behaviors associated with stuttering. Thus, the reader is cautioned to take with a grain of salt conclusions about antecedents versus consequences of stuttering. For if we are still struggling to meet the criteria for establishing the cause of stuttering, we are certainly going to struggle to distinguish between that which is antecedent to and that which is the consequence of stuttering. Or, as Voltaire reminds us, "Doubt is not a comfortable condition, but certainty is absurd."

2.9.3 The Diagnosis versus the Behavior of Stuttering

To date, much of the research into the cause(s) of stuttering has involved comparing two groups of people: individuals who stutter and a comparable (e.g., in age and sex) group of individuals who do not. Results from these investigations have been helpful, informative, and insightful regarding possible causes of/contributors to stuttering (as well its nature). Such research can and should continue, particularly when used as an initial investigation into a promising line of investigation. However, knowing something about stuttering, the diagnostic category, is not quite the same as knowing something about stuttering, the behavior. The diagnostic category is based on a variety of objective and subjective measurements of stuttering (e.g., measuring the frequency and severity of stuttering; measuring their level of articulatory, vocabulary, or language development; asking the parents of a child who may or may not be stuttering about the child's speech, language, or fluency; or asking the person who stutters about their behavior and experiences with stuttering). These measures help the clinician know or understand a variety of things about the client, for example, whether the child is stuttering and, if so, their risk of continuing to stutter; how stuttering is impacting a teen's or adult's academic, emotional, social, and vocational lives; and so forth. Fine, such information is important and needed knowledge for clinical practice. However, one should probably not equate knowing how to diagnose stuttering with knowing how/why instances of stuttering occur. Certainly, knowledge about diagnosis of stuttering is *related* to knowledge about how/why instances of stuttering occur, but knowledge about one is not *identical* to knowledge about the other.

Risking redundancy, our understanding of the causal contributors to stuttering would be stronger if there were available data that showed that when X variable is present or active, instances of stuttering occur, or that more stuttering occurs when there is evidence that a cognitive, emotional, linguistic, or motor process known to be associated with stuttering occurs with more frequency or strength. Stronger or more data-supported levels of knowledge does not imply, of course, *absolute* as much as simply *greater* knowledge.

In essence, more direct, observable measurement of possible connections between a causal variable and instances of stuttering is what is needed. However, this may be easier said than done considering that some processes are currently difficult, if not impossible, to measure on a moment-by-moment basis. For example, it is not clear how one would measure whether someone was having difficulty retrieving a lexical item or motor plan at exactly the same time an instance of stuttering occurred. And, even if one could measure these exceedingly rapid events,

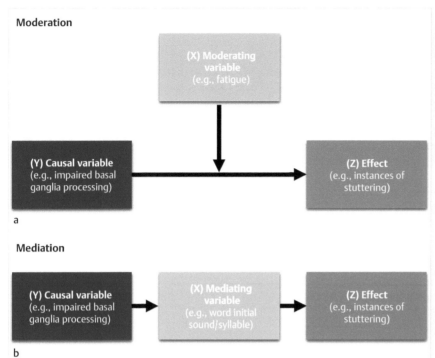

Moderation

Mediation

a

b

Fig. 2.1 Hypothetical *moderating* and *mediating* variables. To make the concepts of moderating and mediating variables more tangible, we hypothetically assumed that Y causes Z. **(a)** In the case of *moderation*, X (fatigue) conditions, influences, or moderates the relation between Y and Z. **(b)** In the case of *mediation*, X (word initial sound/syllable) determines or mediates, to a large degree, whether Y will cause Z.

it would be nearly impossible to know if what is observed is an antecedent or a consequence of stuttering itself. For example, perhaps an instance of stuttering that resulted from something other than what is being measured interfered with the retrieval of the lexical item or motor plan. Keeping that in mind, it is possible that the connection between a seeming causal variable and stuttering might be either *moderated* or *mediated* by a third variable. *Hypothetical* examples of such interactions are demonstrated in ▶ Fig. 2.1. In ▶ Fig. 2.1a, a third or X *moderating* variable (i.e., fatigue) conditions, influences, or moderates the relation between Y, the causal variable (i.e., impaired basal ganglia processing), and Z, the effect (i.e., instance of stuttering). For example, if the person who stutters is fully rested in the beginning of the day, the basal ganglia process may have minimal impact on the speaker's fluency, but far more at the end of the day when the speaker is more tired.

In ▶ Fig. 2.1b, a third or X *mediating* variable (i.e., word-initial sound/syllable) determines or mediates, to a large degree, the relation between Y causal variable (i.e., impaired basal ganglia processing) and Z effect (i.e., instance of stuttering). For example, stuttering would be most prominent on word-initial sounds or syllables, and less so during other portions of the word. Again, moderation and mediation are *hypothetical* examples of how a third variable might impact the relation between a purported or known causal variable and an instance of stuttering.

Whether moderated, mediated, or not, it would be a significant move forward to know, based on data or evidence, that when alleged causal agent occurs, so too does an instance of stuttering. Certainly, a causal agent could act in concert with other agents and/or be "activated" or "set into motion" by other processes or events. Nothing is off the table when it comes to considering causal activities, agents, or events associated with stuttering.

Of course, singular, data-based knowledge about stuttering is helpful; it provides a pretty good, decent start. For example, it

is helpful to know that judgments of instances of stuttering are often associated with particular aspects of speech (dis)fluency, for example, sound/syllable repetition or sound prolongations. Yes, such basic knowledge is a start to a data-based understanding of stuttering. Likewise, in terms of variables associated with the diagnosis of stuttering, for example, we know that more boys than girls are apt to be diagnosed as stuttering. Again, such knowledge is all well and good, but what does such knowledge tell us about instances of stuttering and/or the diagnosis of stuttering, whether we measure variables like disfluency types or gender quantitatively or qualitatively?

Perhaps we could extend such knowledge by building upon known, singular facts in a more "stair-step" fashion. For example, assume that several rigorously conducted empirical studies involving many people who stutter report that utterance-initial words act like a magnet to attract the iron filings of instances of stuttering. Starting with such findings might lead us to develop additional, reasonable, hypotheses. Such hypotheses might, in turn, guide empirical testing to determine, for example, if utterance-initial word position acts alone or in concert with other concurrent variables (e.g., sentence length). This sort of a "stair-step" approach, done rigorously and systematically, allowing the findings to guide each step, would seem to have potential for furthering our knowledge of stuttering, and, by doing so, contribute to the development of a comprehensive, data-based understanding of instances of stuttering, the diagnosis of stuttering, and so forth.

2.9.4 Nature, Nurture, and Their Interaction

Some of the aforementioned theories, such as the diagnosogenic theory, lend themselves to a predominantly nurture, learned, or environmental explanation of stuttering. Other theories (e.g., the DIVA family of theories) lend themselves to a predominantly nature, constitutional, genetic, or neural processes explanation of stuttering. Obviously, these explanations cannot be both right, or can they?

Perhaps the truth lies in the fusion of both approaches. For example, one might speculate that a nature perspective best explains the basic, essentially universal speaking disruption associated with judgments stuttering (e.g., sound/syllable repetitions and sound prolongations). Conversely, a nurture perspective may best explain individual differences in related behavioral, cognitive, and/or emotional processes (e.g., some children who stutter are quieter, whereas others are quite talkative). Such a nature–nurture account is unlikely to come about unless those who are adamant that stuttering is solely a product of nature and, likewise, those who are steadfast in their belief that it is solely a product of nurture can collaborate, communicate, and work together. For in the end, that which looks purely genetic may be shown, with further research, to be subject to experience and learning. Similarly, that which appears purely experiential may be shown, with further research, to be inherited as well. Whatever the case, pushing the two ends—nature and nurture—toward the middle would ultimately help people who stutter and their families, the ones who must ultimately contend with, in their daily lives, the interactions between the two extremes.

2.9.5 Different Measurements, Different Results

There is an old saying that if one's only tool is a hammer, everything looks like a nail. Translated to theories of stuttering: if one only views stuttering from an anatomical perspective, everything about stuttering looks like bone, cartilage, ligament, muscle, etc. The notion of *parallax* is an apt proxy for differing perspectives that occur when trying to tell time by viewing the hands of an old-fashioned (analog) clock. If one person "measures" the hands of an analog clock when directly facing the clock, they will get perspective A. This perspective will differ, somewhat, from perspective B, when another person looks at the same hands telling the same time, but this time they are standing nearly 90 degrees to the right of the clock face. Yet another person will get perspective C when they stand nearly 90 degrees to the left of the clock face. All three viewers have a slightly different perspective regarding the time displayed on the clock face, but each is correct from their differing perspectives or forms of "measurement" of time.

In other words, different ways of measuring or observing provide different perspectives of the same constructs. In our clock analogy above, the different perspectives would probably correlate with one another, but that is not always the case. For example, our perception of a speech sound is one thing, the acoustic "profile" of the sound another, and the physiological movements of the lips, lower jaw, tongue, soft palate, and larynx still another. Their relation may be less than perfect, but they are still accurate representations of the same event, just based on different measures which, in turn, may lead to different perspectives.

So too are our findings relative to stuttering based on examiner observation, parental report, electrophysiology, brain imaging, acoustic analysis, psychophysical measures, and so forth. Each

"type of measurement/observation" provides information, just from different perspectives. Indeed, converging these divergent indices onto a single behavior, construct, event, or problem would be one excellent, comprehensive means to better understand that single "issue." That is true, even if some of the indices do not correlate with one another or when more of index X is associated with less of index Y. Hence, having *more than one* means of measurement in our methodological toolbox, whether one is a researcher or a clinician, is wise if one is to achieve a truly comprehensive understanding of stuttering.

2.9.6 A Varying Effect, an Unvarying Cause

Johnson[72] stated that "…a varying effect may not be accounted for by reference to an unvarying cause" (p.5). In short, this statement makes apparent something often overlooked, but fundamental, about stuttering: *it varies.* Indeed, for many, if not most, people who stutter, their speech is more fluent than it is stuttered. At the least, a fixed or *nonvariable* "cause" is highly unlikely to be the one and only cause of a *variable* problem like stuttering. It is more likely that a stable variable in a chain of variables converges to create instances of stuttering, provided that the other variables change in a similar manner to instances of stuttering. In other words, the nonvarying variable may only be a factor during certain conditions—for example, beginning an utterance—and not others.

Whatever the case, in any of the theories described earlier, as well as other extant theories not covered or may yet to be developed and put forth, the notion that stuttering varies must be recognized and accounted for. Yes, it is an inconvenient truth, but the truth, nonetheless. Again, we quote Aldous Huxley, who said "facts do not cease to exist because they are ignored."

2.10 Conclusions

This chapter presented a brief overview of some of the more prominent theories of stuttering of the 20th and earlier 21st centuries. In so doing, it also provided, some of the antecedents to as well as context and background surrounding these theories. Furthermore, it briefly covered some of the challenges and issues that *all* theories must account for and/or deal with. In general, all theories have pluses and minuses, but taken as a whole, they provide a framework within which readers may view the onset, development, and maintenance of stuttering. Indeed, theories might be likened to cooking recipes and ingredients.

2.10.1 Recipes/Ingredients

One might suggest that theories help narrow the number of ingredients that need to be considered when we think about the cause of stuttering. However, each theory leverages a different recipe to bring those ingredients together in a manner thought to cause stuttering. Where the challenge remains is not with the various recipes and their array of ingredients. Instead, the challenge is that theoretical recipe A may exclude some ingredients of theoretical recipe B. Conversely, theory B may exclude some of the key ingredients of theoretical recipe A! Both theories might reflect attempts to account for stuttering but do so based on different sets of constructs, behaviors, or processes. However, to paraphrase the late U.S. Senator, Daniel Patrick Moynihan, "You are entitled to your own opinion. But you are not entitled to your own facts." Thus, the reader should attempt to discern what the sets of facts may be, the actual documented evidence for such facts, and form their opinions accordingly.

Our confidence in "facts" increases (or at least it should) as the number of peer reviewed reports from different sources attest to their existence, occurrence, presence, etc. Keep in mind, though, that some differences between theories relate to the context that surrounds their development. For example, some differences can, and often do, reflect the (1) general and specific state of knowledge *at the time* that each theory was developed, (2) the quantity and quality of the available technology and methodology to test the theory, and (3) the prevailing clinical and research perspectives at the time the theory was developed. We can hardly fault, for example, the 1700s theorists proposing a theory that ignores bacteria, microbes, neurotransmitters, and viruses if during that long-ago time there was little or no knowledge of bacteria, microbes, neurotransmitters, and viruses! When a country's only forms of transportation are oxen and horses, it seems inappropriate to fault that country for not having gas stations.

2.10.2 Divergent Approaches to Same Topic

Returning to our recipe/ingredient metaphor, from the outside looking in, there is the tendency to think that too many cooks spoil the broth. Perhaps, but empirically studying the same construct (e.g., fear) using divergent perspectives and methods can be, and generally is, a strength rather than weakness. It can provide a more comprehensive, multifaceted understanding of a given construct rather than one whose view is constricted by personal, philosophical, or theoretical blinders. Ideally, divergent scientific approaches and specialties should come together to, at the least, determine that something exists, is present, and observable. Present and observable, however, does not mean understood. Likewise, employing an equally divergent approach helps ensure that meaningful contributors to stuttering are not ignored or left out of the purview of clinicians and researchers alike.

2.10.3 The Only Certainty is That Nothing is Certain

Although a divergent approach to stuttering may provide a breadth and comprehensiveness to our understanding of stuttering, it may also engender uncertainty. And although such uncertainty may indeed occur, to be absolutely certain that only X is worthy of study seems strange when applied to an uncertain problem such as stuttering. Indeed, as the old saying goes, the only certainty is that nothing is certain. Perhaps, a more middle-ground approach is to suggest that both certainty and uncertainty are relative in nature. For example, multiple studies have made it increasingly clear that a significant number of children who begin to stutter will recover from stuttering without the assistance of formalized treatment.[73] We can, therefore, be relatively certain that within a group of children who are initially diagnosed with stuttering, more than a few will recover without treatment.

Such "relative" certainty should come, however, with more than a little doubt or uncertainty. For example, why does recovery occur for some children but not others? Can we identify, from the very beginning, those who will and those who will not recover? Should we treat all such children regardless of whether they will recover without treatment? Such questions grow out of the petri dish of uncertainty. Suffice it to say that it is doubt not certainty that more often helps energize our attempts to advance our knowledge about the onset, development, and maintenance of stuttering. And advancing such knowledge is one of the creative and important accomplishments achieved by the theoreticians reviewed in this chapter.

2.10.4 Facts Are the Foundation

Facts are pesky things. They simply refuse to go away no matter the strength of our theoretical disinfectant. For example, certain tests are routinely employed to evaluate the frequency, impact, and severity of stuttering. Fine, but the "authority" implied by the consistent, widespread use of such tests should not thwart attempts, based on systematic collection and analysis of relevant data, to advance, refine, or even replace such tests. Certainly, these consistently used tests tell us about important parts of stuttering. But parts do not necessarily constitute a whole. Indeed, present and future methods, especially in the area of measuring elements associated with instances of stuttering[74] or factors that contribute to individual differences in stuttering,[75,76] may lead us to question our understanding of stuttering. And by raising such questions, they make us a bit less complacent and certain about what we know about stuttering. This, in turn, should help us to develop different perspectives, which may more accurately trace the contours of reality, no matter how jagged they may be. Without these different perspectives, which are often fostered by new information or old information viewed in a new way, it will be quite difficult to advance our understanding of stuttering beyond that of the present. Fortunately, most clinicians, researchers, and students who read these words are the offspring of the age of enlightenment. As such, these individuals are likely to expect that the old and new theories and perspectives will be evaluated based on relevant data, evidence, and facts. Such evaluation, of course, will find that some theories are not supported, whereas others are supported by data, evidence, and facts. And although these same individuals may regret the former's demise, it is hoped that they will employ the latter to help build present and future theories of stuttering upon a foundation of fact more so than fancy.

"Begin at the beginning," the King said, very gravely, "and go on till you come to the end: then stop."

Lewis Carroll (b. 1832, d. 1898)

2.11 Definitions

Approach-avoidance conflict theory: A psychological (nurture) theory that proposes that stuttering resulted from opposing drives or tendencies to both speak and refrain from speaking.

Causality: The relationship between a cause and its result or consequence (an effect).

Causality conditions: Three conditions are necessary for establishing causality: temporal precedence (X must come before Y), covariation (if more of X, more of Y), and elimination of alternative causes (no other variable is responsible for the relationship between X and Y).

Cerebral dominance theory: A physiological (nature) theory that posits that children stutter have ambiguous or uncertain laterality of cortical dominance, resulting in conflict between the left and right hemispheres for control of the speech musculature.

Classical conditioning: A form of learning, sometimes called "Pavlovian conditioning" after the Russian experimenter Ivan Pavlov who is generally credited as the originator of this model of learning. Classical conditioning involves a learning process that occurs when two stimuli are repeatedly paired; a response that is at first elicited by the second stimulus is eventually elicited by the first stimulus alone.

Demands and capacities model: A multifactorial model that suggests that stuttering occurs when the "demands" (social or otherwise) that are being placed on a child for fluent speech exceed the child's "capacities" (social-emotional maturity, language formulation, cognitive skills, and/or speech motor) for producing fluency.

Diagnosogenic theory: A psychosocial (nurture) theory that proposes that stuttering developed because a listener, usually a parent, erroneously labeled a child's normal disfluencies (i.e., repetitions of sound, syllables, words, and phrases) as stuttering.

Diathesis: A constitutional predisposition or vulnerability (sometimes referred to as "weakness") that can take the form of biological, genetic, psychological, or situational factors.

Dual-diathesis stressor model: A multifactorial model that suggests that stuttering develops from an interaction between speech-language and/or emotional diatheses and stressors associated with environmental factors.

Feedback: One means for controlling a system, of which there are two types: negative and positive feedback. Negative feedback occurs when the end results of an action *decrease* that action from continuing to occur. Positive feedback occurs when the end results of an action *increases* that action to continue to occur.

Feedforward: Another means for controlling a system. A mechanism in a system that monitors performance inputs rather than outputs. This mechanism reacts to maintain a specified state, thus preventing or minimizing problems *before* they occur. Both feedback and feedforward can coexist, often do, and concurrently function within one system.

Humor: A bodily fluid. Humors were involved with a very early theory that a person's health came from balance between the bodily liquids. Disease and disorders were to happen to when an imbalance occurred between a person's humors.

Humoralism: An ancient/early system of medicine sometimes referred to as the humoral theory or humoralism. This system detailed the supposed makeup and workings of the human body. This theory originated with ancient Greek and Roman physicians and philosophers but was widely practiced in western medicine into the 19th century. Humorism began to fall out of favor in the 1850s with the advent of germ theory, which put forth the idea that many diseases previously thought to be humoral were in fact caused by pathogens.

Interactive perspective: It refers to the interaction of both nature (genetic) and nurture (environmental) factors associated with human development.

Mediating variable: A variable that explains how or why there is a relationship between two variables—a cause and an effect—in a causal chain.

Moderating variable: A variable that affects the strength and/ or direction of a relationship between two variables.

Multifactorial dynamic pathways theory: A multifactorial theory that proposes that motor, linguistic, and emotional factors variables interact with an unstable speech motor system to result in stuttering.

Multifactorial theories: Theories that propose that traits and conditions are caused by the interaction of more than one factor.

Nature perspective: Refers to genetic and biological factors associated with human development.

Nurture perspective: Refers to environmental, learned, and psychosocial factors associated with human development.

Operant conditioning: A form of learning, sometimes called instrumental conditioning. Operant conditioning (also called instrumental conditioning) is a type of associative learning process through which the strength of a behavior is modified by reinforcement or punishment. It is also a procedure that is used to bring about such learning.

Operant conditioning theory: A psychological (nurture) theory that suggested that stuttering is learned or established through response-contingent reinforcement.

Parallax: An effect that occurs when the position or direction of an object appears to differ when viewed from different positions.

Physiological theories: Theories that emphasize a biological basis for a condition or disorder.

Psychological theories: Theories that emphasize a psychological or emotional basis or a condition or disorder.

Scientific method: A method of research in which a problem is identified, relevant data are gathered, a hypothesis is formulated from these data, and the hypothesis is tested.

Directions Into Velocities of Articulators (SimpleDIVA): A neural network model of speech motor development and production.

Stressor: A biological, chemical, environmental condition, or an external stimulus or event seen as causing stress to an organism. Psychologically speaking, a stressor can be events or environments that individuals might consider demanding, challenging, and/or threatening to individual safety.

Two-factor theory of stuttering: A psychological (nurture) theory that proposed that instances of stuttering were developed through classical conditioning and secondary behaviors through operant conditioning.

References

[1] Duffy J. From humors to medical science: A history of American medicine. 2nd ed. Champaign: University of Illinois Press; 1993

[2] Rieber RW, Wollock J. The historical roots of the theory and therapy of stuttering. J Commun Disord. 1977; 10(1)(–)(2):3–24

[3] Van Riper C. The Treatment of stuttering. Englewood Cliffs, NJ: Prentice Hall; 1973

[4] Morens DM. Death of a president. N Engl J Med. 1999; 341(24):1845–1849

[5] Fletcher JM. An experimental study of stuttering. Am J Psychol. 1914; 25: 201–255

[6] Orton S. Studies in stuttering: introduction. Arch Neurol Psychiatry. 1927; 18 (5):671–672

[7] Orton ST, Travis LE. Studies in stuttering: IV. Studies of action currents in stutterers. Arch Neurol Psychiatry. 1929; 21(1):61–68

[8] Orton ST. A physiological theory of reading disability and stuttering in children. N Engl J Med. 1928; 199(21):1046–1052

[9] Travis LE. Speech pathology. New York, NY: Appleton and Co.; 1931

[10] Geschwind N, Behan P. Laterality, hormones, and immunity. In: Geschwind N, Galaburda A, eds. Cerebral Dominance. Cambridge, MA: Harvard University Press; 1984:217

[11] Brown S, Ingham RJ, Ingham JC, Laird AR, Fox PT. Stuttered and fluent speech production: an ALE meta-analysis of functional neuroimaging studies. Hum Brain Mapp. 2005; 25(1):105–117

[12] Chang S-E, Erickson KI, Ambrose NG, Hasegawa-Johnson MA, Ludlow CL. Brain anatomy differences in childhood stuttering. Neuroimage. 2008; 39(3): 1333–1344

[13] Sowman PF, Crain S, Harrison E, Johnson BW. Lateralization of brain activation in fluent and non-fluent preschool children: a magnetoencephalographic study of picture-naming. Front Hum Neurosci. 2014; 8:354

[14] Johnson W. The Indians have no word for it: I. Stuttering in children. Q J Speech. 1944; 30(3):330–337

[15] Johnson W. A study of the onset and development of stuttering. In: Johnson W, Leutenegger R, eds. Stuttering in Children and Adults. Minneapolis, MN: University of Minnesota Press; 1955a:37–73

[16] Johnson W. The time, the place, and the problem. In: Johnson W, Leutenegger R, eds. Stuttering in Children and Adults. Minneapolis, MN: University of Minnesota Press; 1955:3–24

[17] Kraft SJ, Yairi E. Genetic bases of stuttering: the state of the art, 2011. Folia Phoniatr Logop. 2012; 64(1):34–47

[18] Sheehan JG. Theory and treatment of stuttering as an approach-avoidance conflict. J Psychol. 1953; 36(1):27–49

[19] Sheehan J. Conflict theory of stuttering. In: Eisenson J, ed. Stuttering: A Symposium. New York, NY: Harper & Row; 1958:121–166

[20] Bloodstein O, Bernstein N. A handbook on stuttering. 6th ed. Clifton Park, NY: Thomson-Delmar; 2008

[21] Brutten EJ, Shoemaker DJ. The modification of stuttering. Englewood Cliffs, NJ: Prentice-Hall; 1967

[22] Brutten G, Shoemaker D. Stuttering: the disintegration of speech due to conditioned negative emotion. In: Gray B, England G, eds. Stuttering and the Conditioning Therapies. Monterey, CA: Monterey Institute of Speech and Hearing; 1969:57–68

[23] Conture EG, Kelly EM. Young stutterers' nonspeech behaviors during stuttering. J Speech Hear Res. 1991; 34(5):1041–1056

[24] Wolpe J. Psychotherapy by reciprocal inhibition. Stanford, CA: Stanford University Press; 1958

[25] Hull CL. Principles of behavior: an introduction to behavior theory. New York, NY: Appleton-Century-Crofts; 1943

[26] Janssen P, Brutten GJ. The differential effects of punishment of oral prolongations. In: Lebrun Y, Hoops R, eds. Neurolinguistic Approaches to Stuttering. The Hague: Mouton; 1973:337–344

[27] Oelschlaeger ML, Brutten GJ. The effect of instructional stimulation on the frequency of repetitions, interjections, and words spoken during the spontaneous speech of four stutterers. Behav Ther. 1976; 7(1):37–46

[28] Brutten GJ. The effect of punishment on a factor I stuttering behavior. J Fluency Disord. 1980; 5(2):77–85

[29] Costello JM, Hurst MR. An analysis of the relationship among stuttering behaviors. J Speech Hear Res. 1981; 24(2):247–256

[30] Flanagan B, Goldiamond I, Azrin N. Operant stuttering: the control of stuttering behavior through response-contingent consequences. J Exp Anal Behav. 1958; 1(2):173–177

[31] Shames GH, Sherrick CE, Jr. A discussion of nonfluency and stuttering as operant behavior. J Speech Hear Disord. 1963; 28(1):3–18

[32] Ingham RJ, Andrews G. Behavior therapy and stuttering: a review. J Speech Hear Disord. 1973; 38(4):405–441

[33] Ingham RJ. Stuttering and behavior therapy. San Diego, CA: College-Hill Press; 1984

[34] Skinner BF. Science and human behavior. New York, NY: Macmillan; 1953

[35] Siegel GM. Punishment, stuttering, and disfluency. J Speech Hear Res. 1970; 13(4):677–714

[36] Onslow M, Packman A, Harrison E. The Lidcombe program of early stuttering intervention: a clinician's guide. Austin TX: Pro-Ed; 2003

[37] Jones M, Onslow M, Packman A, et al. Randomised controlled trial of the Lidcombe programme of early stuttering intervention. BMJ. 2005; 331 (7518):659

[38] Starkweather CW. Fluency and Stuttering. Englewood Cliffs, NJ: Prentice-Hall, Inc.; 1987

[39] Adams MR. The demands and capacities model: I. Theoretical elaborations. J Fluency Disord. 1990; 15(3):135–141

[40] Starkweather CW, Gottwald SR. The demands and capacities model II: clinical applications. J Fluency Disord. 1990; 15(3):143–157

[41] Yaruss JS. The role of performance in the demands and capacities model. J Fluency Disord. 2000; 25(4):347–358

[42] Bosshardt HG. Cognitive processing load as a determinant of stuttering: summary of a research programme. Clin Linguist Phon. 2006; 20(5):371–385

[43] Postma A, Kolk H. The covert repair hypothesis: prearticulatory repair processes in normal and stuttered disfluencies. J Speech Hear Res. 1993; 36 (3):472–487

[44] Kolk H, Postma A. Stuttering as a covert repair phenomenon. In: Curlee R, Siegel G, eds. Nature and Treatment of Stuttering: New Directions. 2nd ed. Boston, MA: Allyn & Bacon; 1997:182–203

[45] Yaruss JS, Conture EG. Stuttering and phonological disorders in children: examination of the covert repair hypothesis. J Speech Hear Res. 1996; 39(2): 349–364

[46] Singer CM, Hessling A, Kelly EM, Singer L, Jones RM. Clinical characteristics associated with stuttering persistence: a meta-analysis. J Speech Lang Hear Res. 2020; 63(9):2995–3018

[47] Anderson JD, Conture EG. Sentence-structure priming in young children who do and do not stutter. J Speech Lang Hear Res. 2004; 47(3):552–571

[48] Pellowski MW, Conture EG. Lexical priming in picture naming of young children who do and do not stutter. J Speech Lang Hear Res. 2005; 48(2):278–294

[49] Melnick KS, Conture EG, Ohde RN. Phonological priming in picture naming of young children who stutter. J Speech Lang Hear Res. 2003; 46(6):1428–1443

[50] Byrd CT, Conture EG, Ohde RN. Phonological priming in young children who stutter: holistic versus incremental processing. Am J Speech Lang Pathol. 2007; 16(1):43–53

[51] Howell P, Au-Yeung J. The EXPLAN theory of fluency control applied to the diagnosis of stuttering. In: Fave E, ed. Pathology and Therapy of Speech Disorders. Amsterdam: John Benjamin; 2002:75–94

[52] Howell P. Assessment of some contemporary theories of stuttering that apply to spontaneous speech. Contemp Issues Commun Sci Disord. 2004; 31 (Spring):122–139

[53] Howell P, Dworzynski K. Reply to letter to the editor: planning and execution processes in speech control by fluent speakers and speakers who stutter. J Fluen Disord. 2005; 30:343–354

[54] Conture EG, Walden T. Dual diathesis-stressor model of stuttering. In: Theoretical Issues of Fluency Disorders. Moscow: National Book Centre; 2012:94–127

[55] Walden TA, Frankel CB, Buhr AP, Johnson KN, Conture EG, Karrass JM. Dual diathesis-stressor model of emotional and linguistic contributions to developmental stuttering. J Abnorm Child Psychol. 2012; 40(4):633–644

[56] Choi D, Conture EG, Walden TA, Jones RM, Kim H. Emotional diathesis, emotional stress, and childhood stuttering. J Speech Lang Hear Res. 2016; 59 (4):616–630

[57] Monroe SM, Simons AD. Diathesis-stress theories in the context of life stress research: implications for the depressive disorders. Psychol Bull. 1991; 110 (3):406–425

[58] Rocha MS, Yaruss JS, Rato JR. Temperament, executive functioning, and anxiety in school-age children who stutter. Front Psychol. 2019; 10:2244

[59] Smith A, Kelly E. Stuttering: a dynamic, multifactorial model. In: Curlee R, Siegel G, eds. Nature and Treatment of Stuttering: New Directions. 2nd ed. Boston, MA: Allyn & Bacon; 1997

[60] Smith A, Weber C. How stuttering develops: the multifactorial dynamic pathways theory. J Speech Lang Hear Res. 2017; 60(9):2483–2505

[61] MacPherson MK, Smith A. Influences of sentence length and syntactic complexity on the speech motor control of children who stutter. J Speech Lang Hear Res. 2013; 56(1):89–102

[62] Usler ER, Walsh B. The effects of syntactic complexity and sentence length on the speech motor control of school-age children who stutter. J Speech Lang Hear Res. 2018; 61(9):2157–2167

[63] Kearney E, Nieto-Castañón A, Weerathunge HR, et al. A simple 3-parameter model for examining adaptation in speech and voice production. Front Psychol. 2020; 10:2995

[64] Guenther FH. Cortical interactions underlying the production of speech sounds. J Commun Disord. 2006; 39(5):350–365

[65] Guenther FH, Ghosh SS, Tourville JA. Neural modeling and imaging of the cortical interactions underlying syllable production. Brain Lang. 2006; 96(3):280–301

[66] Guenther FH. Neural Control of Speech (▶ Chapter 8). Cambridge, MA: MIT Press; 2016

[67] Bohland JW, Bullock D, Guenther FH. Neural representations and mechanisms for the performance of simple speech sequences. J Cogn Neurosci. 2010; 22(7):1504–1529

[68] Civier O, Bullock D, Max L, Guenther FH. Computational modeling of stuttering caused by impairments in a basal ganglia thalamo-cortical circuit involved in syllable selection and initiation. Brain Lang. 2013; 126(3):263–278

[69] Daliri A, Wieland EA, Cai S, Guenther FH, Chang SE. Auditory-motor adaptation is reduced in adults who stutter but not in children who stutter. Dev Sci. 2018; 21(2):e12521

[70] Garnett EO, Chow HM, Nieto-Castañón A, Tourville JA, Guenther FH, Chang S-E. Anomalous morphology in left hemisphere motor and premotor cortex of children who stutter. Brain. 2018; 141(9):2670–2684

[71] Chang S-E, Guenther FH. Involvement of the cortico-basal ganglia-thalamocortical loop in developmental stuttering. Front Psychol. 2020; 10:3088

[72] Johnson W. The Onset of Stuttering: Research Findings and Implications. Minneapolis, MN: University of Minnesota Press; 1959

[73] Shimada M, Toyomura A, Fujii T, Minami T. Children who stutter at 3 years of age: a community-based study. J Fluency Disord. 2018; 56:45–54

[74] Amir O, Shapira Y, Mick L, Yaruss JS. The Speech Efficiency Score (SES): a time-domain measure of speech fluency. J Fluency Disord. 2018; 58:61–69

[75] Ntourou K, DeFranco EO, Conture EG, Walden TA, Mushtaq N. A parent-report scale of behavioral inhibition: validation and application to preschool-age children who do and do not stutter. J Fluency Disord. 2020; 63:105748

[76] Ntourou K, Anderson JD, Wagovich SA. Executive function and childhood stuttering: parent ratings and evidence from a behavioral task. J Fluency Disord. 2018; 56:18–32

Section II

Processes Associated with Stuttering

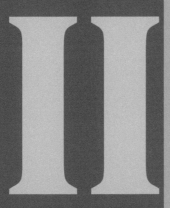

3 Genetic Processes

Shelly Jo Kraft and Jennifer E. Below

Abstract

In this chapter, we review basic concepts of genetics, describe what is known about how genetics impact risk of stuttering, and discuss directions for future study. The chapter begins with a review of the concept of heritability and how the familial nature of stuttering has been used to learn about the genes that impact its risk. Next, we introduce key concepts in human molecular genetics including how deoxyribonucleic acid (DNA) is inherited, how genes are transcribed as ribonucleic acid (RNA) and translated into protein, and how the characteristics of these molecules, which differ from person to person, can help us understand risk of stuttering on a cellular level. Then we will learn about the genes linked to stuttering that have been identified thus far, explore the limitations of these studies, and consider the kinds of future research that will be needed to understand three primary, but still incompletely understood, questions, in stuttering: *(1) Why are some people and families at greater risk of stuttering? (2) What genes and genetic variants have been identified in studies of developmental stuttering to date? and (3) How are the genetics of stuttering related to the genetics of other traits and how can these relationships help us understand and treat stuttering?* Finally, we will discuss future steps in genomics that are poised to inform the design and development of effective therapies for stuttering and empower people who stutter with information about how genetic factors may underlie their conditions.

Keywords: genome-wide association studies (GWAS), family-based linkage analysis, medical genetics, biobanks

3.1 Introduction

The central goal of classical epidemiology is to understand patterns of disease occurrence in human populations and the factors, or "exposures," that influence these patterns. In genetic epidemiology, genetic variation is the factor of interest. Genetic variation has some important qualities: because the DNA you are born with typically does not change over the course of your life, it is an exposure that is intrinsic to the individual; and although some genetic variation can be causal for disease, many diseases and disorders are the consequence of a constellation of genetic and environmental effects. In general, it is fair to say that research findings to date characterize developmental stuttering as an example of one such disorder. Thus, the goal of genetic epidemiology as applied to developmental stuttering is to assess the contribution of genetic and environmental factors to better understand the cause (etiology), distribution, and treatment of stuttering in families and populations. To apply genetic epidemiology to stuttering, the central steps are:

1. Establish that there is a genetic component to the stuttering by assessing its heritability.
2. Establish the relative size of that genetic influence (effect) in relation to other factors impacting disease risk (i.e., environmental effects).
3. Identify the gene(s) responsible for the genetic component of stuttering risk.

Genetic epidemiology enhances our understanding of the pathogenesis of disease, while medical genetics is the branch of medicine that utilizes what is known about the genetic causes to diagnose and treat hereditary disorders. Together, these fields can help us understand the molecular and cellular basis of stuttering risk and utilize the knowledge to improve treatment and outcomes for people who stutter. Today, active areas of research in genetic epidemiology and medical genetics include studies of the inheritance of diseases and disorders in families, mapping genetic risk factors within the genome in populations and families, analyzing and understanding the molecular processes that lead to disease, and diagnosing and treating genetic diseases and disorders. Medical genetics as a field has only existed for about 60 years, beginning around the time of the first X-ray photograph of DNA taken by Rosalind Franklin and Raymond Gosling in 1952. When we compare this to many other medical or scientific specialties, it is still in its infancy, and this is reflected in our rapidly growing and evolving understanding of human genetics generally, and the genetics of developmental stuttering specifically.

3.1.1 Heritability of Stuttering

Stuttering occurs more often in some families; many individuals who stutter have a family member who also stutters. Clues as to the heritability of developmental stuttering emerged when Dr. Mildred Berry, a pioneer in the field of speech pathology, surveyed a thousand families in 1937 and discovered that twinning occurred more frequently in families that stuttered; moreover, stuttering also occurred more frequently in twins than siblings.[1] More recent familial incidence studies report familial stuttering in 30 to 60% of probands (the first affected family member being studied) compared to less than 10% in families of control probands.[2,3] For example, in 1993 Ambrose et al evaluated a sample of 69 preschool children who stuttered, determining that 45% of probands had relatives who stutter in their immediate family (parents and siblings) and 71% of probands had relatives who stutter in their extended family (grandparents, first cousins, avuncular relationships).[4] Although genetics is one explanation, there can be multiple reasons stuttering occurs more often in family members of people who stutter, including nongenetic factors such as the environment and random chance, and gene–environment interactions can play a role as well.

Because stuttering is enriched in families, we can hypothesize that there might be shared environmental and/or genetic factors that explain the enrichment. Heritability is a measure of the variance in a trait that can be explained by genetic factors. Studies of the differing rates of stuttering among family members provide one way to measure the proportion of risk that comes from genetics. For example, if we assume that environmental effects impact identical (monozygotic) twins and fraternal (dizygotic) twins similarly, then any differences in concordance rates (the percentage of cases in which both twin pairs exhibit a given disorder or trait) between monozygotic and dizygotic twins can be assumed to be due to their differences in genetic sharing: monozygotic twins share 100% of their DNA while dizygotic twins, on average, share only 50% of their DNA. The genetic heritability of a trait can be calculated from the difference between concordance rate of monozygotic twins and the concordance rate of dizygotic twins. Since Berry's seminal study, published estimates of the genetic heritability of stuttering have fluctuated with recent studies reporting heritability estimates as low as 42%[5] and as high as 81 to 84% (▶ Table 3.1).[6,7,8] Nevertheless, many studies of other complex disorders (e.g., type 2 diabetes,[9] serum lipid levels,[10] Parkinson's disease,[11] Alzheimer's disease[12]) with similar or smaller genetic heritability estimates have discovered genetic risk factors essential to understanding the molecular basis of the disease. However, note that even in monozygotic twins there is not complete concordance of stuttering, indicating that although there is a strong genetic component to developmental stuttering, nongenetic factors play an important role in an individual's risk as well. Indeed, most phenotypes (the measurable characteristics of an individual) range from highly heritable (genetic) to highly plastic (nongenetic), and are influenced by a combination of genetic, environmental, and completely random factors.

The fact that genetic factors are contributing to much of the interindividual variability in risk for stuttering does not tell us anything about the specific genetic factors that affect risk of stuttering, nor does knowing that environmental and random factors also substantially contribute to stuttering tell us what those factors might be. Well-powered genetic and epidemiological studies are required to identify the specific genetic and nongenetic risk factors for stuttering. Given that researchers have established that stuttering is heritable and have estimated the proportion of variance that is explained by genetics, the next step is to identify the specific regions of the genome that contribute to stuttering risk. To map these regions (step 3 of the central process listed above) researchers utilize the data, concepts, and approaches central to genetic epidemiology that are reviewed below.

3.2 Introduction to Basic Genetics

Genetics is the field of study investigating how traits are inherited from parents to offspring. In 1865, Gregor Mendel investigated characteristics of green peas, such as their shape and size, and demonstrated that these characteristics were inherited. More recent molecular experiments have shown that DNA is the hereditary material and within the last 20 years the complete human genome was sequenced. The central dogma of genetics is as follows: DNA encodes molecular instructions, which are transcribed into a messenger molecule, ribonucleic acid (RNA), which is translated into protein, which in turn form the building blocks of all cellular functions.

3.2.1 DNA

DNA resides in the nucleus and mitochondria of cells and is present in most cells in your body. The fundamental role of DNA is to encode all the information necessary to create the

Table 3.1 Summary of heritability estimates in stuttering from the literature

Study	Source	H2	DZ concord	MZ concord	Notes
Andrews et al, 1991	Australian Twin Registry, born between 1893 and 1964	0.711	3.5% (3/85)	20% (10/50)	Assumed additive genetic model; reported **pairwise** concordance
Felsenfeld et al, 2000	Australian Twin Registry, twins born between 1964 and 1971	0.7	12%/26%	29%/62%	Assumed additive genetic model for H2; interviewed individuals passed more stringent case criteria (vs. self-report screening concordance calculations); reporting proband-wise concordance
Ooki et al, 2005	Japanese Twin Database, aging from infant to 15 years at time of data collection	0.8 (males)/ 0.85 (females)	11% (6/56)	52% (54/104)	Structural equation modeling to calculate the proportion of phenotypic variance explained by genetics; DZ proband-wise concordance in same-sex twins was 12%; whereas, for female-male siblings it was 9% 2/23; reporting proband-wise concordance
Dworzynski et al, 2007	Twins Early Development Study, a longitudinal UK-based study of all twins born between 1994 and 1996	0.65	12%	32%	Reporting proband-wise concordance; H2 estimate for 4-year-old children; longitudinal study looking at participants at 2, 3, 4, and 7 years
Beijsterveldt et al, 2010	Netherlands Twin Register	0.42	26–36%	53–61%	Parents evaluated their children's speech fluency via questionnaires around their fifth birthday; additive genetic model
Fagnani et al, 2011	Danish twins	0.84 (males)/ 0.81 (females)	4–16% (same sex only)	38–62%	Nation-wide questionnaire answers for phenotype
Rautakoski et al, 2012	Finnish twins, born between 1961 and 1989	0.82	27%	74%	Structural equation modeling to calculate the proportion of phenotypic variance explained by genetics

Abbreviations: DZ, dizygotic twins; H2, calculated heritability (i.e., the difference between concordance rate of monozygotic twins and the concordance rate of dizygotic twins); MZ, monozygotic twins.

vast array of proteins required for cellular function. DNA is a polymer of nucleotides, each consisting of a deoxyribose, a phosphate group, and a base. Nucleotides are often noted by shorthand using the first letter of the base—adenine (A), thymine (T), guanine (G), and cytosine (C). The nitrogenous bases pair with each other (adenine pairs via two hydrogen bonds with thymine, and guanine via three hydrogen bonds with cytosine) forming a double helix of two strands of DNA. The exact sequence of these bases specifies the proteins that can be built.

3.2.2 Chromosomes

Each long strand of DNA is called a chromosome. Each human chromosome has a short arm ("p" for "petit") and long arm ("q" for "queue"), separated by a centromere. The ends of the chromosome are called telomeres. Ploidy is the number of complete sets of chromosomes in a cell. Humans are diploid, meaning your genetic code is in pairs of chromosomes with one set of 23 chromosomes inherited from each parent. Mutations that occur in somatic cells can affect the individual but are not passed to offspring. On the other hand, reproductive cells called gametes, namely, sperm and egg cells in humans, are haploid, meaning they contain only one set of chromosomes, and mutations present in these cells may be passed to offspring. Chromosomes are visible through a microscope when condensed before cell division ("chromosome" comes from the Greek words for "colored bodies"); the number and visual appearance of the chromosomes are called a karyotype (see ▶ Fig. 3.1).

The study of the number and morphology of chromosomes, called cytogenetics, is common in clinical diagnostic labs and is useful for identifying large abnormalities. The detection of many chromosomal abnormalities is made possible by staining chromosomes with a dye, which creates the appearance of horizontal black and white stripes called cytogenetic bands. Each chromosome has its own unique pattern which can be analyzed for abnormalities and used as a map for the location of genes on chromosomes. ▶ Fig. 3.1 depicts stained chromosomes, with visible cytogenetic bands.

3.2.3 Genes

Genes are functional units of the genome that are often transcribed into RNA, which is then usually translated into protein. Genome refers to the complete set of genetic material present in an organism. In 2003, The Human Genome Project completed a 13-year-long international collaboration between thousands of investigators to assess the content of a complete human genome comprising approximately 3 billion base pairs and made these data immediately available to the public. The scientists set out with the anticipation to find between 50,000 and 140,000 genes but were surprised to identify only between 20,000 and 25,000. The task of identifying these genes remains challenging, and it is likely that more will be found. Technological advancements that have made assessing the content of genomes efficient and inexpensive have resulted in a tidal wave of data and propelled the field of genetics into new territory.

3.2.4 RNA

An essential activity for RNA is protein synthesis, a universal function in which RNA molecules direct the synthesis of proteins. Inside the nucleus, DNA is transcribed into mRNA, a type of nucleic acid that is chemically similar to DNA, which is then shuttled out of the nucleus and is subsequently translated into protein on ribosomes. In translation, mRNA forms a template for the synthesis of proteins. Amino acids cannot bind directly to the mRNA, rather the interaction is mediated by molecules called transfer RNA (tRNA), a cloverleaf shaped molecule of RNA that contains an amino acid on the "stem" and a three-base region opposite the stem called an anticodon. A ribosome slides along the mRNA strand using tRNA to assemble a growing string of amino acids into a polypeptide chain that may

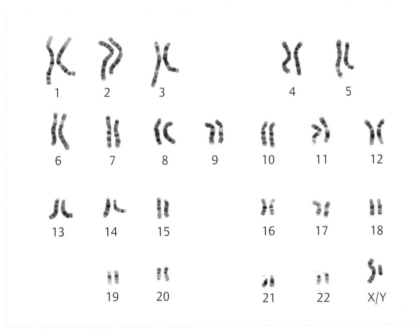

Fig. 3.1 A karyotype refers to the number and visual appearance of chromosomes for an organism or species. (Courtesy: National Human Genome Research Institute, public domain, via Wikimedia Commons.)

eventually become a functional protein in the cell. As a result of this process, every three bases in an exon (the nucleotide sequences that bond to create mature mRNA) translates to a single amino acid in a protein. Thus, a single swap of one nucleotide for another (one kind of mutation) in a gene can result in a change of an amino acid in the resulting protein, potentially altering its function and subsequently impacting risk of a disease, modifying a trait, or changing behavior.

As we have already discussed, approximately 99% of DNA is never transcribed into RNA. Similarly, although the function of many RNA molecules is providing a template for building proteins, most RNAs are *never translated into protein*: approximately 97% of the transcriptional output is nonprotein-coding in humans! Although it has been known for some time that proteins can regulate gene expression, it turns out that some noncoding RNA (ncRNA), such as microRNAs, long ncRNAs, and enhancer RNAs, can also play a range of functional roles in translation and gene regulation.

3.3 Genetic Variation

Through collective study of a range of human genomes, a consensus reference genome was established. As additional large samples of people have been studied, public databases of observed differences from the reference genome, as well as how often these differences are observed in populations (their frequency), have become available. Today millions of alterations from the reference genome have been recorded including chromosome abnormalities, single nucleotide changes (or SNPs, for "single nucleotide polymorphisms"), insertions, deletions, inversions, and copy number changes, in which a segment of the genome is repeated a different number of times relative to the reference (also called CNV for "copy number variant"). A given variant can be extremely common in populations or so rare that it has only ever been observed in a single person. Because of natural selection, although any genetic variant can have an impact on disease or effect a condition, often common variants have more modest effects, while very rare variants can be highly deleterious.

Because most of the genome is nonprotein coding, much of the variation in the genome is of uncertain consequence. This facilitates rare events in which gene segments are shuffled, or genes or chromosomal segments are duplicated, creating redundancy and the opportunity for mutations to differentiate their functions in new ways, such as becoming new members of a gene family or whole new kinds of genes. Genetic variation can have no effect at all (silent variation), change the content of protein (coding variation), or change the amount of RNA or protein that is expressed (regulatory variation). On average, your personal genome differs by only about 1% from any other human on earth, and studies of human populations have demonstrated that the amount of genetic variation within populations is markedly greater than variation between populations. Because people from different populations can be more genetically similar to each other than to other members of their own populations, caution is necessary when using labels for groups of people in biomedical settings, including in personalized medicine and pharmacogenetics. In this context, it is important to stress that race is a social construct, not a biological one, and human variation is continuous across geographic clines within and across continents.

In this section, we focus on two kinds of genetic variation: chromosomal abnormalities and SNPs. We briefly review how they are measured and how we can establish the effect they can have on human health generally and stuttering specifically.

3.3.1 Chromosomal Abnormalities

Atypical karyotypes are often referred to as chromosomal abnormalities and are the cause of a wide array of conditions. They can take several forms including complete duplications or deletions of whole or partial chromosomes, or translocation of a portion (or entirety!) of one chromosome to another chromosome. Like all genetic variation, chromosomal abnormalities can occur in all or just a portion of cells in the affected individual. Although many abnormalities are possible, most large abnormalities are inconsistent with life.

For example, Prader-Willi is a syndrome typically caused by deletion of a part of chromosome 15 passed down by the father. Trisomy, having three copies of a chromosome, is only observed on 13 (Patau syndrome), 18 (Edwards syndrome), and 21 (Down syndrome), and sex chromosomes (X and Y). Notably, speech disfluencies are more often observed in people with several chromosomal abnormalities including Down syndrome, fragile X syndrome, Prader-Willi syndrome, and Turner syndrome than in the general population.[13] Although the exact genetic mechanism of increased risk is not yet known, the estimated prevalence of stuttering in individuals with Down syndrome has been reported to range from 15 to 45%, much higher than the general population prevalence.[14] These findings suggest that there may be genes that reside on these chromosomes that impact risk of stuttering and other speech disfluencies.

3.3.2 Another Variation in the Human Genome: Single Nucleotide Polymorphism (SNP)

Although variation in the human genome can take several forms, SNPs (pronounced "snip") are the most common. A SNP is a DNA sequence variation that occurs when a single nucleotide (adenine, thymine, cytosine, or guanine) in the genome sequence is altered.

On average, SNPs occur once in every 1,000 base pairs throughout a person's DNA, resulting in roughly 4 to 5 million SNPs in any given person's genome.[15] Today, more than 781 million SNPs and 62 million short insertion/deletion variants have been found across humans from multiple populations.[16]

Most SNPs reside in portions of the genome that have undefined functionality and have no measurable effect. Even SNPs located within genes may have no impact on the amount or type of protein made. For example, many intronic SNPs have no effect on gene expression or resulting protein. Synonymous SNPs do not result in a change to the amino acid sequence in the resulting protein. These are often referred to as "silent" in that they cause no difference in the polypeptide sequence of the resulting protein. On the other hand, nonsynonymous SNPs do lead to alterations in the resulting protein by swapping one amino acid for another. Additionally, so-called "nonsense" SNPs can cause the transcription machinery to stop early, leading to a truncated protein. SNPs at the junction of introns and exons can impact the splicing process in which introns (a portion of a gene that does not code for amino acids) are cut out of mRNA ahead of transcription, leading to changes in the protein that can be made from a single gene. Finally, SNPs that reside in transcription factor binding sites or enhancer regions can lead to changes in the amount of protein made. SNPs such as these, which are associated with the expression of genes, are called expression quantitative trait loci, or eQTLs.

3.4 Strategies for Measuring Genetic Variation

To identify genetic changes that are too small to visibly alter chromosomal banding patterns, geneticists have developed technologies which measure the exact pattern of nucleotides in the genome such as microarray-based genotyping and genome or exome sequencing. The specific genetic variants that are observed in a given site in the genome, such as a gene or base pair position, are called alleles. If you have the same allele at a given location in the human genome (or locus) on both chromosomes, you are said to be a homozygote, and if your alleles are different from one another, you are a heterozygote. The exact combination of alleles in a given locus is called a genotype.

There are two main techniques for analyzing DNA. One uses genotyping microarrays, which are a collection of microscopic spots of single-stranded DNA of known sequence (called probes) tacked down to a solid surface called an array. By detecting the probes that have become bound to sample DNA, the genetic content of the sample can be determined. Next generation sequence technology, on the other hand, determines the exact order of nucleotides in entire genomes or targeted regions, such as the exomes (all exons within the genome) of DNA or RNA. Although sequencing remains comparatively expensive ($200–$300 for high-quality whole-exome sequencing and $500–$800 for high-quality whole-genome sequencing) it can capture extremely rare alleles and even new mutations.

3.4.1 Epigenetic Factors in the Expression of DNA

Although genes play a critical role in our health and development, so do our experiences and the environment in which we live. Epigenetics is the study of how behavioral and environmental factors alter the expression of DNA without changing the DNA sequence itself. Three epigenetic mechanisms have been identified: DNA methylation which can essentially turn off gene expression, histone modification which can change the accessibility of portions of the genome to the transcriptional machinery, and ncRNA-associated gene silencing in which small pieces of RNA bind to DNA and block it from being expressed. Although changes to the sequence of DNA (e.g., mutation) occur rarely, social and environmental conditions can lead to big changes in epigenetic factors, with profound effects on traits and disease. In this way, nongenetic factors such as diet, exercise, social interactions, infectious disease exposures, drugs, economic status, stress, exposure to pollution or toxins, among many others can interact with a person's specific genotype to influence the risk for a trait like stuttering.

3.5 Transmission Models of Inheritance

As defined earlier, a phenotype is an observable characteristic resulting from the interaction of an individual genotype with the environment (see Definitions). When a particular phenotype is observed at a higher rate within a family than in the general population, it suggests a genetic or environmental factor is putting that family at greater risk. Therefore, one way to find genetic factors linked to a disorder such as stuttering is to study the inheritance patterns of the disorder in families (▶ Fig. 3.2). Tracking the inheritance of a disorder alongside the inheritance of DNA allows geneticists to identify regions of the genome which may contribute to risk.

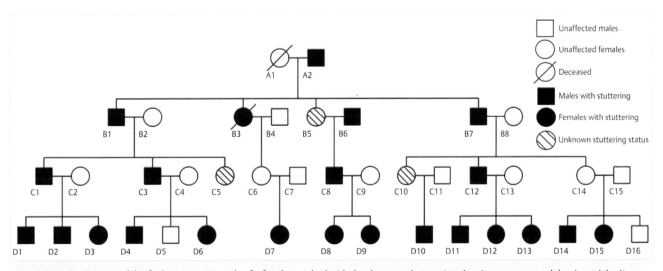

Fig. 3.2 Transmission models of inheritance. Example of a family enriched with developmental stuttering showing an autosomal dominant inheritance pattern with incomplete penetrance.

Many genetic diseases are caused by a mutation in a single gene. As of this writing, the Online Mendelian Inheritance in Man resource (http://omim.org) lists nearly 7,000 phenotypes with a known molecular genetic basis including more than 4,500 genes with a known phenotype-causing mutation. The pattern of inheritance of single-gene disorders in families depends on whether the mutation is autosomal (carried on chromosomes 1–22) or X-linked (carried on the X chromosomes) and the model of inheritance.

3.5.1 Autosomal Dominant Inheritance

In an autosomal dominant inheritance model, a single copy of the disease-causing allele, inherited from either the mother or the father, is sufficient to result in an affected offspring. Autosomal dominant inheritance is characterized by vertical transmission of the resulting phenotype through a family with a 50% chance that an affected parent will have an affected offspring.

3.5.2 Autosomal Recessive Inheritance

In a recessive model of inheritance, both copies of the disease-causing allele are required for the phenotype to be expressed. A recessive disease allele *will not* typically result in a disease phenotype in a heterozygous carrier. An exception to this rule occurs when a person carries two different disease-causing mutations impacting the function of the same gene or molecular pathway. When two different mutations lead to recessive disease in this way, the carrier is said to be a compound heterozygote. Recessive inheritance is characterized by clustering of disease among siblings, without a requirement that the disease is observed in the parents or other family members. Recessive diseases are observed with greater frequency in the presence of consanguinity (inbreeding).

In addition, some homozygous carriers of recessive disease alleles and some heterozygous carriers of dominant disease alleles may not express the associated disease. The rate of affection in people with a disease-causing genotype is called penetrance. Penetrance may be altered by other modifying genetic or environmental factors. Additionally, not all genetic disorders are expressed from birth; age-dependent penetrance refers to the changing rate of expression of a phenotype in people carrying the disease-causing genotype by age, such as Alzheimer's disease. In stuttering, because many people recover at an early age, stuttering may exhibit reduced penetrance in families due to true lack of stuttering in mutation carriers or due to transient stuttering that was not clinically noted.

3.5.3 Approaches to Mapping Disease Genes: Linkage Analysis

Two common approaches to mapping disease genes are linkage analysis and association study. In linkage analyses, given a specific genetic model, the co-transmission of disease and genomic segments through a pedigree is measured to find regions of the genome that are "linked" to disease.

Because each transmission event (meiosis) in a family contributes to the statistical evidence for or against linkage, linkage is exceptionally well-powered to find causal genes in large families or by summing together the evidence from multiple smaller families in which causal variants fall in the same locus.

Genome-wide significance can be achieved in a single family with as few as 12 people. Because very rare or even private genetic variants are frequent within a given family, linkage is exceptionally well-powered to detect even the rarest genetic risk factors, and because evidence of linkage of different mutations in the same gene region can be combined across families, linkage is well-powered even when different families carry different causal mutations in the same gene (allelic heterogeneity).

Several factors can severely limit the success of linkage studies. First, families enriched for disease are often difficult and expensive to ascertain. Second, if the transmission model is miss-specified, the analysis can be confounded leading to a failure to detect the causal variant. Linkage can be performed without specifying a model of inheritance (so-called nonparametric linkage); however, these studies are considerably less well-powered than parametric linkage in which the transmission model (e.g., dominant or recessive) is accurately specified. Third, reduced disease penetrance and age-dependent penetrance both dramatically reduce power in linkage analyses. Fourth, linkage is highly sensitive to phenotypic miss-specification—a single case labeled as a control or vice versa can severely impact evidence of linkage at the causal variant. And finally, linkage has very little power to detect disorders that are caused by multiple different genes within or across families (genetic heterogeneity). ► Fig. 3.3 depicts results of a linkage analysis for stuttering.

3.5.4 Association Studies

In an association study, genetic variants are tested for a statistical relationship with a disease or trait in a sample from a general population. If an allele occurs more frequently in people affected with a disease than it does in the general population, the variant is said to be *associated* with the disease. When variants from across the entire genome are tested, the analysis is called a genome-wide association study (GWAS). Unlike linkage studies, GWAS is much less sensitive to model miss-specification (most assume an additive model where each additional copy of a variant confers equal additional risk), tolerates some degree of case/control mislabeling without large losses in power, and is not impacted by genetic heterogeneity—GWAS can detect risk associations from multiple genes and variants in the genome. GWAS is typically performed on very dense genetic data (millions of SNPs), with the hope that the causal variant itself, or a variant in close physical proximity to the causal variant will be tested. However, although GWAS can identify genes and variants that contribute only modestly to risk of disease or trait, GWAS requires much larger samples to reach genome-wide significant levels of association. Today, it is not uncommon for GWAS to comprise samples of over a million people. GWAS is also markedly susceptible to bias due to patterns of ancestry or relatedness within the sample.

3.6 Genetic Studies of Stuttering

To date, published literature investigating genetic contributions to developmental stuttering has primarily drawn on family-based analyses and studies of population isolates, yet for developmental stuttering, identifying the causal gene(s) within and across families has proven challenging. Below, we review the findings of genetic analyses of stuttering in families that have been published to date, which are also listed in ► Table 3.2.

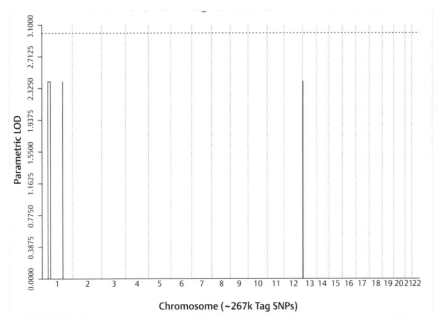

Fig. 3.3 Example of parametric multipoint logarithm of the odds (LOD) score for familial stuttering linkage analysis. Dotted line indicates a LOD score reaching genome-wide significance (3.0). The first peak spans chr1: 34136452–56798308 with 1,581 genes found in that region; the second peak spans chr1: 178927427–178938964 with no genes found in that region. The third peak spans chr13:19314519–21804021 with 118 found in that region. SNPs, single nucleotide polymorphisms.

Table 3.2 Summary of genetic findings in stuttering

Study	Year	Chromosome	Region	Statistical strength	Chromosome:bp (build 38)	Population architecture
Shugart et al	2004	Chr 18	18q11.2–21.1	Suggestive	chr18:21,500,000–50,700,000	68 outbred families with persistent stuttering in North America and England
Riaz et al*	2005	Chr 12	12q23.3	Significant	chr12:103,500,000–108,600,000	46 consanguineous Pakistani families
Suresh et al	2006	Chr 9	9p	Suggestive	chr9:0–43,000,000	100 families of European descent
Wittke-Thompson et al	2007	Chr 13	13q21	Suggestive	chr13:54,700,000–72,800,000	One 232-person genealogy with 48 affected (Hutterites population in South Dakota)
Lan et al[a]	2009	Chr 11	DRD2	Significant	chr11:113,409,605–113,475,398	Case-control (gender-matched controls) association study focusing specifically on dopaminergic gene haplotypes and allele frequencies among SNPs in the Han Chinese population
Raza et al[b]	2010	Chr 3	3q13.2-13.33	Significant	chr3:111,600,000–122,200,000	One consanguineous family (three cousin matings in F3 generation) from Pakistan; study performed a two-point linkage analysis, modeling autosomal recessive stuttering
Kang et al	2010	Chr 12	12q23.3	Significant	chr12:103,500,000–108,600,000	77 unrelated Pakistani individuals who stutter plus unrelated cases from 46 Pakistani families (see Suresh et al), 270 affected unrelated individuals from N. America and England *Follow-on study
Raza et al[b]	2012	Chr 16	16q	Significant	chr16:36,800,000–90,338,345	One consanguineous family from Pakistan
Raza et al[b] **	2013	Chr 2, 15	2p +15q	Significant	chr2:0–93,900,000; chr15:19,000,000–101,991,189	71 individual family from Cameroon comprised of 33 affected members
Domingues et al[b]	2014	Chr 10	10q21	Significant	chr10:51,100,000–68,800,000	43 Brazilian families; **2 families** with genome-wide significance after modeling dominant inheritance
Raza et al	2015	Chr 15	AP4E1	Significant	chr15:50,908,683–51,005,895	Cameroonian family +probands from Cameroon, Pakistani, and N. America **Follow-on study
Mohammadi et al[a]	2017	Chr 10	CYP17A1	Significant	chr10:102,830,531–102,837,472	Case-control (age and ethnic background matched) study of Kurdish population aged 3–9 years from western Iran

Table 3.2 (*Continued*) Summary of genetic findings in stuttering

Study	Year	Chromosome	Region	Statistical strength	Chromosome:bp (build 38)	Population architecture
Kazemi et al	2018	Chr 12, 16	*GNPTAB, GNPTG, NAGPA*	Significant	chr12:101,745,499– 101,830,959; chr16:1,351,931– 1,364,113; chr16:5,024,844– 5,034,141	25 Iranian families with at least two first-degree, related, nonsyndromic stutterers

Abbreviation: SNPs, single nucleotide polymorphisms.
Notes: [a] Results not replicated in follow-on literature.
[b] Results for only one or two families.
Suggestive: Findings did not reach genome-wide significance.
Significant: Findings reached genome-wide significance.
* The study, Kang et al. 2010, included some of the same Pakistani families investigated by Riaz et al. 2005
** The study, Raza et al. 2015, included some of the same Cameroonian families investigated by Raza et al. 2013

3.6.1 Stuttering Risk: *GNPTAB* and Lysosomal Transport Genes

In 2005, Riaz et al[17] performed linkage analyses in 46 consanguineous (i.e., common ancestry) Pakistani families where stuttering occurred in at least two generations and diagnosis was confirmed independently by two different clinicians. They discovered a region with developmental stuttering in a single family but failed to pinpoint a causal gene. After 5 years in 2010, Kang et al[18] reported the results from a follow-up study of 77 unrelated Pakistani individuals who stutter plus unrelated cases from the same 46 Pakistani families included in the study by Riaz et al in 2005.[17] Their investigation identified three genes that likely contribute to the risk of developmental stuttering: *GNPTAB*, *GNPTG*, and *NAGPA*. *GNPTAB* produces the enzyme that works to prepare lysosomes for transportation. In 2018, Kazemi and colleagues performed sequencing and gene mapping in 25 Iranian families with high prevalence of developmental stuttering and identified an additional three gene variants in *GNPTAB* and *GNPTG* that co-segregated (i.e., transmitted on the same chromosome) with stuttering.[19]

3.6.2 *DRD2*: A Potential Role for Dopamine in Stuttering Risk

Research has identified three additional candidate risk genes for stuttering: *DRD2*,[20] *AP4E1*,[21] and *CYP17A1*.[22] Familial studies of stuttering in patients with Tourette's syndrome had previously implicated *DRD2*[23] and more than 10 years later Lan et al published an association study focusing specifically on dopaminergic gene haplotypes and allele frequencies in stuttering cases and controls from a population of Han Chinese in which both risk and protective alleles were identified in *DRD2*.[20] These results were not replicated in 2011 study by Kang et al[24] in a case-control cohort from Brazil and western Europe.

DRD2 encodes a dopamine receptor. Dopamine is a type of chemical messenger (neurotransmitter) that the nervous system uses to send messages between nerve cells and plays a role in how people feel and experience pleasure. As a key player in cellular response of dopamine, it is hypothesized that *DRD2* plays a role in reinforcing and rewarding behaviors by altering how we feel after stimulation. As with most biological systems, there are genetic variants that can make typical function go awry, and the same is true here. For example, variants in *DRD2* have been associated with addictive behaviors,[25,26,27,28,29,30] but have also been implicated in neurologic disorders such as Tourette's syndrome, post-traumatic stress disorder,[31] and schizophrenia.[32] In addition, *DRD2* variants have been implicated in Parkinson's disease[33] and movement disorders. Although the evidence of a role for *DRD2* as a risk factor for stuttering is far from conclusive, the idea that neurotransmitters may be involved is alluring because it opens the doors for development of targeted pharmacologic approaches in treatment.

3.6.3 *AP4E1*: Intercellular Trafficking and Stuttering Risk

In 2015, Raza et al[21] identified two heterozygous *AP4E1* variants linked with persistent developmental stuttering in a large Cameroonian family (using the same family as published in their earlier work from 2013[34]); they also observed these same two variants in unrelated Cameroonians with persistent stuttering. Although Raza et al[21] also reported 23 additional rare variants (including loss-of-function variants) within *AP4E1* among unrelated stuttering individuals from Cameroon, Pakistan, and North America, their findings have yet to be replicated by another group. *AP4E1* is a member of a protein complex that plays a key role in intercellular trafficking by sorting and organizing membrane proteins. Recessive mutations in *AP4E1* cause a type of slow progressing neurodegenerative disorder called spastic paraplegia.[35] People with spastic paraplegia usually have developmental delay, moderate to severe intellectual disability, impaired or absent speech, small head size (microcephaly), seizures, and progressive motor symptoms.

3.6.4 Hormone Regulation May Explain Biological Sex Differences in Stuttering Risk

In 2017, Mohammadi et al[22] performed a case-control study of the Kurdish population aged 3 to 9 years from western Iran, specifically focusing on the sexually dimorphic nature of stuttering and identified an allelic polymorphism associated with stuttering susceptibility in *CYP17A1*, a gene integral for the synthesis of steroid hormones. *CYP17A1* encodes a key enzyme in the pathway that produces the hormones progestin, mineralocorticoid, glucocorticoid, androgen, and estrogen. As reported by Domingues et al in 2019, these results were not replicated in an independent case and population-matched control association study from the United States, Brazil, Pakistan, and Cameroon.[36,37]

3.6.5 Introducing Genetic Mutations into Animal Models of Stuttering

After Kang et al pinpointed three genes critical for the lysosomal targeting pathway (*GNPTAB*, *GNPTG*, and *NAGPA*) in Pakistani individuals who stutter, the mechanism of why specific mutations in these genes might cause stuttering remained obscure.[18] To investigate plausible mechanisms, the authors worked to build a mouse model of stuttering. In 2005, Shu et al successfully demonstrated that introducing human *FOXP2* mutations into the orthologous Foxp2 gene in mice altered ultrasonic vocalizations in mice, mimicking vocalizations observed in humans with the *FOXP2* mutation, which set the precedent for using mice as a model of human speech and language traits.[38] In 2016, Barnes et al developed a mouse model of stuttering for mice carrying a human stuttering mutation in *GNTAB* in the orthologous mouse GNPTAB gene and found differences in the timing of vocalizations, namely, increased pauses between bouts of syllables and abnormally long pauses in homozygous mutant mice when compared to control mice.[39] Several years later in 2019, they introduced another human mutation in GNPTAB into mice and once again demonstrated that the mutant mice displayed vocalization abnormalities compared to control mice.[40] Moreover, they compared brain images from the mutant and control mouse groups and saw a decrease in the number of astrocytes in the corpus callosum of mutant mice, suggesting a role for neurological cell deficit in the genesis of persistent developmental stuttering.

Although intriguing biological processes have been highlighted by these analyses, there is a remarkable lack of consensus across studies, and the molecular underpinnings of developmental stuttering in general populations remain obscure. Taken together, these studies suggest that there is no single gene or molecular pathway that explains the risk of developmental stuttering in families or populations. Rather, it appears that different families have different genetic risk factors and not everyone in a family who carries the risk genotype stutters. We can conclude that stuttering is likely a complex trait, meaning that risk of stuttering in general does not follow simple Mendelian inheritance patterns. Instead, it is likely that the prevalence of stuttering in general populations is polygenic, meaning that risk effects combine across many genes and may be modified by the environment.

As we have learned, complex, polygenic traits are challenging to study with family-based designs. Instead, approaches that are well-powered in the presence of genetic heterogeneity and can identify variants with modest effect sizes such as GWAS are needed to identify the genetic variants at play. But, as discussed earlier, GWAS often requires thousands or even millions of study participants to identify genetic risk factors, posing a significant challenge for investigators. Building such a cohort for the study of stuttering from scratch would likely take many years and cost many millions of dollars. In the following section, we describe some sources of genetic data for thousands or millions of people for the purpose of understanding risks of stuttering.

3.7 Sources of Large-Scale Genetic Data from People Who Stutter

3.7.1 The International Stuttering Project

The International Stuttering Project (ISP) formed a global collaboration to study stuttering at a population level. Investigators collected DNA specimens from a diverse global population of individuals who stutter and then performed a case-control GWAS.[41] Published in 2021, this inaugural population-level study of almost 1,500 stuttering cases and about 6,800 controls identified one significant variant. This genetic variant occurred in *SSUH2*, a gene previously reported to play a role in tooth formation (association results from the study are summarized in ▶ Fig. 3.4).[36] Although it remains unclear how this genetic association might impact stuttering risk this study found an enrichment of top genes, including *SSUH2*, involved in biological processes including extracellular matrix and structure organization, cell adhesion, anatomical structure development, nervous system development, ossification, neurogenesis, cell migration, and bone morphogenesis. Studies to replicate this finding and understand its function are ongoing.

3.7.2 Biobanks

Under traditional genetic study designs, investigators usually acquire case data by directly recruiting subjects with a phenotype of interest. This process can often be time intensive, cost inefficient, and result in small sample sizes that are insufficiently powered for genetic discovery in complex traits. Biobanks are large repositories of biological specimens, often suitable for genotyping, that can facilitate genetic analysis. Some biobanks have been linked to participant's electronic medical records making them especially powerful for biomedical research. These resources provide unmatched sample sizes (with some biobanks exceeding 500,000 participants) and a quick and comparatively cost-efficient method for identifying relationships between patient genetics and any phenotypes of interest. Additionally, these large-scale health record sets can provide an agonistic approach to studying relationships between conditions (e.g., in analyses to identify) and genotype–phenotype relationships across the entire set of medical traits (phenome).

3.7.3 Phenome Wide Association Studies (PheWAS)

In direct recruitment studies, investigators typically define and measure all comorbidities they will study. This hypothesis-driven approach limits the relationships that can be established. Research into comorbidities of stuttering prior to 2020 performed analysis on only a handful of hypothesis-driven phenotypes, typically motivated by prior literature, such as neurological conditions (autism, motor coordination, etc.). Because electronic health records include notation of all medical billing through a health system, comorbidity analyses in these data allow for the discovery of potentially novel disease associations that were previously unstudied.

In direct recruitment studies, enrolled participants must meet the phenotypic definitions of the study. When utilizing electronic

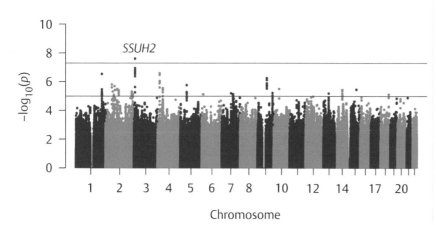

Fig. 3.4 Manhattan plot summarizing stuttering genome-wide association study (GWAS) results. In this GWAS, genetic variants were tested for a statistical relationship with stuttering status (case or control). Variants represent a specific nucleobase at a location in the human genome (e.g., adenine or "A," guanine or "G"). Each assessed variant is plotted as a dot by chromosome/position (x-axis) against log transformed p-values (y-axis) from the association analysis. Blue and red lines denote suggestive (α = 5.0e-6) and genome-wide (α = 5.0e-8) significance respectively. Genome-wide significance threshold was set according to field standards, which assumes that α = 0.05 and is then corrected for each independent test (α = 0.05/1,000,000 or 5.0e-8). The field assumes there are approximately one million independent variants genome-wide. The suggestive threshold (α = 5.0e-6) assumes an expectation of one false positive association per GWAS (i.e., one/total number of independent variants). This plot revealed that a variant on chromosome 3 within the gene *SSUH2* reached genome-wide significance in this analysis of clinically validated stuttering cases collected through the International Stuttering Project and self-reported stuttering cases collected from The National Longitudinal Study of Adolescent to Adult Health (Add Health).

health records to define cases and controls, investigators derive case and control information from the hospital billing codes, clinical notes, and laboratory results. For many pathologies that are likely to be noted in a medical setting, this is a straightforward process; however, identifying a robust case cohort for stuttering in health record data is difficult for a number of reasons: (1) identification and treatment of stuttering typically occurs in speech pathology clinics and schools rather than in a medical setting, and consequently, records of stuttering evaluation and treatment are not often included in medical databases; (2) because severity of stuttering can vary greatly from subject to subject, stuttering may be unnoticed or considered irrelevant by medical practitioners; (3) most people who stutter (approximately 80%) fully recover by adolescence, meaning any visit to the doctor after this period will not result in a clinical diagnosis. This challenge disproportionately impacts identification in health records of females who stutter because of their elevated rate of recovery and often reduced severity in stuttering relative to males. For example, although stuttering is a relatively common condition, affecting roughly 5 to 10% of the population at some point during their lifetime, within Vanderbilt University Medical Center's heath record, only 0.01% of subjects have a diagnostic code for stuttering. As a result, in 2020, investigators turned toward comorbidities of stuttering that are better captured within these databases to understand the biology of stuttering.

3.7.4 Additional Considerations: Analyzing Comorbidities Associated with Stuttering

A comorbidity is an additional health condition that occurs concurrently with another diagnosis. Comorbid conditions exist simultaneously but independently of the primary diagnosis, in contrast to a syndrome where several symptoms occur together that characterize a specific disease. Greater understanding of stuttering comorbidities may not only improve clinical care, but also our understanding of causes of stuttering.

Historically, investigations of stuttering comorbidities have focused on the presence of co-occurring speech and language impairments, or behavioral or psychological conditions like ADHD, anxiety, and social anxiety.[42,43] However, it can be difficult to disentangle the cause-and-effect relationship between stuttering and other comorbid conditions. For example, social anxiety may be caused by feared speaking situations due to stuttering or may exist fully independent of stuttering. Mapping comorbidities through common genetic factors is one way to reveal shared pathways between stuttering and other conditions.

Understanding comorbidities can be particularly important if concurrent disorders predict clinical outcomes or influence risk for a condition. Although medical conditions outside the realm of speech-language pathology are not routinely discussed with a speech pathologist, electronic health records offer a depth and breadth of medical information experienced throughout a lifetime. Using these records, we can attempt to replicate previously identified comorbidities and explore latent, unstudied comorbidities.

A recent study utilizing electronic health records identified potential novel comorbid conditions for developmental stuttering.[44] In the study by Pruett et al, medical records of people who stutter were significantly enriched with 38 distinct clinical phenotype groups.[44] These included broad phenotype groups that encompass traits noted in prior literature as associated with stuttering such as developmental delays and disorders,[42,45,46] tics and stuttering,[7] hearing loss,[47] sleep disorders,[48] and a variety of codes related to the skin and lung inflammation.[49,50]

Other statistically significant comorbidities included previously unreported comorbidities such as infections, neurological deficits, aphasia/speech disturbance, obesity, metabolism, and measures of development. Some of these comorbidities are no doubt surprising to see. Importantly, this approach detects associations, so we cannot make assumptions about causality from these data, but it serves to generate new hypotheses about how complex traits manifest clinically and lays the groundwork for future studies designed to validate these associations and determine causality.

In addition to providing biological insight to the pathophysiology of stuttering, these comorbidities can be utilized to amass the sample sizes required to provide meaningful results from a GWAS within large-scale genetic biobanks. In 2021, Shaw et al built a stuttering prediction machine-learning model based on the Pruett et al stuttering-associated clinical diagnoses that uses diagnostic history of patients to identify clusters of symptoms that predict stuttering.[51] With this prediction algorithm, they were able to infer cases and controls for an analysis of stuttering in approximately 100,000 participants in Vanderbilt University's biobank, BioVU. The algorithm predicted that approximately 10% of participants stutter, resulting in a sample size of >9,000 genotyped stuttering samples to be analyzed through GWAS. In addition, using a comorbidity-based GWAS, Shaw et al identified two genetic variants that were associated with the predicted stuttering phenotype.[51] These variants mapped to two genes: *FAM49A* on chromosome 2 for subjects of European ancestry and *ZMAT4* on chromosome 8 for stuttering in subjects of African ancestry. Neither *ZMAT4* or *FAM49A* had been previously implicated in developmental stuttering.

ZMAT4 is a zinc finger protein highly expressed in the brain. Zinc finger proteins work to maintain the health of neurons. The specific functions of this protein family are extraordinarily diverse. They act to facilitate transcription, lipid binding, and regulation of cell death. *ZMAT4* has been previously implicated in African Americans for nearsightedness and higher fasting blood glucose levels. *FAM49A* is a signaling protein and is also abundantly expressed in the brain regions. Previous studies of *FAM49A* in Asian and Brazilian populations have found associations with cleft palate.

3.7.5 Summary of Findings from Genetic Studies in Stuttering

Because they represent population-level genetic effects derived from well-powered case-control studies from genome-wide analyses, the identification of *SSUH2*, *ZMAT4*, and *FAM49A* are key discoveries in developmental stuttering genetics. These studies did not strongly replicate the effects seen in prior genes, but this is expected since the variants in those genes linked to stuttering were extremely rare mutations unlikely to be present in general populations with sufficient frequency to be detected by association analysis. However, independent replication of effects of very rare mutations in *GNPTG* in an unrelated cohort as well as animal models have provided additional support, and the field is beginning to make headway. Like the initial findings from linkage studies, these newly identified genes from GWAS require further study in independent datasets. The nature and function of these genes are complex and diffuse, acting on a wide variety of systems within the body. Investigating network pathology, comorbidities, and the function of solute carriers, zinc finger proteins, signaling proteins, and the lysosomal targeting pathway will hopefully yield some answers to the biology that underlies stuttering.

3.8 Applying Research Findings to Models and Characteristics of Stuttering

Identifying the genes and variants that may contribute to risk of stuttering in families and in populations is a landmark advance for the field to be sure, but how much have we really learned about the cause of stuttering? How can we apply this new knowledge to predict who might stutter or improve speech and quality of life for people who stutter? Below, we review several exciting approaches to interpret and apply the findings of genetic studies of stuttering.

3.8.1 Modeling Polygenic Risk of Stuttering

For most of the population, we have learned that genetic risk of stuttering is driven by a large set of small effect variants rather than a small number of mutations with large effect. Recently, geneticists have used data generated from GWAS to measure complex genetic risk through an approach that summarizes all the effects from across the genome in a person into a single, individual risk score. To do this, geneticists develop polygenic risk score (PRS) models, which are calculations of an individual's disease liability or risk based on the individual's genetic code.

As previously discussed, most phenotypes, including stuttering, cannot be fully explained by a single mutation within our genetic code. Instead, genetic heritability of these phenotypes is explained by multiple genetic variants. It is important to note that not all variants equally impact stuttering. Although there do exist regions of our genetic code where one mutation can result in drastic changes in a person's phenotype, most variants have a low impact on someone's phenotypic status. Although these effects can be small, if many of these low impact variants are present within a patient's genetic code, the combined impact could be substantial, resulting in an altered phenotype. Simply put, this equation can quantify the overall impact of all the variants in the genome to assess a person's genetic risk of a disease or condition.

Although the development of PRS models is an important step toward understanding the role that genetics play in the development of stuttering, it is critical to understand that these models are never used to diagnose stuttering, or for that matter used in any clinical context in their current state. They simply provide an additional means to study the collective effects of the genome on an individual's risk of stuttering, and therefore can be very informative in a research context. Like the comorbidity-based imputation approach discussed above, developing stuttering PRS models within one dataset allows us to infer the phenotypic status based on individual genetic risk in other datasets. For example, Shaw et al used this approach to show that a PRS developed in the GWAS results from Vanderbilt University's biobank could significantly predict case/control

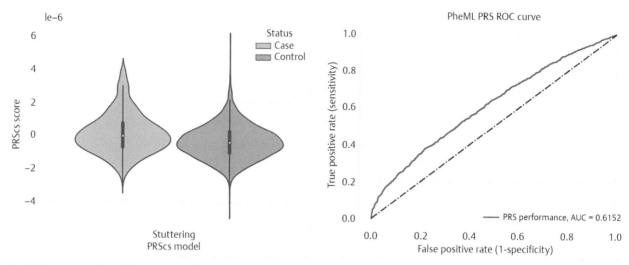

Fig. 3.5 Polygenic-risk models are developed from genome-wide association study (GWAS) summary statistics. This specific model was developed from the association results from the imputed stuttering analysis and applied to a subject set consisting of clinically evaluated stuttering patients (cases) and population controls from the International Stuttering Project. The violin plot to the left shows that the case set (*green violin*) scored higher according to these polygenic risk score models compared to controls (*red violin*). This means that the model captures polygenic risk of stuttering (i.e., stuttering cases have a higher burden of genetic risk for stuttering compared to controls). The receiver operator curve (ROC) (right plot) shows the classification performance of the model, demonstrating that the model performance (*solid red line*) does better than randomly assigning stuttering status (*dashed black line*). The area under the curve (AUC) calculated from these ROC plots indicate how well the model can guess stuttering status of individuals. These model performance scores range from perfect performance (AUC = 1) to being no better than random chance (AUC = 0.5). An AUC = 0.6152 indicates moderate model performance.

status in the International Stuttering Project dataset (▶ Fig. 3.5). Even in the absence of a stuttering diagnosis, PRS allows investigators to utilize biobanks where stuttering is underreported to estimate genetic risk of stuttering and then study the diagnostic history of subjects with higher risk and compare to those with lower genetic risk.

Importantly, most PRS models are built around GWAS results and capture common, low-effect genetic predictors, and therefore generally do not model rare or family-specific mutations which can drive the stuttering phenotype within pedigrees. With PRS models in stuttering, we can also identify scenarios where people who do stutter have a low PRS. These interesting cases may be explained by (1) the model not adequately capturing all the common genetic effects associated with stuttering, (2) these subjects may carry a rare, higher impact variant, or (3) other environmental effects are contributing to their stuttering phenotype. Using PRS models to identify cases of stuttering with low genetic risk can therefore help researchers identify people for further follow-up by exome sequencing or deeper assessments of other potential nongenetic risk factors.

3.8.2 Correlations between Stuttering Risk and Related Traits

In a yet unpublished data, researchers have found that PRS models developed from GWAS of other traits can predict stuttering. For example, a soon-to-be published study by Niarchou et al identified SNPs associated with a person's ability to keep rhythm and showed a genetic correlation of rhythm with breathing function, motor function, processing speed, and chronotype.[52] Analysis of a PRS model developed to predict rhythm ability applied in the International Stuttering Project

data shows that those who stutter are genetically predicted to have significantly worse rhythm than those who do not, illustrating a shared genetic architecture across these two traits and an as-yet uncharacterized underlying biological mechanism connecting them. Indeed, these findings are supported by and provide a molecular basis for prior work that reported a rhythm perception deficit in children who stutter.[53] Identifying the specific genetic loci driving this correlation will be key to understanding the common genetic etiology of rhythm and stuttering. Still, demonstrating that PRS models can predict genetic liability in alternative phenotypes and establishing shared etiology have immediate relevance for new research avenues that may lead to therapeutic advances.

3.9 Conclusions

Today, the genomes of many millions of people from around the world have been studied, enabling discovery of associations between regions of the genome and human traits. These sophisticated new technologies have helped us unravel the genetic bases of complex diseases and disorders like language impairment, autism, and stuttering. Genetics has come a long way! At the same time, there is a long way yet to go in unraveling the complexity and specific mechanisms that underlie stuttering, but as laid out in this chapter, we have already learned a tremendous amount.

We know that stuttering often runs in families and have estimated the proportion of variance in stuttering that comes from genetics. We have mapped rare mutations in genes that may be the cause of some familial forms of stuttering and have explored the effects of these mutations in other populations and animal models. We have also established from these analyses that there is no single gene or mutation that explains all cases of stuttering, but rather we have searched for genetic risk factors throughout the genome in GWAS of population-based clinically ascertained stuttering case and control data and found an array of common variants that are associated with stuttering. We have also used large-scale existing biobank data to study comorbidities of stuttering and built predictive models to identify people who are likely to stutter, even in the absence of a clinical record of stuttering, and found additional genetic variants associated with this trait. We have seen that polygenic risk scores that summarize the genome-wide genetic risk of stuttering into a single genetic liability score can predict people who stutter and established genetic correlations between stuttering risk and rhythm ability. Thanks to the efforts of the participants and researchers who worked together on these studies, the remarkable steps that have been made toward characterizing the genetic basis of stuttering pave the way forward for future research that will shape how stuttering is perceived, managed, and prevented.

Understanding the heritability and molecular basis of stuttering can alleviate stress or worry that individuals or families may have about the cause of stuttering. For example, some individuals who stutter (and the parents of children who stutter as well) may believe that stuttering is caused by a genetic abnormality leading to low intelligence, mood, or personality disorders (nature). On the other hand, parents of children who stutter may believe that their parenting style or other aspects of the environment are to blame. When these concerns are expressed in the clinical setting, speech-language pathologists can say with confidence that findings from different lines of research, including genetics, point to stuttering as a complex and polygenic trait caused by an array of genes and variants, as well as environmental and even random factors. Simply put, stuttering can best be considered as the result of a complex interaction between the environment and what the child brings to it. Even so, there is much yet to learn about the genetic factors that underlie the high heritability of stuttering. Nonetheless, it is worthwhile to envision what possibilities exist for treatment approaches and prevention strategies built around the function of the genetic risk factors identified to date. For example, given the correlation with rhythm, future research will be needed to explore whether an intervention to strengthen rhythm abilities may be associated with an increased recovery rate or prevention of stuttering in those at risk. Furthermore, the positive identification of genes is monumental to people who themselves stutter, their families, and the community. Genetic discoveries can provide answers, reduce stigma, shame, or blame that often results from not knowing the cause of developmental stuttering.

Acknowledgments

Many thanks to Dr. Nancy Cox, Dr. Heather Highland, Dr. Hung-Hsin Chen, Ms. Hannah Polikowsky, and Mr. Douglas Shaw, who contributed essential expert feedback, content, and revisions to this chapter.

3.10 Definitions

Allele: One of two or more alternative forms of a nucleotide or gene that arise by mutation and are found at the same location on a chromosome.

Centromere: A special sequence of DNA in a chromosome to which microtubules attach during cell division.

Chromosome: A cellular unit made up of a long DNA molecule.

Cytogenetic bands

Cytogenetics: The study of the number and morphology of chromosomes.

Dizygotic twins: Fraternal twins sharing approximately 50% of their genomes.

DNA: Deoxyribonucleic acid is a molecule composed of two strings of nucleic acids that coil around each other to form a double helix. DNA contains genetic instructions for the development, function, growth, and reproduction of all known organisms and many viruses.

Effect: A statistical value measuring the strength of the relationship between two variables.

eQTLs: Expression quantitative trait loci are genetic variants that have been associated with gene expression levels in a given tissue.

Etiology: The cause or set of causes of a disease or condition.

Frequency: The rate of observing an allele or genotype in a given population.

Gamete: Reproductive cell; in humans these are the egg and sperm which are haploid.

Gene: A functional and heritable unit of DNA, typically translated into RNA which may or may not later be translated into protein.

Genotype: The precise combination of alleles in a given locus.

Heritability: A measure of the variance in a trait that can be explained by genetic factors.

Heterozygote: Individuals who inherited different alleles from their mother and their father at a given locus.

Homozygote: Individuals who inherited the same allele from their mother and their father at a given locus.

Karyotype: The number and visual appearance of the chromosomes.

Locus: A specific site in the genome, usually referred to by chromosomal band or physical location.

Monozygotic twins: Identical twins with identical genomes.

Mutation: An alteration in the nucleotide sequence of the genome.

Nucleotide: A subunit of DNA, consisting of a deoxyribose, a phosphate group, and a base, that is often noted by shorthand using the first letter of the base contained in the subunit—adenine (A), thymine (T), guanine (G), and cytosine (C).

Penetrance: In Mendelian disease genetics, the rate of affection in people with a disease-causing genotype.

Phenotype: The observable characteristics of an individual resulting from the interaction of its genotype with the environment. Phenotypes can be continuous (e.g., weight or height) or discrete (you have it or you don't; e.g., color blindness, autism, or a stutter) in nature.

Ploidy: The number of complete sets of chromosomes in a cell—diploid refers to a cell with two sets of chromosomes, haploid refers to a cell with one set of chromosomes.

RNA: Ribonucleic acid is an essential molecule involved in gene expression, with key roles in translation, transcription, and regulating gene expression. Like DNA, RNA comprises strings of nucleic acids.

Single nucleotide polymorphism: A type of genetic variation involving the substitution of one nucleotide for another at a specific position in the genome.

Somatic cell: Nonreproductive cell; in human somatic cells are diploid.

Telomere: A region of repetitive sequences of noncoding DNA that occurs at the ends of a chromosome and protect the chromosome from damage.

References

[1] Berry MF. A common denominator in twinning and stuttering. J Speech Disord. 1938; 3(1):51–57

[2] Kraft SJ, Yairi E. Genetic bases of stuttering: the state of the art, 2011. Folia Phoniatr Logop. 2012; 64(1):34–47

[3] Yairi E, Ambrose N, Cox N. Genetics of stuttering: a critical review. J Speech Hear Res. 1996; 39(4):771–784

[4] Ambrose NG, Yairi E, Cox N. Genetic aspects of early childhood stuttering. J Speech Hear Res. 1993; 36(4):701–706

[5] van Beijsterveldt CE, Felsenfeld S, Boomsma DI. Bivariate genetic analyses of stuttering and nonfluency in a large sample of 5-year-old twins. J Speech Lang Hear Res. 2010; 53(3):609–619

[6] Fagnani C, Fibiger S, Skytthe A, Hjelmborg JV. Heritability and environmental effects for self-reported periods with stuttering: a twin study from Denmark. Logoped Phoniatr Vocol. 2011; 36(3):114–120

[7] Ooki S. Genetic and environmental influences on stuttering and tics in Japanese twin children. Twin Res Hum Genet. 2005; 8(1):69–75

[8] Rautakoski P, Hannus T, Simberg S, Sandnabba NK, Santtila P. Genetic and environmental effects on stuttering: a twin study from Finland. J Fluency Disord. 2012; 37(3):202–210

[9] Mahajan A, Go MJ, Zhang W, et al. DIAbetes Genetics Replication And Meta-analysis (DIAGRAM) Consortium, Asian Genetic Epidemiology Network Type 2 Diabetes (AGEN-T2D) Consortium, South Asian Type 2 Diabetes (SAT2D) Consortium, Mexican American Type 2 Diabetes (MAT2D) Consortium, Type 2 Diabetes Genetic Exploration by Nex-generation sequencing in muylti-Ethnic Samples (T2D-GENES) Consortium. Genome-wide trans-ancestry meta-analysis provides insight into the genetic architecture of type 2 diabetes susceptibility. Nat Genet. 2014; 46(3):234–244

[10] Willer CJ, Schmidt EM, Sengupta S, et al. Global Lipids Genetics Consortium. Discovery and refinement of loci associated with lipid levels. Nat Genet. 2013; 45(11):1274–1283

[11] Nalls MA, Pankratz N, Lill CM, et al. International Parkinson's Disease Genomics Consortium (IPDGC), Parkinson's Study Group (PSG) Parkinson's Research: The Organized GENetics Initiative (PROGENI), 23andMe, GenePD, NeuroGenetics Research Consortium (NGRC), Hussman Institute of Human Genomics (HIHG), Ashkenazi Jewish Dataset Investigator, Cohorts for Health and Aging Research in Genetic Epidemiology (CHARGE), North American Brain Expression Consortium (NABEC), United Kingdom Brain Expression Consortium (UKBEC), Greek Parkinson's Disease Consortium, Alzheimer Genetic Analysis Group. Large-scale meta-analysis of genome-wide association data identifies six new risk loci for Parkinson's disease. Nat Genet. 2014; 46(9):989–993

[12] Gatz M, Pedersen NL, Berg S, et al. Heritability for Alzheimer's disease: the study of dementia in Swedish twins. J Gerontol A Biol Sci Med Sci. 1997; 52(2):M117–M125

[13] Van Borsel J, Tetnowski JA. Fluency disorders in genetic syndromes. J Fluency Disord. 2007; 32(4):279–296

[14] Eggers K, Van Eerdenbrugh S. Speech disfluencies in children with Down syndrome. J Commun Disord. 2018; 71:72–84

[15] Auton A, Brooks LD, Durbin RM, et al. 1000 Genomes Project Consortium. A global reference for human genetic variation. Nature. 2015; 526(7571):68–74

[16] Taliun D, Harris DN, Kessler MD, et al. NHLBI Trans-Omics for Precision Medicine (TOPMed) Consortium. Sequencing of 53,831 diverse genomes from the NHLBI TOPMed Program. Nature. 2021; 590(7845):290–299

[17] Riaz N, Steinberg S, Ahmad J, et al. Genomewide significant linkage to stuttering on chromosome 12. Am J Hum Genet. 2005; 76(4):647–651

[18] Kang C, Riazuddin S, Mundorff J, et al. Mutations in the lysosomal enzyme-targeting pathway and persistent stuttering. N Engl J Med. 2010; 362(8):677–685

[19] Kazemi N, Estiar MA, Fazilaty H, Sakhinia E. Variants in GNPTAB, GNPTG and NAGPA genes are associated with stutterers. Gene. 2018; 647:93–100

[20] Lan J, Song M, Pan C, et al. Association between dopaminergic genes (SLC6A3 and DRD2) and stuttering among Han Chinese. J Hum Genet. 2009; 54(8):457–460

[21] Raza MH, Mattera R, Morell R, et al. Association between rare variants in AP4E1, a component of intracellular trafficking, and persistent stuttering. Am J Hum Genet. 2015; 97(5):715–725

[22] Mohammadi H, Joghataei MT, Rahimi Z, et al. Sex steroid hormones and sex hormone binding globulin levels, CYP17 MSP AI (-34T:C) and CYP19 codon 39 (Trp:Arg) variants in children with developmental stuttering. Brain Lang. 2017; 175:47–56

[23] Comings DE, Wu S, Chiu C, et al. Polygenic inheritance of Tourette syndrome, stuttering, attention deficit hyperactivity, conduct, and oppositional defiant disorder: the additive and subtractive effect of the three dopaminergic genes—DRD2, D beta H, and DAT1. Am J Med Genet. 1996; 67(3):264–288

[24] Kang C, Domingues BS, Sainz E, Domingues CE, Drayna D, Moretti-Ferreira D. Evaluation of the association between polymorphisms at the DRD2 locus and stuttering. J Hum Genet. 2011; 56(6):472–473

[25] Ariza M, Garolera M, Jurado MA, et al. Dopamine genes (DRD2/ANKK1-TaqA1 and DRD4-7R) and executive function: their interaction with obesity. PLoS One. 2012; 7(7):e41482

[26] Chen D, Liu F, Shang Q, Song X, Miao X, Wang Z. Association between polymorphisms of DRD2 and DRD4 and opioid dependence: evidence from the current studies. Am J Med Genet B Neuropsychiatr Genet. 2011; 156B(6):661–670

[27] Joutsa J, Hirvonen MM, Arponen E, Hietala J, Kaasinen V. DRD2-related TaqIA genotype is associated with dopamine release during a gambling task. J Addict Med. 2014; 8(4):294–295

[28] Kranzler HR, Zhou H, Kember RL, et al. Genome-wide association study of alcohol consumption and use disorder in 274,424 individuals from multiple populations. Nat Commun. 2019; 10(1):1499

[29] Liu M, Jiang Y, Wedow R, et al. 23andMe Research Team, HUNT All-In Psychiatry. Association studies of up to 1.2 million individuals yield new insights into the genetic etiology of tobacco and alcohol use. Nat Genet. 2019; 51(2):237–244

[30] Stolf AR, Cupertino RB, Müller D, et al. Effects of DRD2 splicing-regulatory polymorphism and DRD4 48 bp VNTR on crack cocaine addiction. J Neural Transm (Vienna). 2019; 126(2):193–199

[31] Zhang K, Wang L, Cao C, et al. A DRD2/ANNK1-COMT interaction, consisting of functional variants, confers risk of post-traumatic stress disorder in traumatized Chinese. Front Psychiatry. 2018; 9:170

[32] Li Z, Chen J, Yu H, et al. Genome-wide association analysis identifies 30 new susceptibility loci for schizophrenia. Nat Genet. 2017; 49(11):1576–1583

[33] Planté-Bordeneuve V, Taussig D, Thomas F, et al. Evaluation of four candidate genes encoding proteins of the dopamine pathway in familial and sporadic Parkinson's disease: evidence for association of a DRD2 allele. Neurology. 1997; 48(6):1589–1593

[34] Raza MH, Gertz EM, Mundorff J, et al. Linkage analysis of a large African family segregating stuttering suggests polygenic inheritance. Hum Genet. 2013; 132(4):385–396

[35] Abou Jamra R, Philippe O, Raas-Rothschild A, et al. Adaptor protein complex 4 deficiency causes severe autosomal-recessive intellectual disability, progressive spastic paraplegia, shy character, and short stature. Am J Hum Genet. 2011; 88(6):788–795

[36] Xiong F, Ji Z, Liu Y, et al. Mutation in SSUH2 causes autosomal-dominant dentin dysplasia type I. Hum Mutat. 2017; 38(1):95–104

[37] Frigerio Domingues CE, Grainger K, Cheng H, Moretti-Ferreira D, Riazuddin S, Drayna D. Are variants in sex hormone metabolizing genes associated with stuttering? Brain Lang. 2019;191:28–30

[38] Shu W, Cho JY, Jiang Y, et al. Altered ultrasonic vocalization in mice with a disruption in the Foxp2 gene. Proc Natl Acad Sci U S A. 2005; 102(27):9643–9648

[39] Barnes TD, Wozniak DF, Gutierrez J, Han TU, Drayna D, Holy TE. A mutation associated with stuttering alters mouse pup ultrasonic vocalizations. Curr Biol. 2016:S0960–9822(16)30179–8

[40] Han TU, Root J, Reyes LD, et al. Human GNPTAB stuttering mutations engineered into mice cause vocalization deficits and astrocyte pathology in the corpus callosum. Proc Natl Acad Sci U S A. 2019; 116(35):17515–17524

[41] Polikowsky HG, Shaw DM, Petty LE, et al. Population-based genetic risk of developmental stuttering. HGG Advances. 2022; 3(1):100073

[42] Arndt J, Healey EC. Concomitant disorders in school-age children who stutter. Lang Speech Hear Serv Sch. 2001; 32(2):68–78

[43] Donaher J, Richels C. Traits of attention deficit/hyperactivity disorder in school-age children who stutter. J Fluency Disord. 2012; 37(4):242–252

[44] Pruett DG, Shaw DM, Chen HH, et al. Identifying developmental stuttering and associated comorbidities in electronic health records and creating a phenome risk classifier. J Fluency Disord. 2021; 68:105847

[45] Blood GW, Ridenour VJ, Qualls CD, Hammer CS. Co-occurring disorders in children who stutter. J Commun Disord. 2003; 36(6):427–448

[46] Scott KS. Dysfluency in autism spectrum disorders. Procedia Soc Behav Sci. 2015; 193:239–245

[47] Arenas RM, Walker EA, Oleson JJ. Developmental stuttering in children who are hard of hearing. Lang Speech Hear Serv Sch. 2017; 48(4):234–248

[48] Macey PM, Henderson LA, Macey KE, et al. Brain morphology associated with obstructive sleep apnea. Am J Respir Crit Care Med. 2002; 166(10):1382–1387

[49] Strom MA, Silverberg JI. Asthma, hay fever, and food allergy are associated with caregiver-reported speech disorders in US children. Pediatr Allergy Immunol. 2016; 27(6):604–611

[50] Strom MA, Silverberg JI. Eczema is associated with childhood speech disorder: a retrospective analysis from the National Survey of Children's Health and the National Health Interview Survey. J Pediatr. 2016; 168:185–192.e4

[51] Shaw DM, Polikowsky HP, Pruett DG, et al. Phenome risk classification enables phenotypic imputation and gene discovery in developmental stuttering. Am J Hum Genet. 2021; 108(12):2271–2283

[52] Niarchou M, Gustavson DE, Sathirapongsasuti F, et al. Genome-wide association study of musical beat synchronization demonstrates high polygenicity. bioRxiv 836197

[53] Wieland EA, McAuley JD, Dilley LC, Chang SE. Evidence for a rhythm perception deficit in children who stutter. Brain Lang. 2015; 144:26–34

4 Speech, Language, and Cognitive Processes

Julie D. Anderson, Katerina Ntourou, and Stacy Wagovich

Abstract

The objective of this chapter is to provide a concise overview of speech, language, and cognitive processes in developmental stuttering. We will begin with an introduction to the topic, followed by a discussion of linguistic constraints on stuttering—that is, linguistic factors that influence which words and/or utterances are likely to be stuttered. The speech and language abilities of individuals who stutter will then be considered, along with the potential impact of executive function and attention. By the end of this chapter, the reader will have a basic understanding of these tripartite processes as they relate to the onset and development of stuttering, as well as some of the theory that undergirds our knowledge of the interrelationships among stuttering, speech, language, and cognition. We will also consider the extent to which our knowledge of these processes assists with clinical decision-making, setting the stage for ▶ Chapter 13 Language and Phonological Considerations.

Keywords: stuttering, fluency disorder, language, phonology, articulation, cognition, executive function, attention

4.1 Introduction

Humans speak to communicate, a process that occurs quite rapidly. In fact, speakers produce, on average, about two to four words per second. Since the average word has more than two phonemes, this translates to about 10 to 15 phonemes per second or upward of 1,000 phonemes per minute![1] The rate at which humans can produce speech is quite remarkable considering the complexity of the speech and language production process that must take place to produce a single word.

Most psycholinguists agree that word production involves at least four stages: semantic processing, lexical processing, phonological processing, and speech-motor programming and execution[2] (▶ Fig. 4.1). Word production begins with the initial intent to communicate. For example, let us say that a speaker is thinking about a cat and wants to say something about it. This thought triggers the retrieval of the conceptual features associated with a cat, such as furry, whiskers, tail, four legs, meows, etc. (this is what is called *semantic processing*). These features collectively distinguish it from other similar concepts (e.g., dog), leading to the selection of the word that best matches the description: cat (*lexical processing*). Once the word has been selected, the individual sounds (i.e., phonemes) associated with it—[k æ t]—must be retrieved and linked together (*phonological processing*). These phonemes serve as input to the motor system, which produces the programs that eventually enable us to articulate the intended word (*speech-motor programming and execution*; see ▶ Chapter 5 for more information about speech-motor programming and execution). Throughout this process, speakers can *monitor* the accuracy and appropriateness of their speech both before and after they produce it. If a speaker detects an error, then they can repair it by interrupting ongoing speech.[1]

This model is simplistic in that it only illustrates how single words are spoken; the process is considerably more complex when multiple words must be retrieved and strung together to

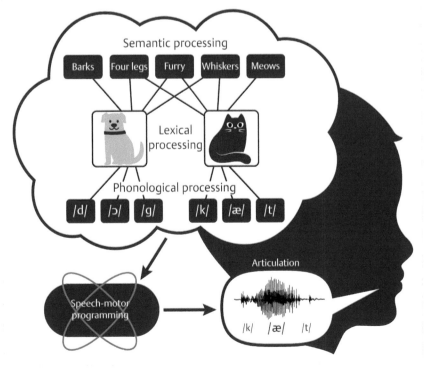

Fig. 4.1 A simplified model of word production. Source: Image created by Jared Sinclair.

form sentences that conform to the rules of language (**syntactic processing**). When preparing multiword utterances, speakers can vary the amount of time between the phonological processing of a word (i.e., when the sounds are chosen and joined) and its articulation, such that sometimes they may produce the word immediately and at other times, they may hold it in storage (also known as buffering) until it is time to produce the word.[3] The more speech that is planned in advance, the more likely it is that the utterance will be fluent,[4] but this also increases demands on working memory (the ability to temporarily store and manage information in mind).[5] Thus, planning an utterance in advance safeguards fluency. This implies that when a speaker does not plan ahead, disfluencies are more likely to result.

Most of the time, we use our speech system seamlessly to produce fluent speech. This is true not only for individuals who do not stutter but also for those who do. Occasionally, however, glitches occur somewhere in the system, resulting in a disfluency. Although disfluencies can have causes that are unrelated to the speech production system (e.g., lapses in attention, holding the floor during a conversational exchange, etc.[6]), many disfluencies—namely, interjections or filled pauses, unfilled (silent) pauses, revisions, and repetitions—have long been associated with difficulties in semantic, lexical, or phonological processing and cognitive control (i.e., executive function;[7] see ▶ Chapter 1 for a description of different types of disfluencies).

Whether or not these struggles could also be responsible for the disfluencies associated specifically with stuttering—that is, part-word repetitions, sound prolongations, and blocks—is not clear. Nevertheless, given how quickly we can speak, it seems reasonable that even a slight delay or disruption in semantic, lexical, and/or phonological processing could disrupt the forward flow of speech. For example, it has been estimated to take 75 milliseconds to select a single word during lexical processing.[8] Thus, if a speaker experienced a 200-millisecond delay in this process due to, for example, difficulty suppressing competing semantically related lexical items (e.g., if the target word is cat, other semantically related words, such as dog, would need to be inhibited), then this might disrupt ongoing speech, resulting in a disfluency.

Linguistic demands can influence a person's ability to be fluent, as we discuss later. However, whether speech and/or language difficulties are *directly* implicated in the onset and development of stuttering is less clear. Cognitive processes—namely, executive function and attention—may also play a role in some yet unknown way. It is important to note that when we refer to cognitive processes, we do not mean intelligence. That is, there is no evidence to suggest that children who stutter (CWS) or adults who stutter (AWS) are less intelligent than those who do not stutter; studies have been consistent in showing that the intelligence quotients of people who stutter fall well within the average range for the population.[9]

In the following sections, we will explore linguistic constraints on stuttering, the speech and language abilities of individuals who stutter, and cognitive factors associated with stuttering. We will also consider the theoretical, diagnostic, and treatment implications of these findings. We will focus mainly on CWS, as the onset of stuttering generally occurs in childhood, but, where relevant, we will also consider research findings for adults.

4.2 Linguistic Constraints on Stuttering

As indicated in ▶ Chapter 1, stuttering is not a randomly occurring event. Rather, there is marked consistency both in *where* stuttering is likely to occur within an utterance and in the *types of words* that are more likely to be stuttered. Among the earliest observations were that adults are more likely to stutter on (1) content words (nouns, verbs, adjectives, or adverbs); (2) longer words (five or more letters); (3) sentence-initial words (the first three words); and (4) words beginning with a consonant.[10] Subsequent research revealed that these characteristics also hold true for children, with one possible exception. Although older children, adolescents, and adults are more likely to stutter on content words, some have noted that young children tend to stutter disproportionally on function words (e.g., determiners, conjunctions, prepositions, pronouns).[11] This tendency on the part of young English-speaking children, however, may be more related to sentence position than grammatical class, since function words are also more likely to occur at the beginning of a sentence.[12]

Since the early work of Brown[10] with AWS, researchers have identified many other phonological, lexical, and syntactic constraints on instances of stuttering. ▶ Table 4.1 summarizes findings in this area. As noted in the table, some language factors have been observed only in children or only in adults. For example, syntactic complexity appears to have less of an effect on stuttering over time, as some studies have failed to find any relationship between syntactic complexity and stuttering in adolescents and AWS.[13] It should be noted that ▶ Table 4.1 features the constraints observed across the literature, capturing results of *most* studies; we do not imply that findings of *every* study reveal these overall patterns. For that matter, many of these constraints also apply to individuals who do not stutter. For example, like CWS, children who do not stutter (CWNS) are more likely to be disfluent on newly emerging and/or more complex sentence structures.[14]

Why is stuttering more likely to occur on certain word types and places within utterances? The first possibility is that linguistic constraints simply make some words and sentences more challenging to produce and therefore more vulnerable to disruption. That is, they place more cognitive and linguistic demands on the speaker. For example, take the following sentences: "Donkeys are good" and "Dogs are good." A speaker would be much more likely to stutter on the word *donkeys* than *dogs* because the former does not occur frequently in language, making it harder to retrieve, and it has more phonemes, requiring additional phonological processing and speech-motor programming. For a young child in the midst of early language development, the increase in demand associated with using more complex language may result in disfluency as more resources are diverted away from fluency and directed toward language processing.[16]

Another possibility is that individuals who stutter have difficulty with speech-language processing (i.e., semantic, lexical, phonological, and/or syntactic processing), so when they experience challenges to this already vulnerable system, the result is stuttering rather than a typical, nonstuttered disfluency. If CWS have difficulties with speech-language processing (discussed in

Table 4.1 Linguistic characteristics of words/utterances and their likelihood of eliciting stuttering (more likely to elicit stuttering > less likely to elicit stuttering)

Lexical factors	
Familiarity	Less familiar words > more familiar words
Grammatical class	Content words > function words (older) Function words > content words (younger)
Word length	Longer words (5 or more letters) > shorter words
Phonological factors	
Phoneme position	Initial position > middle or final position
Frequency	Low-frequency words > high-frequency words
Neighborhood density[a]	Sparse neighborhoods > dense neighborhoods (adults)
Neighborhood frequency[b]	Low-frequency neighbors > high-frequency neighbors
Stress	Stressed syllables > unstressed syllables
Syntactic factors	
Acquisition	Newly acquired sentences > established sentences (children)
Complexity	More complex sentences > less complex sentences (children)
Sentence length	Longer utterances > shorter utterances
Grammatical errors	Utterances with more grammatical errors > utterances with fewer grammatical errors
Utterance- or clause-initial	Beginning of an utterance/clause > middle or end of an utterance/clause
Syntactic boundaries (e.g., noun or verb phrase)	Before a major syntactic boundary > during or after a major syntactic boundary

[a] Words are thought to be organized into phonologically similar "neighborhoods."[15] For example, the neighbors of the target word cat would include rat, mat, cattle, gnat, bat, etc. Some words have many (dense) neighbors, whereas others have few (sparse) neighbors.
[b] Neighborhood frequency refers to the average frequency of a word's neighbors.

the following sections), the places in which stuttering occurs could point to specific areas of greater processing difficulty for the child. For example, stuttering at the beginning of a long, complex dependent clause could reflect difficulty with syntactic processing. In fact, there is some evidence that specific processing limitations may result in distinct types of disfluency. In several studies, researchers found evidence to suggest that part-word repetitions and sound prolongations may be related to difficulty with phonological processing, whereas single-syllable word repetitions may result from disruptions in other nonphonological processing operations, such as lexical processing.[17]

Although one or both possibilities could explain why certain words and sentences tend to be more susceptible to stuttering, we currently do not have a definitive answer to this question. Nevertheless, the fact that there are linguistic constraints on stuttering does suggest, more generally, that developmental stuttering is related—indirectly or directly—to the process of language planning.

4.3 Speech and Language Abilities and Stuttering

As noted in ▶ Chapter 1, the average age of stuttering onset is 33 months, and can range widely between 30 and 60 months. Thus, children typically do not begin to stutter until they are able to string words together to form phrases or sentences. During this period, children are also rapidly developing their speech and language skills, prompting some to consider whether stuttering could be a consequence of difficulties with speech and language development.

Speech and language skills in CWS can be examined in several ways. First, we can consider how CWS perform on formal standardized, norm-referenced tests of speech and language and/or in informal spontaneous language samples. Second, we can examine children's linguistic processing abilities using experimental tasks that are designed to "tap into" different semantic, lexical, phonological, and syntactic processes. For example, children might complete a picture–word interference task in which they name a target picture in the presence or absence of a semantic or phonological prime (e.g., seeing the target picture *dog* while hearing the word *cat*), to examine the extent to which the prime impacts processing. Observable measures from tasks like this include accuracy (e.g., correctly saying *dog* vs. incorrectly saying *cat*), reaction time (e.g., how long it took to name the picture), or neural activity (e.g., event-related potentials). Experimental tasks like this allow us to look beyond static measures of performance, such as language tests, to explore underlying processes. We might learn, for example, that CWS perform similarly to CWNS on a particular language test and perhaps even on an experimental task of language processing, but it takes them much longer to do so or they arrive at answers in a different way. In this way, experimental tasks are better at identifying subtle differences in language abilities than standardized tests.

Although findings from some studies have suggested that CWS may be more likely to exhibit concomitant speech and language disorders (e.g., having both stuttering and a phonological disorder) than their typically fluent peers,[18,19] a recent study showed that this was not the case.[20] (For further discussion of the topic of concomitant speech and language disorders in CWS, see ▶ Chapter 13). For the remainder of this chapter, we will be focusing on CWS who do *not* have concomitant speech and language disorders. That is, we will be considering the speech and language abilities of CWS who are otherwise within normal limit. We will first turn our attention to examining the articulation/phonological abilities of young CWS and then consider their vocabulary/morphosyntactic abilities.

4.3.1 Articulation and Phonology
Formal and Informal Measures

The relationship between articulation/phonology and childhood stuttering has been a topic of interest among investigators and clinicians alike for well over 30 years. In this discussion, we will use the terms articulation and phonology interchangeably, even though they are not synonymous, with the former referring to the motoric processes of speech production (i.e., phonetic) and the latter to linguistic processes (i.e., phonemic). We use these terms interchangeably because they have not always been differentiated in the stuttering literature.

Most of the investigations that have used standardized, norm-referenced tests of articulation (e.g., the *Goldman–Fristoe Test of Articulation-2*)[21] to compare the speech sound production of young CWS and CWNS have failed to detect differences,[22,23,24,25,26] although this is not true of all studies.[27] Most of this research, however, was not explicitly designed to examine speech sound production; rather, these studies had different goals and were simply ruling out the possibility of phonological difficulties prior to exploring the goals of interest. Therefore, measures were designed to screen performance rather than fully explore children's phonological skills.

CWS who otherwise do not have clinically significant coexisting speech sound disorders appear to perform similarly to CWNS on tests of articulation/phonology. There does appear to be a relationship between articulation/phonological development and whether children recover naturally from stuttering, however. That is, young CWS who have weaker articulation/phonological skills have a greater risk for stuttering persistence than CWS who have stronger abilities (see ▶ Chapter 7).[28]

Only a handful of studies have examined phonological awareness, or the ability to analyze the speech sound structure of oral language, in CWS and CWNS using standardized tests such as the *Phonological Awareness Test–Second Edition*.[29] Common tasks that assess children's phonological awareness require them to segment words (e.g., cupcake) into their constituent syllables (e.g., cup-cake) or sounds/phonemes (e.g., c-u-p-c-a-k), contrast words that sound similar (e.g., seat–sheet), or blend syllables (e.g., snow-man = snowman) or sounds/phonemes (e.g., a-p-l = apple) to make words. These tasks are important because they provide a window into children's phonological representations (i.e., how phonological information about words is stored and accessed in long-term memory). Findings from studies that have investigated these skills in CWS have been mixed. Some studies have reported significantly lower phonemic awareness skills in younger (5- to 6-year-old)[30] and older (10- to 14-year-old)[31] CWS compared to their typically fluent peers, but other studies have not observed differences.[32,33]

Experimental Measures

To date, research that has focused on the phonological processing abilities of CWS is relatively limited and results have been mixed. These studies use a range of experimental procedures, including phoneme elision (i.e., repetition of a nonword or a real word with the omission of a phoneme), auditory rhyming judgment (i.e., deciding whether auditorily presented words rhyme or not), and phonological priming (i.e., hearing the first phoneme /b/ of a picture [bed] just before naming it), to name a few. This is a burgeoning area of study, and conclusions should be reached with caution. Nonetheless, two observations based on this work are the following:

- Young (5-year-old) CWS may rely on a developmentally less mature phonological processing system than their typically fluent peers.[23,34]
- There may be subgroups of school-age CWS who have difficulty with phonological processing.[35,36]

There is some suggestion that AWS may have difficulty with phonological processing as well, especially when cognitive processing demands are high.[37,38,39] However, findings are inconsistent, as some studies have not found differences between AWS and adults who do not stutter.[40]

4.3.2 Vocabulary and Morphosyntax
Formal and Informal Measures

Language weakness can impact speech fluency. In fact, as a group, children with developmental language disorders have been shown to produce substantially more disfluencies—both stuttered and nonstuttered—in their spontaneous speech than children who do not exhibit developmental language disorder.[41,42] These disfluencies, however, are often quantitatively and qualitatively different from those associated with developmental stuttering in that they may be produced without tension or struggle, secondary behaviors, or avoidances. Further, not all children with language disorders show a pattern of greater disfluencies relative to their peers. Thus, while language weaknesses can impact speech fluency, this relationship is not observed in all children.

Since language weakness can impact speech fluency, a relevant question is whether CWS are more likely to exhibit weaknesses in language. Some studies have explicitly examined whether CWS differ from CWNS on standardized, norm-referenced measures of expressive or receptive language, and, for the most part, have revealed that CWS perform more poorly on these measures than their typically fluent peers.[26,27,43,44,45] These results are also consistent with a meta-analysis (including some of these studies) in which CWS were found to score lower than CWNS in receptive and expressive language, as well as vocabulary.[46]

Not only have CWS shown weaker language skills on average, but also their performance reveals dissociations (i.e., imbalances or mismatches) across speech and language areas. For example, a child with a dissociation might have above-average overall expressive language skills coinciding with average to below-average expressive vocabulary skills. CWS are at least three times more likely to exhibit these dissociations in their speech and language skills than their normally disfluent peers.[43,47] Observations of dissociations among CWS reveal that language weaknesses are more complex than a single language score indicates. Rather, the language weaknesses observed in CWS reflect the interrelationships among different components of the speech and language system.

It is much less clear whether CWS differ from peers in spontaneous language. Using measures such as lexical diversity and mean length of utterance, some studies have revealed differences, with CWS scoring lower than CWNS.[46] Further, some investigations have reported that CWS score near or above age-level expectations compared to CWNS.[48,49] Taken together, research findings using informal measures of spontaneous speech and language are somewhat conflicting, making it difficult to draw conclusions. Although this is the case, the findings related to formal testing suggest that, on average, CWS perform less well compared to their nonstuttering peers. What might account for between-group differences in performance observed in formal versus informal language testing? It may be that formal testing is a more robust evaluation of children's language skills. Although language samples are more functional measures of language ability, in some cases they may not be sensitive enough to detect more subtle weaknesses relative to peers. For example, a child's lexical diversity in a conversation with a parent might not fully tap the extent of the child's expressive vocabulary, as the context may be limiting in detecting this knowledge.

When considering these findings, there are several points to keep in mind. First, even when research findings reveal that CWS perform more poorly than CWNS, results still show that, in general, the performance of both groups is within normal limits. That is, CWS do not have clinically significant language delays or disorders.*

Rather, observed language difficulties are more subtle in nature. Second, not all CWS have weaknesses in their language skills or present with dissociations across language areas. Indeed, some CWS have stronger language skills than their typically fluent peers! Therefore, in sum, CWS, as a group, are more prone to such weaknesses and dissociations, although subgroups displaying different patterns may be evident, as well.

Experimental Measures

Far fewer studies have examined the language processing abilities of CWS using experimental and/or electrophysiological measures. Although findings from these studies have been inconsistent, two broad conclusions are warranted:

- CWS may be delayed in their ability to develop more complex or adultlike approaches to language processing.[50,51]
- CWS appear to be slower than CWNS in processes associated with lexical and/or syntactic processing.[22,25,51]

Like studies with children, studies of AWS have yielded inconsistent results. However, it would seem that whatever difficulties CWS have in their language processing skills may persist in some form into adulthood.[39,52] Some studies have found that the language processing systems of AWS may be more vulnerable to increases in timing and/or cognitive demands (e.g., they may have more difficulty formulating utterances when being rushed to speak or when trying to avoid, by way of circumlocution, saying a feared word).[37] Thus, it may be that any difficul-

ties AWS have with language processing may not be evident until they are under conditions of high cognitive demand.

4.3.3 Summary

All aspects of speech and language processing (phonological, lexical, and syntactic) have been implicated as a potential source of difficulty for both CWS and AWS. However, when one considers that stuttering typically does not develop until children begin to string words together to form phrases or sentences, it is likely that syntactic processes are involved to at least some extent—either in the way they interact with phonological and lexical processes (e.g., difficulty accessing or organizing words in sentences) or as a source of linguistic demand (i.e., processing linguistic stimuli concurrently).

It is also clear that studies conducted by different research groups have yielded inconsistent results, with some finding differences between CWS and AWS and their peers in speech and language and others not. Some of these disparities may simply be due to differences in the way the studies were conducted. For example, some studies may have relied on small sample sizes or used tasks that were not sensitive enough to detect differences. It is important to note that the assumption that underlies all of these studies is this: If children or adults have problems with speech or language processes, such difficulties should be apparent at all times in all tasks. One might ask whether such an assumption is reasonable given differences in the communicative demands across a range of contexts.

Consider that we all produce disfluencies in our speech—both nonstuttered and stuttered—and most of us do not have a diagnosis of stuttering. As indicated in the introduction to this chapter, nonstuttered disfluencies can have many different causes. They may allow us to maintain the floor during a conversational exchange, or they may signal to the listener that we are having language processing difficulties (e.g., having trouble finding a specific word). In addition to these typical disfluencies, individuals who do not stutter also occasionally produce stuttered disfluencies.

Why are disfluencies produced? Many years of research have shown that this is a complex question to answer. There are explanations that focus on the linguistic processing limitations we all experience to a greater or lesser extent. For example, an individual may have difficulty with word retrieval (i.e., lexical processing) or planning the grammar of a sentence (i.e., syntactic processing). Although those who stutter may experience these difficulties more often, all of us share them to a degree. Challenges in different aspects of language processing may lead to a disruption that "freezes" the forward flow of speech, resulting in disfluent speech. The nature of the difficulty (i.e., whether the disruption occurs during semantic, lexical, phonological, or syntactic processing) could also result in different types of stuttered disfluencies.[17] This linguistic explanation could be used to explain the disfluencies experienced by all of us but especially by those with a fluency disorder.

Both stuttering and typical disfluency are complex phenomena, and it is unlikely that strictly linguistic models are adequate to explain the full range of speech disruptions observed in individuals who stutter and those who are typically fluent. In the next section, we examine the role of cognitive

---

* Note that in these studies, children who do not perform within normal limits are excluded from participation

processes, foundational for speech and language, as a way to provide a more robust explanation of the development and occurrence of stuttering.

4.4 Cognitive Processes and Stuttering

4.4.1 Executive Function

Executive function refers to a set of cognitive skills that are critical for learning and performing goal-directed tasks in everyday life (e.g., searching for information about a product on the computer).[53] Although the nature of executive function continues to be debated, there is some consensus that at least three components are involved: inhibition, working memory, and cognitive flexibility.[54] ▶ Table 4.2 provides definitions and examples of these three executive function components.

Executive function emerges during infancy and continues to develop throughout adolescence; however, exponential growth in these skills occurs during the preschool years.[58] Executive function helps children control their thoughts, emotions, and behaviors so they can plan, solve problems, and complete tasks.[59] For example, let us say that a little girl is playing with a kitchen set, while her brother and sister are playing patty-cake in the background. The child must focus on what she is doing while also ignoring her siblings; she must remember the steps involved in "cooking" play food and use objects in a different way when needed (e.g., using a paper towel roll as a rolling pin). If a parent tells the child that it is time for dinner, the child must also resist the desire to keep on playing and shift her attention to the new activity. See ▶ Fig. 4.2 for another example of executive function processes at work in a child's everyday life.

The importance of executive function during early development cannot be overstated; it is a factor in virtually all aspects

Table 4.2 Definitions and examples of the three major components of executive function[55,56,57]

Inhibition	
The ability to ignore irrelevant information or suppress a response	• Ignoring a distraction in the environment • Not blurting out an answer in class before raising a hand • Waiting until someone gets done speaking before talking • Asking for permission before taking something
Working memory	
The ability to temporarily store (short-term memory) and manipulate information	• Remembering and integrating information from more than one conversational partner and formulating a response • Listening to a story while trying to understand what it means • Listening to, remembering, and following multistep directions • Adding two numbers spoken to you by another person in your head
Cognitive flexibility	
The ability to switch from one perspective, representation, or rule to another	• Switching from one topic to another in conversation • Adjusting to a change in plans or routines • Lining up inside a building when it is cold and rainy but outside when it is warm and dry • Using a stick or coat hanger to reach something that is under a bed • Taking off shoes when entering the house but leaving them on when entering the classroom • Encountering a roadblock when walking to school and devising an alternate route • Following different rules about talking when at the library versus the park

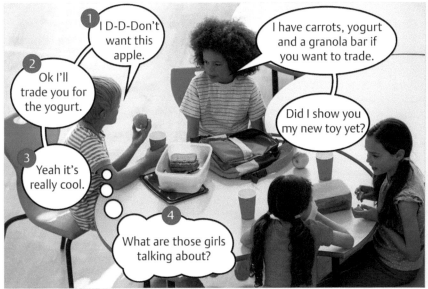

Fig. 4.2 Depiction of executive function and attention demands for Sam, a boy who stutters, during a typical conversational interaction. Sam talks with his friend (1, 2, 3; selective attention) while ignoring environmental distractions (e.g., girls chatting in proximity) and inhibiting any action related to his thought "what are those girls talking about?" (4; inhibition). Furthermore, Sam held in memory the list of foods that his friend said he could have as a trade while considering his choices and picking his favorite item (2; working memory). Finally, Sam was able to readily switch from the topic "food" to "toy" when his friend asked him whether he had shown him his new toy (3; cognitive flexibility). Source: Image created by Jared Sinclair.

of development from learning language to acquiring motor skills.[59] Furthermore, a wide variety of childhood disorders have been associated with difficulties in executive function, such as anxiety disorder, attention deficit hyperactivity disorder, autism spectrum disorder, deafness, developmental language disorder, and speech sound disorder.[60,61,62,63,64] This suggests that weaknesses in executive function may be a common characteristic of many neurodevelopmental disorders.[65]

Although at first glance it may seem odd to consider executive function as a factor in stuttering, it is a foundational skill that supports all of the processes that have been implicated in the development of stuttering—namely, language, motor, sensory, and emotional processes. Therefore, understanding executive function in CWS should lead to a richer understanding of the disorder itself. Findings from studies that compared CWS to their peers in executive function have been conflicting. To some extent, contradictory findings are to be expected. This is especially true because of the variability in sample size across studies, as well as the measures used, the modality in which the stimuli are presented (auditory vs. visual), the domain being assessed (verbal vs. nonverbal), the outcome measure (accuracy vs. speed), the context in which the child is being examined (naturalistic vs. laboratory experiment), the level of task difficulty, and the response modality (manual vs. verbal). However, when we consider the studies collectively, most evidence points toward CWS having lower levels of inhibition, short-term memory (a component of working memory), and cognitive flexibility compared to CWNS (see ▸ Table 4.2 for examples).[66,67] Some studies have also shown that CWS are up to seven times more likely than their peers to have clinically significant deficits in executive function.[68]

Although more research is clearly needed, it is interesting to consider how executive function (and attention) might theoretically play a role in developmental stuttering. We will expand on this idea later, but for now, it is important to emphasize that the relationship between executive function and the processes associated with language, motor, sensation, and emotion is thought to be bidirectional.[69] This means that weaknesses in language and/or motor function, for example, could lead to weaknesses in executive function and vice versa. Furthermore, since executive function is shared across the different domains (i.e., language, motor, etc.), it is also possible for a weakness in one process (e.g., language) to affect other processes (e.g., motor) by way of these shared cognitive resources.

4.4.2 Attention

In 1890, the psychologist William James declared that "everyone knows what attention is."[70] Indeed, we all have an intuitive understanding as to what attention is; however, researchers who study it for a living cannot always agree on a working definition for the purpose of careful study of the construct. Nevertheless, investigators have made progress in identifying different types of attention, of which there are many.[71] Some have suggested that attention may be best described as "attentions," meaning that there is likely more than one type of attention and, consequently, any attempt to arrive at a single definition will be fruitless.

It is beyond the scope of this chapter to discuss all the variants of attention; rather, we will focus on those that have been examined within the developmental stuttering literature. There are three types of attention that undergo substantial growth during the period in which stuttering typically develops: sustained attention, selective attention, and alternating/shifting attention. Attention is crucial to the development of executive function, as it allows children to exercise more control over what they pay attention to and how much attention they devote to it.[55] The different aspects of attention also become more integrated throughout the preschool years. ▸ Table 4.3 provides definitions and examples of the three types of attention.

Attention has been shown to predict a variety of cognitive, language, academic, and social skills in typically developing children, such as executive functioning, narrative production, academic achievement, mathematical abilities, literacy, verbal ability, knowledge attainment, social competence, and emotion regulation.[82,83,84] Likewise, deficits in attention have been reported in children with developmental language disorder, speech sound disorder, and autism spectrum disorder.[85,86,87]

Table 4.3 Definitions and examples of sustained, selective, and alternating attention

Sustained attention	
The ability to maintain alertness for prolonged periods of time	• Working on a puzzle • Listening to a story • Watching a movie • Coloring a picture of a cat • Building a Lego house • Looking at a picture of a barnyard and pointing to and naming the cow, horse, sheep, duck, etc. • Riding a tricycle down a street without bumping into a mailbox
Selective attention	
The ability to focus on select information while ignoring irrelevant information	• Listening to a parent talk while ignoring other conversations in the room • Working on a puzzle while other children are playing in the background • Counting all the cats in a picture containing images of cats and dogs • Reading in a loud classroom while filtering out the noise from a plane that is flying overhead • Playing a game while ignoring the dog barking outside
Alternating attention	
The ability to disengage attention from one activity or task to another	• Playing musical chairs • Alternating reading directions and following them, step by step • Making a caterpillar out of play dough, taking a break to talk to grandma on the phone, finishing the conversation, and then returning to making the caterpillar

Of course, clinically significant attention difficulties are observed in children diagnosed with attention deficit hyperactivity disorder.

Given the importance of attention for a variety of outcomes and behaviors, it is perhaps not surprising that investigators have examined the attention skills of CWS. There is some suggestion that CWS may be more prone to clinical or subclinical attention deficit hyperactivity disorder, which is characterized by symptoms of inattention and hyperactivity/impulsivity.[88] Direct observation and parental report have also found that CWS tend to perform more poorly than their peers on behavioral tasks of sustained and/or selective attention, and alternating attention.[67,89,90]

Not all CWS have problems with attention. Indeed, many do not. But for those who do, the question is, what does attention have to do with stuttering? At this point, there is no clear answer to this question. However, we do know that, like executive function, attention is crucial to the development of a wide range of skills in early childhood, including speech and language. Children learn the sounds and words of their native language and how to create sentences by listening and attending to those around them. If speech production involves planning an utterance and monitoring it for errors prior to production, attention skills may impact these processes, resulting in the production of speech that is not fully "ready" for execution and is therefore produced disfluently. Of course, this suggestion is speculative but may explain, in part, the link between attention and stuttering. Alternatively, symptoms of inattention and hyperactivity/impulsivity could lead to behavioral difficulties that are known to exacerbate fluency, such as difficulty with turn-taking and topic maintenance.

4.4.3 Summary

Although the findings of studies are sometimes contradictory, much of the evidence suggests that, like children with other neurodevelopmental disorders, CWS have subtle to not so subtle difficulties with executive function and attention. The mechanism by which these cognitive processes contribute to developmental stuttering, however, is less than clear. Nevertheless, it has been suggested that differences in executive function and attention could help explain the multifactorial nature and heterogeneity of stuttering.[66]

Multifactorial models of stuttering posit no single cause of stuttering (see ▶ Chapter 2 for more in-depth discussion). Rather, multiple factors (e.g., linguistic, motor, sensory, cognitive, and emotion) are thought to come together in divergent ways to contribute to the onset and/or development of stuttering. These models embrace individual differences, recognizing that the factors that contribute to stuttering in one individual may not be the same as those that contribute to another individual's stuttering. Multifactorial models have emerged because individuals who stutter have been shown to display differences, usually subtle ones, in a wide range of skills, yet the etiology of stuttering has remained elusive. Indeed, if there were gross disturbances in the speech, language, motor, and other processes of individuals who stutter, the cause of stuttering would, no doubt, have been revealed long ago, as researchers have intensely scrutinized and compared them to those of typically fluent speakers for many years. Regardless, one important

question remains: how could individuals who stutter have weaknesses in so many different processes?

The answer to this question is complex. Recall that emerging research has revealed that, like CWS, children who have primary deficits in specific domains (e.g., a sensory deficit in deafness, a language deficit in developmental language disorder, etc.) also have weaknesses in other domains (e.g., motor skills), including executive function and attention. We see deficits in other domains, both in CWS and those with other speech-language disorders, likely because processes that are domain specific (i.e., those having to do with a single process, such as language, motor, sensation, or emotions) are interconnected with the domain-general cognitive processes of executive function and attention (see ▶ Fig. 4.3 for a visual depiction of the relationship).[69] For example, it is possible for weaknesses in executive function to impact motor performance and conversely for weaknesses in language to impact executive function. Moreover, limitations in language processing could affect motor processing and vice versa by way of their shared cognitive processes. To put it another way, these processes do not exist in isolation; what influences one process can influence another.

In short, then, weaknesses in executive function and/or attention are good candidates for explaining the multifactorial nature of stuttering, that is, limitations in cognitive processes could result in modest deficiencies in a wide range of skills (e.g., semantics, auditory processing, etc.), given that these cognitive processes are shared across multiple domains. Of course, as noted earlier, whatever "weaknesses" CWS have in executive function and/or attention need not be clinically significant or even substantially different from that of CWNS. Rather, a CWS could have strong executive function and/or attention skills relative to other children his or her age, but weaker skills relative to the child's other domain-specific strengths. This disconnect across domains could, theoretically, contribute to difficulty maintaining fluent speech production.

4.5 Implications for Theory and Clinical Practice

4.5.1 Theoretical

As a result of evidence suggesting that CWS and AWS may have atypical or depressed linguistic abilities, as well as findings that the linguistic characteristics of stuttering events in children and adults are highly predictable, theorists have speculated that stuttering may result from difficulties with language processing. Some psycholinguistic theories, such as the covert repair hypothesis[91] and the vicious circle hypothesis,[92] associate fluency breakdowns with difficulties in language processes (e.g., phonological processing) or the speech monitoring system. Other theories, such as the EXPLAN theory,[93] neuropsycholinguistic theory,[94] suprasegmental sentence plan alignment Model,[95] and fault-line hypothesis,[96] attribute stuttering to dyssynchronies in timing within or between speech-language production processes.

Of the theories that have been proposed, the covert repair hypothesis[91] has garnered the most attention. This theory acknowledges that all speakers, regardless of whether they stutter or not, occasionally produce errors during language processing. If speakers detect an error before speech is

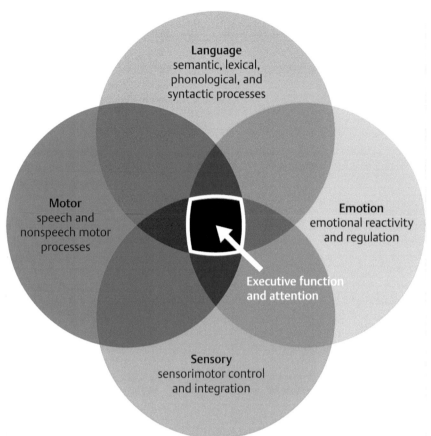

Fig. 4.3 A schematic representation of the relationships among the domain-specific (language, motor, sensory, emotion) and domain-general (executive function, attention) processes that are implicated in developmental stuttering. Executive function and attention are shared resources (thus centered in the diagram) that are essential for the development and proper functioning of domain-specific processes, which are likewise interconnected. Weaknesses in one or more of these domain-specific processes could contribute to stuttering by way of their interconnection with domain-general processes. Source: Image created by Jared Sinclair.

produced, they can correct it by interrupting speech. It is this process of correcting the error prior to speaking that results in both normal and stuttered disfluencies. Individuals who stutter, however, differ from individuals who do not stutter in that their phonological processing systems are thought to be impaired. As a result, they will produce more errors during language processing. The resulting increase in errors will, in turn, create more error correction opportunities, resulting in even more disfluencies.

The vicious circle hypothesis[92] also proposes that stuttering occurs when internal errors in language processing are repaired. However, instead of asserting that individuals who stutter produce more errors, this theory suggests that they are hyper vigilant in their attempt to identify errors; consequently, even slight errors, which would otherwise go unnoticed by typically fluent individuals, are repaired. In fact, even the disfluencies themselves may be identified as errors, serving to further aggravate the situation (hence the "vicious circle"). Thus, it is the internal speech monitoring system that is presumed to be impaired, not the phonological processing system.

Some theorists have suggested that disfluencies may result from a dyssynchrony between utterance planning and assembly,[96] whereas others have alluded to the possibility of dyssynchrony in the alignment of a revised utterance with its original suprasegmental (i.e., rhythm, melody, and stress) plan.[95] The neuropsycholinguistic theory,[94] however, speculates that disfluencies result from dyssynchrony between linguistic (i.e., lexical and phonological) and suprasegmental components of the language

system. The resulting disfluency will only become stuttered, however, if the speaker experiences time pressure to continue speaking and the sensation of "loss of control."

According to the EXPLAN theory,[93] the dyssynchrony associated with disfluency and stuttering is between language planning and motor execution: when language planning processes are slower than the rate at which speech is executed, disfluencies ensue, as the delay leaves the speaker with no speech to execute. Thus, to "buy time" for further processing, typically fluent speakers will adopt a "stalling process" in which they repeat the previously executed word or insert a filled or unfilled pause until they are ready to proceed. People who stutter, however, are thought to adopt an "advancing process" where they repeat fragments of a word that is currently being processed, leading to part-word repetitions, blocks, and presumably sound prolongations.

There is both support and conflicting evidence for nearly all these psycholinguistic models/theories, but none have gained widespread acceptance. This is partly because many of these theories do not lend themselves to experimental manipulation, although some are more testable than others. It is also the case that many of these theories are lacking in their ability to account for the marked variability of stuttering within and between individuals, as well as its onset and development, spontaneous or unassisted recovery, and many other phenomena associated with stuttering. These problems, however, are not unique to psycholinguistic theories; rather, they are endemic to all etiological accounts of stuttering.

4.5.2 Diagnostic

When we assess and treat an individual for stuttering, or any other communication disorder for that matter, we should do so based on our knowledge of the problem, which should, of course, be up-to-date and evidence based. In other words, what a clinician does, both diagnostically and therapeutically, is explicitly and/or implicitly based on their understanding of the disorder.

We have emphasized in this chapter that CWS, as a group, may have weaknesses in speech, language, and/or cognitive processes and some of these children may even have clinically significant difficulties in these areas (i.e., disorders that co-occur with stuttering). Thus, when children with suspected fluency disorders are evaluated, clinicians should always assess the other speech and language skills of these children and, if needed, screen executive function and/or attention, especially when parents express concern. That is, they should be evaluating more than just the fluency characteristics of the child's speech and his or her cognitive and affective reactions hereto.

For a child who is suspected of stuttering, the assessment of speech and language skills (1) helps the clinician determine if the child has other concomitant disorders (e.g., phonological disorder, language impairment, etc.) that also need to be addressed in treatment and (2) informs the clinician about aspects of the child's speech or language that could be contributing to his or her disfluency. For example, perhaps the child stutters more when producing syntactically complex utterances or has word finding problems that interfere with his or her ability to maintain fluent speech production. The reader is referred to ▶ Chapter 8 for additional discussion of the benefits of comprehensive assessment of the speech and language skills of CWS.

Although speech-language clinicians cannot diagnose executive dysfunction and/or attention deficit hyperactivity disorder, screening these skills in children, when needed, can serve as a basis for referral to a licensed pediatric psychologist or neuropsychologist for further assessment and diagnosis. If a child has clinical or subclinical disturbances in executive function and/or attention, the clinician needs to be aware that they can negatively impact the intervention process and treatment outcomes[88,97] (see ▶ Chapter 4.5.3 for more information). Children's executive function and attention skills can be screened using behavioral observation and rating scales.

Behavioral observation is one tool that clinicians can use to gain some insight into children's executive function and attention skills. When administering a standardized speech or language test, for example, the clinician can observe how well the child follows verbal instructions even with reminders (working memory), the percent of time the child is able to attend to the test (sustained attention), how many times the child speaks out of turn (inhibition), and how the child responds as the test becomes more difficult (cognitive flexibility). When administering multiple tests, the clinician can also observe how well the child shifts from one test to another (cognitive flexibility).

Behavioral rating scales of executive function and/or attention, which are completed by observers (parents and/or teachers) or the child (depending on his or her age), can be easily incorporated into an assessment. These scales provide information about a child's executive function and attention skills in everyday "real-world" contexts. A variety of behavioral rating scales of

Table 4.4 Behavioral rating scales of executive function and/or attention

Preschool

- Behavior Rating Inventory of Executive Function—Preschool[72]
- Brown Executive Function/Attention Scales (ages 3–7 y)[73]
- Child Behavior Checklist (ages 1.5–5 y)[74]
- Conners Early Childhood[75]
- Early Childhood Inventory, 5th edition[76]

Children and adolescents

- Barkley Deficits in Executive Function Scale—Children and Adolescents[77]
- Behavior Rating Inventory of Executive Function, 2nd edition[78]
- Brown Executive Function/Attention Scales (ages 8–12 and 13–18 y)[73]
- Child Behavior Checklist[79]
- Comprehensive Executive Function Inventory[80]
- Conners, 3rd edition[81]

executive function and attention have been developed for children and adolescents and are shown in ▶ Table 4.4.

Behavioral rating scales have several limitations. For example, results may represent the biases of the observer. Many studies have also demonstrated that the results of behavioral rating scales do not always correspond well with the results of performance-based tests. This is likely because the behavioral rating scales and performance-based measures are measuring the same skills (e.g., inhibition) but in dissimilar contexts where they are exhibited differently.[67,68] For this reason, it has been suggested that executive function and attention should be assessed using a variety of different measures, with performance-based tests administered by a psychologist or other professionals with appropriate credentials and expertise.

4.5.3 Treatment

There are three implications for treatment based on the speech and language research discussed in this chapter. First, if a child who stutters is determined to have a concomitant speech and/or language disorder, the clinician will need to treat not only the stuttering but also the other concern(s) (see ▶ Chapters 11 and 13 for treatment suggestions). Second, many of the parent-focused intervention approaches (see ▶ Chapter 10) that clinicians use to treat early childhood stuttering are implicitly based on the notion that stuttering is associated with a mismatch between the child's *capacities* for fluent speech production (e.g., speech motor, language) and the internal or external *demands* placed on them for speech fluency. For example, when we encourage parents to use a slower rate of speech or to speak using shorter, less complex utterances, we are assuming that these strategies reduce the time pressure and/or linguistic demands on the child. Thus, if parents give the child more time to plan and produce speech and/or reduce the language load of utterances the child hears or is expected to produce, the child will be more likely to be fluent. Third, when working directly with CWS, clinicians should consider the speech and language demands of the material they are using to teach children either fluency shaping or stuttering modification techniques. Based on a hierarchy of increasing complexity (see ▶ Fig. 4.4 for an example), the clinician would introduce a technique using reduced communicative demand and gradually increase linguistic complexity as the child progresses (see ▶ Chapters 11 and 13 for further discussion).

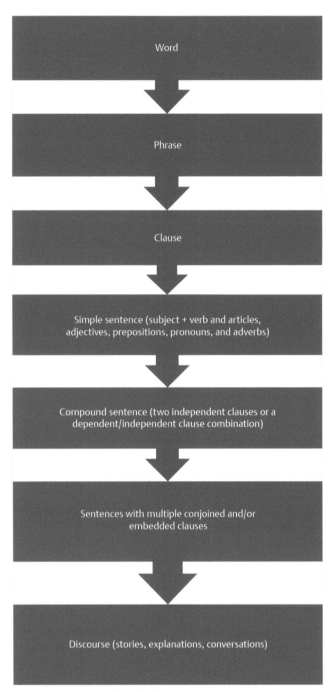

Word

Phrase

Clause

Simple sentence (subject + verb and articles, adjectives, prepositions, pronouns, and adverbs)

Compound sentence (two independent clauses or a dependent/independent clause combination)

Sentences with multiple conjoined and/or embedded clauses

Discourse (stories, explanations, conversations)

Fig. 4.4 Example of a linguistic hierarchy.

Earlier in the chapter, we considered the literature on executive function and attention in childhood stuttering, noting that CWS may have weaknesses in these cognitive processes. Even so, we may need to consider these skills when planning treatment, even when the child does *not* present with suspected or diagnosed concomitant executive function and/or attention difficulties. Executive function and attention do not have to be clinically significant to be clinically relevant and worthy of consideration in treatment planning.

For preschool children, some of the suggested indirect treatment modifications (e.g., turn-taking, parents pausing between phrases, etc.) not only reduce time pressure and linguistic demand but also executive function and/or attention demands. For example, as illustrated in ▶ Table 4.5, when parents insert pauses at sentence boundaries, it can reduce working memory demands on the child and facilitate language comprehension. Some indirect treatment approaches may even promote executive function and attentional skills. For example, in many parent-focused intervention approaches, parents are instructed to wait for 1 to 2 seconds before responding to their child's question or comment and children are encouraged to do likewise (e.g., "listen while others are talking," "wait your turn while others are talking," and "be quiet while others are talking"). This behavior not only gives the child more time to formulate a response but also promotes the development of sustained attention and inhibition.

When older children acquire and use fluency shaping and stuttering modification techniques in treatment, they are also drawing on executive function and attention skills. For example, pausing, phrasing, slow rate of speech, and cancellations all require inhibition, as children must overcome the natural tendency to speak as they typically do. When children use these techniques outside the therapy room, they must also be more vigilant and engage in a higher level of self-monitoring. Helping children change their thoughts about stuttering requires cognitive flexibility, whereas high levels of worry and anxiety about talking and stuttering can tax working memory. The point here is that clinicians need to be aware that stuttering therapy can pose a challenge for children, particularly those who have clinically significant weaknesses in executive function and/or attention.

Finally, if children have clinical or subclinical symptoms of attention deficit hyperactivity disorder, clinicians need to consider that these symptoms can exacerbate stuttering and, if needed, address them in therapy.[98] Some of these symptoms include rapid rate of speech, difficulty with conversational turn-taking, and production of long utterances that often lack clarity, organization, and cohesion. Clinicians should also be mindful of how to keep the child with clinical or subclinical attention deficit hyperactivity disorder engaged, motivated, interested, and focused during therapy sessions by establishing predictable routines, creating visual reminders, using concise and simple instructions, repeating instructions frequently, incorporating topics that are interesting and motivating to the child, and introducing frequent practice blocks during the session.

4.6 Future Directions

The astute reader will no doubt realize that despite having made progress, researchers still have much to learn about speech, language, and cognitive processes in developmental stuttering. Such progress is undoubtedly hampered by the fact that individuals who stutter are, by nature, heterogeneous and stuttering is a complicated disorder. Nevertheless, this should not be construed as a weakness, as science often progresses incrementally. Yet with each new study, the field continues to move forward, even if slowly.

There are several specific areas of research that would contribute to our knowledge base and help us better understand how speech, language, and cognitive processes contribute to

Table 4.5 Examples of indirect stuttering treatment strategies and their impact on executive function and attention

Pausing between conversational turns: Parents wait for 1–2 seconds before responding to their child's question or comment	Reduces attention and working memory demands on the child, giving them more time to process the message and formulate their response. Learning to pause and wait for their turn also promotes the development of sustained attention and inhibition
Balancing utterance ratio: Parents maintain a balance between the number of spoken utterances they produce and the number of utterances their child produces during each conversational turn (~1:1)	Reduces working memory demands on the child
Adjusting language input: Parents use language that is within their child's range of linguistic competence (e.g., shorter and/or less complex language)	Reduces working memory demands on the child
Modifying questioning: Parents avoid asking frequent rapid-fire questions and questions that require complex, lengthy responses	Reduces working memory and cognitive flexibility demands on the child, especially if questions are about different topics
Following the child's lead: Parents talk about what their child is doing and respond to the child's conversation topic of interest	Fosters sustained attention and, when talking about the "here and now" (instead of something more abstract), reduces working memory demands
Maintaining conversation topic: Parents avoid introducing multiple conversational topics during the same interaction	Decreases cognitive flexibility demands on the child
Pausing between phrases/clauses: Parents insert short pauses between phrases or clauses (e.g., "Please come here [pause] I need your help.")	Reduces working memory demands on the child, giving them more time for information storing and processing

developmental stuttering. Areas of future research include the way in which language and cognitive factors interact with stuttering persistence and biological sex. First, it is important to determine whether executive function and/or attention influences stuttering persistence. As previously indicated, research suggests that CWS who have weaker articulation/phonological skills have a higher risk of being among the 20 to 30% of children whose stuttering persists.[28] There is also evidence to suggest that persistence may be higher for CWS with weaker expressive and/or receptive language skills[99] and lower attention spans.[28] Although we have some knowledge of the impact of articulation/phonology, language, and attentional skills on stuttering persistence, research on the effect of executive function on persistence lags far behind.

A second area of future research is examining the impact of biological sex on speech, language, and cognitive processes in CWS and CWNS. Few studies have examined biological sex differences in developmental stuttering, which is somewhat surprising given that it is well known that boys are more likely to persist in stuttering than girls. Nevertheless, without more research, we cannot simply assume that girls who stutter are the same as boys who stutter. In fact, the findings of one recent study suggest that they may not be entirely the same in at least some skills. In this study, the investigators found that boys who stutter were more impulsive than boys who do not stutter, but there was no difference between the girls who do and do not stutter.[100] These findings illustrate the need for further study of biological sex differences in developmental stuttering.

The ongoing study of speech, language, and cognitive processes in individuals who stutter is also critical for the development and/or delivery of effective therapies. As previously indicated, given that fluency shaping and stuttering modification techniques utilize executive function and attention skills, it stands to reason that if a child has clinical or subclinical deficiencies in these areas, it will negatively affect the extent to which they may benefit from treatment. Only a few studies have examined this possibility, both of which demonstrated that CWS who have more attentional difficulties require more treatment sessions to achieve typical fluency[88] and have reduced treatment outcomes.[97] Clearly,

more studies are needed to further examine how executive function and attention might impact treatment outcomes and, perhaps, the efficacy of the techniques that children use to achieve fluency and/or modify their stuttering.

4.7 Conclusions

The production of words and multiword utterances requires a complex series of events, beginning with the retrieval of the semantic features associated with the intended word(s) and ending with the articulation of the selected word(s). Given the rapid rate at which these events unfold, it seems as if breakdowns in fluency should occur for all of us more often than they do! For millions of individuals who stutter, this is indeed the case. Disfluencies are not random; some words and locations within an utterance are more likely to be disfluent, reflecting increased cognitive and linguistic demands on the speaker or vulnerabilities in the speech-language production system.

Although findings from studies of the articulation/phonology and language abilities of CWS have been mixed, we can make several broad conclusions from this work. First, while CWS do not appear to appreciably differ from CWNS on tests of articulation/phonology, they do tend to perform more poorly (albeit still within normal limits) on standardized, norm-referenced tests of language. Second, the phonological and language processing abilities of at least some CWS may be slower and/or developmentally less mature than CWNS. Psycholinguistic theories of stuttering point to dyssynchronies in the simultaneous timing of different aspects of speech-language production. Further, there is growing evidence that cognitive processes may play a role in developmental stuttering, with some studies reporting that CWS have subtle to not so subtle difficulties with executive function and attention. Therefore, speech, language, and cognitive factors should be considered when evaluating and treating a CWS.

Although much progress has been made in our understanding of the role of speech, language, and cognitive processes in developmental stuttering, more work needs to be done. Speech production is as complex as the neural systems that subserve it, making it likely that any quest to attribute a single cause to stuttering will remain elusive. In fact, in his classic textbook, Charles Van Riper[101] described stuttering as "…a puzzle, the pieces of which lie scattered on the tables of speech pathology, psychiatry, neurophysiology, genetics, and many other disciplines… we suspect that some of the essential pieces are not merely misplaced but still missing." These words are just as apt today as they were in 1971, for even though stuttering has been studied extensively, its puzzling and enigmatic nature is and will continue to be a worthy challenge for students, clinicians, and researchers, now and for the foreseeable future.

4.8 Definitions

Alternating/shifting attention: The ability to disengage attention from one activity or task to another.

Cognitive flexibility: The ability to switch from one perspective, representation, or rule to another.

Covert repair hypothesis: A psycholinguistic theory of stuttering proposing that disfluencies result from the speaker's attempt to covertly repair errors arising at the level of phonological encoding before those errors are overtly produced.

Executive function: A set of cognitive skills that are critical for learning and performing goal-directed tasks in everyday life.

EXPLAN theory: A psycholinguistic theory of stuttering proposing that disfluencies result from a timing mismatch/dyssynchrony between language planning and motor execution processes.

Inhibition: The ability to ignore irrelevant information or suppress a response.

Lexical processing: The stage of word production during which the word is selected among others with competing/similar semantic features (e.g., dog).

Linguistic constraints on stuttering: Linguistic factors that influence which words and/or utterances are likely to be stuttered.

Linguistic dissociations: Imbalances/mismatches among different components of the speech-language system.

Neuropsycholinguistic theory: A psycholinguistic theory of stuttering proposing that disfluencies result from dyssynchrony between phonetic and prosodic components of the language system and when the speaker is under time pressure.

Phonological awareness: The ability to manipulate units of speech (words, syllables, phonemes).

Phonological processing: The stage of word production during which the sound structure of the selected word is retrieved (e.g., /k/, /æ/, /t/).

Phonological processing abilities: The skill of distinguishing and manipulating the sound units of language. This term encompasses other metalinguistic skills such as phonological awareness and phonological working memory.

Psycholinguistic theories of stuttering: Theories of stuttering (e.g., covert repair hypothesis, vicious circle hypothesis) that propose disruptions in language processing (e.g., phonological encoding and/or monitoring) as a causal variable in stuttering.

Semantic processing: The stage of word production during which the conceptual features (e.g., furry four-legged feline) of the intended word are retrieved (e.g., cat).

Speech-motor programming and execution: The stage of word production during which the abstract linguistic (phonological) code of the selected word is transformed into motor programs leading to the articulation of the word.

Selective attention: The ability to focus on select information while ignoring irrelevant information.

Sustained attention: The ability to maintain alertness for prolonged periods of time.

Syntactic processing: Multilevel process involving word retrieval and construction of syntactic frames that conform to the rules of language.

Vicious circle hypothesis: A psycholinguistic theory of stuttering proposing that individuals who stutter perceive an excessive number of internal errors in language processing and their disfluencies are a by-product of the repair of those perceived errors.

Working memory: The ability to temporarily store (short-term memory) and manipulate information.

References

[1] Levelt WJM. Relations between speech production and speech perception: some behavioral and neurological observations. In: Dupoux E, ed. Language, Brain, and Cognitive Development: Essays in Honor of Jacques Mehler. Cambridge, MA: MIT Press; 2001:241–256

[2] Ferreira VS, Pashler H. Central bottleneck influences on the processing stages of word production. J Exp Psychol Learn Mem Cogn. 2002; 28(6):1187–1199

[3] Ferreira F, Swets B. How incremental is language production? Evidence from the production of utterances requiring the computation of arithmetic sums. J Mem Lang. 2002; 46(1):57–84

[4] Griffin ZM, Bock K. What the eyes say about speaking. Psychol Sci. 2000; 11 (4):274–279

[5] Spieler DH, Griffin ZM. The influence of age on the time course of word preparation in multiword utterances. Lang Cogn Process. 2006; 21(1–3):291–321

[6] Engelhardt PE, McMullon MEG, Corley M. Individual differences in the production of disfluency: a latent variable analysis of memory ability and verbal intelligence. Q J Exp Psychol (Hove). 2019; 72(5):1084–1101

[7] Roelofs A. Goal-referenced selection of verbal action: modeling attentional control in the Stroop task. Psychol Rev. 2003; 110(1):88–125

[8] Indefrey P. The spatial and temporal signatures of word production components: a critical update. Front Psychol. 2011; 2:255

[9] Bloodstein O, Bernstein-Ratner N. A Handbook on Stuttering. 6th ed. Clifton Park, NY: Thomson-Delmar; 2008

[10] Brown SF. The loci of stutterings in the speech sequence. J Speech Disord. 1945; 10(3):181–192

[11] Bernstein NE. Are there constraints on childhood disfluency? J Fluency Disord. 1981; 6:341–350

[12] Choi D, Sim H, Park H, Clark CE, Kim H. Loci of stuttering of English- and Korean-speaking children who stutter: preliminary findings. J Fluency Disord. 2020; 64:105762

[13] Logan K. The effect of syntactic complexity upon the speech fluency of adolescents and adults who stutter. J Fluency Disord. 2001; 26(2):85–106

[14] Rispoli M, Hadley P. The leading-edge: the significance of sentence disruptions in the development of grammar. J Speech Lang Hear Res. 2001; 44(5):1131–1143

[15] Charles-Luce J. The interaction of semantics and lexical properties in speech production. Univ Buffalo Work Pap on Lang Percept. 2002; 1:380–423

[16] Wagovich SA, Hall NE, Clifford BA. Speech disruptions in relation to language growth in children who stutter: an exploratory study. J Fluency Disord. 2009; 34(4):242–256

[17] Anderson JD. Phonological neighborhood and word frequency effects in the stuttered disfluencies of children who stutter. J Speech Lang Hear Res. 2007; 50(1):229–247

[18] Blood GW, Ridenour VJ, Qualls CD, Hammer CS. Co-occurring disorders in children who stutter. J Commun Disord. 2003; 36(6):427–448

[19] Shimada M, Toyomura A, Fujii T, Minami T. Children who stutter at 3 years of age: a community-based study. J Fluency Disord. 2018; 56:45–54

[20] Unicomb R, Kefalianos E, Reilly S, Cook F, Morgan A. Prevalence and features of comorbid stuttering and speech sound disorder at age 4 years. J Commun Disord. 2020; 84:105976

[21] Goldman R, Fristoe M. Goldman-Fristoe Test of Articulation. 2nd ed. Circle Pines, MN: American Guidance Service, Inc.; 2000

[22] Anderson JD, Conture EG. Sentence-structure priming in young children who do and do not stutter. J Speech Lang Hear Res. 2004; 47(3):552–571

[23] Byrd CT, Conture EG, Ohde RN. Phonological priming in young children who stutter: holistic versus incremental processing. Am J Speech Lang Pathol. 2007; 16(1):43–53

[24] Clark CE, Conture EG, Walden TA, Lambert WE. Speech sound articulation abilities of preschool-age children who stutter. J Fluency Disord. 2013; 38 (4):325–341

[25] Pellowski MW, Conture EG. Lexical priming in picture naming of young children who do and do not stutter. J Speech Lang Hear Res. 2005; 48(2):278–294

[26] Ratner NB, Silverman S. Parental perceptions of children's communicative development at stuttering onset. J Speech Lang Hear Res. 2000; 43(5):1252–1263

[27] Anderson JD, Conture E. Language abilities of children who stutter: a preliminary study. J Fluency Disord. 2000; 25(4):283–304

[28] Singer CM, Hessling A, Kelly EM, Singer L, Jones RM. Clinical characteristics associated with stuttering persistence: a meta-analysis. J Speech Lang Hear Res. 2020; 63(9):2995–3018

[29] Robertson C, Salter W. The Phonological Awareness Test: Examiner's Manual. 2nd ed. East Moline, IL: LinguiSystems; 2007

[30] Pelczarski KM, Yaruss JS. Phonological encoding of young children who stutter. J Fluency Disord. 2014; 39(1):12–24

[31] Sasisekaran J, Brady A, Stein J. A preliminary investigation of phonological encoding skills in children who stutter. J Fluency Disord. 2013; 38(1):45–58

[32] Gerwin K, Brosseau-Lapré F, Brown B, Christ S, Weber C. Rhyme production strategies distinguish stuttering recovery and persistence. J Speech Lang Hear Res. 2019; 62(9):3302–3319

[33] Sasisekaran J, Byrd CT. A preliminary investigation of segmentation and rhyme abilities of children who stutter. J Fluency Disord. 2013; 38(2):222–234

[34] Melnick KS, Conture EG, Ohde RN. Phonological priming in picture naming of young children who stutter. J Speech Lang Hear Res. 2003; 46 (6):1428–1443

[35] Sasisekaran J, Byrd C. Nonword repetition and phoneme elision skills in school-age children who do and do not stutter. Int J Lang Commun Disord. 2013; 48(6):625–639

[36] Weber-Fox C, Spruill JE, III, Spencer R, Smith A. Atypical neural functions underlying phonological processing and silent rehearsal in children who stutter. Dev Sci. 2008; 11(2):321–337

[37] Bosshardt H-G, Ballmer W, de Nil LF. Effects of category and rhyme decisions on sentence production. J Speech Lang Hear Res. 2002; 45(5):844–857

[38] Coalson GA, Byrd CT. Metrical encoding in adults who do and do not stutter. J Speech Lang Hear Res. 2015; 58(3):601–621

[39] Maxfield ND, Pizon-Moore AA, Frisch SA, Constantine JL. Exploring semantic and phonological picture-word priming in adults who stutter using event-related potentials. Clin Neurophysiol. 2012; 123(6):1131–1146

[40] Vincent I, Grela BG, Gilbert HR. Phonological priming in adults who stutter. J Fluency Disord. 2012; 37(2):91–105

[41] Guo LY, Tomblin JB, Samelson V. Speech disruptions in the narratives of English-speaking children with specific language impairment. J Speech Lang Hear Res. 2008; 51(3):722–738

[42] Finneran DA, Leonard LB, Miller CA. Speech disruptions in the sentence formulation of school-age children with specific language impairment. Int J Lang Commun Disord. 2009; 44(3):271–286

[43] Choo AL, Burnham E, Hicks K, Chang SE. Dissociations among linguistic, cognitive, and auditory-motor neuroanatomical domains in children who stutter. J Commun Disord. 2016; 61:29–47

[44] Luckman C, Wagovich SA, Weber C, et al. Lexical diversity and lexical skills in children who stutter. J Fluency Disord. 2020; 63:105747

[45] Zaretsky E, Lange BP, Euler HA, Robinson F, Neumann K. Pre-schoolers who stutter score lower in verbal skills than their non-stuttering peers. Buck J Lang Linguist. 2017; 10(0):96–115

[46] Ntourou K, Conture EG, Lipsey MW. Language abilities of children who stutter: a meta-analytical review. Am J Speech Lang Pathol. 2011; 20(3):163–179

[47] Anderson JD, Pellowski MW, Conture EG. Childhood stuttering and dissociations across linguistic domains. J Fluency Disord. 2005; 30(3):219–253

[48] Watts A, Eadie P, Block S, Mensah F, Reilly S. Language ability of children with and without a history of stuttering: a longitudinal cohort study. Int J Speech Lang Pathol. 2015; 17(1):86–95

[49] Watkins RV, Yairi E, Ambrose NG. Early childhood stuttering III: initial status of expressive language abilities. J Speech Lang Hear Res. 1999; 42(5):1125–1135

[50] Usler E, Weber-Fox C. Neurodevelopment for syntactic processing distinguishes childhood stuttering recovery versus persistence. J Neurodev Disord. 2015; 7(1):4

[51] Weber-Fox C, Hampton Wray A, Arnold H. Early childhood stuttering and electrophysiological indices of language processing. J Fluency Disord. 2013; 38(2):206–221

[52] Maxfield ND, Huffman JL, Frisch SA, Hinckley JJ. Neural correlates of semantic activation spreading on the path to picture naming in adults who stutter. Clin Neurophysiol. 2010; 121(9):1447–1463

[53] Baggetta P, Alexander PA. Conceptualization and operationalization of executive function. Mind Brain Educ. 2016; 10(1):10–33

[54] Karr JE, Areshenkoff CN, Rast P, Hofer SM, Iverson GL, Garcia-Barrera MA. The unity and diversity of executive functions: a systematic review and re-analysis of latent variable studies. Psychol Bull. 2018; 144(11):1147–1185

[55] Garon N, Bryson SE, Smith IM. Executive function in preschoolers: a review using an integrative framework. Psychol Bull. 2008; 134(1):31–60

[56] Diamond A. Executive functions. Annu Rev Psychol. 2013; 64(1):135–168

[57] Zelazo PD, Blair CB, Willoughby MT. Executive Function: Implications for Education (NCER 2017–2000). Washington, DC: US Dept of Education, Institute of Education Sciences, National Center for Education Research; 2016

[58] Wiebe SA, Espy KA, Charak D. Using confirmatory factor analysis to understand executive control in preschool children: I. Latent structure. Dev Psychol. 2008; 44(2):575–587

[59] McClelland MM, Cameron CE. Developing together: the role of executive function and motor skills in children's early academic lives. Early Child Res Q. 2019; 46:142–151

[60] Craig F, Margari F, Legrottaglie AR, Palumbi R, de Giambattista C, Margari L. A review of executive function deficits in autism spectrum disorder and attention-deficit/hyperactivity disorder. Neuropsychiatr Dis Treat. 2016; 12:1191–1202

[61] Kapa LL, Plante E, Doubleday K. Applying an integrative framework of executive function to preschoolers with specific language impairment. J Speech Lang Hear Res. 2017; 60(8):2170–2184

[62] Pisoni DB, Cleary M. Measures of working memory span and verbal rehearsal speed in deaf children after cochlear implantation. Ear Hear. 2003; 24(1) Suppl:106S–120S

[63] Shi R, Sharpe L, Abbott M. A meta-analysis of the relationship between anxiety and attentional control. Clin Psychol Rev. 2019; 72:101754

[64] Torrington Eaton C, Ratner NB. An exploration of the role of executive functions in preschoolers' phonological development. Clin Linguist Phon. 2016; 30(9):679–695

[65] Zelazo PD. Executive function and psychopathology: a neurodevelopmental perspective. Annu Rev Clin Psychol. 2020; 16(1):431–454

[66] Anderson JD, Ofoe LC. The role of executive function in developmental stuttering. Semin Speech Lang. 2019; 40(4):305–319

[67] Ofoe LC, Anderson JD, Ntourou K. Short-term memory, inhibition, and attention in developmental stuttering: a meta-analysis. J Speech Lang Hear Res. 2018; 61(7):1626–1648

[68] Ntourou K, Anderson JD, Wagovich SA. Executive function and childhood stuttering: parent ratings and evidence from a behavioral task. J Fluency Disord. 2018; 56:18–32

[69] Pisoni DB, Conway CM, Kronenberger W, Horn DL, Karpicke J, Henning S. Efficacy and effectiveness of cochlear implants in deaf children. In: Marschark M, Hauser P, eds. Deaf Cognition: Foundations and Outcomes. New York, NY: Oxford University Press; 2008

[70] Mancas M. What is attention? In: Mancas M, Ferrera VP, Riche N, Taylor JG, eds. From Human Attention to Computational Attention: A Multidisciplinary Approach, Springer Series in Cognitive and Neural Systems. Vol. 10. New York, NY: Springer; 2016:9–20

[71] Strayer DL, Drews FA. Multitasking in the automobile. In: Kramer AF, Wiegmann DA, Kirlik A, eds. Attention from Theory to Practice. New York, NY: Oxford University Press; 2007:121–133

[72] Gioia GA, Espy KA, Isquith PK. Behavior Rating Inventory of Executive Function-Preschool Version (BRIEF-P). Odessa, FL: Psychological Assessment Resources; 2003

[73] Brown TE. Brown Executive Function/Attention Scales (Manual). Bloomington, MN: Pearson; 2018

[74] Achenbach TM, Rescorla LA. Manual for the ASEBA Preschool Forms & Profiles. Burlington, VT: University of Vermont, Research Center for Children, Youth, and Families; 2000

[75] Conners CK. Conners Early Childhood. Toronto, ON, Canada: Multi-Health Systems; 2009

[76] Sprafkin K, Gadow KD. Early Childhood Inventory-5 Norms Manual. Stony Brook, NY: Checkmate Plus; 2017

[77] Barkley RA. Barkley Deficits in Executive Function Scale: Children and Adolescents. New York, NY: Guilford Press; 2012

[78] Gioia GA, Isquith PK, Guy SC, Kenworthy L. Behavior Rating Inventory of Executive Function (BRIEF-2). 2nd ed. Odessa, FL: Psychological Assessment Resources; 2015

[79] Achenbach TM, Rescorla LA. Manual for the ASEBA School-Age Forms & Profiles. Burlington, VT: University of Vermont, Research Center for Children, Youth, and Families; 2001

[80] Naglieri J, Goldstein S. Comprehensive Executive Function Inventory: Adult. Torrance, CA: WPS; 2017

[81] Conners CK. Conners. 3rd ed. Toronto, ON, Canada: Multi-Health Systems; 2008

[82] Andrade BF, Brodeur DA, Waschbusch DA, Stewart SH, McGee R. Selective and sustained attention as predictors of social problems in children with typical and disordered attention abilities. J Atten Disord. 2009; 12(4):341–352

[83] Johansson M, Marciszko C, Gredebäck G, Nyström P, Bohlin G. Sustained attention in infancy as a longitudinal predictor of self-regulatory functions. Infant Behav Dev. 2015; 41:1–11

[84] Muller U, Jacques S, Brocki K, Zelazo PD. The executive functions of language in preschool children. In: Winsler A, Fernyhough C, Montero I, eds. Private Speech, Executive Functioning, and the Development of Verbal Self-Regulation. New York, NY: Cambridge University Press; 2009:53–68

[85] Allen G, Courchesne E. Attention function and dysfunction in autism. Front Biosci. 2001; 6:D105–D119

[86] Murphy CFB, Pagan-Neves LO, Wertzner HF, Schochat E. Auditory and visual sustained attention in children with speech sound disorder. PLoS One. 2014; 9(3):e93091

[87] Tomas E, Vissers C. Behind the scenes of developmental language disorder: time to call neuropsychology back on stage. Front Hum Neurosci. 2019; 12:517

[88] Druker K, Hennessey N, Mazzucchelli T, Beilby J. Elevated attention deficit hyperactivity disorder symptoms in children who stutter. J Fluency Disord. 2019; 59:80–90

[89] Eggers K, De Nil LF, Van den Bergh BRH. The efficiency of attentional networks in children who stutter. J Speech Lang Hear Res. 2012; 55(3):946–959

[90] Wagovich SA, Anderson JD, Hill MS. Visual exogenous and endogenous attention and visual memory in preschool children who stutter. J Fluency Disord. 2020; 66:105792

[91] Postma A, Kolk H. The covert repair hypothesis: prearticulatory repair processes in normal and stuttered disfluencies. J Speech Hear Res. 1993; 36 (3):472–487

[92] Vasic N, Wijnen F. Stuttering as a monitoring deficit. In: Hartsuiker RJ, Bastiaanse R, Postma A, Wijnen F, eds. Phonological Encoding and Monitoring in Normal and Pathological Speech. New York, NY: Psychology Press; 2005:226–247

[93] Howell P, Au-Yeung J. The EXPLAN theory of fluency control applied to the treatment of stuttering. In: Fava E, ed. Pathology and Therapy of Speech Disorders. Amsterdam: John Benjamins; 2002:75–94

[94] Perkins WH, Kent RD, Curlee RF. A theory of neuropsycholinguistic function in stuttering. J Speech Hear Res. 1991; 34(4):734–752

[95] Karniol R. Stuttering, language, and cognition: a review and a model of stuttering as suprasegmental sentence plan alignment (SPA). Psychol Bull. 1995; 117(1):104–124

[96] Wingate M. Stuttering: A Psycholinguistic Analysis. New York, NY: Springer-Verlag; 1988

[97] Riley G, Riley J. A revised component model for diagnosing and treating children who stutter. Contemp Issues Commun Sci Disord. 2000; 27: 188–199

[98] Donaher J, Richels C. Traits of attention deficit/hyperactivity disorder in school-age children who stutter. J Fluency Disord. 2012; 37(4):242–252

[99] Leech KA, Bernstein Ratner N, Brown B, Weber CM. Preliminary evidence that growth in productive language differentiates childhood stuttering persistence and recovery. J Speech Lang Hear Res. 2017; 60 (11):3097–3109

[100] Ofoe LC, Anderson JD. Complex nonverbal response inhibition and stopping impulsivity in childhood stuttering. J Fluency Disord. 2021; 70:105877.

[101] Van Riper C. The Nature of Stuttering. Englewood Cliffs, NJ: Prentice-Hall; 1971

Further Readings

Anderson JD, Ofoe LC. The role of executive function in developmental stuttering. Semin Speech Lang. 2019; 40(4):305–319

Druker K, Hennessey N, Mazzucchelli T, Beilby J. Elevated attention deficit hyperactivity symptoms in children who stutter. J Fluency Disord. 2019; 59:80–90

Eggers K, De Nil LF, Van den Bergh BRH. The efficiency of attentional networks in children who stutter. J Speech Lang Hear Res. 2012; 55(3):946–959

Leech KA, Bernstein Ratner N, Brown B, Weber CM. Preliminary evidence that growth in productive language differentiates childhood stuttering persistence and recovery. J Speech Lang Hear Res. 2017; 60(11):3097–3109

Ntourou K, Conture EG, Lipsey MW. Language abilities of children who stutter: a meta-analytical review. Am J Speech Lang Pathol. 2011; 20(3):163–179

Ofoe LC, Anderson JD, Ntourou K. Short-term memory, inhibition, and attention in developmental stuttering: a meta-analysis. J Speech Lang Hear Res. 2018; 61(7): 1626–1648

Sasisekaran J. Exploring the link between stuttering and phonology: a review and implications for treatment. Semin Speech Lang. 2014; 35(2):95–113

5 Neural and Physiological Processes

Deryk Beal, Evan Usler, and Anna Tendera

Abstract

Over the past century, investigations into the underlying mechanisms of developmental stuttering have advanced considerably to reveal a complex neurophysiology. A greater understanding of the neural and physiological processes associated with stuttering is relevant not only for those with a natural curiosity of the theoretical neurophysiological underpinnings of the disorder but also for those who seek to improve client education and treatment. A clear description of the neurophysiology of stuttering will shed light on potential causes, developmental trajectories, and may improve the effectiveness of stuttering treatment. The purpose of this chapter is to describe and discuss the neural and physiological processes underlying developmental stuttering. The chapter begins with an introduction to how the brain controls stuttering, followed by a multileveled analysis across the various levels of physiology: (1) perceptual disfluency; (2) articulatory, laryngeal, and respiratory dynamics; (3) neuromuscular activation; (4) electrocortical activation; and (5) brain regions and networks. The chapter concludes with a discussion of the theoretical and treatment implications of these findings, as well as a glance into potential future research directions regarding the neural and physiological processes of developmental stuttering.

Keywords: stuttering, fluency disorder, speech motor control, neuroanatomy, neurophysiology

5.1 Introduction

Developmental stuttering is a neurodevelopmental and multifactorial fluency disorder whose neural mechanisms remain unclear. In other words, we know its characteristics quite well, but we are less certain about how and why the brain and body produce stuttering behavior. Speech fluency is the product of the consistent, smooth, and rapid movement of the speech motor system, even in the face of linguistic, cognitive, and emotional demands. To achieve these movements, the brain must rapidly and accurately execute various neural and physiological processes associated with speech motor control.

Developmental stuttering has been considered by some to be primarily a disorder of speech motor control and coordination.[1] From this perspective, we will focus on how the brain controls movement, a process that assumes that the brain stores representations of movement sequences, commonly known as motor programs, in memory.[2] Speech motor programs allow for the quick selection of learned, sequential movements that facilitate the production of phonemes and syllables.[3] Thus, according to this viewpoint, difficulty with the timing and/or sequencing of these programs, which are also influenced by cognitive and linguistic abilities, would result in the production of stuttering disfluencies (sound/syllable repetitions, prolongations, and blocks), the most salient symptom of the disorder.[3,4]

Developmental stuttering is a disorder that is often misunderstood because its neurophysiological nature is complex, and stuttering behaviors often differ across people who stutter (PWS) and even within a person over time. As shown in ▶ Fig. 5.1, PWS may appear fluent in one situation but not another. Others may only have difficulty saying certain sounds or words. This variability in stuttering behaviors makes it challenging for researchers to elucidate the neurophysiological underpinnings of developmental stuttering. Nevertheless, to improve the well-being and diverse needs of PWS, it is helpful for clinicians to have at least some understanding of the complex neurophysiological events associated with stuttering.

Almost a century ago, Lee Travis and his colleagues at the University of Iowa proposed that developmental stuttering was associated with a lack of cerebral dominance.[5] As discussed in

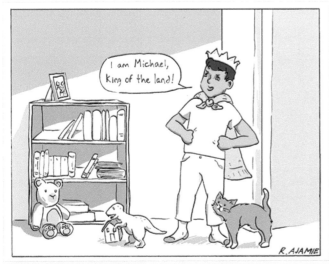
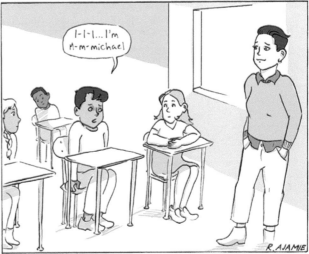

Fig. 5.1 The situational variability of developmental stuttering. Source: Image created by Rae Ajamie.

▶ Chapter 2, the cerebral dominance theory of stuttering posited that if one hemisphere failed to dominate over the other, the two hemispheres would function independently, resulting in poor synchronization of the speech musculature. During this time, many left-handed children were forced to write with their right hand. This change in handedness was thought to prevent the development of a dominant hemisphere for speech and language, thereby contributing to the emergence of stuttering. This early theory was largely incorrect, in part, because most children who were forced to change handedness did not develop stuttering, but the notion that biases in hemispheric activation were associated with stuttering would turn out to be influential.

Over the past five decades, neurophysiological explanations have implicated areas of the brain responsible for the control of speech-language production in the development of the disorder and/or the elicitation of stuttering behaviors.[6] Empirical research has revealed considerable neural and physiological differences between PWS and their fluent peers, including atypical brain anatomy and connectivity. To make sense of these findings and interpretations, we will describe the multiple interrelated levels of neural and physiological processes underlying developmental stuttering (▶ Fig. 5.2).

5.2 Level 1: Perceptual Disfluency

As stated in ▶ Chapter 1, stuttering disfluencies are perceptual disruptions in the acoustic speech signal, often characterized by type, frequency, and duration. PWS may also exhibit secondary behaviors (such as lesser eye contact or circumlocutions), covert behaviors for avoidance or escape from feared speaking situations, and/or atypical habits to produce certain words. Analysis of these behaviors provides useful information about overall severity, but it tells us relatively little about the neural and physiological processes underlying the disorder. A nice analogy

by Smith[7] is that studying when and how often disfluencies occur is similar to studying the flow of lava coming out of a volcano. Although we are not volcanologists, it seems self-evident that understanding plate tectonics and other activity under the earth's surface would give us more valuable information on when and why a volcanic eruption will occur, compared to just studying surface phenomena such as the speed and direction of flowing lava. Thus, let us dig a little deeper into the subsystems of speech in our investigation about what underlying factors play a role in stuttering.

5.3 Level 2: Articulatory, Laryngeal, and Respiratory Dynamics

As mentioned earlier, stuttering disfluencies may occur when difficulties in the initiation and execution of speech motor programs disrupt the coordination of the articulatory, laryngeal, and respiratory subsystems necessary for fluent speech. Measuring the movement of these speech subsystems allows for a quantification of speech motor control processes beyond what we can normally perceive with our eyes and ears. Research using speech acoustics and kinematics, which measure speech movements, has revealed that PWS exhibit speech motor systems that operate differently from their fluent peers, particularly during times of increased cognitive-linguistic demands or environmental stress. For example, even during perceptually fluent speech (speech that sounds fluent), PWS exhibit higher articulatory variability across utterances compared to fluent peers, particularly under increased task demands.[8] Interestingly, some adults who stutter may also adopt more restricted articulatory movements when producing utterances, perhaps as a way to safeguard speech fluency.[9]

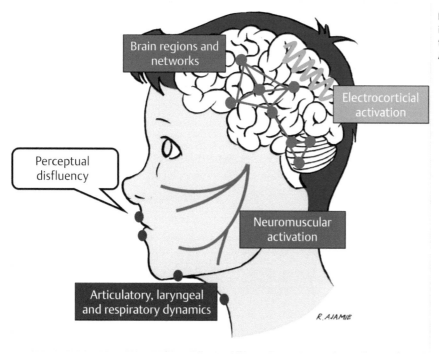

Fig. 5.2 The multiple levels of neural and physiological processes associated with developmental stuttering. Source: Image created by Rae Ajamie.

Young children who stutter, and males in particular, have also been shown to exhibit deficits in articulatory movement compared to typically developing children.[10] Increased articulatory variability also distinguishes school-age children with persistent stuttering compared to peers who had previously recovered.[11] Finally, as a measure of motor learning across utterance repetitions, articulatory variability of adults who stutter has been shown to decrease from early to later utterances. This dynamic was not observed in fluent controls.[12] These reported deficits in the control of articulation may represent an underlying instability of the speech motor control processes in PWS.[4]

In addition to articulation, stuttering has also been related to disruptions in laryngeal and respiratory muscle coordination. Acoustic measures of laryngeal function, such as fundamental frequency, jitter, and shimmer, are different in PWS compared to their fluent counterparts.[13,14] Stuttering has also been associated with discoordination in respiratory movements, resulting in difficulty maintaining constant levels of subglottal pressure during speech.[15] Even when fluent, adults who stutter exhibit atypical levels of subglottal pressure compared to fluent adults.[16]

In sum, atypical articulatory, laryngeal, and respiratory dynamics appear to contribute not only to stuttering behaviors but also to the perceptually fluent speech of PWS. However, these differences in respiratory, phonatory, and articulatory control are subtle. That is, there are no gross or obvious abnormalities in the speech subsystems of PWS. Furthermore, it is difficult to determine if these physiological differences are causally associated with stuttering or are a symptom of or a reaction to the stuttering.

5.4 Level 3: Neuromuscular Activation

When the moment of stuttering is described by PWS, they often report feeling tension in facial, mandibular, and laryngeal muscles.[17] This characteristic of the disorder has been long known and suggests that stuttering may be the result of aberrant muscle physiology. The disruptions in speech coordination that were summarized earlier in ► Chapter 5.3 Level 2: Articulatory, Laryngeal, and Respiratory Dynamics can also be measured at the level of the muscles themselves using electromyography (EMG). Depicted in ► Fig. 5.3, EMG is a technique for recording electrical activity, usually from electrodes placed on the skin, produced during muscle contraction.[18] Although some have suggested that stuttering disfluencies may result from atypical contraction of the facial, mandibular, and/or laryngeal muscles,[19,20] activity recorded by EMG does not appear to differ during fluent and disfluent speech in PWS.[21,22] This indicates that aberrant muscle physiology is not likely to play a causal role in stuttering disfluencies.

A little understood behavior associated with stuttering is an involuntary, rhythmic movement (i.e., tremor) that can be measured across the muscles of the jaw, lip, and larynx during stuttering disfluencies.[23,24] Tremor is not observed in young children who stutter, nor is it universally present in all adults who stutter or in every instance of disfluency.[24] The reason why some PWS develop tremor and whether it could be related to anxiety remains unclear. Nevertheless, given that tremor

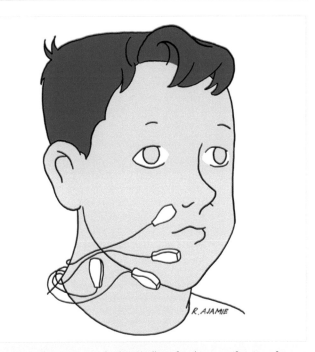

Fig. 5.3 Electromyography (EMG) allows for the quantification of speech muscle activity associated with developmental stuttering. Source: Image created by Rae Ajamie.

emerges in later childhood—years after the typical onset of stuttering[25]—it is clear that tremor does not cause stuttering.

A greater understanding of how neuromuscular activation may differ between PWS and their fluent peers may be achieved by examining the brain. Transcranial magnetic stimulation is a noninvasive method that can be used to explore the interaction between the left and right hemispheres and the excitability of the brain. The use of this technique has revealed that adults who stutter exhibit decreased motor excitability in left hemisphere brain areas associated with speech and language production, while fluent speakers present with the opposite pattern (i.e., increased excitability).[26,27] Although evidence is still being accumulated, it seems that PWS may have atypical neuromuscular activation from the motor cortex to the speech muscles. However, to fully appreciate the neuromotor processes involved in stuttering, we must have a better understanding of how the brain controls speech.

5.5 Level 4: Electrocortical Activation

If, as stated in the Introduction, stuttering disfluencies are the result of aberrant timing and sequencing of motor programs, processes within the brain must play a central role. Fluent speech requires the rapid coordination of multiple brain regions that have distinct, yet related processing tasks. According to psycholinguistic models, it takes approximately half a second from the conceptualization of a word to its articulation (see ► Chapter 4).[28] Stuttering disfluencies emerge during this short, dynamic period of time. How do we study this fleeting activity in a noninvasive way? Electroencephalography (EEG) measures brain function by directly recording electrical activity in the

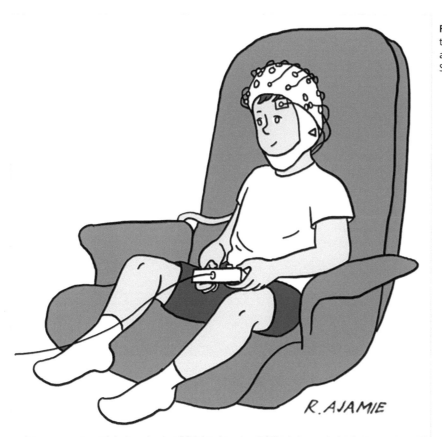

Fig. 5.4 Electroencephalography (EEG) allows for the quantification of electrocortical activation associated with developmental stuttering. Source: Image created by Rae Ajamie.

cortex (▶ Fig. 5.4), while magnetoencephalography (MEG) detects magnetic fields that are associated with electrical brain activity. Both EEG and MEG, which are recorded from electrodes on the scalp, have a high temporal resolution. This means that these methods are very sensitive to millisecond changes in brain activity associated with speech. A limitation of EEG and MEG is that both provide relatively low spatial resolution, meaning that it is difficult to know exactly where the brain activity is occurring.

Two EEG/MEG approaches that have been used to study stuttering are time-frequency analyses and event-related potentials (ERPs) or event-related fields (ERFs). Time-frequency analyses reflect changes in the strength of ongoing electrical activity, which are referred to as modulations. Studies that have examined modulations both before the onset of speech and during its execution have revealed that adults who stutter may have reduced coordination in the motor system relative to their fluent peers.[29,30]

If an event (such as auditory or visual stimuli) is repeatedly presented to a participant, EEG/MEG activity can be time locked (i.e., lined up in time) to this event and averaged across trials. This averaging process creates an ERP waveform, which can reveal important information about brain processes associated with sensory perception (detecting and interpreting sensory information from the environment), sensorimotor prediction (predicting the sensory consequences of speech), speech monitoring (monitoring the accuracy of speech before and during its production), and other cognitive activities (e.g., remembering, paying attention, etc.).

ERPs/ERFs elicited after seeing or hearing a stimulus (i.e., before speech is produced) have revealed that adults who stutter demonstrate abnormalities in auditory–motor integration and preverbal speech monitoring (they may perceive their speech plans as incorrect even if they are correct).[31,32] ERP studies have also revealed that PWS may have difficulties with various cognitive processes, such as inhibitory control (see ▶ Chapter 4).[33,34] A particular type of ERP, the contingent negative variation (CNV), may be generated by the basal ganglia and is a measure of cortical excitability associated with the preparation of speech.[35] Although previous findings have been mixed, the CNV measured right before speech appears to be greater in adults who stutter compared to fluent peers and this effect is largest for adults with severe stuttering.[36] Furthermore, CNV amplitude was observed to be increased before fluent words compared to stuttered words.[37] These differences in the CNV suggest that the basal ganglia may be overactivated during speech motor preparation in adults who stutter, which may represent a successful, albeit taxing, cognitive strategy for producing fluent speech.[37] ERPs/ERFs that are elicited to a sound, also known as auditory evoked potentials, have been used to examine the interactions between auditory processing and speech in PWS and their fluent peers.[38,39] Although both PWS and their peers demonstrate reduced brain activity during speech when compared to passive listening, adults who stutter exhibit shorter auditory evoked potential latencies in the right hemisphere during speech.[40] In other words, differences in cortical activation associated with auditory processes may contribute to stuttering.

5.6 Level 5: Brain Regions and Networks

Although the neuroanatomical and neurophysiological basis of speech production is not fully understood, we know that speech production is driven by a complex network of brain regions. This speech network plans, coordinates, and executes articulatory movements and connected speech sounds (see Levels 1 and 2). In the broadest of terms, the brain can be segmented into its two hemispheres. The brain network for speech and language spans both hemispheres, as regions across both are active during typical speech and language tasks. However, subtle differences in anatomic landmarks and brain function, especially for language, indicate that the networks are largely lateralized to the left hemisphere. In fact, approximately 94% of right-handed people and 84% of left-handed people are left-hemisphere dominant for language.[41] The lateralization of brain activity in PWS has been of interest since the 1920s, with early theories (e.g., the cerebral dominance theory) positing that stuttering was caused by an abnormal hemispheric imbalance in the speech production network. However, most modern views, informed by the latest in neuroimaging data, recognize the complex characteristics of brain activation across the speech networks and that hemispheric differences in PWS are likely dependent on the experimental task used and when the data are collected (i.e., childhood vs. adulthood).[42]

Here we briefly summarize current knowledge of typical speech production. The speech network spans the brain and includes several cortical and subcortical gray matter regions (composed of nerve cell bodies and dendrites) that are interconnected by numerous white matter fiber pathways (composed of myelinated axons). ▶ Fig. 5.5 displays the left hemisphere of the brain. The key speech and language areas are color coded and labeled accordingly. There is a large degree of overlap in the brain networks that support speech and language, and it is very difficult to tease them apart. Some studies have attempted to

examine only speech-motor control by creating stimuli with minimal linguistic information for production, such as simple syllables. Based on work using stimuli like this, a minimal speech production network has been identified that relies on the integration of motor, somatosensory, and auditory information.[43,44] The cortical areas that contribute to speech motor control, precise timing, and prosody of speech sounds include the inferior frontal gyrus (IFG), motor cortex, supplementary motor area, supramarginal gyrus, and superior temporal gyrus. Subcortical areas (e.g., basal ganglia and thalamus) and the cerebellum also play a role.

A widely cited neurocomputational model of speech production, named the Directions Into Velocities of Articulators (DIVA) model (see ▶ Chapter 2), posits that when we start speaking, neurons in the posterior IFG activate a representation of the sound and create an articulatory map that specifies, for example, where the sound is made in the mouth and whether the vocal folds vibrate, the sounds in a word or utterance that we want to produce.[45] This articulatory representation is then passed to neurons in the motor areas that send signals to the articulatory muscles, which initiate speech vocalizations. The supplementary motor area, cerebellum, and basal ganglia control the sequencing and timing of the speech sounds. When sounds are articulated, the superior temporal gyrus and supramarginal gyrus receive the articulatory representation and then forward it to the posterior IFG, which monitors the quality of production and detects potential errors.[46]

Advances in noninvasive neuroimaging over the past 30 years, especially magnetic resonance imaging (MRI; see ▶ Fig. 5.6), have allowed for an unprecedented surge in our ability to observe human brain structure and function. Structural imaging techniques allow us to visualize the size and shape of the brain to determine whether abnormalities are present, whereas functional imaging measures patterns of brain activity associated with perceptual, cognitive, behavioral, and emotional processes. Much of what we have learned is based on observations averaged across groups of PWS who volunteer to participate in

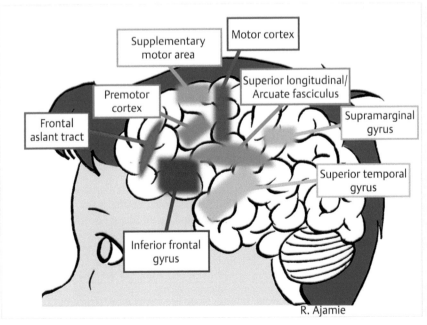

Fig. 5.5 Cortical areas of the brain associated with developmental stuttering. Source: Image created by Rae Ajamie.

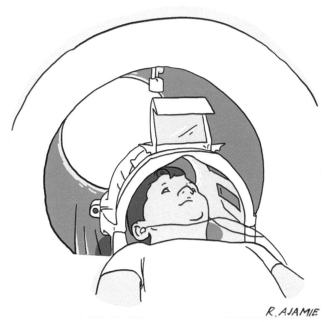

R. AJAMIE

Fig. 5.6 Magnetic resonance imaging (MRI) allows for the quantification of structural and functional brain characteristics associated with developmental stuttering. Source: Image created by Rae Ajamie.

neuroimaging studies. It is important to note that there is currently no known "stuttering spot" in the brain that causes developmental stuttering. That is, there is no single region in the brain that is grossly abnormal in any given individual who stutters or across all PWS. To obtain most of the observations discussed below, quantitative metrics must be averaged across many participants to reveal differences. At the group level, we have learned that there are differences between PWS and fluent speakers in various gray matter regions and white matter tracts.

5.6.1 Structural Differences in Brain Regions and Networks of PWS

Gray Matter

Structural MRI has been widely used to collect images of the brain with high spatial resolution. When we say that MR images of the brain have high spatial resolution, it means that more anatomical details are visible. Structural MRI measures of the brain commonly include gray matter volume and thickness. Accumulating evidence indicates that the parts of the brain that are associated with speech planning processes have reduced gray matter volume in PWS.[47,48] A study of cortical thickness across development in male school-age children who stutter revealed an abnormal pattern of development in the left IFG.[49] Specifically, typical development of cortical thickness in this area involves a peak in thickness in childhood with a slow and steady decline with age. These patterns are thought to reflect maturational processes in gray matter related to the growth and increased efficiency of neuronal networks. Incredibly, the pattern of left IFG thickness in the males who stutter was flat,

indicating that, unlike their peers who do not stutter, these children did not experience the typical burst in left IFG development, which may be related to their stuttering behaviors. A similar abnormal pattern of cortical thickness development has been found in the left premotor cortex, which lies just posterior to the IFG, in school-aged children who stutter.[50]

These developmental differences are not necessarily causal but may reflect changes in how the speech network matures. Other important brain regions for speech production have also been found to differ in structure in PWS relative to fluent peers.[51] For example, children who stutter have been shown to have increased gray matter volume in the middle prefrontal gyrus, postcentral gyrus, superior temporal gyrus, and the inferior parietal lobule and motor cortex in the right hemisphere relative to their fluent peers.[52]

Taken together, it is evident that structural differences occur across several critical regions involved in speech production in PWS relative to people who do not stutter. As one considers these differences across various gray matter regions in the speech network, it is only natural to wonder how these regions are connected structurally and then ultimately how they function together. The current view is that cognitive, linguistic, emotional, and speech-motor processes and their interactions across regions may be of more interest than the individual brain regions themselves. However, the posterior IFG, premotor cortex, and motor cortex are important for integrating auditory information (i.e., what you heard yourself say) and motor information (i.e., what you planned to say) and timing the movements of the speech articulators. In the following sections, we will discuss how these brain regions are connected and function for these important processes.

White Matter

Examining structural differences in the integrity or volume of the white matter pathways that connect the gray matter regions of the brain in individuals who stutter is also important. The gray matter of the brain network for speech is interconnected via the underlying white matter pathways. These pathways are analogous to a system of highways, roads, and streets for automobile traffic in that they merge into major pathways to carry information over long distances in the brain and diverge into smaller regional pathways before reaching their destination. Fractional anisotropy is a common measure used to infer information about the "integrity" or myelination of the white matter pathways linking language and speech motor regions of the brain. Using this measure, several studies have shown that both adults and children who stutter have decreased white matter integrity in the parts of the brain (e.g., left arcuate fasciculus, superior longitudinal fasciculus) that are thought to be involved in the mapping of speech sounds to motor plans.[6,53] Smaller volumes of white matter in these brain areas may reduce the efficiency of the language and speech mechanisms that are necessary for fluent speech.

5.6.2 Functional Differences in Brain Regions and Networks of PWS

Differences in brain structure may be related to how speech is produced in PWS. Brain activity can be measured using various functional imaging techniques, such as positron emission tomography and functional magnetic resonance imaging (fMRI). These techniques commonly detect changes in blood flow, glucose consumption, or oxygen utilization, for when the brain is active, more blood, glucose, and oxygen are needed for it to function properly. To date, several studies have reported anomalous brain function in PWS during speech and/or nonspeech tasks, indicating that stuttering may be associated with atypical speech and language planning processes.[54,55] For example, there is evidence that the motor cortex, which is responsible for motor execution, is engaged earlier than the IFG in stuttering, which is the opposite of the typical speech production process.[56] Similarly, atypical activity in the IFG, which is also important for language, has been found in adolescents and adults who stutter during speech production tasks.[52,57]

Reminiscent of the cerebral dominance theory of stuttering (see ▸ Chapter 5.2 Introduction above and ▸ Chapter 2), some investigators have argued that stuttering may be associated with an imbalance in hemispheric functioning during speech production.[58] Indeed, findings from some studies have revealed that the typical left lateralization of the motor cortex during speech preparation may not be present in adults who stutter.[59] Other studies have reported hemispheric differences in the activity of the right IFG, with more activity occurring in this area during stuttered speech and less activity following fluency shaping treatment.[48] However, it remains unclear if these differences in hemispheric activation are a compensatory mechanism that facilitates speech production.

Aberrant activity in subcortical structures—namely, the basal ganglia-thalamo-cortical motor circuit—that are important for making smooth transitions between syllables and words has also been reported in adults who stutter (see ▸ Fig. 5.7 for an image of the structures associated with this circuit).[60,61] To compensate for this aberrant activity, the cerebellum, which fine-tunes the timing of motor commands during speech production, may become more activated. Indeed, in adults who stutter, increased activity in the cerebellum has been associated with fluently produced utterances and the completion of

fluency shaping therapy.[48,62] Taken together, neuroimaging techniques have given us the tools with which to investigate the neural pathways involved in stuttering. These studies have demonstrated an array of possible abnormalities in the neural network for speech production in PWS. However, more research is clearly needed to better understand the neural and physiological processes of developmental stuttering.

5.7 Discussion

5.7.1 Theoretical Implications

The heterogeneity of stuttering behaviors across PWS, the situational variability in the elicitation of stuttering disfluencies, and the multiple levels of neurophysiological processes implicated in the disorder should underscore its intrinsic complexity. Despite the complexity, a growing consensus among researchers has resulted in several empirically supported assumptions about the etiology of developmental stuttering. First, empirical research of neural and physiological processes supports the view that developmental stuttering may be a disorder of speech motor performance, although influenced by multiple internal and external factors. The linguistic processes underlying fluent speech involve a complex series of events including the selection and retrieval of words from the mental lexicon, the retrieval and linking together of phonemes associated with the words, and the construction of syntactic phrase structure (see ▸ Chapter 4). All this must occur before the initiation of speech production. The motor control processes underlying fluent speech involve the retrieval of a learned representation of articulatory targets (commonly referred to as a motor program), the continuous and smooth articulation of these motor programs, and the online updating of these motor programs via sensorimotor adaptation.[63] The motor skills necessary for fluent speech are acquired through protracted practice during childhood, resulting in refined, efficient, and stable movement patterns that are predictable over a wide range of environmental conditions.[64]

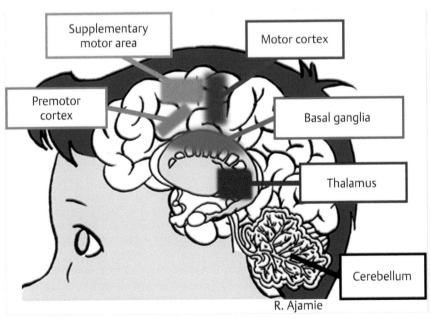

Fig. 5.7 Function of the basal ganglia-thalamo-cortical motor circuit appears to be associated with developmental stuttering. Source: Image created by Rae Ajamie.

Despite the complexities of speech, the seemingly little effort most individuals expend to produce fluent speech is due, in part, to increasing psychomotor efficiency—that is, better motor execution using fewer brain resources.[65] For novices (i.e., very young children and adults learning a new language), limitations in speech motor performance are most evident when capacity is stressed under increased processing demands. In the case of PWS, we speculate that these demands may disrupt the timing and sequencing of neural representations of articulatory movement commands (i.e., motor programs) to the speech muscles. To this point, some scientists have posited that PWS may reside on the lower end of a spectrum of speech motor skills.[66] The functioning of speech-language processes in PWS may be indistinguishable to people who do not stutter under optimal conditions; however, PWS may exhibit a "fragile" speech motor system that breaks down under environmental stressors. This dynamic would account for the multileveled disruptions across neural and physiological processes described in this chapter. This dynamic would also be consistent with multifactorial theories of developmental stuttering and therapeutic approaches that aim to increase capacities and reduce demands in children who stutter.[4,67]

Second, empirical research of neural and physiological processes supports the view that developmental stuttering may be a disorder of dysfunction within the basal ganglia-thalamo-cortical motor circuit.[3,68] This includes brain areas whose function includes the appropriate timing and initiation of speech sounds (or motor programs), which are then driven by the motor cortex to motor neuron pools in the brainstem, and then to the articulatory muscles. The potential instability of the speech motor system in PWS, even when perceptually fluent and revealed during articulation (see Level 2), may be related to how speech motor programs were learned in early childhood.[4] More specifically, a model of speech sound sequencing related to the DIVA model, the Gradient Order Directions Into Velocities of Articulators (GODIVA; see ► Chapter 2), proposes that a lack of white matter integrity within the basal ganglia-thalamo-cortical motor circuit may hinder the appropriate timing and sequencing of motor programs.[69] Interestingly, the produced acoustic output from computational simulations of such a brain deficit is similar to some stuttering disfluencies.[70]

Third, empirical research of neural and physiological processes supports the view that developmental stuttering may be a neurodevelopmental and multifactorial disorder. Neurodevelopmental disorders reflect atypical growth processes in the brain and are represented by individuals with autism spectrum disorder, fragile X syndrome, Williams syndrome, dyslexia, developmental language disorder, and developmental stuttering.[71] Across the multiple levels of neurophysiological processes explored, a consistent finding is that (1) PWS are a very heterogeneous population, (2) stuttering behaviors can change in an individual both suddenly and sometimes over years of exhibiting the disorder, and (3) some of these changes in young children represent neurodevelopmental trajectories toward recovery or persistence. Thus, there is a need to understand both the nature of risk factors for persistence and the mechanisms by which they may be related to stuttering in young children. Stuttering is thought by some to emerge from a complex combination of factors (e.g., motor, linguistic, emotional) and their

interactions that ultimately lead to breakdowns in speech-motor processes and speech fluency (i.e., it is multifactorial).

5.7.2 Treatment Implications and Future Directions

Current and future research in neural and physiological processes may contribute to the innovation of new treatments that target excitation or inhibition of key brain areas (e.g., IFG, premotor cortex, motor cortex, supplementary motor area, supramarginal gyrus, and superior temporal gyrus) in stuttering. Understanding the precise characteristics of the neurophysiology of developmental stuttering can yield causal insights into speech disfluencies and lead to a new generation of neuromodulation treatments for PWS. Noninvasive neuromodulation techniques, such as transcranial electrical stimulation or transcranial magnetic stimulation, alter nerve activity by applying electrical stimulation to the brain, spinal cord, nerves, or muscles. Although neuromodulation applications for developmental stuttering have not been extensively studied, there is some evidence to suggest that focal stimulation may improve speech fluency as a stand-alone treatment or in combination with behavioral techniques.[72,73,74] Such treatments may reduce stuttering severity and/or increase chances for recovery in children and facilitate more effective compensatory brain activity to alleviate stuttering disfluencies in adults. Future studies may also use transcranial alternating current stimulation to boost EEG activation at targeted frequencies (see Section "Level 4: Electrocortical Activation") to enhance brain activity associated with speech-motor processes. However, more research studies and ethical deliberation are needed to determine if these treatments are appropriate for children.

The most salient characteristic of developmental stuttering is, of course, the occurrence of stuttering disfluencies during speech production. If, as we suggest, these disfluencies represent disruptions in speech motor programming that result from interactions between neural systems for cognitive, linguistic, and emotional processes, it makes sense that some PWS may exhibit atypical abilities in these nonmotoric domains. As revealed in ► Chapters 4 and 6, PWS often demonstrate difficulties in executive function (e.g., working memory), linguistic processes, and emotion regulation. Considerable work has been done to understand how these processes may affect the speech motor systems of PWS, as described in Level 2. Still, much work remains to better understand the multitude of variables that contribute to stuttering, especially at the individual level. Speech is a complex and highly variable phenomenon and understanding the neural and physiological processes that affect, or are affected by, this disorder requires much ingenuity and perseverance among professionals with wide-ranging expertise who are dedicated to helping individuals with developmental stuttering. For example, research into the neurophysiology of stuttering has expanded beyond speech science and speech-language pathology, with new lines of research focusing on computational models, genetics/genomics (see ► Chapter 3), pharmacology (see ► Chapter 15), and animal modeling.[70,75,76,77]

Stuttering severity is often exacerbated in situations of high stress or when cognitive or linguistic complexity is high. These intertangled processes may stem from the atypical interaction of complex neurophysiological systems. The previously discussed research findings demonstrate that stuttering is likely a multifactorial problem. Neurophysiological research in stuttering often focuses on specific brain areas or systems. However, there is still a lack of large-scale studies that compare speech and nonspeech brain functions in PWS and fluent speakers. Furthermore, to better understand speech production in stuttering, future studies should use a whole-brain analysis or a combination of neurophysiological research methods to reveal differences at multiple levels (e.g., articulatory, neuromuscular, electrocortical, etc.). For example, combining EEG/ERP and fMRI methods would provide an analysis of both electrocortical and neural activation of the brain simultaneously.

Another important issue that needs to be addressed is the relation between neurophysiological abnormalities and how they may change over time. As discussed earlier, neurophysiological differences are evident in childhood; however, most findings rely on cross-sectional studies where data are collected at a given moment in time. It is still unclear whether these abnormalities persist in the long term and which play a role in recovery versus persistence. Longitudinal studies that track the development of children who stutter are likely to reveal more insights into the maturation processes in stuttering and its recovery.

5.8 Conclusion

The purpose of this chapter was to provide the reader with an overview of the neural and physiological processes that are associated with stuttering. Of course, there are disagreements among neuroscientists, speech scientists, speech-language pathologists, and other researchers on the exact nature of stuttering neurophysiology. This is the dynamic nature of science, especially when trying to understand the complexity of human social behavior of which stuttering is a part. Still, our knowledge of the neural and physiological basis of stuttering is increasing faster than ever before, with theoretical perspectives moving away from simple, univariate, homogeneous explanations to those that are more complex, multifactorial, and heterogeneous.

Revealing every scientific finding concerning neural and physiological processes is beyond the scope of this chapter, but we hope that this summary has shown that stuttering behaviors extend beyond the perceptible moments, such as stuttering disfluencies. Beyond the surface are a multitude of neural processes underlying speech, language, cognition, and emotion that contribute to the disorder, processes that may not be evident using behavioral measures alone. In our view, it is not adequate to simply say that stuttering is a "mystery" or that the "cause of stuttering is unknown." Rather, we believe that stuttering disfluencies may result from aberrant timing and sequencing of neural representations for speech within the basal ganglia-thalamo-cortical motor circuit and interactions between linguistic, cognitive, and emotional neural systems. Because of the dynamic, multifactorial, and complex nature of the disorder, stuttering behaviors may be dependent on the specific characteristics and capacities of the individual within their environment. For the clinician, understanding the neurophysiological bases of developmental stuttering may elucidate the development of the disorder, the likelihood of

recovery or persistence, and the potential for neuroplastic changes with treatment. Future advances in the treatment of developmental stuttering are likely to be influenced by new knowledge of its neural and physiological basis.

5.9 Definitions

Auditory evoked potential: An event-related electroencephalographic (EEG) potential recorded from the scalp and time locked to an acoustic stimulus.

Arcuate fasciculus: A fiber tract or bundle of axons that connect the temporal and frontal brain regions associated with speech and language.

Basal ganglia: A group of neurons underneath the cortex that includes the globus pallidus and striatum. The basal ganglia, associated with speech motor programming and learning, are connected to areas of the cortex, thalamus, and brainstem.

Cerebellum: Area of the posterior brain that contributes to speech motor control and other functions, including coordination and timing of movement.

Contingent negative variation (CNV): Event-related potential (ERP) elicited between a "warning" and "go" signal that is associated with speech motor preparation and control.

Diffuse tensor imaging: A method of magnetic resonance imaging used to measure fractional anisotropy of the white matter pathways in the brain.

Directions Into Velocities of Articulators (DIVA): A computational and neuroanatomical model of speech production that includes feedforward and feedback control processes.

Electrocortical activation: Electrical activity that can be recorded from the collected firing of action potentials from the cortex, often in response to a stimulus.

Electroencephalography (EEG): A method of recording of electrical brain activity using electrodes placed on the scalp.

Electromyography (EMG): A method of recording of electrical activity from muscle tissue using electrodes inserted into the muscle or placed on the skin surface.

Event-related potential or field (ERP/ERF): A time-locked and averaged EEG or magnetoencephalography (MEG) signal, respectively, related to a specific cognitive, linguistic, or motoric process and that is usually evoked by a relevant stimulus.

Fractional anisotropy: A scalar measure of density and myelination of white matter pathways in the brain.

Frontal aslant tract: A fiber tract or bundle of axons that connect the lateral inferior frontal gyrus and supplementary motor areas.

Functional imaging: Techniques such as EEG/MEG and functional magnetic resonance imaging (fMRI) that are used to measure neurophysiological changes in the brain.

Functional magnetic resonance imaging (fMRI): An indirect measure of brain activity, with high spatial resolution, using the detection of changes in cerebral blood flow (hemodynamic response).

Gradient Order Directions Into Velocities of Articulators (GODIVA): A computational model of speech production associated with neural processes for the initiation and sequencing of speech.

Gray matter: Areas of neuronal cell bodies in the brain whose activation is associated with speech-language processes.

Inferior frontal gyrus (IFG):   Gyrus in the lower frontal lobe that facilitates speech-language production.

Inferior parietal lobule: Area of the parietal lobe associated with language and other cognitive processes.

Magnetoencephalography (MEG):   A method of recording electrical brain activity from the scalp using generated magnetic fields.

Magnetic resonance imaging (MRI):   An imaging technique that uses a magnetic field to produce three-dimensional detailed anatomical images of brain structure.

Middle prefrontal gyrus: Gyrus or ridge of gray matter within the prefrontal cortex or frontal lobe.

Motor cortex: Area in the frontal lobe associated with the control and execution of movement.

Motor program: An abstract representation of movement in the brain.

Neuromuscular activation: The sending of motor commands from the brain to muscles.

Positron emission tomography: A brain imaging method that uses a radioactive drug (tracer) to show brain activity.

Postcentral gyrus: Gyrus or ridge of gray matter in the parietal lobe; location of the sensory cortex.

Premotor cortex: Area of the cortex that is anterior to the motor cortex and associated with speech motor programming.

Putamen: A subcortical structure of the basal ganglia, involved in the selection and initiation of movement sequences.

Structural imaging: Techniques such as MRI that are used to measure the structure of the brain.

Superior longitudinal fasciculus: A fiber tract or bundle of axons that connects the frontal, temporal, parietal, and occipital lobes, connecting areas of the brain associated with speech and language.

Superior temporal gyrus: Gyrus or ridge of gray matter in the temporal lobe; location of the auditory cortex.

Supplementary motor area: Part of the cerebral cortex, in front of the motor cortex that contributes to motor control.

Supramarginal gyrus: Gyrus or ridge of gray matter in the parietal lobe that is associated with language processes.

Thalamus: A subcortical area of gray matter that acts as a relay center for signaling between the cortex and basal ganglia associated with motor control.

Transcranial electrical stimulation: Neuromodulatory application of a low-intensity electrical current at a chosen frequency to stimulate the brain through electrodes placed on the scalp. Transcranial direct current stimulation involves the application of a constant, low-intensity electrical current. Transcranial alternating current stimulation involves the application of a current at a chosen frequency.

Transcranial magnetic stimulation: A method that uses magnetic fields to stimulate brain activity.

White matter: Tracts or connections of myelinated nerve fibers (i.e., axons) that send electrical impulses known as action potentials between areas of gray matter.

References

[1] Ludlow CL, Loucks T. Stuttering: a dynamic motor control disorder. J Fluency Disord. 2003; 28(4):273–295, quiz 295

[2] Summers JJ, Anson JG. Current status of the motor program: revisited. Hum Mov Sci. 2009; 28(5):566–577

[3] Chang S-E, Guenther FH. Involvement of the cortico-basal ganglia-thalamocortical loop in developmental stuttering. Front Psychol. 2020; 10:3088

[4] Smith A, Weber C. How stuttering develops: the multifactorial dynamic pathways theory. J Speech Lang Hear Res. 2017; 60(9):2483–2505

[5] Travis LE, Johnson W. Stuttering and the concept of handedness. Psychol Rev. 1934; 41(6):534–562

[6] Etchell AC, Civier O, Ballard KJ, Sowman PF. A systematic literature review of neuroimaging research on developmental stuttering between 1995 and 2016. J Fluency Disord. 2018; 55:6–45

[7] Smith A. Stuttering: A unified approach to a multifactorial, dynamic disorder. In: Ratner NB, Healey EC, eds. Stuttering Research and Practice: Bridging the Gap. New York, NY: Psychology Press; 1999:27–44

[8] Kleinow J, Smith A. Influences of length and syntactic complexity on the speech motor stability of the fluent speech of adults who stutter. J Speech Lang Hear Res. 2000; 43(2):548–559

[9] Jackson ES, Tiede M, Beal D, Whalen DH. The impact of social-cognitive stress on speech variability, determinism, and stability in adults who do and do not stutter. J Speech Lang Hear Res. 2016; 59(6):1295–1314

[10] Walsh B, Mettel KM, Smith A. Speech motor planning and execution deficits in early childhood stuttering. J Neurodev Disord. 2015; 7(1):27

[11] Usler E, Smith A, Weber C. A lag in speech motor coordination during sentence production is associated with stuttering persistence in young children. J Speech Lang Hear Res. 2017; 60(1):51–61

[12] Walsh B, Smith A, Weber-Fox C. Short-term plasticity in children's speech motor systems. Dev Psychobiol. 2006; 48(8):660–674

[13] Hall KD, Yairi E. Fundamental frequency, jitter, and shimmer in preschoolers who stutter. J Speech Hear Res. 1992; 35(5):1002–1008

[14] Subramanian A, Yairi E, Amir O. Second formant transitions in fluent speech of persistent and recovered preschool children who stutter. J Commun Disord. 2003; 36(1):59–75

[15] Zocchi L, Estenne M, Johnston S, Del Ferro L, Ward ME, Macklem PT. Respiratory muscle incoordination in stuttering speech. Am Rev Respir Dis. 1990; 141(6):1510–1515

[16] Peters HF, Boves L. Coordination of aerodynamic and phonatory processes in fluent speech utterances of stutterers. J Speech Hear Res. 1988; 31(3):352–361

[17] Tichenor S, Leslie P, Shaiman S, Yaruss JS. Speaker and observer perceptions of physical tension during stuttering. Folia Phoniatr Logop. 2017; 69(4):180–189

[18] Kazamel M, Warren PP. History of electromyography and nerve conduction studies: a tribute to the founding fathers. J Clin Neurosci. 2017; 43:54–60

[19] Shapiro AI. An electromyographic analysis of the fluent and dysfluent utterances of several types of stutterers. J Fluency Disord. 1980; 5(3):203–231

[20] Freeman FJ, Ushijima T. Laryngeal muscle activity during stuttering. J Speech Hear Res. 1978; 21(3):538–562

[21] Smith A. Neural drive to muscles in stuttering. J Speech Hear Res. 1989; 32(2):252–264

[22] Walsh B, Smith A. Oral electromyography activation patterns for speech are similar in preschoolers who do and do not stutter. J Speech Lang Hear Res. 2013; 56(5):1441–1454

[23] Fibiger S. Stuttering explained as a physiological tremor. STL-QPSR. 1971; 2(3):1–24

[24] Denny M, Smith A. Gradations in a pattern of neuromuscular activity associated with stuttering. J Speech Hear Res. 1992; 35(6):1216–1229

[25] Kelly EM, Smith A, Goffman L. Orofacial muscle activity of children who stutter: a preliminary study. J Speech Hear Res. 1995; 38(5):1025–1036

[26] Alm PA, Karlsson R, Sundberg M, Axelson HW. Hemispheric lateralization of motor thresholds in relation to stuttering. PLoS One. 2013; 8(10):e76824

[27] Barwood CHS, Murdoch BE, Goozee JV, Riek S. Investigating the neural basis of stuttering using transcranial magnetic stimulation: preliminary case discussions. Speech Lang Hear. 2013; 16(1):18–27

[28] Indefrey P, Levelt WJM. The spatial and temporal signatures of word production components. Cognition. 2004; 92(1)(–)(2):101–144

[29] Jenson D, Reilly KJ, Harkrider AW, Thornton D, Saltuklaroglu T. Trait related sensorimotor deficits in people who stutter: an EEG investigation of μ rhythm dynamics during spontaneous fluency. Neuroimage Clin. 2018; 19:690–702

[30] Mersov A-M, Jobst C, Cheyne DO, De Nil L. Sensorimotor oscillations prior to speech onset reflect altered motor networks in adults who stutter. Front Hum Neurosci. 2016; 10:443

[31] Daliri A, Max L. Electrophysiological evidence for a general auditory prediction deficit in adults who stutter. Brain Lang. 2015; 150:37–44

[32] Daliri A, Max L. Modulation of auditory responses to speech vs. nonspeech stimuli during speech movement planning. Front Hum Neurosci. 2016; 10: 234

[33] Arnstein D, Lakey B, Compton RJ, Kleinow J. Preverbal error-monitoring in stutterers and fluent speakers. Brain Lang. 2011; 116(3):105–115

[34] Piispala J, Määttä S, Pääkkönen A, Bloigu R, Kallio M, Jansson-Verkasalo E. Atypical brain activation in children who stutter in a visual Go/Nogo task: an ERP study. Clin Neurophysiol. 2017; 128(1):194–203

[35] Prescott J. Event-related potential indices of speech motor programming in stutterers and non-stutterers. Biol Psychol. 1988; 27(3):259–273

[36] Vanhoutte S, Santens P, Cosyns M, et al. Increased motor preparation activity during fluent single word production in DS: a correlate for stuttering frequency and severity. Neuropsychologia. 2015; 75:1–10

[37] Vanhoutte S, Cosyns M, van Mierlo P, et al. When will a stuttering moment occur? The determining role of speech motor preparation. Neuropsychologia. 2016; 86:93–102

[38] Beal DS, Cheyne DO, Gracco VL, Quraan MA, Taylor MJ, De Nil LF. Auditory evoked fields to vocalization during passive listening and active generation in adults who stutter. Neuroimage. 2010; 52(4):1645–1653

[39] Beal DS, Quraan MA, Cheyne DO, Taylor MJ, Gracco VL, De Nil LF. Speech-induced suppression of evoked auditory fields in children who stutter. Neuroimage. 2011; 54(4):2994–3003

[40] Sowman PF, Crain S, Harrison E, Johnson BW. Lateralization of brain activation in fluent and non-fluent preschool children: a magnetoencephalographic study of picture-naming. Front Hum Neurosci. 2014; 8:354

[41] Mazoyer B, Zago L, Jobard G, et al. Gaussian mixture modeling of hemispheric lateralization for language in a large sample of healthy individuals balanced for handedness. PLoS One. 2014; 9(6):e101165

[42] Beal DS, Lerch JP, Cameron B, Henderson R, Gracco VL, De Nil LF. The trajectory of gray matter development in Broca's area is abnormal in people who stutter. Front Hum Neurosci. 2015; 9:89

[43] Bohland JW, Guenther FH. An fMRI investigation of syllable sequence production. Neuroimage. 2006; 32(2):821–841

[44] Sörös P, Sokoloff LG, Bose A, McIntosh AR, Graham SJ, Stuss DT. Clustered functional MRI of overt speech production. Neuroimage. 2006; 32(1): 376–387

[45] Tourville JA, Guenther FH. The DIVA model: a neural theory of speech acquisition and production. Lang Cogn Process. 2011; 26(7):952–981

[46] Guenther FH. Cortical interactions underlying the production of speech sounds. J Commun Disord. 2006; 39(5):350–365

[47] Beal DS, Gracco VL, Brettschneider J, Kroll RM, De Nil LF. A voxel-based morphometry (VBM) analysis of regional grey and white matter volume abnormalities within the speech production network of children who stutter. Cortex. 2013; 49(8):2151–2161

[48] Kell CA, Neumann K, von Kriegstein K, et al. How the brain repairs stuttering. Brain. 2009; 132(Pt 10):2747–2760

[49] Garnett EO, Chow HM, Nieto-Castañón A, Tourville JA, Guenther FH, Chang S-E. Anomalous morphology in left hemisphere motor and premotor cortex of children who stutter. Brain. 2018; 141(9):2670–2684

[50] Chang S-E, Erickson KI, Ambrose NG, Hasegawa-Johnson MA, Ludlow CL. Brain anatomy differences in childhood stuttering. Neuroimage. 2008; 39(3): 1333–1344

[51] Sommer M, Koch MA, Paulus W, Weiller C, Büchel C. Disconnection of speech-relevant brain areas in persistent developmental stuttering. Lancet. 2002; 360(9330):380–383

[52] Watkins KE, Smith SM, Davis S, Howell P. Structural and functional abnormalities of the motor system in developmental stuttering. Brain. 2008; 131(Pt 1):50–59

[53] Belyk M, Kraft SJ, Brown S. Stuttering as a trait or state - an ALE meta-analysis of neuroimaging studies. Eur J Neurosci. 2015; 41(2):275–284

[54] Metzger FL, Auer T, Helms G, et al. Shifted dynamic interactions between subcortical nuclei and inferior frontal gyri during response preparation in persistent developmental stuttering. Brain Struct Funct. 2018; 223(1):165–182

[55] Walsh B, Tian F, Tourville JA, Yücel MA, Kuczek T, Bostian AJ. Hemodynamics of speech production: an fNIRS investigation of children who stutter. Sci Rep. 2017; 7(1):4034

[56] Salmelin R, Schnitzler A, Schmitz F, Freund HJ. Single word reading in developmental stutterers and fluent speakers. Brain. 2000; 123(Pt 6): 1184–1202

[57] Neef NE, Bütfering C, Anwander A, Friederici AD, Paulus W, Sommer M. Left posterior-dorsal area 44 couples with parietal areas to promote speech fluency, while right area 44 activity promotes the stopping of motor responses. Neuroimage. 2016; 142:628–644

[58] Braun AR, Varga M, Stager S, et al. Altered patterns of cerebral activity during speech and language production in developmental stuttering. An H2(15)O positron emission tomography study. Brain. 1997; 120(Pt 5):761–784

[59] Neef NE, Hoang TNL, Neef A, Paulus W, Sommer M. Speech dynamics are coded in the left motor cortex in fluent speakers but not in adults who stutter. Brain. 2015; 138(Pt 3):712–725

[60] Harrewijn A, Schel MA, Boelens H, Nater CM, Haggard P, Crone EA. Children who stutter show reduced action-related activity in the rostral cingulate zone. Neuropsychologia. 2017; 96:213–221

[61] Neef NE, Anwander A, Bütfering C, et al. Structural connectivity of right frontal hyperactive areas scales with stuttering severity. Brain. 2018; 141(1): 191–204

[62] Neumann K, Preibisch C, Euler HA, et al. Cortical plasticity associated with stuttering therapy. J Fluency Disord. 2005; 30(1):23–39

[63] Houde JF, Jordan MI. Sensorimotor adaptation in speech production. Science. 1998; 279(5354):1213–1216

[64] Green JR, Nip ISB. Some organization principles in early speech development. In: Maassen B, van Lieshout P, eds. Speech Motor Control: New developments in basic and applied research. Oxford: Oxford University Press; 2010:171–188

[65] Hatfield BD. Brain dynamics and motor behavior: a case for efficiency and refinement for superior performance. Kinesiol Rev (Champaign). 2018; 7(1): 42–50

[66] Namasivayam AK, van Lieshout P. Speech motor skill and stuttering. J Mot Behav. 2011; 43(6):477–489

[67] Walden TA, Frankel CB, Buhr AP, Johnson KN, Conture EG, Karrass JM. Dual diathesis-stressor model of emotional and linguistic contributions to developmental stuttering. J Abnorm Child Psychol. 2012; 40(4):633–644

[68] Alm PA. Stuttering and the basal ganglia circuits: a critical review of possible relations. J Commun Disord. 2004; 37(4):325–369

[69] Bohland JW, Bullock D, Guenther FH. Neural representations and mechanisms for the performance of simple speech sequences. J Cogn Neurosci. 2010; 22(7):1504–1529

[70] Civier O, Bullock D, Max L, Guenther FH. Computational modeling of stuttering caused by impairments in a basal ganglia thalamo-cortical circuit involved in syllable selection and initiation. Brain Lang. 2013; 126(3):263–278

[71] Karmiloff-Smith A. Atypical epigenesis. Dev Sci. 2007; 10(1):84–88

[72] Yada Y, Tomisato S, Hashimoto R-I. Online cathodal transcranial direct current stimulation to the right homologue of Broca's area improves speech fluency in people who stutter. Psychiatry Clin Neurosci. 2019; 73(2):63–69

[73] Garnett EO, Chow HM, Choo AL, Chang S-E. Stuttering severity modulates effects of non-invasive brain stimulation in adults who stutter. Front Hum Neurosci. 2019; 13:411

[74] Chesters J, Möttönen R, Watkins KE. Transcranial direct current stimulation over left inferior frontal cortex improves speech fluency in adults who stutter. Brain. 2018; 141(4):1161–1171

[75] Maguire GA, Nguyen DL, Simonson KC, Kurz TL. The pharmacologic treatment of stuttering and its neuropharmacologic basis. Front Neurosci. 2020; 14:158

[76] Chow HM, Garnett EO, Li H, et al. Linking lysosomal enzyme targeting genes and energy metabolism with altered gray matter volume in children with persistent stuttering. Neurobiol Lang. 2020; 1(3):365–380

[77] Kubikova L, Bosikova E, Cvikova M, Lukacova K, Scharff C, Jarvis ED. Basal ganglia function, stuttering, sequencing, and repair in adult songbirds. Sci Rep. 2014; 4:6590

Further Readings

Chang SE, Garnett EO, Etchell A, Chow HM. Functional and neuroanatomical bases of developmental stuttering: current insights. Neuroscientist. 2019; 25(6):566–582

Etchell AC, Civier O, Ballard KJ, Sowman PF. A systematic literature review of neuroimaging research on developmental stuttering between 1995 and 2016. J Fluency Disord. 2018; 55:6–45

Guenther FH. Neural control of speech. Cambridge, MA: MIT Press; 2006

Smith A, Weber C. How stuttering develops: the multifactorial dynamic pathways theory. J Speech Lang Hear Res. 2017; 60(9):2483–2505

6 Temperamental and Emotional Processes

Robin Jones, Kurt Eggers, and Hatun Zengin-Bolatkale

Abstract

The purpose of this chapter is to describe and discuss temperamental and emotional processes that are associated with developmental stuttering. In doing so, the chapter will provide a definition, brief history, and broad overview of temperament, as well as emotional reactivity and regulation processes, serving as the foundation for readers to better understand the relation between these processes and stuttering. Building on this foundation, the chapter will review empirical evidence and theoretical perspectives on the role of temperamental and emotional processes in developmental stuttering along with potential clinical considerations for assessment and treatment. At the outset, it should be noted that while this chapter is designed to cover the lifespan, it will primarily focus on children because this age range has been studied the most with regard to temperamental and emotional processes.

Keywords: stuttering, fluency disorder, temperament, emotion, regulation

6.1 Brief Overview of Temperament and Emotional Processes

6.1.1 Temperament

Historical Perspective on Temperament

The construct of temperament has been considered throughout history. The ancient Greeks, for example, used a temperament model to explain behavioral characteristics. According to this view, behavior was the result of biological differences in bodily fluids, referred to as the four humors (blood, yellow bile, black bile, and phlegm). Individual differences in behavior resulted from the balance or imbalance of these humors, leading to four behavioral types: melancholic (sad), choleric (irritable), sanguine (optimistic), and phlegmatic (calm; ▶ Fig. 6.1). Thus, according to this typology, individual differences in behavior were linked to underlying physiological mechanisms.[1] Recent studies on the biological basis of temperament, showing the relation between emotions and the endocrine system,[2,3] have provided support for this ancient conceptualization.

Depiction of Temperamental Typologies

In the 20th century, there was renewed interest in studying temperament. Some researchers tried to explain individual differences in terms of physiological constructs, based on a wide range of empirical studies,[4] whereas others concentrated on maturational aspects, which supported the role of heredity, separate from environmental influences.[5] In the latter half of the 20th century, the nature-versus-nurture debate emerged in response to increased emphasis on individual differences in behavior. Scholars who supported the *nature* perspective

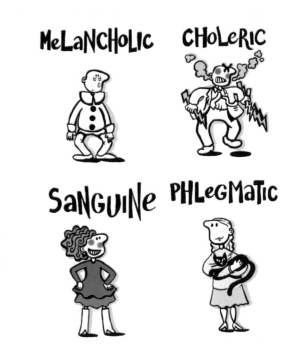

Fig. 6.1 This figure depicts the fourfold temperament typology that is, melancholic (sad), choleric (irritable), sanguine (optimistic), and phlegmatic (calm) that was used to explain the different behavioral types. Source: Image created by Lucia Fabiani.

argued that individual differences were a product of genetics and biology, whereas those who embraced the *nurture* point of view stressed the importance of early environmental influences on behavior.[6] Both, however, acknowledged that the behavioral expression of temperament characteristics is influenced by situational factors.

During the last few decades, temperament has been conceptualized in different ways, depending on the perspective of the researchers. For example:

- Thomas and Chess viewed temperament as representing individual differences in behavior (e.g., activity level, attentional characteristics, adaptability, mood, approach/withdrawal).[7]
- Buss and Plomin defined temperament as differences in emotionality, activity, and sociability.[8]
- Goldsmith and Campos characterized temperament from an emotion-oriented point of view—namely, individual differences in the experience and expression of emotions, such as distress, fear, anger, sadness, pleasure, and surprise.[9]
- Kagan's concept of temperament referred to inherited behavioral and biological profiles that underlie reaction patterns, primarily focusing on inhibited (e.g., shy, reserved, timid) and uninhibited (e.g., social, spontaneous, low fear) temperaments.[2]

Although some of these conceptualizations focus mainly or even exclusively on emotion-oriented traits and others on behavioral style, they are similar in that they all refer to characteristics in which individuals differ.

Contemporary Perspective on Temperament

At present, most theorists agree that temperament refers to biologically based individual differences that are relatively stable over time, and appear early in development.[10] Recent models further acknowledge that temperament develops over time,[11,12] incorporates motivational and self-regulatory systems,[13] and is influenced by environmental interactions.[14,15]

Rothbart's temperament model, which defines temperament as constitutionally based individual differences in reactivity and self-regulation, has gained much popularity among child-oriented researchers.[12,16] *Reactivity* refers to the arousability of physiological and sensory response systems (e.g., getting frustrated about something), and *self-regulation* are processes that can modulate (facilitate or inhibit) one's reactivity (e.g., shifting one's attentional focus away from the frustrating stimulus). *Constitutional* refers to the biological basis of temperament (i.e., it is something you are born with), which is influenced over time by genetics, maturation, and experience. In other words, the temperament structure changes over time, from a

predominantly reactivity-driven concept in infants to a structure with more emphasis on self-regulatory processes in older children. For example, when infants are distressed, they will cry, much to the dismay of their parents; older children, on the other hand, can deal with distress using a broader range of tools, such as shifting their attention away from that which they find distressing.[17]

Rothbart[12] developed a framework specifying the role and interactional patterns of reactivity and self-regulation (▶ Fig. 6.2). When a child is confronted with a stimulus, this stimulus might lead to positive (e.g., smiling) or negative (e.g., fear, anger) reactivity within the child. As the child grows older, he or she will be able to consciously (hence the term "effort" in the figure) modulate this reactivity by using self-regulation processes to increase positive reactivity and/or decrease negative reactivity. Note that an increase in positive reactivity does not necessarily correspond with a decrease in negative reactivity and vice versa. Children can, for example, become less fearful without smiling and laughing. Self-regulation processes include executive attention variables (e.g., consciously driven attention shifting) and effortful control (the ability to inhibit a dominant [motor] response in order to perform a subdominant response, detect errors, and engage in planning).[18]

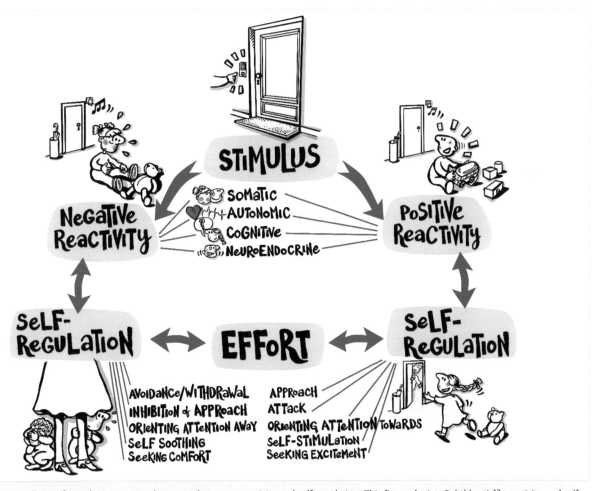

Fig. 6.2 Framework specifying the interactional patterns between reactivity and self-regulation. This figure depicts Robthbart's[12] reactivity and self-regulation framework. Children with more positive reactivity and strong self-regulation skills may become excited and approach the door when the doorbell rings. On the other hand, children with negative reactivity and strong self-regulation skills may stand behind mom when the doorbell rings. Source: Image created by Lucia Fabiani.

Positive and negative reactivities are expressed via somatic (e.g., facial expressions), autonomic (e.g., increase in heart rate), cognitive (e.g., alerting), and neuroendocrine (e.g., cortisol release) reactions and can be experienced as pleasure or distress. When the intensity of the stimulus is high, children who are more prone to react negatively will experience greater distress, whereas children who are less likely to react negatively will experience feelings of pleasure. These reactions (i.e., somatic, autonomic, cognitive, and neuroendocrine) do not follow the same time course:[19] cognitive reactions may be initiated within a few milliseconds, whereas neuroendocrine reactions take anywhere from a few minutes to a few hours.[12]

Children have different levels of reactivity—some react with more intense feelings of distress or pleasure, whereas others react more mildly. Children also differ in the ease with which they are able to apply attentional (e.g., looking toward [attentional orienting] or away from [attentional shifting] an exciting or distressing event) and motor control processes (e.g., self-soothing by thumb sucking) to regulate their reactivity.[12,20] Self-regulation is triggered by the positive or negative reactions experienced by a child (e.g., negative reactivity elicits withdrawal, while positive reactivity elicits approach) and by stimulus characteristics (such as high vs. low intensity). These self-regulatory processes will, in turn, modulate (facilitate or inhibit) reactivity, showing a bidirectional relationship between these two processes.

6.1.2 Measurement of Temperament

Since there is no consensus among researchers as to how temperament should be defined, there is no commonly accepted view of how temperament should be measured.[1] Several approaches have been used to measure temperament in children, including caregiver/parent questionnaires and surveys, self-reports for older children, (semi-) structured interviews, home observational measures and laboratory measures, and psychophysical and psychophysiological measures. Every method has its relative advantages and disadvantages,[21,22] which underscores the benefit of using multiple approaches to assess temperament (▸ Table 6.1).

Rothbart et al developed a set of validated temperament questionnaires (caregiver report or self-report depending on age group), such as the *Children's Behavior Questionnaire* (CBQ) [16] aimed at 3- to 7-year-old children. The CBQ consists of 15 scales (▸ Table 6.2), clustering under the three broad dimensions of Rothbart's temperament model, labeled as extraversion/surgency (or positive reactivity), negative affectivity (or negative reactivity), and effortful control (or self-regulation). As we describe later, these measures have been used in the empirical study of developmental stuttering and can also be used in the clinical assessment of stuttering.

Temperament plays an important role in the experience and expression of emotions such as distress, fear, anger, sadness, pleasure, and surprise. How easily does a child get frustrated? How does a child respond to frustration? Does he or she use physical aggression, cry, or seek help? Temperament relates to children's in-the-moment emotional states, and their emotional states determine their behavior. Therefore, it is important to investigate emotions, emotional reactivity and regulation, and how they relate to behavior.

6.1.3 Emotion

Emotions are critical for survival and adaptation as they motivate human behavior. Although there is no consensus on a single definition, the present most widely accepted view is that emotions are neurally based affective states that involve conscious experience and overt or internal physical responses that facilitate or inhibit behaviors.

Historical theories are important for our present understanding of emotions as they guide how the empirical work in the field of psychology has been conducted in the past century. In this section, we will briefly discuss some of the more prominent ones, including the James–Lange theory and Papez circuit. According to the James–Lange theory, which was developed in the 19th century, emotions result from changes in physiological arousal.[23] For example, when we see a snake while out hiking, our pupils will dilate, our heart rate will go up, and we will start running away. These physiological changes lead to the subjective experience of fear.

Considerable progress has been made in the field of psychology after Papez improved and expanded on the earlier theories and proposed a set of structures, known as the "Papez circuit," that are responsible for the emotional experience.[24] Papez suggested that sensory input concerning emotional stimuli is transmitted from the thalamus into two streams: the upstream ("thought stream") and the downstream ("feeling stream"). The *upstream* directs the sensory input to the parts of the brain that transform the sensation into perceptions, thoughts, and memories. The *downstream* conveys the sensory input to the body for emotional expression.[24,25]

Researchers also started taking cognitive interpretations into consideration in the emotional experience after Schachter and Singer[26] proposed that emotions involved two key components: physiological arousal and cognitive label. For example, if you saw a burglar enter your home, your heart rate would begin to race, and you might start to sweat. This physiological response, however, can also occur in other situations, such as when you catch sight of someone you are in love with. So, why do you experience fear when you see the burglar and not happiness? The answer, according to Schachter and Singer, is that your brain must also determine *why* the physiological arousal is

Table 6.1 Examples of advantages and disadvantages of measurement approaches used to study temperament

	Parent questionnaires	Home observation	Laboratory measures
Advantages	Based on parental knowledge of child over a long period of time and across many situations	Potentially higher level of objectivity of the measurement of the child's behavior	Researchers are able to precisely control the context of the child's behavior
Disadvantages	Potentially biased by subjective factors (e.g., perceptual bias of the informant)	Often unable to capture all relevant behaviors in a somewhat restricted observation	Limited to the types of behaviors elicited by the laboratory task and measures

Table 6.2 Children's behavior questionnaire (CBQ) scale definitions and sample items[16]

CBQ-scale	Definition (sample item)
Factor 1: extraversion/surgency	
Activity level	The level of gross motor activity including rate and extent of locomotion. *Sample item: moves about actively (runs, climbs, jumps) when playing in the house*
Approach/positive anticipation	The amount of excitement and positive anticipation for expected pleasurable activities. *Sample item: becomes very excited while planning for trips*
High-intensity pleasure	The amount of pleasure or enjoyment related to situations involving high stimulus intensity, rate, complexity, novelty, and incongruity. *Sample item: likes to play so wild and recklessly that he or she might get hurt*
Impulsivity	The speed of response initiation. *Sample item: usually rushes into an activity without thinking about it*
Shyness (negative loading)	Slow or inhibited approach in situations involving novelty or uncertainty. *Sample item: sometimes prefers to watch rather than join other children playing*
Smiling and laughter	The amount of positive affect in response to changes in stimulus intensity, rate, complexity, and incongruity. *Sample item: laughs a lot at jokes and silly happenings*
Factor 2: negative affectivity	
Anger/frustration	The amount of negative affect related to interruption of ongoing tasks or goal blocking. *Sample item: gets quite frustrated when prevented from doing something he or she wants to do*
Discomfort	The amount of negative affect related to sensory qualities of stimulation, including intensity, rate or complexity of light, movement, sound, or texture. *Sample item: is quite upset by a little cut or bruise*
Falling reactivity and soothability	The rate of recovery from peak distress, excitement, or general arousal. *Sample item: calms down quickly following an exciting event*
Fear	The amount of negative affect, including unease, worry, or nervousness related to anticipated pain or distress, and/or potentially threatening situations. *Sample item: is afraid of loud noises*
Sadness	The amount of negative affect and lowered mood and energy related to exposure to suffering, disappointment, and object loss. *Sample item: becomes upset when loved relatives or friends are getting ready to leave following a visit*
Factor 3: effortful control	
Attentional focusing	The tendency to maintain attentional focus upon task-related channels. *Sample item: when picking up toys or other jobs, usually keeps at the task until it is done*
Inhibitory control	The capacity to plan and to suppress inappropriate approach responses under instructions or in novel or uncertain situations. *Sample item: can easily stop an activity when he or she is told "no"*
Low-intensity pleasure	The amount of pleasure or enjoyment related to situations involving low stimulus intensity, rate, complexity, novelty, and incongruity. *Sample item: enjoys "snuggling up" next to a parent*
Perceptual sensitivity	The amount of detection of slight, low-intensity stimuli from the external environment. *Sample item: is quickly aware of some new items in the living room*

occurring—that is, a cognitive label must be applied to the situation (e.g., "the burglar is scary"). It is the cognitive label that determines which emotion is experienced.[25]

Current theories of emotion propose that multiple components are involved: physiological changes, feelings and thoughts, and expressive behavior (▶ Fig. 6.3). Therefore, the American Psychological Association defines emotion as "a complex reaction pattern, involving experiential, behavioral, and physiological elements."[27] Emotional arousal to external stimuli can result in significant physiological changes in the body such as increased heart rate, increased sweating, and pupil dilation. Emotional arousal (i.e., reactivity) also involves feelings and thoughts about the impact of the external stimuli (e.g., perceiving it as a reward or punishment) and how it makes us feel depending on the context (e.g., anxious, threatened, thrilled, nervous, etc.). Apart from physiological changes, emotional arousal can also result in overt behavioral responses such as running, freezing, or facial responses such as frowning, smiling, and grimacing.

Types of Emotions

There has been much debate in the psychology literature over the classification of emotions. The two major models used to classify the types of emotions are dimensional models and categorical models. Dimensional models categorize emotions based on two or three dimensions. Schlosberg[28] and colleagues, for instance, suggested that emotions are defined according to three dimensions: (1) pleasantness–unpleasantness, (2) level of activation/arousal (sleep–tension), and (3) acceptance–rejection. For example, "disgust" and "depressed" are both unpleasant emotions that differ in level of activation/arousal (*depressed* is closer to "sleep" and *disgust* is closer to "tension") and acceptance-rejection (*depressed* is closer to "acceptance" and *disgust* is closer to "rejection").[29]

Categorical models of emotions are based on discrete emotion theory, which proposes that there is a set of *basic emotions* that are universally experienced by all humans: *anger, disgust, fear, sadness, happiness,* and *surprise.*[30] All other emotions experienced result from various combinations of these emotions. These basic emotions are not only cross-cultural but are observed in other animals as well. Categorical models also posit that emotions and dimensions of temperament and personality traits are highly related to each other.[31] Further, it is proposed that each of the basic emotions impacts cognition[32] (e.g., executive functions, thoughts) and behavior in particular ways and individual differences in "emotion thresholds"

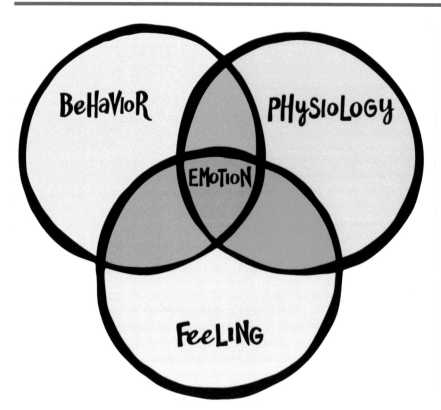

Fig. 6.3 Components of emotion. This figure depicts the multiple components of emotion, which include physiological changes, feelings and thoughts, and expressive behavior. Source: Image created by Lucia Fabiani.

yield different patterns of behavior and thinking that shapes one's personality.[31,33]

At present, it is widely accepted that both models of categorizing emotions contribute to understanding and studying emotions, and the adoption of one of these models does not negate the other.[34] Further, although there is abundant evidence to support the existence of cross-cultural emotions, it is also acknowledged that certain emotions are influenced by cultural norms and practices. For example, for people who grew up in America, happiness is a high-arousal positive emotional state, while people who grew up in China tend to associate happiness with low-arousal positive emotional states, feeling solemn, and reserved.[35]

Emotional Development and Regulation

An important concept regarding emotion relates to regulation. Emotion regulation, also referred to as self-regulation, relates to "the ways individuals influence which emotions they have, when they have them, and how they experience and express these emotions" (p.557).[36] There are several ways emotions can be regulated. Some of the most popular emotional regulation strategies are (1) the *cognitive-linguistic strategy*, which involves reappraising a stimulus or condition in a different/more positive light; (2) the *suppression* of negative emotions and reduction of associated physiological and behavioral reactivity; and (3) *distraction*, which refers to directing attention away from emotional stimuli.

The successful use of these emotional regulation strategies is highly dependent on age and maturation,[37] given that they depend on the development of the prefrontal cortex, executive function skills (e.g., inhibitory control),[38] and linguistic skills.[39] The use of the cognitive-linguistic strategy tends to appear at around 5 years of age; infants and toddlers rely more on distraction and social support from others.[40] Preschool-age children use simple regulation strategies such as suppression, while children older than 5 years of age use the cognitive-linguistic strategy, which further develops with increasing age.[37] Between childhood and adulthood, during mid-adolescence, there is a temporary decline in the use of advanced emotion regulation strategies, such as cognitive-linguistic strategy and social support seeking, and more reliance on suppression and dysfunctional rumination.[41] This is thought to be associated with greater emotional instability due to intense neurological and hormonal changes, greater desire to please peers, and increased conflicts with parents.[42] For example, when dealing with sadness or anger, adolescents might be less likely to choose an adaptive emotion regulation strategy, such as social support seeking, due to their perceived lack of support from their family or their desire to maintain a strong, positive social image among peers. Further, there are significant gender differences in the development of emotion regulation, with females being more likely to successfully use various emotion regulation strategies earlier than males.[37,41]

Measurement of Emotions

Although there are plenty of standardized measures available for the assessment of cognitive and linguistic skills, emotional measures are relatively scarce. The measurement of emotions in children is significantly more challenging than assessment in adults. Nevertheless, a growing base of evidence and advances in technology has enabled emotions to be measured from infancy through adulthood. Given the multidimensional and complex nature of emotions, various methods have been used to measure emotions—namely, self-report measures, behavior observations, and psychophysiology.[43]

Self-report measures in the form of paper-and-pencil or online surveys or interviews are used to assess emotional *traits* (i.e., dispositions) or *states*,[44] such as subjective experiences, thoughts, and feelings. Self-report measures have good face validity and are cheaper and easier to administer than other methods. However, they also require a high level of self-awareness, which may be difficult for young children, and depend on the individual's ability and willingness to truthfully and openly report their emotional experiences.[45] Another method of assessing emotions is by observing individuals' *nonverbal behaviors* such as their vocal characteristics (e.g., higher levels of arousal has been associated with higher-pitched voice),[46] body movements and gestures (e.g., greater pride associated with bigger and more expansive body posture and movements),[47] and facial expressions (e.g., coding emotions based on anatomical landmarks and associated muscle movements such as raising of the eyebrows, upward movement of the lips, etc.).[48] Behavioral observations can be particularly useful when participants are not able or willing to report their emotional experiences, but they can be impractical and expensive, as well as time-consuming.[44]

It has become increasingly popular to measure emotions via *psychophysiology*, such as measurement of autonomic and central nervous system activity. The autonomic nervous system is primarily responsible for the "fight or flight" response and it consists of sympathetic (responsible for activation/reactivity) and parasympathetic (responsible for relaxation/regulation) activity.[43,44] As discussed earlier, the brain is responsible for both somatic arousal and emotional experience. Therefore, measuring central nervous system activity[43] using tools such as electroencephalography and neuroimaging is getting increasingly popular. For an example of the experimental setup for the psychophysiological measurement of emotion, see ▸ Fig. 6.4.

Psychophysiological measures of emotion can provide objective, stable, and reliable information. They are particularly useful when an individual is not able or willing to openly provide accurate representations of their emotional experience. However, like behavioral observations, these methods can also be impractical, time-consuming, and expensive.

6.1.4 Role of Temperament and Emotion

Temperament exerts an important influence on the child's social-emotional development, personality development, and family system.[49] It also has a profound effect on the way in which children interact with their environments.[50] First, a child's temperament shapes how other people in the environment react to them. Children high in negative emotions, for example, tend to evoke more negative parental attempts to exert control, whereas extraverted, self-controlled children are more likely to elicit parental warmth.[51] Second, environmental experiences are interpreted by children in different ways depending on their temperament. For example, children who are high in anger/frustration tend to perceive negative events in their lives as more threatening compared to children with lower levels of negative emotions. Temperament traits can also make some life outcomes more or less likely to occur. For example, children who are more inhibited have a somewhat greater chance of developing social anxiety or depression, while children who are high in effortful control tend to develop more

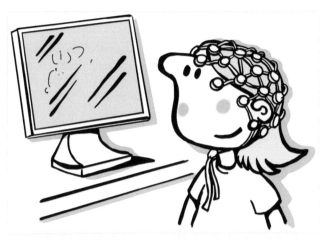

Fig. 6.4 This figure depicts the experimental set-up to measure the emotion-related physiological responses of cortical activity. Source: Image created by Lucia Fabiani.

social competence and are less likely to develop behavior problems.[51,52]

To better understand the relation between temperament and emotions, consider the following analogy: emotions are to temperament as weather is to seasons. We expect more rainy or stormy weather during winter, whereas summer typically brings forth more bright and sunny weather. Accordingly, we would expect children who have temperament profiles of high anger/frustration (i.e., negative affectivity; *winter*) to be more likely to experience emotional outbursts (i.e., rain and storms) than those who exhibit temperament profiles associated with extraversion/surgency (i.e., positive affectivity; *summer*).

6.2 The Association between Temperamental and Emotional Processes and Developmental Stuttering

To date, there have been several reviews of the relation between temperament, emotions, and developmental stuttering.[53,54,55] For a broad overview of the main "takeaways" from these reviews, see ▸ Table 6.3. Notably, each review concluded that there is likely an association between temperamental and emotional processes and developmental stuttering, although the exact nature of this association is less than clear. Since these reviews were published, more studies have been conducted, the results of which are briefly described below. We begin with a discussion of the findings of studies that have compared people who stutter to people who do not stutter, with a specific focus on young children. We then discuss research on the association of temperamental and emotional processes with stuttering frequency and severity (i.e., the behavior of stuttering) within people who stutter. These two lines of investigation provide multiple points of view on the potential contributions of temperamental and emotional processes to stuttering and have implications for clinical management, as discussed in the Section "Theoretical and Clinical Implications."

Table 6.3 Overview of the main "takeaways" from past reviews of temperamental and emotional processes associated with developmental stuttering in children

Review article	Review focus	Main takeaways	Implications
Alm[53]	Anxiety, temperament, and personality	Review of 14 studies revealed significant differences between CWS and CWNS in inattention and hyperactivity/impulsivity, but not in temperamental traits related to shyness or social anxiety	Proposed that there are likely subgroups characterized by inattention and hyperactivity/impulsivity
Jones et al[54]	Temperament and emotion	Findings from 19 studies indicated that preschool-aged CWS exhibit differences in temperament and emotion compared to CWNS	Proposed that temperament and emotion may be a causal contributor to developmental stuttering within the context of a multifactorial disorder
Kefalianos et al[55]	Temperament and anxiety	Although the findings from 10 studies were inconsistent, there were consistently reported differences between CWS and CWNS in adaptability, attention span/persistence, and mood	Suggested that firm conclusions are premature, given the modest scope of the work, and temperament and emotion would be best ascertained by studying longitudinal cohorts prior to stuttering onset

Abbreviations: CWS, children who stutter; CWNS, children who do not stutter.

6.2.1 Differences between People Who Stutter and People Who Do Not Stutter

The main findings of studies that have examined emotional reactivity and regulation in people who do and do not stutter, based on data from caregiver reports and behavioral and psychophysiological measures, are shown in ▶ Table 6.4. To date, findings pertaining to *reactivity* have indicated that young children who stutter, compared to young children who do not stutter, may be more emotionally reactive and exhibit more negative emotions.[56,57,58,59,60,61,62,63] These processes may also be associated with persistence.[64,65] Relative to *regulation*, a growing body of studies have demonstrated that children who stutter have lower emotion regulation than children who do not stutter[58,60,66] as well as difficulties in the processes that support regulation, such as shifting/focusing attention and inhibitory control.[56,58,67,68,69,70] Therefore, while there is no perfect consensus (i.e., several studies[71,72] have not found group differences), there is a growing body of evidence to suggest salient differences between children who stutter and children who do not stutter in temperamental and emotional processes, with children who stutter having increased reactivity and more difficulty with regulation.

Emerging research on temperament and emotion in adults has demonstrated lower positive affect scores in adults who stutter than those who do not.[73] Physiological processes have been studied in the adult population with mixed results. Some studies have indicated that adults who stutter exhibit increased reactivity,[74] while others have reported no differences.[75] During speaking tasks, adults who stutter have demonstrated *less* marked physiological responses than adults who do not stutter.[76,77,78] Although this may seem paradoxical, Alm[79] argued that these findings may represent "anticipatory anxiety resulting in a freezing response" prior to and/or during speaking. As we mentioned at the outset, there are fewer studies on temperament and emotion in adults who stutter and further research is necessary to draw more firm conclusions.

6.2.2 Association with Stuttering Frequency and Severity

In addition to studying between-group differences, the study of the association between stuttering behaviors and emotional processes is of interest, given that it potentially links emotions directly to moments of stuttering. ▶ Table 6.5 provides an overview of the findings from studies that have investigated the relation between *reactivity* and *regulation* and stuttering frequency and severity. Numerous studies have shown that *increased reactivity*, both positive and negative, is associated with *increased stuttering frequency and/or stuttered utterances (compared to fluent)*.[57,78,80,81,82,83,84] In a similar vein, empirical studies on *regulation* have found that *decreased regulation* is associated with *increased stuttering frequency and/or severity*.[59,85,86,87,88] Taken together, these findings provide evidence that temperamental and emotional processes may be importantly linked to stuttering, which may in turn impact an individual's communication, thus providing motivation for speech-language pathologists to consider these processes in assessment and treatment.

6.2.3 Summary of Empirical Evidence and Takeaways

As indicated by the above review, there is substantial evidence to support an association between temperamental and emotional processes and developmental stuttering. Taking the broadest view, these can be summarized as follows: (1) children who stutter, compared to children who do not stutter, may exhibit increased reactivity and decreased regulation and (2) increased reactivity and decreased regulation appear to be associated with increased stuttering severity and/or frequency for children who stutter. However, this broad view certainly does not tell the whole story. There are areas for which there are many studies and replicated findings (e.g., differences in negative emotion and/or attention), other areas that are newly emerging (e.g., cortical reactivity differences), and still others where there are no differences or insufficient evidence to make

Table 6.4 Main findings from empirical studies comparing reactivity and regulation of people who do and do not stutter

Reactivity components	
Approach	CWS scored higher on the approach scale than CWNS[56]
Anger/frustration	CWS scored higher on the anger/frustration scale than CWNS[56]
Emotional reactivity	CWS were more emotionally reactive than CWNS[58]
Negative emotion	CWS exhibited more negative emotional expressions after receiving an undesirable gift[57] and during a frustrating task than CWNS,[59] but in other studies CWS were found to be less negative.[127] Persistent CWS exhibited higher negative affect than recovered CWS and CWNS[64]
Behavioral inhibition	No between-group differences, but more CWS exhibited extremely high behavioral inhibition than extremely low behavioral inhibition[80]
Positive emotion	AWS exhibited lower positive affect scores than AWNS[73]
Hormone stress response	CWS exhibited no significant differences in salivary cortisol[128] than CWNS[72]
Acoustic startle	AWS exhibited an increased acoustic startle response compared to AWNS.[74] Other studies have not found differences[75,129]
Autonomic nervous system reactivity	CWS exhibited higher skin conductance during a fast-paced picture naming task (3-year-old)[63] and a positive speaking condition[60] than CWNS. CWS also exhibited increased reactivity during various (non) speech tasks than CWNS.[61] Persistent CWS exhibited higher skin conductance during a fast-paced naming task than CWS who recovered.[65] Further, AWS and AWNS exhibit increased physiological reactivity during various (stressful) speaking tasks, with some responses being less marked for AWS[76,77,78]
Cortical reactivity	CWS exhibited greater late positive potential (cortical index of emotional reactivity) when viewing unpleasant pictures than CWNS[62] but not differences when viewing peer facial expressions[71]
Regulation components	
Attention control and shifting	CWS had more caregiver-reported problematic attention abilities,[130] lower attention shifting,[56] lower attention regulation,[58] and lower attentional focusing than CWNS.[70] Further, CWS had more difficulty flexibly shifting their attention[67] and were less efficient in selective attention than CWNS[68]
Inhibitory control	CWS exhibited lower caregiver-reported and behavioral indices of inhibitory control than CWNS[56,69]
Adaptability	CWS exhibited less adaptability than CWNS[66]
Emotion regulation	CWS exhibited lower emotion regulation than CWNS[58]
Autonomic nervous system regulation	CWS exhibited lower baseline physiological regulation than CWNS,[60] which serves as an index of regulation capacity when faced with challenges

Abbreviations: CWS, children who stutter; CWNS, children who do not stutter; AWS, adults who stutter; AWNS, adults who do not stutter.

Table 6.5 Main findings from studies examining the association between components of reactivity and regulation and stuttering frequency and severity in people who stutter

Reactivity components	
Positive emotion	Higher positive emotional reactivity[81] and emotions were associated with increased stuttering frequency in CWS
Emotional reactivity	Increased emotional reactivity and decreased emotion regulation were associated with increased stuttering in CWS[82]
Negative emotion	CWS with a higher negative emotional reactivity exhibited higher stuttering frequency during positive emotion conditions[81]
Behavioral inhibition	CWS with very high levels of behavioral inhibition exhibited increased stuttering frequency[80]
Autonomic nervous system reactivity	The stuttered utterances of CWS[83] and AWS[78] were higher in physiological reactivity than the fluent utterances
Regulation components	
Attention control and shifting	CWS who shifted their attention away from frustrating stimuli exhibited reduced stuttering during subsequent narrative speaking tasks[59]
Effortful control	Increased regulation was linked to decreased stuttering in CWS,[87,88] although this was not confirmed in all studies[56,125]
Emotion regulation	Increased use of behavioral strategies for emotion regulation was associated with decreased stuttering frequency[85]
Autonomic nervous system regulation	Decreased physiological regulation was associated with increased stuttering frequency for CWS with lower effortful control[86]

Abbreviations: CWS, children who stutter; CWNS, children who do not stutter; AWS, adults who stutter; AWNS, adults who do not stutter.

a strong determination. Also, these findings apply to groups, not individuals, an important consideration given that people who stutter tend to be heterogeneous.[64,89] Therefore, while there have been many advancements since previous reviews on this topic were published, continued study, replication, and extension are necessary to develop a better understanding of the nature of temperamental and emotional processes in developmental stuttering.

6.3 Theoretical and Clinical Implications

6.3.1 Directionality of the Effect

An often discussed and still unresolved issue regarding the contributions of temperamental and emotional processes to developmental stuttering is that of the *directionality of the effect* (for a comprehensive discussion, see Conture et al[90]). Said another way, are temperamental and emotional processes causal contributors to developmental stuttering, or are differences in these processes caused by experiences with stuttering? There are several alternative possibilities as well. First, a bidirectional relationship may exist whereby temperamental and emotional processes contribute to stuttering, but experiences with stuttering also influence an individual's temperament and/or emotional responses. Second, temperament and emotion may be associated with developmental stuttering by virtue of a "third-order" variable, such as sex (e.g., more males stutter and males may be more likely to exhibit certain temperamental characteristics).

Considering the nature of temperament—namely, that it is a genetically influenced set of individual differences[19,22,91]—it would seem unlikely that experiences with stuttering would be solely responsible for differences in young preschool-age children who do and do not stutter, as these children are close to the age of stuttering onset and have relatively little experience with stuttering.[56,60,65,66] However, it also seems unlikely that temperament and emotional processes would be completely immune to experiences associated with stuttering. This is especially true for school-age children and adults who have been stuttering for many years, a perspective that is generally supported by evidence of increased (speech-related and/or social) anxiety in adolescents and adults who stutter.[92,93] Therefore, we suggest that a bidirectional association (i.e., temperament and emotion impacting stuttering and vice versa) that varies by the individual's characteristics is the most likely to be true, at least based on our current understanding of the evidence.

6.3.2 Theoretical Implications

Conture and Walden's recent *Dual Diathesis-Stressor Model of Stuttering* is arguably the most contemporary theoretical account that includes temperament and emotion as potential causal factors in developmental stuttering.[94] Specifically, this model suggests that some children who stutter have emotion-related vulnerabilities (i.e., *diathesis*), such as heightened negative emotional reactivity and decreased regulation, that can be activated by challenging environmental situations or events (i.e., *stressors*) and that these processes contribute to the onset and development of stuttering. Children who exhibit emotional

diatheses may be more likely to have their attention and other cognitive resources diverted during emotionally arousing speaking situations (social-emotional stressor) and, consequently, be more likely to stutter. These children may also be more likely to react to difficulties with speech production, leading to a worsening of stuttering. Although temperament and emotion are central in this model, the authors recognize the heterogeneity of stuttering and specify that for some children these processes may play little to no role in stuttering.

The *Multifactorial Dynamic Pathways Theory of Stuttering* by Smith and Weber[95] also posits that temperament and emotion may play a key role in the onset, development, and/or persistence of stuttering. This model focuses on the interaction between speech-motor, linguistic, and emotional processes, emphasizing the concurrent development of these processes over the period when stuttering first emerges and pathways of persistence and recovery are developing. They note that while the precise role of temperament and emotion in the onset and development of stuttering is not clear, one possibility is that negative emotion related to speech disruption may further destabilize speech motor performance, thereby contributing to stuttering.

In sum, this brief overview demonstrates how temperamental and emotional processes could potentially contribute to stuttering. Some perspectives suggest that these processes play a causal role (at least for some people who stutter) in the onset and development of stuttering, whereas others suggest that these processes may serve to worsen or exacerbate stuttering caused by other factors (e.g., speech-motor, linguistic, etc.). Regardless, there is significant justification to consider these processes in comprehensive etiological accounts of developmental stuttering.

6.3.3 Diagnostic Implications

Although speech disfluencies are the most characteristic symptom of stuttering, the assessment of stuttering involves more than these overt (behavioral) symptoms. Rather, covert aspects of stuttering, such as underlying emotional and cognitive reactions, and the impact that stuttering has on the client's day-to-day functioning also need to be assessed. This is crucial because behavioral symptoms may fluctuate (e.g., depending on the situation), resulting in an (overt) stuttering severity that may not fully capture the severity and impact of the disorder on the individual client.[96]

Covert symptoms refer to feelings and thoughts, such as high levels of concern for listener reactions, fear of stuttering, frustration when stuttering, anxiety related to specific speaking situations, and feelings of guilt and shame. These reactions to stuttering often result in an increase in secondary behaviors, including struggling, avoidance, or postponement. It is often assumed that this mainly occurs with older clients and that young children are not aware of their stuttering. The extent to which children who stutter are aware of their stuttering and how they emotionally react to it are highly variable;[97] however, some studies[98,99] have shown that, prior to 3 years of age, children may have some awareness that their speech is different from that of other children. Although some children may respond in very subtle ways to their speech difficulty by withdrawing from speaking or the speaking situation (e.g., very outgoing, talkative at first but now much quieter, whispering), with only mild noticeable emotional reactions, other children react more visibly by becoming emotionally frustrated and demonstrating struggle behaviors. The extent and nature of a child's response to his or her stuttering is likely related to his or her temperament (e.g., see Manning[100]), since it plays a crucial role in emotional regulation.

The assessment of a child who stutters should, therefore, include the evaluation of affective (feelings, emotions, etc.), behavioral (tension, struggle, avoidance, etc.), and cognitive (thought processes) reactions to stuttering. Understanding how a child reacts in certain situations and how he or she regulates these emotions provides the clinician and parents with important insights into why their child may react strongly to moments of stuttering and develop secondary behaviors and/or more negative speech attitudes.

Assessing emotions and temperament can be done informally during an interview, or more formally using surveys and questionnaires. For preschool children, an informal gathering of information is based on parent interview, parent–child interaction, and/or child–clinician interaction. See ▸ Table 6.6 for example interview questions probing emotional reactions and temperament. Those working with older children may choose to interview the child directly, instead of or in addition to interviewing parents, and possibly teachers as well. Although interviewing has many advantages, it can be time-consuming and inconsistent because parents vary in how much detail they provide when answering questions. Parents may also present biased information about their children and answer questions for social desirability.[6] Parent–child or child–clinician interactions may overcome some of these concerns, but they can also be very time-consuming and limited in that they can only provide information about reactions in the clinic, not other contexts.

Because of the limitations of interviews and observations, more formalized procedures, such as surveys and questionnaires, have been developed, not only for the evaluation of the client's beliefs and feelings about his stuttering[101,102,103,104,105] but also for temperament.[16,106] For example, the Communication Attitude Test for Preschool and Kindergarten Children Who Stutter (KiddyCAT)[103] is a questionnaire developed to assess communication attitudes in preschool-age children who stutter, and the Overall Assessment of the Speaker's Experience of Stuttering (OASES)[107] measures similar constructs as well as the functional and emotional "impact" of stuttering in adults. As we have already mentioned, the CBQ[16] is useful in measuring temperament. There are also shorter versions of the CBQ available, versions available for various age ranges (e.g., adults[108]), and alternative brief options (for an alternative option, see Kristal[6]). The Short Behavioral Inhibition Scale (SBIS) has recently been used to study temperament in young children who stutter, is readily available, and easy to score, representing a viable option to assess behavioral inhibition.[109]

6.3.4 Treatment Implications

Until the underlying mechanisms associated with temperament, emotions, and stuttering have been fully unraveled, formulating treatment recommendations based on these associations may be premature. However, several approaches developed for working with children's temperaments[6] are applicable to children who stutter.[110] Examples are strategies for creating a better parent–child alliance such as anticipating how children will react in certain circumstances and changing/adjusting environmental contexts, or providing problem-solving/coping strategies (e.g., teaching parents to co-regulate the child's emotions—in the case of limited frustration tolerance, a parent may encourage a child to count while waiting, think of something fun instead, or vent emotions). In the past, some authors in the field of stuttering have emphasized the importance of evaluating and improving the child's vulnerabilities and reducing emotional stressors, such as high expectations and sensitivity.[111,112] More recent, evidence-based approaches have described different ways of working with temperament and emotions in young children who stutter.[113,114] For example, clinicians can work on desensitizing children to moments of stuttering, using problem-solving strategies to decrease emotional arousal to stressors, counseling and training parents to react appropriately to stressors, and evaluating and changing parenting styles. Druker et al[115] demonstrated that training parents to improve self-regulation in their children contributed to the successful management of fluency and the emotional impacts of the disorder.

Perhaps somewhat more speculative, but in line with findings in other populations,[116] temperament may impact treatment outcomes. Preliminary data[117] have shown that children with more "expressive temperaments" (i.e., lower behavioral inhibition) exhibited greater long-term decreases in stuttering frequency following indirect treatment than children with less "expressive temperaments" (i.e., higher levels of behavioral inhibition).

Table 6.6 Example informal interview questions probing emotional reactions and temperament

A clinician probing a child's *emotional reactions* could ask the parent(s):

- "Has your child shown signs of being concerned or embarrassed about the way he speaks?"
- "Does he sometimes get frustrated when he cannot get the words out?"
- "Is he avoiding or acting fearful in certain speaking situations?"

A clinician probing to gain more insight into a preschool child's *temperament* could ask the parent(s):

- "Is he easily distracted by surrounding activities or can he get so focused on an activity that all else is blocked out?"
- "Is he more hesitant with new situations, people, or things—or does he dive right in, seeking out novelty?"
- "When he is building a tower with Lego blocks and it falls down, how does he react—does he persist and start building the tower again, does he ask for help, or does he become angry and frustrated and quit if it is too difficult?"
- "If he is watching a cartoon and you ask him to turn off the TV because you have to go somewhere, can he easily do that and switch his attention to putting on his shoes and jacket or does he have difficulty with that?"

6.4 Future Directions

As we have discussed, there have been significant advances in our empirical, theoretical, and clinical understanding of the role of temperamental and emotional processes in developmental stuttering, especially over the past 10 years. As is often the case, new research questions have emerged as well as areas of potential interest for clinical practice. Below, we briefly discuss some of these research and clinically related future directions.

From a research perspective, researchers should use a comprehensive, diverse multimethod approach for studying temperamental and emotional processes in developmental stuttering. Such an approach will advance our knowledge in areas of empirical and theoretical interest. The following two areas of research exemplify ongoing efforts designed to further our understanding of the link between temperament, emotion, and developmental stuttering:

- One emerging research effort that has begun to receive attention is on emotion-related mechanisms that may help us to understand *how* emotions and temperament contribute to stuttering. For example, it has been speculated that changes in emotional processes may impact the planning and production (i.e., linguistic, cognitive, and speech-motor) processes that are necessary for fluent speech. Research in both young children[118] and adults who stutter[119,120,121,122] has demonstrated that emotion impacts their speech-motor processes to a greater degree than in similarly aged nonstuttering participants. This emerging research is important because it may lead to novel insights into the mechanisms by which emotional processes contribute to stuttering—advancing our understanding of the nature of stuttering and development of treatment approaches.

- Another emerging area of research has focused on the influence of temperamental and emotional processes on the *impact* of stuttering and *speech-related anxiety*. Temperament influences how children adapt to life[20] and cope with stressors,[18] thereby impacting their overall well-being.[123] Thus, it may come as no surprise that some studies have shown that adolescents[124,125] and adults[73,126] who stutter who exhibit more negative reactivity are not only more anxious but also more impacted by their stuttering. In contrast, adolescents who have more positive reactivity are less impacted by their stuttering and have lower anxiety. These studies, which demonstrate that temperament and emotion may play a role in how individuals respond to stuttering, have the potential to lead to advances in clinical management. For example, techniques may be developed to support the ability of individuals to better cope with stuttering based on their unique temperament profile.

From a clinical perspective, clinicians should expect to see studies of temperament and emotions to continue to emerge in the stuttering literature. As is always the case with new research, clinicians should cautiously interpret these findings and carefully consider how best to apply, if at all, the results to practice. From the authors' perspective, there are at least a few areas of development that would significantly advance the translation of research findings to clinical practice. First, it is imperative that researchers continue to use methodological approaches that can also be employed in the clinic—for example, using caregiver report and behavioral measures in addition to psychophysiological, neuroanatomical measures, etc.—because the latter approaches are not readily accessible to most clinicians. A comprehensive approach such as this will not only facilitate our understanding of stuttering but also provide insight into which clinically accessible measures relate to laboratory-based approaches (physiology, neuroanatomy) and which do not. Second, systematic assessment of individual differences and subtypes in temperamental and emotional processes could potentially yield significant advances to clinical practice. For example, as has been speculated,[54] some children may respond differently to different types of intervention based on their temperamental profiles. Finally, future work should strive to identify and develop guidelines for the application of temperament- and emotion-related diagnostic and treatment tools (e.g., establish cutoffs for high/low values of reactivity and regulation) to facilitate their clinical utility and potential for application.

6.5 Conclusions

In the 21st century, there have been significant advances to the empirical study, theoretical understanding, and potential clinical application of temperamental and emotional processes to developmental stuttering. From 2000 to 2010, this work was newly emerging and focused, almost predominantly, on caregiver report of temperament. Beginning in 2010 and extending to the present day, this work has focused on using a broad range of methodological approaches to comprehensively study temperamental and emotional processes in developmental stuttering. Both past and present works have provided evidence to suggest that increased reactivity and decreased regulation are associated with developmental stuttering. Despite these advances, there are still many theoretical and empirical applications that must be pursued to further our understanding of the role of temperamental and emotional processes in developmental stuttering and translate these advances to clinical practice.

6.6 Definitions

Arousal: A state of physiological or psychological excitation in response to an external or internal stimuli.

Attention regulation: Attention regulation refers to the ability to self-monitor one's deployment of attention, which includes maintaining attention, ignoring distracting or irrelevant stimuli, staying alert to task goals, and coordinating one's attention during a task.

Behavioral inhibition: A term introduced by Kagan that refers to a temperamental trait characterized by the tendency to show reluctance, withdrawal, and fearfulness especially when encountering novel situations, objects, or people.[131]

Effortful control (or self-regulation): A temperament dimension indicated by the capacity to refrain from a desired or dominant behavior while also maintaining attention on a task and resisting distraction.

Emotion: Affective states with neurological underpinnings involving conscious experience. Emotions may lead to internal or overt physical responses and they may inhibit or facilitate behaviors.

Endocrine system: The glands/organs that make hormones and release them directly into the blood so they can travel all over the body.

Extraversion/surgency (or positive reactivity): A temperament dimension indicated by impulsivity, intense pleasure seeking, high activity level, and low levels of shyness.

Negative affectivity (or negative reactivity): A temperament dimension indicated by mood instability, angry reactivity, and dysregulated negative emotions.

Parenting style: The levels of expectations, performance demands, attentiveness, and style of discipline parents use in child rearing. Different styles can lead to different child development and child outcomes.

Physiology: Functioning of the systems, organs, and tissues of the body.

Psychophysiological measures: Measures studying the relationship between physiological and psychological phenomena.

Reactivity: Responsiveness to an external or internal stimuli. Emotional reactivity may be experienced as internal physiological states or overt physical responses.

Reappraisal: Reinterpretation of internal or external stimuli under a different light.

Regulation: Changes that may be in the form of suppressing (decreases) or intensifying (increases). Emotional regulation refers to changes in the intensity, valence, or duration of emotional activation for the internal emotional states or physiological processes.

Rumination: Negative perseverative thinking that can result in emotional or physiological stress.

Somatic: Relating to or affecting the body.

Suppression: Downregulation, reducing the intensity or duration of emotional states or physiological responses.

Temperament: Constitutionally based individual differences in reactivity and self-regulation.

References

[1] Strelau J. Temperament: a psychological perspective. New York, NY: Plenum Press; 1998

[2] Kagan J. Biology and the child. In: Eisenberg N, ed. Handbook of Child Psychology: Social, Emotional, and Personality Development. Vol. 3. 5th ed. New York, NY: Wiley; 1998:177–235

[3] Strelau J. The role of temperament as a moderator of stress. In: Wachs TD, Kohnstamm GA, eds. Temperament in Context. Mahwah, NJ: Lawrence Erlbaum Associates; 2001:153–172

[4] Bodunov MV. Studies on temperament in Russia: after Teplov and Nebylitsyn. Eur J Pers. 1993; 7(5):299–311

[5] Gesell A, Ames LB. Early evidences of individuality in the human infant. Sci Mon. 1937; 45(3):217–225

[6] Kristal J. The temperament perspective: working with children's behavioral styles. New York, NY: Paul H Brookes Publishing; 2005

[7] Thomas A, Chess S. Temperament and development. New York, NY: Brunner/Mazel; 1977

[8] Buss AH, Plomin R. Temperament: early developing personality traits. Hillsdale, NJ: Erlbaum; 1984

[9] Goldsmith HH, Campos JJ. The structure of temperamental fear and pleasure in infants: a psychometric perspective. Child Dev. 1990; 61(6):1944–1964

[10] Goldsmith HH, Buss AH, Plomin R, et al. Roundtable: what is temperament? Four approaches. Child Dev. 1987; 58(2):505–529

[11] Plomin R, Dunn J, Eds. The Study of Temperament: Changes, Continuities and Challenges. Hillsdale, NJ: Lawrence Erlbaum Associates; 1986

[12] Rothbart MK. Temperament in childhood: a framework. In: Kohnstamm G, Bates J, Rothbart MK, eds. Temperament in Childhood. Chichester, UK: Wiley; 1989:59–73

[13] Posner MI, Rothbart MK. Attention, self-regulation and consciousness. Philos Trans R Soc Lond B Biol Sci. 1998; 353(1377):1915–1927

[14] Halverson CF, Deal JE. Temperamental change, parenting and the family context. In: Wachs TD, Kohnstamm GA, eds. Temperament in Context. Mahwah, NJ: Lawrence Erlbaum Associates; 2001:61–80

[15] Saudino KJ. Behavioral genetics and child temperament. J Dev Behav Pediatr. 2005; 26(3):214–223

[16] Rothbart MK, Ahadi SA, Hershey KL, Fisher P. Investigations of temperament at three to seven years: the Children's Behavior Questionnaire. Child Dev. 2001; 72(5):1394–1408

[17] Putnam SP, Ellis LK, Rothbart MK. The structure of temperament from infancy through adolescence. In: Eliasz A, Angleitner A, eds. Advances/Proceedings in Research on Temperament. Lengerich, Germany: Pabst Scientist Publishers; 2001:165–182

[18] Rueda MR, Rothbart MK. The influence of temperament on the development of coping: the role of maturation and experience. New Dir Child Adolesc Dev. 2009; 2009(124):19–31

[19] Rothbart MK, Derryberry D. Development of individual differences in temperament. In: Lamb ME, Brown AL, eds. Advances in Developmental Psychology. Vol. 1. Mahwah, NJ: Lawrence Erlbaum Associates; 1981:37–86

[20] Rothbart MK. Becoming Who we are: temperament and personality in development. New York, NY: Guilford Press; 2011

[21] Joyce J. Essentials of temperament assessment. Hoboken, NJ: John Wiley & Sons, Inc.; 2010

[22] Rothbart MK, Bates JE. Temperament. In: Eisenberg N, ed. Handbook of Child Psychology: Social, Emotional, and Personality Development. Vol. 3. 5th ed. New York, NY: Wiley; 1998:105–176

[23] Cannon WB. The James-Lange theory of emotions: a critical examination and an alternative theory. Am J Psychol. 1927; 39(1/4):106–124

[24] Papez JW. A proposed mechanism of emotion. Arch Neurol Psychiatry. 1937; 38(4):725–743

[25] Dalgleish T. The emotional brain. Nat Rev Neurosci. 2004; 5(7):583–589

[26] Schachter S, Singer JE. Cognitive, social, and physiological determinants of emotional state. Psychol Rev. 1962; 69(5):379–399

[27] VandenBos GR. APA Dictionary of Psychology. Washington, DC: American Psychological Association; 2007

[28] Schlosberg H. Three dimensions of emotion. Psychol Rev. 1954; 61(2):81–88

[29] Engen T, Levy N, Schlosberg H. The dimensional analysis of a new series of facial expressions. J Exp Psychol. 1958; 55(5):454–458

[30] Ekman P. An argument for basic emotions. Cogn Emotion. 1992; 6(3–4):169–200

[31] Izard CE, Libero DZ, Putnam P, Haynes OM. Stability of emotion experiences and their relations to traits of personality. J Pers Soc Psychol. 1993; 64(5):847–860

[32] Dolcos F, Iordan AD, Dolcos S. Neural correlates of emotion-cognition interactions: A review of evidence from brain imaging investigations. J Cogn Psychol (Hove). 2011; 23(6):669–694

[33] Izard CE. Organizational and motivational functions of discrete emotions. In: Lewis M, Haviland JM, eds. Handbook of Emotions. New York, NY: Guilford Press; 1993:631–641

[34] Harmon-Jones E, Harmon-Jones C, Summerell E. On the importance of both dimensional and discrete models of emotion. Behav Sci (Basel). 2017; 7(4):66

[35] Lu L, Gilmour R. Culture and conceptions of happiness: individual oriented and social oriented SWB. J Happiness Stud. 2004; 5(3):269–291

[36] Gross JJ. Emotion regulation: past, present, future. Cogn Emotion. 1999; 13(5):551–573

[37] Gullone E, Hughes EK, King NJ, Tonge B. The normative development of emotion regulation strategy use in children and adolescents: a 2-year follow-up study. J Child Psychol Psychiatry. 2010; 51(5):567–574

[38] Carlson SM, Wang TS. Inhibitory control and emotion regulation in preschool children. Cogn Dev. 2007; 22(4):489–510

[39] Sala MN, Pons F, Molina P. Emotion regulation strategies in preschool children. Br J Dev Psychol. 2014; 32(4):440–453

[40] Ekas NV, Braungart-Rieker JM, Messinger DS. The development of infant emotion regulation: time is of the essence. In: Cole PM, Hollenstein T, eds. Emotion Regulation: A Matter of Time. New York, NY: Routledge; 2018:49–69

[41] Zimmermann P, Iwanski A. Emotion regulation from early adolescence to emerging adulthood and middle adulthood: age differences, gender differences, and emotion-specific developmental variations. Int J Behav Dev. 2014; 38(2):182–194

[42] Somerville LH, Jones RM, Casey BJ. A time of change: behavioral and neural correlates of adolescent sensitivity to appetitive and aversive environmental cues. Brain Cogn. 2010; 72(1):124–133

[43] Mauss IB, Robinson MD. Measures of emotion: a review. Cogn Emotion. 2009; 23(2):209–237

[44] Kaplan S, Dalal RS, Luchman J. Measurement of emotions. In: Sinclair RR, Wang M, Tetrick LE, eds. Research Methods in Occupational Health Psychology: State of the Art in Measurement, Design, and Data Analysis. New York, NY: Routledge; 2013:61–75

[45] Simoës-Perlant A, Lemercier C, Pêcher C, Benintendi-Medjaoued S. Mood self-assessment in children from the age of 7. Eur J Psychol. 2018; 14(3): 599–620

[46] Scherer KR, Banse R, Wallbott HG, Goldbeck T. Vocal cues in emotion encoding and decoding. Motiv Emot. 1991; 15(2):123–148

[47] Stepper S, Strack F. Proprioceptive determinants of emotional and nonemotional feelings. J Pers Soc Psychol. 1993; 64(2):211–220

[48] Ekman P, Friesen WV, Hager JC. Facial action coding system. Salt Lake City, UT: Research Nexus; 2002

[49] Rothbart MK, Derryberry D, Hershey K. Stability of temperament in childhood: laboratory infant assessment to parent report at seven years. In: Molfese VJ, Molfese DL, eds. Temperament and Personality: Development across the Life Span. Mahwah, NJ: Lawrence Erlbaum Associates; 2000

[50] Shiner RL, Caspi A. Temperament and the development of personality traits, adaptations, and narratives. In: Zentner M, Shiner RL, eds. Handbook of Temperament. New York, NY: Guilford Press; 2012

[51] Caspi A, Shiner RL. Personality development. In: Damon W, Lerner R, Eisenberg N, eds. Handbook of Child Psychology: Social, Emotional, and Personality Development. New York, NY: Wiley; 2006:300–365

[52] Kagan J. The structure of temperament. In: Emde RM, Hewitt JK, eds. Infancy to Early Childhood: Genetic and Environmental Influences on Developmental Change. Oxford: Oxford University Press; 2001:45–51

[53] Alm PA. Stuttering in relation to anxiety, temperament, and personality: review and analysis with focus on causality. J Fluency Disord. 2014; 40:5–21

[54] Jones R, Choi D, Conture E, Walden T. Temperament, emotion, and childhood stuttering. Semin Speech Lang. 2014; 35(2):114–131

[55] Kefalianos E, Onslow M, Block S, Menzies R, Reilly S. Early stuttering, temperament and anxiety: two hypotheses. J Fluency Disord. 2012; 37(3): 151–163

[56] Eggers K, De Nil LF, Van den Bergh BR. Temperament dimensions in stuttering and typically developing children. J Fluency Disord. 2010; 35(4): 355–372

[57] Johnson KN, Walden TA, Conture EG, Karrass J. Spontaneous regulation of emotions in preschool children who stutter: preliminary findings. J Speech Lang Hear Res. 2010; 53(6):1478–1495

[58] Karrass J, Walden TA, Conture EG, et al. Relation of emotional reactivity and regulation to childhood stuttering. J Commun Disord. 2006; 39(6):402–423

[59] Ntourou K, Conture EG, Walden TA. Emotional reactivity and regulation in preschool-age children who stutter. J Fluency Disord. 2013; 38(3):260–274

[60] Jones RM, Buhr AP, Conture EG, Tumanova V, Walden TA, Porges SW. Autonomic nervous system activity of preschool-age children who stutter. J Fluency Disord. 2014; 41:12–31

[61] Walsh B, Smith A, Christ SL, Weber C. Sympathetic nervous system activity in preschoolers who stutter. Front Hum Neurosci. 2019; 13:356

[62] Zengin-Bolatkale H, Conture EG, Key AP, Walden TA, Jones RM. Cortical associates of emotional reactivity and regulation in childhood stuttering. J Fluency Disord. 2018; 56:81–99

[63] Zengin-Bolatkale H, Conture EG, Walden TA. Sympathetic arousal of young children who stutter during a stressful picture naming task. J Fluency Disord. 2015; 46:24–40

[64] Ambrose NG, Yairi E, Loucks TM, Seery CH, Throneburg R. Relation of motor, linguistic and temperament factors in epidemiologic subtypes of persistent and recovered stuttering: Initial findings. J Fluency Disord. 2015; 45:12–26

[65] Zengin-Bolatkale H, Conture EG, Walden TA, Jones RM. Sympathetic arousal as a marker of chronicity in childhood stuttering. Dev Neuropsychol. 2018; 43(2):135–151

[66] Anderson JD, Pellowski MW, Conture EG, Kelly EM. Temperamental characteristics of young children who stutter. J Speech Lang Hear Res. 2003; 46(5):1221–1233

[67] Bush A. Effects of childhood stuttering on attention regulation in emotionally arousing situations. VURJ. 2006; 2:1–14

[68] Eggers K, De Nil LF, Van den Bergh BRH. The efficiency of attentional networks in children who stutter. J Speech Lang Hear Res. 2012; 55(3): 946–959

[69] Eggers K, De Nil LF, Van den Bergh BRH. Inhibitory control in childhood stuttering. J Fluency Disord. 2013; 38(1):1–13

[70] Embrechts M, Ebben H, Franke P, van de Poel C. Temperament: a comparison between children who stutter and children who do not stutter. In: Bosshardt HG, Yaruss JS, Peters HF, eds. Nijmegen, The Netherlands: Nijmegen Press; 1998:557–562

[71] Usler ER, Weber C. Emotion processing in children who do and do not stutter: an ERP study of electrocortical reactivity and regulation to peer facial expressions. J Fluency Disord. 2021; 67:105802

[72] Ortega AY, Ambrose NG. Developing physiologic stress profiles for school-age children who stutter. J Fluency Disord. 2011; 36(4):268–273

[73] Lucey J, Evans D, Maxfield ND. Temperament in adults who stutter and its association with stuttering frequency and quality-of-life impacts. J Speech Lang Hear Res. 2019; 62(8):2691–2702

[74] Guitar B. Acoustic startle responses and temperament in individuals who stutter. J Speech Lang Hear Res. 2003; 46(1):233–240

[75] Alm PA, Risberg J. Stuttering in adults: the acoustic startle response, temperamental traits, and biological factors. J Commun Disord. 2007; 40 (1):1–41

[76] Caruso AJ, Chodzko-Zajko WJ, Bidinger DA, Sommers RK. Adults who stutter: responses to cognitive stress. J Speech Hear Res. 1994; 37(4):746–754

[77] Peters HFM, Hulstijn W. Stuttering and anxiety: the difference between stutterers and nonstutterers in verbal apprehension and physiologic arousal during the anticipation of speech and non-speech tasks. J Fluency Disord. 1984; 9:67–84

[78] Weber CM, Smith A. Autonomic correlates of stuttering and speech assessed in a range of experimental tasks. J Speech Hear Res. 1990; 33(4):690–706

[79] Alm PA. Stuttering, emotions, and heart rate during anticipatory anxiety: a critical review. J Fluency Disord. 2004; 29(2):123–133

[80] Choi D, Conture EG, Walden TA, Lambert WE, Tumanova V. Behavioral inhibition and childhood stuttering. J Fluency Disord. 2013; 38(2):171–183

[81] Choi D, Conture EG, Walden TA, Jones RM, Kim H. Emotional diathesis, emotional stress, and childhood stuttering. J Speech Lang Hear Res. 2016; 59 (4):616–630

[82] Walden TA, Frankel CB, Buhr AP, Johnson KN, Conture EG, Karrass JM. Dual diathesis-stressor model of emotional and linguistic contributions to developmental stuttering. J Abnorm Child Psychol. 2012; 40(4):633–644

[83] Walsh B, Usler E. Physiological correlates of fluent and stuttered speech production in preschool children who stutter. J Speech Lang Hear Res. 2019; 62(12):4309–4323

[84] Jones RM, Conture EG, Walden TA. Emotional reactivity and regulation associated with fluent and stuttered utterances of preschool-age children who stutter. J Commun Disord. 2014; 48:38–51

[85] Arnold HS, Conture EG, Key APF, Walden T. Emotional reactivity, regulation and childhood stuttering: a behavioral and electrophysiological study. J Commun Disord. 2011; 44(3):276–293

[86] Jones RM, Walden TA, Conture EG, Erdemir A, Lambert WE, Porges SW. Executive functions impact the relation between respiratory sinus arrhythmia and frequency of stuttering in young children who do and do not stutter. J Speech Lang Hear Res. 2017; 60(8):2133–2150

[87] Jo Kraft S, Ambrose N, Chon H. Temperament and environmental contributions to stuttering severity in children: the role of effortful control. Semin Speech Lang. 2014; 35(2):80–94

[88] Kraft SJ, Lowther E, Beilby J. The role of effortful control in stuttering severity in children: replication study. Am J Speech Lang Pathol. 2019; 28 (1):14–28

[89] Seery CH, Watkins RV, Mangelsdorf SC, Shigeto A. Subtyping stuttering II: contributions from language and temperament. J Fluency Disord. 2007; 32 (3):197–217

[90] Conture EG, Kelly EM, Walden TA. Temperament, speech and language: an overview. J Commun Disord. 2013; 46(2):125–142

[91] Sanson A, Hemphill SA, Smart D. Connections between temperament and social development: a review. Soc Dev. 2004; 13(1):142–170

[92] Craig A, Tran Y. Trait and social anxiety in adults with chronic stuttering: conclusions following meta-analysis. J Fluency Disord. 2014; 40:35–43

[93] Davis S, Shisca D, Howell P. Anxiety in speakers who persist and recover from stuttering. J Commun Disord. 2007; 40(5):398–417

[94] Conture EG, Walden TA. Dual diathesis-stressor model of stuttering. In: Beliakova L, Filatova Y, eds. Theoretical Issues of Fluency Disorders. Moscow: Vlados; 2012:94–127

[95] Smith A, Weber C. How stuttering develops: the multifactorial dynamic pathways theory. J Speech Lang Hear Res. 2017; 60(9):2483–2505

[96] Yaruss JS, Quesal RW. Stuttering and the International Classification of Functioning, Disability, and Health: an update. J Commun Disord. 2004; 37 (1):35–52

[97] Yairi E, Ambrose N. Early childhood stuttering. Austin, TX: Pro-Ed; 2005

[98] Ezrati-Vinacour R, Platzky R, Yairi E. The young child's awareness of stuttering-like disfluency. J Speech Lang Hear Res. 2001; 44(2):368–380

[99] Vanryckeghem M, Brutten GJ, Hernandez LM. A comparative investigation of the speech-associated attitude of preschool and kindergarten children who do and do not stutter. J Fluency Disord. 2005; 30(4):307–318

[100] Manning WH. Clinical decision-making in the diagnosis and treatment of fluency disorders. 3rd ed. Clifton Park, NY: Delmar; 2010

[101] Brutten GJ, Vanryckeghem M. Behavior assessment battery for school-age children who stutter. San Diego, CA: Plural Publishing; 2007

[102] Erickson RL. Assessing communication attitudes among stutterers. J Speech Hear Res. 1969; 12(4):711–724

[103] Vanryckeghem M, Brutten GJ. Communication Attitude Test for Preschool and Kindergarten Children Who Stutter (KiddyCAT). San Diego, CA: Plural Publishing; 2007

[104] Vanryckeghem M, Brutten GJ. The behavior assessment battery for adults who stutter. San Diego, CA: Plural Publishing; 2018

[105] Yaruss JS, Quesal RW. Overall assessment of the Speaker's experience of stuttering. McKinney, TX: Stuttering Therapy Resources; 2016

[106] Carey WB, McDevitt SC, Medoff-Cooper B, Fullard W, Hegvik RL. The Carey Temperament Scales: Professional Practice Set with Test Manual & User's Guide. Scottsdale, AZ: Behavioral-Developmental Initiatives; 2000

[107] Yaruss JS, Quesal RW. Overall Assessment of the Speaker's Experience of Stuttering (OASES): documenting multiple outcomes in stuttering treatment. J Fluency Disord. 2006; 31(2):90–115

[108] Evans DE, Rothbart MK. Developing a model for adult temperament. J Res Pers. 2007; 41(4):868–888

[109] Ntourou K, DeFranco EO, Conture EG, Walden TA, Mushtaq N. A parent-report scale of behavioral inhibition: validation and application to preschool-age children who do and do not stutter. J Fluency Disord. 2020; 63:105748

[110] Eggers K. Working with temperament styles with children who stutter and their families. Preconference workshop presented at the Oxford Disfluency Conference. St Catherine's College, Oxford, UK, September 20–23, 2017

[111] Riley G, Riley J. A revised component model for diagnosing and treating children who stutter. Contemp Issues Commun Sci Disord. 2000; 27:188–199

[112] Starkweather CW. Therapy for younger children. In: Curlee RF, Siegel GM, eds. Nature and Treatment of Stuttering. 2nd ed. Boston, MA: Allyn and Bacon; 1997:257–279

[113] de Sonneville-Koedoot C, Stolk E, Rietveld T, Franken M-C. Direct versus indirect treatment for preschool children who stutter: The RESTART randomized trial. PLoS One. 2015; 10(7):e0133758

[114] Kelman E, Nicholas A. Palin Parent-Child Interaction Therapy for Early Childhood Stammering. 2nd ed. London: Routledge; 2020

[115] Druker KC, Mazzucchelli TG, Beilby JM. An evaluation of an integrated fluency and resilience program for early developmental stuttering disorders. J Commun Disord. 2019; 78:69–83

[116] Rapee RM, Jacobs D. The reduction of temperamental risk for anxiety in withdrawn preschoolers: a pilot study. Behav Cogn Psychother Camb. 2002; 30(2):211–215

[117] Richels CG, Conture EG. Indirect treatment of childhood stuttering: diagnostic predictors of treatment outcome. In: Guitar B, McCauley RJ, eds. Treatment of Stuttering: Established and Emerging Interventions. Baltimore, MD: Lippincott Williams & Wilkins; 2010

[118] Erdemir A, Walden TA, Jefferson CM, Choi D, Jones RM. The effect of emotion on articulation rate in persistence and recovery of childhood stuttering. J Fluency Disord. 2018; 56 Supplement C:1–17

[119] Bauerly KR. The effects of emotion on second formant frequency fluctuations in adults who stutter. Folia Phoniatr Logop. 2018; 70(1):13–23

[120] Bauerly KR, Jones RM, Miller C. Effects of social stress on autonomic, behavioral, and acoustic parameters in adults who stutter. J Speech Lang Hear Res. 2019; 62(7):2185–2202

[121] Jackson ES, Tiede M, Beal D, Whalen DH. The impact of social–cognitive stress on speech variability, determinism, and stability in adults who do and do not stutter. J Speech Lang Hear Res. 2016; 59(6):1295–1314

[122] Lieshout Pv, Ben-David B, Lipski M, Namasivayam A. The impact of threat and cognitive stress on speech motor control in people who stutter. J Fluency Disord. 2014; 40:93–109

[123] Garcia D, Moradi S. Adolescents' temperament and character: a longitudinal study on happiness. J Happiness Stud. 2012; 13(5):931–946

[124] Eggers K, Millard S, Kelman E. (In press). Temperament, anxiety, and depression in school-age children who stutter. Journal of Communication Disorders.

[125] Eggers K, Millard S, Kelman E. Temperament and the impact of stuttering in children aged 8–14 years. J Speech Lang Hear Res. 2021; 64(2):417–432

[126] Bleek B, Reuter M, Yaruss JS, Cook S, Faber J, Montag C. Relationships between personality characteristics of people who stutter and the impact of stuttering on everyday life. J Fluency Disord. 2012; 37(4):325–333

[127] Lewis KE, Golberg LL. Measurements of temperament in the identification of children who stutter. Eur J Disord Commun. 1997; 32(4):441–448

[128] van der Merwe B, Robb M, Lewis JG, Ormond T. Anxiety measures and salivary cortisol responses in preschool children who stutter. Contemp Issues Commun Sci Disord. 2011; 38:1–10

[129] Ellis JB, Finan DS, Ramig PR. The influence of stuttering severity on acoustic startle responses. J Speech Lang Hear Res. 2008; 51(4):836–850

[130] Felsenfeld S, van Beijsterveldt CEM, Boomsma DI. Attentional regulation in young twins with probable stuttering, high nonfluency, and typical fluency. J Speech Lang Hear Res. 2010; 53(5):1147–1166

[131] Kagan J, Reznick JS, Clarke C, Snidman N, Garcia-Coll C. Behavioral inhibition to the unfamiliar. Child Development. 1984;55(6):2212–2225

Further Readings

Temperament

Rothbart MK. Becoming who we are: temperament and personality in development. New York, NY: Guilford Press; 2011

Zentner M, Bates JE. Child temperament: an integrative review of concepts, research programs, and measures. Eur J Dev Sci. 2008; 2:31

Emotion

Dalgleish T. The emotional brain. Nat Rev Neurosci. 2004; 5(7):583–589

Gross JJ. Emotion regulation: past, present, future. Cogn Emotion. 1999; 13(5):551–573

Mauss IB, Robinson MD. Measures of emotion: a review. Cogn Emotion. 2009; 23(2): 209–237

Temperament, Emotion, and Theories of Developmental Stuttering

Conture EG, Walden TA. Dual diathesis-stressor model of stuttering. In: Beliakova L, Filatova Y, eds. Theoretical Issues of Fluency Disorders. Moscow: Vlados; 2012:94–127

Smith A, Weber C. How stuttering develops: the multifactorial dynamic pathways theory. J Speech Lang Hear Res. 2017; 60(9):2483–2505

Reviews of Temperamental and Emotional Processes Associated with Developmental Stuttering

Conture EG, Kelly EM, Walden TA. Temperament, speech and language: an overview. J Commun Disord. 2013; 46(2):125–142

Jones R, Choi D, Conture E, Walden T. Temperament, emotion, and childhood stuttering. Semin Speech Lang. 2014; 35(2):114–131

Clinical Implications

Binns AV, Hutchinson LR, Cardy JO. The speech-language pathologist's role in supporting the development of self-regulation: a review and tutorial. J Commun Disord. 2019; 78:1–17

Druker KC, Mazzucchelli TG, Beilby JM. An evaluation of an integrated fluency and resilience program for early developmental stuttering disorders. J Commun Disord. 2019; 78:69–83

Eggers K, Millard S, Kelman E. Temperament and the impact of stuttering in children aged 8–14 years. J Speech Lang Hear Res. 2021; 64(2):417–432

Kristal J. The temperament perspective: working with children's behavioral styles. New York, NY: Paul H Brookes Publishing; 2005

Section III

Diagnosis of Stuttering

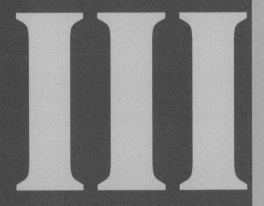

7 Preschool-Age Children

Ellen M. Kelly, Corrin I. Gillis, and Cara M. Singer

Abstract

Stuttering, or childhood-onset fluency disorder, begins in early childhood (between the age of 2 and 5 years) at a time when children are rapidly growing and acquiring skills across speech, language, social, motor, and emotional domains in multiple contexts, most especially within the family. Parents and/or other caregivers play important roles in supporting their children's development by providing models for verbal interactions and support across domains, including communication in all its complexities. In this chapter, we provide the rationales, quantitative and qualitative methods and measures, decision-making guidelines, and possible recommendations we would offer in a comprehensive assessment of preschool stuttering. Tools are provided for analyzing speech disfluencies, interviewing and obtaining questionnaire/survey data from parents/caregivers, evaluating risk for stuttering persistence, interviewing children about talking and stuttering, and discerning "next steps" for each child and family based on the results of the assessment process. Foundational to our methods is a focus on building strong, supportive relationships and therapeutic alliances that will best serve young children who stutter and their families over the short and long-term. We encourage the reader to make use of the tables, figures, and appendices in their own assessments of preschoolers referred to them for stuttering.

Keywords: stuttering, assessment, preschool, children, fluency, fluency disorder

7.1 Purpose

In this chapter, we provide guidelines for a comprehensive assessment of stuttering, related communication skills and challenges, and progress in other significant developmental domains in young children referred for stuttering. Our methods derive from a current understanding of childhood stuttering and of overall child development within the family context. We present methods for interviewing the child and parents/caregivers, gathering information from surveys and questionnaires, and both making observations and conducting formal testing with the child. Suggestions are provided for summarizing and interpreting results to make relevant clinical diagnoses and provide recommendations best suited to the child and family.

7.2 Setting the Stage for Assessing Preschoolers Who Stutter

7.2.1 Multidimensional Assessment of a Multifactorial Disorder

As outlined in ▶ Chapter 1 and expanded upon in subsequent chapters, we know stuttering emerges early in childhood during a period of rapid growth and development, with many factors playing important roles in its onset, development, exacerbation, persistence, and/or improvement.[1] In general, we think of stuttering development as reflecting the interplay between genetic predisposition and its interaction with experience and the environment. Stuttering, genetics, experience, and environment impact and are impacted by the emergence and developmental course of the child's own skills and abilities (e.g., language, speech production, speech motor, speech fluency, temperament, social communication, etc.). In turn, the child develops within the communicative contexts in which they live, learn, and grow (i.e., the family, especially parents/caregivers, and the daily experiences the child has at home, day care, or preschool).[1,2,3] ▶ Fig. 7.1 broadly illustrates the factors that contribute to stuttering in preschool children, suggesting that assessment likewise warrants a multidimensional approach.

Each of these influences will be taken into consideration not only as it relates to the initial appearance of stuttering but also how it may contribute to stuttering that continues into adulthood (i.e., risk for persistence; see ▶ Chapter 10 for more information). Each variable will also be integrated into the content of our assessments, resulting diagnoses, and recommendations to parents/caregivers and other important interactants in children's communicative environments. Under each area are what are commonly called the "ABCs" of stuttering:

- Affective:
  - Emotional makeup of the child and their responses.
- Behavioral:
  - What a child who stutters does (e.g., [dis]fluencies) or does not do (e.g., avoidances).
  - What others do and/or do not do in response to the child's stuttering.
- Cognitive:
  - Thoughts and/or attitudes about stuttering and/or communication, in general.[4]

The ABCs are used as a framework for the assessment process and resulting diagnoses, and shape the recommendations for, and goals and procedures of, any subsequent therapy (▶ Fig. 7.1a). ▶ Fig. 7.2 provides a general outline of the first portion of the assessment process we use for preschoolers who are suspected of stuttering.

7.3 Preschool Stuttering Assessment: Look, Listen, and Learn

7.3.1 Considering "Risk Factors" for Persistent Stuttering

The accumulation of evidence over decades has helped us better understand a number of variables that influence a child's likelihood of natural recovery (i.e., recovery without treatment) from stuttering versus a child's risk for continuing to stutter over time (i.e., stuttering persistence). These have

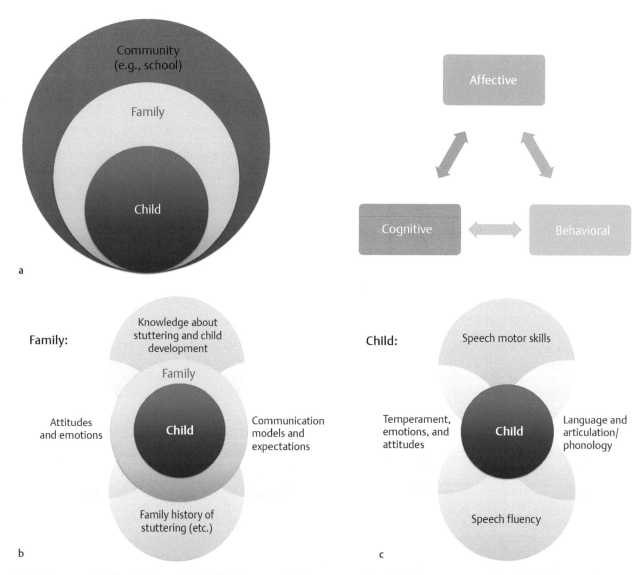

Fig. 7.1 Assessment of the child in context. **(a)** Child in communicative context and the ABCs of communication. **(b)** Familial (e.g., parent/caregiver) factors. **(c)** Child factors.

been identified and explained in earlier chapters and later in ► Chapter 10, and are among the variables we keep in mind when assessing children, counseling parents/caregivers, and making recommendations about "next steps" (e.g., monitoring, reevaluation, treatment, etc.) for preschoolers who are stuttering.[5] To summarize (see ► Chapter 10 for other detail), the current state of our understanding of risk for stuttering persistence indicates that children who are at risk for continuing to stutter are those who:

• are biological males.
• have a family history of stuttering (with some studies suggesting a history of persistent stuttering of greater import).[6,7]
• have been stuttering for more than a year.
• begin to stutter at or after the age of 3.5 years.
• exhibit a trajectory of stuttering that increases over time, fails to decrease, or decreases initially but then continues at levels higher than expected of nonstuttering children.

Further, we know that children who persist in stuttering are more likely than children who recover to show delays, inefficiencies, and/or differences (from nonstuttering children) in speech motor control (i.e., are more variable and imprecise),[8] speech sound articulation (i.e., have less "clear" speech),[9] language comprehension and production (i.e., achieve lower scores on standardized measures),[10,11] speech/language processing (i.e., show slower, less efficient processing),[12] and temperament (i.e., exhibit poorer self-regulation, reactivity, and negative affect).[13] Although the strength of evidence for individual risk factors varies,[14] ► Table 7.1 provides a general checklist for identification of risk-related variables that are important to consider when evaluating stuttering and related speech, language, and temperament variables in young children. Using this checklist reminds us to consider the possible contributors to and maintainers of a child's stuttering, which we will learn more about by obtaining information from parents/caregivers and the children themselves during the evaluation.

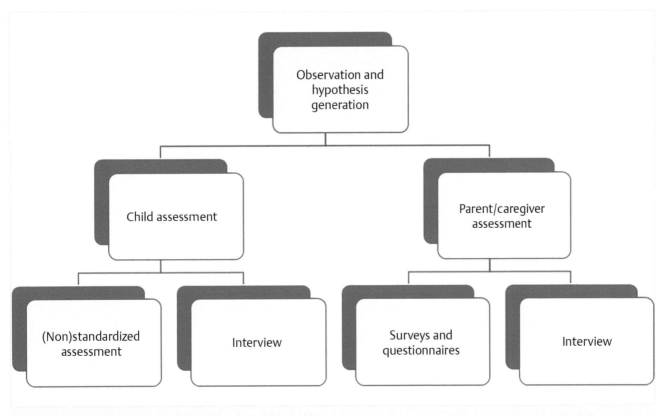

Fig. 7.2 Preschool stuttering assessment overview: look, listen, and learn.

Table 7.1 Checklist of possible risk factors for stuttering persistence

Risk factor	Elevated risk	True for child[a]
Family history of stuttering	Family history of stuttering (especially of persisting stuttering)	
Biological sex	Male	
Age at onset	After age 3.5 y	
Time since onset	Stuttering ≥12 mo	
Stuttering trajectory	Increasing or leveling off after initial decrease	
Biological sex	Male	
Speech articulation skills	Speech sound errors or trouble being understood	
Receptive language skills	Lower listening comprehension	
Expressive language skills	More difficulty verbalizing wants	
Emotional reactivity	More excitable	
Stuttering frequency	More stuttering-like disfluencies (SLDs)	
Speech motor skills	Slower and less coordinated speech motor movements	

Source: Adapted (and updated) from www.stutteringhelp.org/risk-factors.
[a] Place a check next to each that is true for the child.

7.3.2 Assessing the Child

When children suspected to be stuttering are referred for an evaluation, our first step is to "look at, listen to, and learn about" the child's communication skills, abilities, and challenges, at the same time as we observe their verbal interactions with parents or caregivers. We can learn a great deal about not only their stuttering but also other aspects of their communication (e.g., speech sound production, expressive and receptive language, social communication, speech motor structures and functioning, etc.) and developmental attributes (e.g., temperament and, relatedly, behavior and attention, etc.) by observing them interacting with parents/caregivers and with us. Thus, we always begin our assessments by asking parents/caregivers and the child (and sometimes siblings) to play and talk while we observe and record our observations, collect related data, and generate hypotheses about the child's strengths and challenges. In addition, we always engage the child ourselves to help them acclimate to us, the setting, and the assessment process, and to gather valuable data about these same variables.

Collecting and Analyzing Speech Samples

As shown in ▶ Fig. 7.1c, our initial sampling of the child's conversational interactions with parents/caregivers (and/or with us) provides information about the child's speech fluency, language, speech sound production and speech motor skills, temperament (including emotions, attitudes, attention, etc.), and social communication abilities with reference to the ABCs of communication. Initially, we make notes about what we observe. ▶ Table 7.2 includes some of the questions we ask ourselves, and the data we collect at the beginning of our evaluation.

To begin, for many reasons we recommend that students and practitioners take at least 3 to 5 minutes in this initial observation. First, unless we are looking at the child, we are likely to miss subtle and not-so-subtle stuttering behaviors that the child might exhibit (e.g., inaudible sound prolongations or "blocks"; looking away, facial grimaces/tension, stopping or altering talking; gesturing, carrying on undeterred, etc.). Second, a child and/or the child's parents/caregivers may also exhibit visible reactions to the child's stuttering (e.g., leaning in or looking away when the child stutters, finishing the child's sentences or waiting while the child finishes, frowning or smiling, etc.). Third, while watching the child and parent interacting, you will get a "feel" for the child's stuttering pattern, language skills, speech sound production abilities, social communication, and temperament. These observations might include the following: whether the child is initially reluctant to talk and warms up gradually; whether they monologue nonstop and/or are oblivious to others and/or to their own stuttering; whether the child tolerates mistakes in general, and/or with regard to stuttering, or responds negatively to them; whether the child stays with a task until completion in an age-appropriate manner, or quickly changes focus and tasks as if "driven by a motor"; and how the child responds to suggestions or corrections by a parent. These observations allow us to generate initial hypotheses (e.g., whether or not the child stutters, exhibits articulation errors/phonological patterns that interfere with the ability to be understood, has an outgoing/uninhibited temperament, and/or has language skills that appear at or above age-level expectations), and guide our selection and sequencing of follow-up testing, survey/questionnaire administration, and interview procedures.

After the initial 5 minutes or so of looking, listening, and learning, we begin to formally collect samples of the child's conversation for analyses of disfluencies. Using a disfluency count sheet (▶ Fig. 7.3), adapted slightly from Conture[15] and a disfluency count summary chart (▶ Fig. 7.4), we tally the frequencies of stuttering-like disfluencies (SLDs), including *Sound or Syllable Repetitions* (SSRs; e.g., "duh-duh-dog"), *Monosyllabic Whole-Word Repetitions* (Mo-WWRs; e.g., "I-I-I"), *Audible Sound Prolongations* (ASPs; e.g., "mmmmy"), and *Inaudible Sound Prolongations or Blocks* (ISPs; e.g., "...[silent pause]what"), as well as non-stuttering-like disfluencies (NSLDs) including *Multisyllabic Whole-Word Repetitions* (Mu-WWRs; e.g., "wanna-wanna"), *Phrase Repetitions* (PRs; e.g., "I can – I can"), *Interjections* (INTs; e.g., "um"), and *Revisions* (REV; e.g., "I have – I want"). A sample of at least 300 words or syllables of conversation is recommended to capture natural variations occurring in the interactions between the child and others. In general, an average/mean frequency of 3 or more SLDs per 100 words or syllables (i.e., 3% SLDs) is considered indicative of stuttering; however, no one measure, such as frequency of SLDs, should be used in isolation when making a diagnosis of stuttering.

Measuring the duration of SLDs is also recommended, as it provides a more complete picture of a young child's stuttering. For example, we are more concerned if a child prolongs a sound for 2 seconds versus fleetingly, and/or if a child produces four extra units, or iterations of repetition (e.g., **"buh-buh-buh-buh-ball"**) rather than one iteration of an SSR or Mo-WWR. Duration measures may be obtained via stopwatch or timer (e.g., on a smartphone), and by making note of the number of iterations (i.e., extra units of repetition) a child produces during SSRs and Mo-WWRs produced during speaking (e.g., "I-I-I" has two iterations). An important index of duration as well as stuttering severity is the weighted SLD that takes into consideration the average number of iterations of SSRs and Mo-WWRs and the average frequency of ISPs/blocks and ASPs. The formula for calculating the weighted SLD is the following:

$$[(\text{SSRs} + \text{MoWWRs}) \times \text{average no. of iterations of SSRs/MoWWRs}] + [2 \times (\text{ISPs} + \text{ASPs})].$$

It is recommended to include at least 10 instances of SSRs and/or MoWWRs when calculating the average number of iterations.

Duration measures are included in several commercially available stuttering assessment tools, as well. For example, the average duration of the three longest SLDs a child produces are

Table 7.2 Questions guiding initial observations of preschoolers who stutter

Observation area	General questions	Specific questions
Speech fluency	• What is the child's speech (dis)fluency like?	• Does the child stutter? • What is typical of the child's disfluencies? • Are there concomitant behaviors and/or reactions?
Articulation/phonology	• Is the child's speech sound production and phonological development age appropriate?	• What speech sound errors are present? Are they (a)typical? • What phonological processes are present? Are they (a)typical? • How intelligible is the child?
Expressive/receptive language	• Are the child's expressive and receptive language abilities age appropriate?	• Does the child appear to understand language age appropriately? • Are the child's spoken language abilities age appropriate?
Social communication	• Does the child demonstrate typical social communication skills?	• Are the child's social interactions and pragmatic skills (e.g., verbal and nonverbal communication) age appropriate?
Temperament, behavior, attention	• Does the child regulate emotion and behavior while focusing attention and engaging in social interaction?	• How does the child respond (e.g., react) to the testing environment, caregivers, and clinician? • Is the child behaviorally inhibited or outgoing? • Are the child's attentional focusing skills age appropriate?

Disfluency Count Sheet

Client's Name: _____   Clinician's Name: _____

DOB: _____   DOE: _____   Client's Age: _____

Type of Sample: Conversation _____   Reading _____   Words _____   Syllables _____

Sample #1 (100 words or syllables):

TYPE	TOTAL #
SSR	
Mo-WWR	
ASP	
ISP/Block	
TOTAL SLD:	
Mu-WWR	
PR	
INTJ	
REV	
TOTAL NSLD:	
TOTAL ALL:	

Sample #2 (100 words or syllables):

TYPE	TOTAL #
SSR	
Mo-WWR	
ASP	
ISP/Block	
TOTAL SLD:	
Mu-WWR	
PR	
INTJ	
REV	
TOTAL NSLD:	
TOTAL ALL:	

Sample #3 (100 words or syllables):

TYPE	TOTAL #
SSR	
Mo-WWR	
ASP	
ISP/Block	
TOTAL SLD:	
Mu-WWR	
PR	
INTJ	
REV	
TOTAL NSLD:	
TOTAL ALL:	

SSR – sound/syllable repetition; Mo-WWR – Monosyllabic whole-word repetition; ASP – audible sound prolongation. ISP/Block – inaudible sound prolongation or block; PR – phrase repetition; INTJ – interjection; REV – revision; Mu-WWR – multisyllabic whole-word repetition

Fig. 7.3 Disfluency count sheet.

required components of the *Stuttering Severity Instrument, 4th edition* (SSI-4).[16] The SSI-4 combines data on stuttering frequency, duration, and physical concomitants (i.e., nonspeech behaviors associated with moments of stuttering) that equate to a severity rating. Data are gathered from speaking and, when appropriate, reading, including the average frequency of percent syllables stuttered, average duration of the three longest SLDs, and evidence of physical concomitants (i.e., distracting sounds, facial grimaces, head movements, and/or movement of the extremities). Likewise, a judgment of the frequency with which the child repeats a sound or syllable more than once is made when an observer (e.g., parent/caregiver, teacher, speech-language pathologist [SLP]) completes the *Test of Childhood Stuttering Observational Rating Scales* (TOCS ORS; see the section "Obtaining Parent/Caregiver Input" later in the chapter for more information).[17]

Fig. 7.4 Disfluency count summary chart.

DISFLUENCY COUNT SUMMARY CHART

NAME: _____ DATE: _____ AGE: _____

CONVERSATION OR READING: _____ WITH WHOM: _____

SAMPLE SIZE: _____ WORDS OR SYLLABLES: _____

TYPES OF DISFLUENCIES PRODUCED	FREQUENCY SAMPLE 1	FREQUENCY SAMPLE 2	FREQUENCY SAMPLE 3	TOTAL ALL SAMPLES	PERCENTAGE	RANK ORDER
Stutter-Like Disfluencies (SLDs):						
Monosyllabic Whole-Word Repetitions						
Sound/Syllable Repetitions						
Audible Sound Prolongations						
Inaudible Sound Prolongations/Blocks						
TOTAL SLDs:						
Non-Stutter-Like Disfluencies (NSLDs):						
Multi-syllabic Whole-Word Repetitions						
Phrase Repetitions						
Interjections						
Revisions						
TOTAL NSLDs:						
TOTAL ALL DISFLUENCIES:					100%	

AVERAGE ALL DISFLUENCIES = _____   RANGE ALL DISFLUENCIES: _____

AVERAGE SLDs = _____   RANGE SLDs: _____   SLDs % OF TOTAL: _____

AVERAGE NSLDs = _____   RANGE NSLDs: _____   NSLDs % OF TOTAL: _____

DURATION:

ITERATIONS (Extra Units of Repetition):

Average: _____

Range: _____

WEIGHTED SLD:

Number of Iterations:
1. ____   6. ____
2. ____   7. ____
3. ____   8. ____
4. ____   9. ____
5.   10.

PHYSICAL CONCOMITANTS: _____
_____
_____
NOTES: _____
_____
_____
_____
_____

[(Average # MoWWR + Average # SSR) * Average Iterations] + [2 * (Average # ASP + Average # ISP)] = _____

We also make note of any signs of visible tension/struggle or physical concomitants (e.g., eye blinking, head nodding, pressing lips together, craning the neck, etc.) that may accompany SLDs, and any other information that paints a more comprehensive picture of the child's stuttering (e.g., stops talking when stuttering or continues talking whether stuttering or not). Observations about parent/caregiver responses are also noted (e.g., whether eye contact is maintained, corrections are offered [e.g., slow down, take your time, take a deep breath, etc.], empathy is provided [e.g., that's okay, I'm listening], turn taking is positive [e.g., minimizes talking for or "over" the child], language is contingent [e.g., responds to the content of the child's utterances], etc.).

Formal Assessment: Speech Sound Production, Language, Speech Motor, Temperament and Social Communication Skills

Referring back to the questions in ▶ Table 7.2, observation of initial conversational interactions also allows us to note any speech sound production errors and related error patterns, and to evaluate the child's speech intelligibility (i.e., ability to be understood by others). Informal observations of the child's receptive (i.e., comprehension or understanding) and expressive (i.e., production or expression) language abilities, social interactions (e.g., reciprocal conversational exchanges, engagement, etc.), speech motor skills, and temperament (e.g., shy/inhibited, outgoing/uninhibited, fast or slow to warm up, etc.) are also noted.

▶ Table 7.3 contains examples of more formalized assessment tools that may be used to ascertain the child's stuttering, language, speech sound production, speech motor structure/function, and temperament (including behavior and attention). Given the potential risk factors for stuttering persistence as previously outlined (see ▶ Table 7.1), we suggest inclusion of one or more screening or full-scale assessment instruments for each domain in order to provide a comprehensive view of the child's skills and abilities as well as challenges (▶ Table 7.3). We are not suggesting that all of these need to be utilized in every case; observations during the initial interactions with the child will help SLPs select and prioritize the subsequent assessment measures. Individual practitioners will know best which tools

Table 7.3 Preschool stuttering assessment tools and measures

Skill domain	Administered to		
	Child		Parent
Speech fluency	• SSI-4 • KiddyCAT		• TOCS ORS (fluency; consequences) • ECHOS intake (part B) • ISPP • Palin PRS • VRYCS
Speech sound production	• AAPS or GFTA or BBTOP		• Intelligibility in Context Scale (ICS)
Receptive language	• PPVT • TACL • Receptive language portions of PLS, CELF-P, TOLD-P, TELD, etc.		• CELF-P Emerging Literacy Rating Scale
Expressive language	• EVT • Expressive portions of PLS, CELF-P, TOLD-P, TELD, etc. • Conversational sample analyses (e.g., MLU, DSS, etc.)		• CELF-P Emerging Literacy Rating Scale
Speech motor structure/function	• OSMSE and DDK • NRT		• Case history
Temperament (reactivity; self-regulation; behavior; attention)	• Behavioral observation		• SBIS • CBQ-VSF • Parent/caregiver report
Social communication	• Behavioral observation		• CELF-P descriptive pragmatics profile • Parent/caregiver report

Abbreviations: AAPS, Arizona Articulation Proficiency Scale; BBTOP, Bankson–Bernthal Test of Phonology; CBQ-VSF, Children's Behavior Questionnaire (Very Short Form); CELF-P, Clinical Evaluation of Language Fundamentals-Preschool; DDK, diadochokinetic syllable rates; DSS, Developmental Sentence Scoring; ECHOS, Early Childhood Onset Stuttering; EVT, Expressive Vocabulary Test; GFTA, Goldman–Fristoe Test of Articulation; ISPP, Impact of Stuttering on Preschool Children and Parents; KiddyCAT, Communication Attitude Test for Preschool and Kindergarten Children who Stutter; MLU, mean length of utterance; NRT, Nonword Repetition Test; OSMSE, Oral Speech Mechanism Screening Examination; PLS, Preschool Language Scale; PPVT, Picture Peabody Vocabulary Test; SBIS, Short Behavioral Inhibition Scale; SSI-4, Stuttering Severity Instrument, fourth edition; TACL, Test for Auditory Comprehension of Language; TELD, Test of Early Language Development; TOLD-P, Test of Language Development-Primary; VRYCS, Vanderbilt responses to your child's speech.

are suited to the demographics of the child and family (e.g., age, sex, race, ethnicity, background, etc.), the characteristics of the instruments (e.g., standardization norms), and the nature of their clinical settings (e.g., whether parents/caregivers are present), time constraints, and personal preferences.

There are few formal instruments that directly tap children's own perceptions of the ABCs (affective, behavioral, and cognitive) of communication, so most of this information is gleaned from interviewing the child. One exception—a valid, reliable instrument for which normative data are available—is the *Communication Attitudes Test of Preschool and Kindergarten Children Who Stutter* (KiddyCAT).[18] The KiddyCAT includes 12 yes/no questions asked of preschool or kindergarten-age children about their perceptions of, or attitudes about, talking. These questions elicit the child's perceptions of whether talking is hard in general, whether words are hard to say, whether they talk "right," whether or not it is "easy" to talk, whether they like to talk, as well as their perception of how others view their talking. There are also questions that refer specifically to stuttering in that the child is asked whether words sometimes "get stuck" in their mouth, or come out "easily." The child's responses can be compared to those obtained from preschoolers/kindergartners who do and do not stutter. In the initial normative[19] and subsequent replication and extension study,[20] analyses of KiddyCAT results indicated that, on average, young children who stutter (CWS) have more negative attitudes, self-perceptions, and perceptions of others' attitudes toward their talking (i.e., score higher on the KiddyCAT) than do children who do not stutter (CWNS). Most significantly, CWS were more likely

than CWNS to identify speaking as difficult (e.g., talking is hard, words stick in my mouth, words are hard to say, etc.). We often utilize the KiddyCAT as a springboard for conversation about talking and stuttering with the child.

• *Child interview:* While we talk to the child, we learn more about their perceptions of their communication abilities and challenges as well as their stuttering (or whatever they may call it, if they have a name for, or words describing, it). In general, we think of this conversation as having (at least) three parts that proceed from more general to more specific, including (1) learning about the child, (2) learning about the child's communication, and (3) learning about the child's stuttering. We begin by learning about the child—likes, dislikes, favorite things to do, people in the family, friends, etc., as a means for establishing a positive therapeutic relationship, and for learning about the child's makeup and view of the world. Moving toward discussing communication and stuttering, we ask the children why they came to see us. Some children say they do not know, shrug their shoulders, or look at their parents/caregivers for answers, while others tell us that our meeting has something to do with their talking (e.g., they have trouble talking, or "can't talk"), or may say something specifically about their talking difficulties (e.g., can't say their words or "get stuck" when they try to talk), or that they "stutter." We never assume children understand or interpret the word "stutter" or "stuttering" as we do, so we follow their lead and ask what they mean by "stutter" or "stuttering" and if they can show us what happens or what it sounds like. This opens the floor to a conversation about when stuttering occurs (where, with whom), why they think they "stutter" (or whatever word(s) they use), and what they do to help themselves when they do. Conversations like these also provide an opportunity for us to compliment and reinforce how much the child knows (i.e., that they are experts) about themselves, their talking, and their stuttering, thereby modeling for them, and their parents/caregivers, that stuttering is something that can be discussed clearly and openly.

At times, children do not seem to be aware or concerned about the way they talk or their stuttering. At other times, they may say little but indicate nonverbally that they are bothered by or uncomfortable with their stuttering, and/or by others drawing attention to it. This is evidenced by behaviors such as diverting eye contact, changing the subject of a conversation, seeking attention or comfort from a parent, and so forth. A child's reactions to their stuttering may give us indications of both how they are perceiving stuttering and how others perceive and/or react to it. When children seem unaware or unwilling to talk about stuttering, we sometimes wait a bit and then, in the course of play-based interactions, model some easy, effortless SLDs in our own speaking (e.g., SSRs and/or ASPs) and see how the child responds. Sometimes, there is no response. At other times, the child will look at us curiously or show signs of discomfort (e.g., avert their eyes, blush, squirm in their seats, etc.). When children appear to notice, we may then say something like "Oh, I got a little stuck there. I said m-m-my tower has a blue block on top," and leave it there. We may then do it again, adding the comment, "Does that ever happen to you?" For some children, this invites a discussion about their own stuttering and/or speaking difficulties. During one evaluation in our clinic, after modeling some easy SSRs and commenting on them, an alarmed preschooler responded, "Don't do that. Daddy said never do that." A glance at the father revealed a look of embarrassment and uncertainty—something addressed later with him in the context of parents, quite naturally, not knowing how to react to or help their child who is stuttering. During these brief interviews with children, we often hear some very creative explanations about what happens when they stutter (e.g., "My throat locks up and throws away the key"), why they stutter (e.g., "I swallowed a penny when I was a baby"), and what helps (e.g., "I talk like a Jedi"). The information we gather in this manner provides both a broader picture of the child's personal story (in general and with regard to communication and stuttering), and establishes the beginning of positive, supportive relationships with the child and family that will facilitate sharing findings and diagnoses, making recommendations, and providing subsequent therapy services as needed.

Obtaining Parent/Caregiver Input

In addition to the more general or standardized intake form(s) particular to each clinical setting, there are a variety of useful instruments that may be completed by parents to broaden our understanding of their children's skills and abilities across domains, their stuttering and communication in everyday contexts, and parents'/caregivers' own knowledge and/or assumptions about and responses to their children, in general, and with

regard to stuttering (▶ Table 7.3). We may include, exclude, and/or administer any of these orally depending on the parent(s)'/caregiver(s)' language abilities (e.g., if English is a non-primary language for them and/or we are evaluating the child with the help of an interpreter) and literacy skills (as self-reported or observed, e.g., parent/caregiver is struggling to complete a form). We let parents/caregivers know that the forms may contain professional language or terms that are unfamiliar and we would be happy to answer questions or give them more information at any time, making it easier for anyone who may be uncertain or reluctant to ask for assistance.

Our general intake form for parents/caregivers (*Early Childhood Onset Stuttering* [ECHOS] *Intake Form*), includes specific questions (part B) about the child's stuttering behavior at its onset and over time, and any family history of stuttering (see Appendix 7.1). Obtaining this information (along with that pertaining to other familial and developmental variables) facilitates consideration of the risk factors for stuttering persistence. It also informs us of any personal knowledge of and/or experiences with stuttering (or other challenges) in the family that may impact perceptions, reactions, questions, and needs as we assess the child's stuttering and communication, obtain from and provide information to the parents/caregivers, and make collaborative decisions about next steps for the child and family.

There are a variety of helpful parent/caregiver report instruments that help us learn about the child's stuttering and the ways in which parents respond to it. Practitioners may elect to administer one or more of these instruments based on their clinical judgments of what might be most useful for obtaining such information from a particular child and family. When language and/or literacy issues are a factor, instruments may be presented orally (and/or through an interpreter) or omitted in favor of more in-depth parent/caregiver interviews. Of the four described below, the first three (ISPP, Palin Parent Rating Scales [Palin PRS], VRYCS) are cost free:

- *Impact of Stuttering on Preschool Children and Parents (ISPP):* The ISPP,[21] adapted for ease of completion (Appendix 7.2) by Dr. Katerina Ntourou (another contributor to this volume), provides information about parents'/caregivers' perceptions of the impact of stuttering on their child's talking, confidence, play with other children, emotional reactions (e.g., mood changes, withdrawal, frustration), reactions of other children (e.g., teasing, changes in play), and impact on parents/caregivers themselves (e.g., emotionally, knowing/not knowing what to do/say). The 19 questions include items that require selection of "yes" or "no" responses, followed by more specific choices, and open-ended questions requesting parents/caregivers to comment on their observations and perceptions.
- *Palin PRS:* If you have use of a tablet, laptop, or desktop computer, parents (of children of any age who are stuttering) can register online and complete the 19-item *Palin PRS*[22] to rate (1) the impact of stuttering (or "stammering" as it is called in the United Kingdom) on the child, (2) the severity of the child's stuttering and its impact on parents, and (3) parents' knowledge of stuttering and confidence in managing it (https://www.palinprs.org.uk/secure/pprs_connect.php). Results may be used to identify areas of difficulty for the child and related parent concerns, inform counseling and recommendations, and monitor progress over

repeated evaluations and/or the course of therapy. Scores may be compared to those obtained from 259 parents of CWS (ranging in age from 2.6 to 14.6 years) for each of the three factors.

- *Vanderbilt Responses to Your Child's Speech (VRYCS):*[23] Recently, we developed the VRYCS rating scale to obtain parents'/caregivers' perceptions of their own responses to the speech of their children who are stuttering (see Appendix 7.3).[23] The VYRCS contains 18 items pertaining to five factors or categories of parent responses including the following: (1) requesting the child to make changes when speaking (e.g., to think about what he or she is saying, take a deep breath, slow down, or relax); (2) talking for the child (e.g., finish what the child was saying, fill in words for the child); (3) supporting the child's talking (e.g., letting the child lead conversations, waiting for the child to finish, praising what the child said); (4) slowing and/or simplifying their own talking (e.g., pausing before responding, asking simple questions); and (5) responding emotionally (e.g., becoming tense, remaining relaxed, worrying about the child's talking). Parents rate their use of each of the 18 items (e.g., "How often do you ask your child to slow down when talking?") from 0 ("never") to 4 ("always"). Results may be used to compliment and reinforce parents for positive responses (e.g., waiting for the child to finish speaking), discuss and redirect less helpful responses (e.g., filling words in for the child), and inform decisions about recommendations, including the type and content of intervention.

- *TOCS ORS*[17]: The TOCS ORS, including both the *Speech Fluency Rating Scale* (TOCS ORS-Fluency) and the *Disfluency-Related Consequences Rating Scale* (TOCS ORS-Consequences), is a 1-page form to be completed by parents/caregivers (and/or other SLPs or teachers). Using the TOCS ORS-Fluency, respondents score each of nine items on a scale from 0 ("never") to 3 ("always"), reflecting their judgment of how often the child exhibited the behavior over the previous 2 months. Results provide information about the characteristics of the child's stuttering (e.g., repeats parts of words, prolongs sounds, gets stuck or blocked, etc.) and when and with whom it occurs (e.g., when addressing parents, peers, siblings, groups, etc.). The TOCS ORS-Consequences also contains nine items scored by respondents (i.e., using the same 3-point scale) to rate their judgments of the child's physical and emotional reactions to stuttering across the previous 2 months (e.g., becomes tense, runs out of breath, avoids words, becomes concerned, embarrassed, or frustrated, etc.), as well as whether or not the child was rejected by other children because of stuttering. These ratings are used to indicate the severity of the child's stuttering (TOCS ORS-Fluency) and any stuttering-related consequences the child experiences (TOCS ORS-Consequences); however, the published test only contains comparison data for children ranging in age from 7 to 12 years. Because TOCS ORS was developed for children between 7 and 12 years of age, we use the ratings from both questionnaires (fluency and consequences) as a useful inventory of preschoolers' stuttering severity and their responses to it, observed over the past few months in environments outside of the clinical setting. Since variability is a hallmark of stuttering (as discussed elsewhere in this volume), the TOCS ORS gives us a broader understanding of children's stuttering and related behavior in real-world contexts. This is especially important when the child's stuttering on the day of (or even during) our assessment is different from (e.g., less evident and/or severe than) what prompted parents/caregivers to schedule the appointment. Such a mismatch between in- and outside-of-clinic observations can contribute to parent/caregiver concerns that we doubt or disagree with their characterizations of their children's stuttering. By having parents/caregivers complete the TOCS ORS, we acknowledge that (1) we expect their children's day-to-day stuttering and communication, and reactions thereto, to be more varied and complex than what we might observe during our brief assessments; (2) we rely on their input as experts about, and close observers of, their children; and (3) we are seeking a full picture of their children's stuttering in everyday contexts where they communicate naturally (and may be impacted by stuttering).

We use several other instruments, along with our intake form(s) and interviews, to obtain additional parent/caregiver input about children's language, preliteracy, social pragmatic, speech intelligibility, speech motor, and temperament characteristics. Next, we provide a brief discussion of some of these measures, also listed in ▸ Table 7.3.

- *Language/preliteracy skills and social pragmatics*: For language and literacy, we ask parents to complete the Clinical Evaluation of Language Fundamentals Preschool-3 [CELF-P:3] Emerging Literacy Scale), and for social pragmatics abilities, the CELF-P:3 Descriptive Pragmatics Profile.[24] Results are compared to criterion scores for preschool-age children and help us identify areas of possible concern that may require further assessment.

- *Speech intelligibility*: We administer the Intelligibility in Context Scale (ICS),[25] a quick, standardized parent-report measure of functional speech intelligibility, available in 60 different languages (see Appendix 7.4 for the English version). Parents are asked to rate the degree to which different communication partners (i.e., themselves, others in the immediate family, extended family members, friends, acquaintances, teachers, and strangers) are able to understand the child. Ratings of the seven items are made on a 5-point scale from 1 ("never") to 5 ("always"). This indication of children's abilities to be understood in everyday contexts by those with whom they interact most, when added to our own observations, helps us to both provide a better understanding of the child's speech sound production abilities and guide our selection of follow-up questions and additional assessment procedures (e.g., whether a single-word naming articulation test is appropriate and/or sufficient).

- *Speech motor structure and function*: Included in our assessment is examination of the structure and functioning of the child's speech sound production mechanism (e.g., Oral Speech Mechanism Screening Examination [OSMSE-R]).[26] We look for any signs of structural or functional abnormalities when we initially "look, listen, and learn" while the child interacts with parent(s)/caregiver(s) and/or with us, and then look a little more closely at the child's face, neck, lips, teeth, tongue, and soft and hard palates, at rest, during movements (e.g., puffing the cheeks, pursing and puckering the lips, moving the tongue up, down, and side to side, etc.), and during production of vowels and (non)nasal consonants. We also ask the child to produce rapid repetitions of sequences (i.e., diadochokinetic syllable rates or DDKs) of monosyllables (20 repetitions), bisyllables (15 repetitions), and trisyllables (10 repetitions; e.g., "puh," "puhtuh," puhtuhkuh") to further ascertain speed and coordination of oral motor movements.[27] During the DDK task, as children produce the sounds and syllables the clinician can observe (and/or audio/video record to analyze later) the child's productions for discoordination, distortions, motor fatigue, or groping behaviors. Inclusion of the Nonword Repetition Test (NRT)[28] permits more formal examination of speech motor proficiency during the production of novel phonological sequences. We use this test because recent research has shown greater variability and discoordination in speech motor production among some young CWS that does not resolve in those children whose stuttering will persist.[8]

- *Temperament*: We also explore parent(s)'/caregiver(s)' perceptions of their children's temperament, behavior in everyday situations, and attention (e.g., ability to focus, shift attention and to be flexible) by observing and by administering the Short Behavioral Inhibition Scale (SBIS)[28] and the very short form of the Children's Behavior Questionnaire (CBQ-VSF).[29] The SBIS focuses specifically on behavioral inhibition, or the child's tendency to process and respond reluctantly, cautiously, and/or avoidantly to novelty, change, and/or differences in the environment. These tendencies are often seen when the child meets new people (e.g., warming up easily or with difficulty), interacts in a group, or tries out new activities. The parent is asked to consider each of five items in light of their child's behavior during the interval from birth to 4 years of age. Assigned scores range from 1 to 5 for each item (maximum total score = 25), with lower scores reflecting greater behavioral inhibition and higher scores reflecting an unreserved, engaging, or outgoing temperament. Ntourou et al[29] compared results from parents of preschoolers, including 225 CWS and 243 CWNS between the ages of 2.10 and 6.3 years, finding greater behavioral inhibition among CWS. Further, CWS with higher levels of behavioral inhibition stuttered more often (% SLDs) and more severely (SSI-3 or SSI-4 and TOCS ORS-Fluency; see ▶ Chapter 7.3.2), experienced more disfluency-related consequences (TOCS ORS-Consequences), and had more negative communication attitudes (KiddyCAT, see Formal Assessment section), than did CWS with lower levels of behavioral inhibition. We recommend inclusion of all of these measures (SSI-4, TOCS ORS, KiddyCAT, SBIS) in assessments of preschoolers who stutter, allowing for consideration of possible relations between and among variables (see ▶ Table 7.3).

The CBQ-VSF[30] is a 36-item instrument designed to tap three broad domains of temperament including surgency/extraversion (e.g., impulsive, high activity, outgoing, etc.), negative affect (e.g., sadness, fear, anger/frustration, etc.), and effortful control (e.g., inhibition, attentional control, perceptual sensitivity, etc.). It was derived from the more comprehensive, 195-item CBQ.[30] The 36 items describe reactions children may have to various situations (e.g., "seems always in a hurry to get from one place to another," "takes a long time in approaching

new situations," "is quite upset by a little cut or bruise"). Thus, the CBQ-VSF is useful for general screening of temperament, attention, and behavior in 3- to 7-year-old children, and is available in a variety of languages. Parents/caregivers are asked to rate each item on a 7-point scale ranging from 1 ("extremely untrue of your child") to 7 ("extremely true of your child"), based on their observations of the child over the past 6 months.

Knowing how young children respond to situations they may encounter in daily life enriches our understanding of the ways they may react to challenges (positive and negative) they may experience. These challenging situations might include starting a new school year, moving, welcoming a new sibling, getting or not getting their own way, visiting an amusement park, learning new skills, stuttering, having difficulty being understood, and so forth. We typically look for response patterns corresponding to each of the three domains (surgency, negative affect, and effortful control) and note items that are rated as "extremely true" for particular children that may warrant follow-up during the parent/caregiver interview. Children's temperaments not only may impact the ways they respond to what their parents/caregivers (and others) do, or do not do, in response to their stuttering, but also guide our own interactions with them, and inform our recommendations.

By including a variety of instruments, we obtain a comprehensive understanding of the ABCs and impact of stuttering on children and their parents or caregivers within the developmental contexts in which they relate, grow, and learn.

- *Parent/caregiver interview*: We conduct an interview with parents/caregivers after we have had the opportunity to look, listen, and learn as they interact with their child, but before we administer any more comprehensive formal assessment procedures to the child. Interviewing parents or caregivers helps us (1) to obtain additional information and insights that broaden our own observations and hypotheses and inform our selection of assessment tools (e.g., family history of stuttering and/or other communication, developmental, and/or health conditions); (2) to provide opportunities to compliment the parents/caregivers and ask questions about their child and their own interactions (e.g., models of language and communication, parenting styles, presence of communication disorders, e.g., stuttering and/or speech sound production errors); and (3) to discern whether or not what we observed is consistent with their perceptions of and expectations for their child's developmental skills/levels and challenges, communication abilities and concerns, and, specifically, the ABCs of stuttering and their impact on the child and family (▶ Fig. 7.1b).

We begin our interview by thanking parents/caregivers for taking the time to bring their child to see us and to provide an idea of what the child's speech, language, and stuttering is like in interaction with important listeners. This is followed by a general question such as, "How can we be helpful to you and your child today?" or "What do you most want to learn from this assessment?" or "What questions would you like answered as part of today's evaluation?" or "What are your best hopes for our time together today?" That last example is from solution-focused interviewing and therapy, an approach that centers on clients' and/or parent(s)'/caregiver(s)' most important hopes or goals for themselves and their child.[31] Frequently, parents/caregivers talk about their concerns for the child's communication (e.g., stuttering), revealing worries about what may have caused the problem(s) (especially anything that they may have done or failed to do), whether or not the problem will resolve on its own or necessitate therapy, what the impact on the child might be should stuttering continue into the future (e.g., peer relationships, teasing or bullying, academic and/or career impact, etc.), and what they can do to help their child. Oftentimes their best hopes are that the child will overcome stuttering (e.g., grow out of it or resolve it with treatment) and/or that it will not interfere with their future growth and development, relationships, happiness, and life accomplishments. The questions parents/caregivers usually have for us correspond to these same concerns, worries, and hopes for the future as they journey to a better understanding of their child's stuttering and how best to help. For one family where the mother and three of the children stutter, the parents sought evaluations only when they observed their children avoiding speaking and/or exhibiting negative reactions to their stuttering. The parents' perceptions were that it was not the stuttering itself that was problematic, but any impact it might have on their children's social interactions and achievements of academic, career, and life goals.

Once we have an idea of what brought the family to see us, we follow up with questions that our conversation and their responses on the intake form(s) suggest are important, especially about development, health, and/or family history that will help us to better understand the child and the factors that may relate to the onset and development of stuttering. We are especially interested in learning about the onset of the child's stuttering—when, where, how (i.e., what the child's stuttering was like when it was first noticed), and any explanations the parents/caregivers may have for it beginning. We also ask about their child's and their own reactions at that time, those of others, and the progress and/or changes in stuttering that have occurred since then. This conversation includes attention to the potential risk factors for stuttering persistence outlined earlier (see ▶ Table 7.1), especially concerning the trajectory of the problem and whether or not there are others in the child's biological family who stuttered and recovered or who continued to stutter into adulthood. This conversation may involve extended inquiry and include mapping out, on paper, members of the child's biological family (on both the maternal and paternal sides), their relationships to the child (e.g., sibling, parent, aunt, uncle, grandparent, etc.), whether or not they stuttered (and recovered or persisted, if known), and if they have any other health or developmental concerns of note.

If a parent/caregiver stutters, we briefly ask about their own experiences with stuttering (e.g., history, therapy, impact, etc.) and how they think those affect their views of their child's stuttering, as well as their hopes for both our assessment and recommendations for the future (e.g., therapy, school placement, referrals, etc.). As illustrated earlier, we have worked with parents who stutter and are unconcerned about their child's stuttering behavior, but worried that it might interfere with communication, happiness, and future plans. In contrast, we have worked with parents who stutter who hope we can quickly help their child overcome stuttering to prevent any possible negative consequences that might occur in the future,

some of which they may have experienced themselves. For example, one young boy's father recounted being teased, bullied, and ostracized by peers and mocked by teachers as a youngster, contributing to his trying to hide stuttering at all costs and making choices (e.g., about education and career paths) to minimize the necessity of talking. While he supported his son in the short and long-term, he hoped to spare him from the anxiety, negative self-perceptions and communication struggles he experienced himself, and the impact stuttering might have on his child's life choices. We welcome all points of view and use them to guide our presentation of findings and recommendations, especially as they influence our manner and focus in counseling the family and including them in the therapy process. We see the shared experience of stuttering within the family as a positive element of our partnership over the short and longer term.

The information we gain from talking with parents/caregivers helps us to refine our selection of assessment procedures for the child (see ▶ Table 7.3). While we engage the child, we have parents/caregivers complete the parent-report instruments described earlier, letting them know they are free to ask any questions as they proceed. If at all possible, we like to have the parents/caregivers in the same room with us so that they may observe and ask questions. Because they are present in the room, sometimes we have to ask them not to interfere when we are administering a test to their child; for example, by rephrasing questions we ask their child, repeating models or instructions, or adding information to help their child choose the correct answer. At the same time, their presence allows them to learn, along with us, about their child's skills, abilities, and challenges, and gives them an opportunity to think of questions for us, or provide additional information that might be helpful. Once testing is finished, we typically give the family a 10- to 15-minute refreshment and self-care break while we score and compile our results.

7.3.3 Compiling and Synthesizing Results and Making Recommendations

The process of providing parents/caregivers with recommendations includes (1) compiling and synthesizing our assessment results, (2) making differential diagnoses, (3) presenting our findings, (3) delivering our recommendations, (4) providing referral sources, and (5) following up on our recommendations and/or referrals (▶ Fig. 7.5).

- *Assessment*: As shown in ▶ Figs. 7.1, 7.2, and 7.3, the assessment process leads to our understanding of possible risk factors for stuttering persistence (▶ Table 7.1), answers questions about the child's skills and abilities, and helps reveal the ways in which the child and parents/caregivers interact (▶ Table 7.2). It also provides results of formal assessment procedures through conversations with the child, administration of screenings and/or comprehensive testing protocols, completion of intakes and surveys by parents/caregivers, and interviews of the child and parents/caregivers (▶ Table 7.3). When considering our findings, we ask ourselves what communication challenges the child has, if any, when compared to age and culturally appropriate developmental expectations. Throughout our assessment,

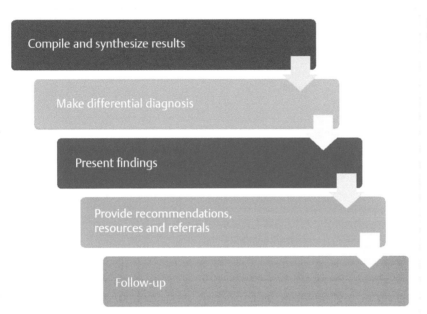

Fig. 7.5 Preschool stuttering assessment overview: part 2.

we have considered the child's speech fluency, language, speech sound production and speech motor skills, temperament (including emotions and attitudes, behavior, attention, etc.), and social communication abilities with reference to the ABCs of communication. We have observed and reflected upon the child's awareness and reactions or responses to communication breakdown, and those of their parents/caregivers, along with parents'/caregivers' knowledge and expectations, concerns and assumptions (e.g., about their own roles), regarding stuttering, communication, and development. In addition to comparing results to objective norms and standards (e.g., cultural, linguistic, etc.), we view our results in light of each child growing and developing within unique family and community environments (▶ Fig. 7.1). Our primary objective is to help the child and family obtain knowledge and tools to foster effective, spontaneous, comfortable, efficient, and joyful communication,[32,33] and reduce negative and enhance positive impacts the child's communication challenges and skills may present now and in the future.

- *Differential diagnoses*: During our assessment we accumulate and analyze a great deal of evidence that forms the basis for our diagnoses of deficits in speech fluency, speech sound production, expressive/receptive language, and/or motor speech coordination, while also gaining a greater understanding of the child's social communication, temperament, and family dynamics. We also discern the concerns, knowledge, assumptions, behaviors, and hopes of parents/caregivers in relation to their child's strengths and challenges. As a result, at the end of the evaluation, we know the deficits or challenges the child has and how they impact and are impacted by the child's developmental skills and trajectory (within and across domains), as well as important elements of family history and interactions. We also have taken the time to forge the beginnings of a strong, confident, and trusting therapeutic relationship with the child and family that will help the parents/caregivers comprehend and

digest our findings and recommendations and facilitate their active partnership with us throughout the therapeutic process. We find most children can be characterized as presenting with typical/age-appropriate fluency skills, a stuttering disorder, or a stuttering disorder with a concomitant speech and/or language disorder. We use ▶ Table 7.4 to summarize our findings and related diagnoses as we prepare to share them with the family.

- *Presenting findings*: Prior to presenting our findings, we thank the parents/caregivers and the child for coming to see us, their participation in the assessment, and for helping us to learn extensively about the child's communication abilities and challenges. We then ask what would be most important for them to know or gain from the time we spent together. Typically, we are asked to share whether or not their child (1) has a problem with stuttering (and/or other challenges); (2) whether the problem(s) will persist; (3) if the child needs therapy and, if so, about the particulars; and (4) how they can best help their child. We begin by answering their questions, from most to least pressing for them, interweaving the results of our assessment. We often highlight those skills that are relative strengths for the child and the family, as this provides an opportunity to share positive findings in anticipation of applying them to addressing diagnoses of delays, disorders, and/or differences and related recommendations for intervention. Most of the time, when we present an area of identified challenge for the child, we are simply confirming what the parents/caregivers have already recognized; at these times, we are able to say, "As you told us, your child...." This confirms their expertise about their child and solidifies our partnership for the present and future.

  After sharing the results and before we offer our recommendations, we ask for any additional questions or other information the parents/caregivers would like to share. We also ask the parents/caregivers what they have learned from the assessment results we have provided. If they lack clarity about and/or misunderstood any of the findings we

Table 7.4 Preschool stuttering assessment results summary form

Domain	Findings	Recommendations
Speech fluency	Disfluencies in conversation: Comments: Means (ranges): SLD: NSLD: TD: Top 3 disfluency types: 1. 2. 3. SSI-4: Comments: Total score: Severity: TOCS ORS: Comments: ORS-fluency: Total score: Severity: ORS-consequences: Total score: Typical or greater than typical	
Risk for persistence	Risks present: Comments:	
Language (expressive and receptive)	Tests/measures and results:	
Speech sound production	Tests/measures and results:	
Oral motor structure/function	Tests/measures and results:	
Temperament/emotion and attitudes	Tests/measures and results:	
Family communication	Comments:	
Other:		

Abbreviations: NSLD, non-stuttering-like disfluency; SLD, stuttering-like disfluency; SSI-4, Stuttering Severity Instrument, fourth edition; TD, total disfluency; TOCS ORS, Test of Childhood Stuttering Observational Rating Scales.

presented and/or their implications, this gives us an opportunity to expand, clarify, and/or rectify any areas, as needed. Most importantly, if parents/caregivers are able to describe to us the content and implications of the findings from their child's assessment, we know they have understood and are ready for specific recommendations about what they can do to help.

- *Making recommendations*: We tailor our recommendations to the results of our collaborative assessment as well as the family's needs and preferences. At times, we are in the position of advising the family that the child is typical/age appropriate in skills/abilities. When this occurs, we provide education about developmental timelines and expectations and how the parents/caregivers have and will continue to play a critical role in their child's healthy development. We always leave the door open for future contacts by telephone or email in case concerns arise and/or they have questions as their child ages.

Treatment is indicated when the child has one or more communication disorders, delays, and/or deficits that are interfering with everyday activities in family, academic, and/or social environments. One, not infrequent, combined diagnosis is that of speech sound disorder or delay and childhood-onset fluency disorder.[34] This co-occurrence requires clinical judgment about the relative impact of each

problem on the child's communication. For some children, their inability to be understood is of major import, while for others, the tension and struggle characteristic of their stuttering, and their negative reactions to it, take precedence. For still others, the two concerns appear to be of equal importance. There are a variety of therapy options to consider with families whose children both stutter and have speech sound deficits. These include group or individual therapy and, within either context, (1) a focus on speech sound errors or error patterns with support for the family with regard to stuttering (e.g., tips for responding positively and supportively to communication and empathizing with any frustration with stuttering); (2) a focus on family-based intervention for stuttering (see ▶ Chapter 10) while also modeling correct speech sound production for the child; or (3) an alternating or cycles approach to providing stuttering and speech sound production therapy.[35,36,37]

- *Providing referral sources*: Another option is to recommend the family return with the child for a reassessment in a set number of months (e.g., 3 or 6 months) or, if indicated, only as needed (i.e., suggest the family contact us if stuttering reemerges or worsens). The length of time until the follow-up assessment is typically selected by mutual agreement between the parents/caregivers and the SLP as they consider the findings we presented, where they are in their thinking given what we have discussed, and the family's schedule and needs over the next 3 to 6 months. This recommendation is appropriate, for example, in cases where there seems to be a known disturbance that led to the stuttering increase.

- *Following up*: When we leave any follow-up assessment unscheduled, it is typically because the child does not show signs of stuttering (e.g., was stuttering at the time the family scheduled the appointment, but it has since resolved) or there has been a downward trajectory in stuttering over time (e.g., stuttering is less severe when it occurs and the interval between episodes is widening; the child is less concerned, or unconcerned, about talking; and/or the parents/caregivers are less concerned than they were earlier in the course of their child's stuttering). As always, we offer the option for parents/caregivers to contact us if the child's stuttering or reactions to it change. Sometimes a phone conversation or e-mail exchange is all that is needed to talk through a "bump in the road," which might include a move, new baby, changes in school, day care or babysitter, or a new school. At these times, the parents/caregivers might be concerned that the child's stuttering will worsen and desire suggestions for how best to help their child through the transition. Sometimes when we suggest reevaluation at a future date, parents express a desire for additional guidance from us for responding to stuttering and/or supporting their child's communication and development in the family context. When this is the case, we may offer them a follow-up visit to spend more time outlining, discussing, and/or modeling recommendations, and/or the option to enroll in a short-term family-based treatment, as described in the next section.

Our assessment results may reveal the child has needs other than those specifically related to stuttering. Some are within our scope of practice (e.g., language, speech sound production, feeding/swallowing, and/or social pragmatic challenges), and we are able to inform the family what is available in our setting, should that be the best option for them, or provided in other settings by SLPs (e.g., at school). Some questions or concerns necessitate connecting the family with other, non-SLP providers. This may include referral to the child's pediatrician for a medical need or question; a mental health professional for evaluation (e.g., when parents suspect a child has an attentional deficit or anxiety disorder) or help with parenting difficulties; a physical or occupational therapist for fine and/or gross motor development challenges, or a developmental preschool or program (e.g., head start), etc. For these purposes, we maintain a list of relevant referral sources within our geographical area. For some families, in-person treatment, when recommended, poses too great a burden for their work, school, transportation, childcare, and other responsibilities. We provide these families with resources closer to home and/or discuss the possibility of services delivered via telepractice, when available.

7.4 Closing the Visit

Our assessments end with our thanking the child and family for coming, asking if they have any other questions they would like addressed now (time permitting) or the next time we connect, what their major "take home" was from the visit, and whether there was anything we could have done to serve them better.

We provide our contact information, resources (e.g., handouts, links, referral information), and an idea of when they can expect to receive a report summarizing our findings.

We do our best to ensure the family leaves with a clear understanding of the "next steps" for their child, especially by confirming recommendations in our conclusory comments. At times, we have provided options to the family to which they are not yet ready to commit. They may want to talk it over with a partner or family member, consider financial resources, or just "sleep on it." We welcome their taking time to discern what is best for their child and family. We learn whether they would like us to contact them (and, if so, when) or if they would prefer to contact us with their decision. If we have offered to follow up on any questions for which we did not yet have an answer (e.g., a particular referral source in their area), we let them know how soon to expect us to reach out to them and discern their contact preferences (e.g., by telephone call, text, or e-mail, and to whom). We also welcome them to contact us if they have questions or concerns when they receive the report summarizing our results and recommendations. By attending to these details, the clarity of the assessment process, results, and recommendations is enhanced, and the client–/family–clinician relationship both forged and strengthened.

For every child, we walk the family through the options, providing descriptions, answering questions, and obtaining family input. If there is a particular option that we do not consider to be potentially helpful to the child, we exclude it from our discussion, and/or help families to understand our decision should it be something they ask about (e.g., an approach they read about on the internet that, given our findings, is not appropriate to their child's needs). Thus, we combine our professional expertise with the input of informed parents/caregivers to determine next steps for the child and family. We have found that including parents/caregivers as key participants in decision-making contributes to their commitment to and engagement in the therapy process, yielding a true partnership that helps bridge the gap between the clinical setting and real-world communication. All early intervention approaches for stuttering include key roles, albeit with different emphases, for parents/caregivers, as is explained in detail in ▶ Chapter 10.

For all preschoolers who are stuttering, we provide some version of family-based support. We consistently provide tips, videos (or links thereto), handouts, and examples of how to respond to stuttering, communication, temperament differences, behavioral and/or attentional challenges, and development, in general, at the conclusion of the assessment. When a course of therapy is warranted, we often begin with what we call our "first line of defense"—a program of family-based intervention that educates and empowers parents to respond to their child's stuttering and communication in helpful ways, and addresses aspects of child development and family interactions, including parenting strategies, that fit the needs of the individual child.[38,39,40]

7.5 Case Studies

The following section provides two case examples describing the stuttering assessment procedures and findings for preschool children.

7.5.1 Case 1: "M"

Speech fluency: M (3.8 years old) was referred for an assessment by her mother after beginning to repeat and prolong sounds at the beginning of words when M started day care. During the evaluation, M produced 3% SLDs, primarily comprised of Mo-WWRs and SSRs.

Speech and language skills: M performed in the average or high-average range for all speech sound production and language testing.

Risk to persist: She began stuttering at 3.6 years, but does not exhibit any other risk factors.

Temperament/attitude: M received a 2 (out of 12) on the KiddyCAT (similar to scores for CWNS) and a 5 (out of 25) on the SBIS, indicating she does not find talking very difficult and is behaviorally inhibited.

Social communication: M's mother reported M expresses her needs effectively to familiar friends and family members, but her day care teacher reports she often plays by herself and rarely talks to other children.

Results and recommendations: Based on the above results, M's stuttering has increased dramatically with acclimation to a new environment (e.g., day care), and the child has an inhibited, slow-to-warm-up temperament. In cases like M's, we might agree that some time (shorter or longer) for adjustment to preschool would give us a better indication of whether speech fluency might naturally improve as M's comfort level increases and she experiences success acclimating to a new environment and new peers and adults. We would provide the family with suggestions for empathizing with, supporting, and guiding M by taking small, manageable, positive steps to foster adjustment to and thriving in her new environment, involving day care personnel in the process. Some of these recommendations include ideas for supporting communication (e.g., focusing on message/content [i.e., what the child is sharing/talking about], rather than manner [i.e., whether the child stuttered or not when speaking], empathizing with any frustration with communication and/or stuttering, etc.), and are presented in greater detail in ▶ Chapter 10. A helpful resource for families that describes and provides relevant examples of positive communication and support is the video, *7 Tips for Talking with the Child Who Stutters*, available, free of charge, from the Stuttering Foundation (https://www.stutteringhelp.org/content/7-tips-talking-child-who-stutters), in English or Spanish, along with pdf documents containing the tips.

7.5.2 Case 2: "J"

Speech fluency: J (4.0 years old) was referred for an assessment by his pediatrician after parents expressed concern that the speech of his peers is becoming easier to understand while his is not and that his stuttering had not resolved since it began 12 months ago. According to the mother, J's stuttering had improved after about 6 months, but not since then. During the evaluation, J produced 7% SLDs, primarily comprised of SSRs, ASPs, and Mo-WWRs. Some of the ASPs were accompanied by a rise in pitch and widening of his eyes.

Speech and language skills: J scored one standard deviation below age-level expectations on standardized assessment of his articulation and phonological skills, was consistent with age-level expectations for receptive and expressive vocabulary and receptive language abilities, and just below average for expressive language (with scoring impacted by omission of final consonants and reduced intelligibility due to articulation errors and phonological processes). His mother noted that she and his older sister are able to understand him better than his father, that peers and teachers have more difficulty, and that unfamiliar adults are unable to understand him.

Risk to persist: J began stuttering at 3.0 years and has continued to stutter for 12 months with an initial decrease and then plateaus in frequency and severity without improvement. His speech articulation skills are below age-level expectations. His mother and brother had therapy for speech sound errors in early elementary school, and his father stuttered briefly at about the same age as J.

Temperament/attitude: J obtained a 6 (out of 12) on the KiddyCAT indicating that he is aware that talking is difficult, does not like how he talks, and thinks others do not like the way he talks. His mother commented that she thought his answers might be related to his difficulties being understood rather than to his stuttering. He received a score of 20 (out of 25) on the SBIS indicating he is behaviorally uninhibited or outgoing.

Social communication: J's mother reported J struggles to express his needs effectively to anyone but her and his sister. J's preschool teacher informed the parents that peers will walk away from J when they cannot understand what he says. His mother commented that he has become less talkative as he has realized that others are having difficulty understanding him.

Results and recommendations: Based on the above results, J both stutters and has speech sound articulation and phonological skills that are below age-level expectations. Combining the results of assessment and parental and teacher input, J's communication is most negatively impacted by his difficulties being understood by peers, teachers, his father, other relatives, and unfamiliar adults. Stuttering is a secondary concern, as it has been present for about a year without resolving. Thus, the first option identified earlier—a focus on speech sound errors or error patterns with support for the family with regard to stuttering (e.g., tips for responding positively and supportively to communication and empathizing with any frustration with stuttering, as well as difficulties being understood)— would be a prudent recommendation to the family. By focusing on improving J's ability to be understood, his communication will be enhanced with familiar and unfamiliar listeners. This may also positively impact his attitudes about speaking and his willingness to do so. Support for the family (e.g., Palin Parent–Child Interaction [PCI] therapy, as presented in detail in ▶ Chapter 10) could be included to simultaneously address stuttering in the context of J's overall communication development. It will be important to reassess J's expressive language abilities once his speech sound production skills improve to ensure age-appropriate skills in this area.

7.6 Conclusions

Assessing young children suspected of stuttering is a complex, multifaceted, and dynamic process. It involves comprehensive analyses of the child's skills and abilities as well as an examination of the child's communication within the context of the family while considering the processes and intricacies of child development. In this chapter, we have provided rationales, steps, tools, and guidance for completing a thorough stuttering assessment, in partnership with the child and family, that will provide all participants with a clear understanding of the preschooler's skills/abilities and challenges, and guidance for the future. At the conclusion of our collaborative assessment, we have the quantitative and qualitative data needed to confidently present the family with our findings, address the questions and concerns that brought them to us, and provide recommendations that will facilitate maximization of the child's communication skills and enjoyment in the family, and other, contexts. In so doing, we have established a partnership with the preschooler and family that fosters mutual trust, cooperation, and teamwork for the short and long-term.

References

[1] Smith A, Weber C. How stuttering develops: the multifactorial dynamic pathways theory. J Speech Lang Hear Res. 2017; 60(9):2483–2505

[2] Adams MR. The demands and capacities model I: theoretical elaborations. J Fluency Disord. 1990; 15(3):135–141

[3] Yaruss JS, Quesal RW. Stuttering and the international classification of functioning, disability, and health: an update. J Commun Disord. 2004; 37(1): 35–52

[4] Conture EG, Walden TA, Arnold HS, Graham CG, Hartfield KN, Karrass J. Communication-emotional model of stuttering. In: Ratner NB, Tetnowski JA, eds. Current Issues in Stuttering Research and Practice. Mahwah, NJ: Lawrence Erlbaum Associates; 2006:17–47

[5] Walsh B, Usler E, Bostian A, et al. What are predictors for persistence in childhood stuttering? Semin Speech Lang. 2018; 39(4):299–312

[6] Ambrose NG, Cox NJ, Yairi E. The genetic basis of persistence and recovery in stuttering. J Speech Lang Hear Res. 1997; 40(3):567–580

[7] Yairi E, Ambrose NG, Paden EP, Throneburg RN. Predictive factors of persistence and recovery: pathways of childhood stuttering. J Commun Disord. 1996; 29(1):51–77

[8] Usler E, Smith A, Weber C. A lag in speech motor coordination during sentence production is associated with stuttering persistence in young children. J Speech Lang Hear Res. 2017; 60(1):51–61

[9] Spencer C, Weber-Fox C. Preschool speech articulation and nonword repetition abilities may help predict eventual recovery or persistence of stuttering. J Fluency Disord. 2014; 41:32–46

[10] Leech KA, Bernstein Ratner N, Brown B, Weber CM. Preliminary evidence that growth in productive language differentiates childhood stuttering persistence and recovery. J Speech Lang Hear Res. 2017; 60(11):3097–3109

[11] Singer CM, Walden TA, Jones RM. Differences in the relation between temperament and vocabulary based on children's stuttering trajectories. J Commun Disord. 2019; 78:57–68

[12] Usler E, Weber-Fox C. Neurodevelopment for syntactic processing distinguishes childhood stuttering recovery versus persistence. J Neurodev Disord. 2015; 7(1):4

[13] Ambrose NG, Yairi E, Loucks TM, Seery CH, Throneburg R. Relation of motor, linguistic and temperament factors in epidemiologic subtypes of persistent and recovered stuttering: Initial findings. J Fluency Disord. 2015; 45:12–26

[14] Singer CM, Hessling A, Kelly EM, Singer L, Jones RM. Singer, Jones, RM. Clinical characteristics associated stuttering persistence: a meta-analysis. J Speech Lang Hear Res. 2020; 63(9):2995–3018

[15] Conture, EG. Stuttering. 2nd ed. Englewood Cliffs, NJ: Prentice Hall; 1990

[16] Riley G, Bakker K. SSI-4: Stuttering Severity Instrument. 4th ed. Austin, TX: Pro-Ed; 2009

[17] Gillam RB, Logan KJ, Pearson NA. TOCS: Test of Childhood Stuttering. Austin, TX: Pro-Ed; 2009

[18] Vanryckeghem M, Brutten EJ. KiddyCAT: Communication Attitude Test for Preschool and Kindergarten Children who Stutter. San Diego, CA: Plural Publishing Incorporated; 2007

[19] Vanryckeghem M, Brutten G, Hernandez L. The KiddyCAT: A comparative investigation of the speech-associated attitude of preschool and kindergarten children who do and do not stutter. J Fluency Disord. 2005; 30:307–318

[20] Clark CE, Conture EG, Frankel CB, Walden TA. Communicative and psychological dimensions of the KiddyCAT. J Commun Disord. 2012; 45(3): 223–234

[21] Langevin M, Packman A, Onslow M. Parent perceptions of the impact of stuttering on their preschoolers and themselves. J Commun Disord. 2010; 43 (5):407–423

[22] Millard SK, Davis S. The Palin Parent Rating Scales: parents' perspectives of childhood stuttering and its impact. J Speech Lang Hear Res. 2016; 59(5): 950–963

[23] White AZ, Kelly EM, Singer, CM, Jones, RM. Validation of the Vanderbilt Responses to Your Child's Speech (VRYCS) rating scale for parents of children who stutter (under review).

[24] Semel E, Wiig EH, Secord WA. Clinical Evaluation of Language Fundamentals-Preschool-3 (CELF-Preschool-3). San Antonio, TX: Psychological Corp.; 2020

[25] McLeod S, Harrison LJ, McCormack J. The Intelligibility in Context Scale: validity and reliability of a subjective rating measure. J Speech Lang Hear Res. 2012; 55(2):648–656

[26] St. Louis KO, Ruscello DM. Oral speech mechanism screening examination. 3rd ed. Austin, TX: Pro-Ed; 2000

[27] Fletcher SG. Time-by-count measurement of diadochokinetic syllable rate. J Speech Hear Res. 1972; 15(4):763–770

[28] Dollaghan C, Campbell TF. Nonword repetition and child language impairment. J Speech Lang Hear Res. 1998; 41(5):1136–1146

[29] Ntourou K, DeFranco EO, Conture EG, Walden TA, Mushtaq N. A parent-report scale of behavioral inhibition: validation and application to preschool-age children who do and do not stutter. J Fluency Disord. 2020; 63:105748

[30] Putnam SP, Rothbart MK. Development of short and very short forms of the Children's Behavior Questionnaire. J Pers Assess. 2006; 87(1):102–112

[31] Rothbart MK, Ahadi SA, Hershey KL, Fisher P. Investigations of temperament at three to seven years: the Children's Behavior Questionnaire. Child Dev. 2001; 72(5):1394–1408

[32] Burns K. Focus on solutions: a health professional's guide. Revised ed. London: John Wiley & Sons; 2016

[33] Sheehan VM, Sisskin V. The creative process in avoidance reduction therapy for stuttering. Perspect Fluen Fluen Disord. 2001; 11(1):7–11

[34] Sisskin V. Avoidance Reduction Therapy for stuttering (ARTs®). In: Amster BJ, Klein ER, eds, More Than Fluency: The Social, Emotional, and Cognitive Dimensions of Stuttering. San Diego, CA: Plural Publishing; 2018:157–186

[35] Wolk L, Edwards ML, Conture EG. Coexistence of stuttering and disordered phonology in young children. J Speech Hear Res. 1993; 36(5):906–917

[36] Conture EG, Louko LJ, Edwards ML. Simultaneously treating stuttering and disordered phonology in children: experimental treatment, preliminary findings. Am J Speech Lang Pathol. 1993; 2(3):72–81

[37] Ratner NB. Treating the child who stutters with concomitant language or phonological impairment. Lang Speech Hear Serv Sch. 1995; 26(2):180–186

[38] Logan KJ, LaSalle LR. Developing intervention programs for children with stuttering and concomitant impairments. Seminars in Speech and Language. 2003; 24(01):013–020

[39] Kelman E, Nicholas A. Palin Parent-child interaction therapy for early childhood stammering. Abingdon, UK: Routledge; 2020

[40] Millard SK, Edwards S, Cook FM. Parent-child interaction therapy: adding to the evidence. Int J Speech Lang Pathol. 2009; 11(1):61–76

Appendix 7.1

EARLY CHILDHOOD ONSET STUTTERING (ECHOS) INTAKE FORM

Vanderbilt Bill Wilkerson Center

Vanderbilt University Medical Center

PART B:

Information about Child's Stuttering:

1. Please provide the month and year that your child's stuttering began: _____ _____

    *If unsure, please provide your best estimate.   Month   Year

2. Did your child's stuttering begin   **suddenly**   or   **gradually**? (Please circle one.)

3. Over time, my child's stuttering has: **increased   decreased   stayed the same   comes and goes** (Please circle one.)

4. What was your child's stuttering like **when it first began**? Please check all that apply.

    _____ Repeated words (*my-my-my*)

    _____ Repeated parts of words (*m-m-m-my*)

    _____ Stretched out sounds (*mmmmmy*)

    _____ Got stuck on a sound and nothing came out (*[silent pause while trying to start sound/word] ... cat*)

    _____ Did anything with his/her face or body when he/she stuttered (*tapping foot, nodding head, grimacing, etc.*)

    _____ Displayed physical tension when he/she stuttered (*straining muscles in neck, pressing lips together hard, etc.*)

5. What is your child's stuttering like **now**? Please check all that apply.

    _____ Repeats words (*my-my-my*)

    _____ Repeats parts of words (*m-m-m-my*)

    _____ Stretches out sounds (*mmmmmy*)

    _____ Gets stuck on a sound and nothing comes out (*... [silent pause while trying to start sound/word] ... cat*)

    _____ Does anything with his/her face or body when he/she stutters (*tapping foot, nodding head, grimacing, etc.*)

    _____ Displayed physical tension when he/she stuttered (*straining muscles in neck, pressing lips together hard, etc.*)

6. Is your child aware of his or her stuttering? (Please circle one.)   **Yes   No**

1

Family History of Stuttering:

Parent/Guardian #1:

Name: _____ Relationship to Child: _____

1. Did you stutter as a child? (Please circle one.) **Yes** **No**   If yes, do you still stutter? (Please circle one.) **Yes** **No**

2. Do you think your child stutters? (Please circle one.) **Yes** **No**

3. On a scale from 0 to 7 where **0 is not at all worried** and **7 is extremely worried** about your child's stuttering, where are you now? (Please circle one.)

0   1   2   3   4   5   6   7

Not at all   Extremely worried

4. On a scale from 0 to 7 where **0 is no stuttering** and **7 is very severe**, how severe is your child's stuttering? (Please circle one.)

0   1   2   3   4   5   6   7

No stuttering   Very severe stuttering

Parent/Guardian #2 (if applicable and parent/guardian #2 is present; otherwise skip to *Biological Family History...*)

Name: _____ Relationship to Child: _____

1. Did you stutter as a child? (Please circle one.) **Yes** **No**   If yes, do you still stutter? (Please circle one.) **Yes** **No**

2. Do you think your child stutters? (Please circle one.) **Yes** **No**

3. On a scale from 0 to 7 where **0 is not at all worried** and **7 is extremely worried** about your child's stuttering, where are you now? (Please circle one.)

0   1   2   3   4   5   6   7

Not at all   Extremely worried

4. On a scale of 0 to 7 where **0 is no stuttering** and **7 is very severe**, how severe is your child's stuttering? (Please circle one.)

0   1   2   3   4   5   6   7

No stuttering   Very severe stuttering

2

Biological Family History of Stuttering:

1. Is there a family history of stuttering on the **biological father's** side of the family? (Please circle one.)

Yes   No   **Unknown**

2. If **yes**, please list all family members on the **biological father's** side of the family who have **ever** stuttered. Please give their **relationship to the child** (e.g., child's uncle, aunt, grandfather, etc.).

1. _____   Does he or she still stutter?   **Yes**   **No**

2. _____   Does he or she still stutter?   **Yes**   **No**

3. _____   Does he or she still stutter?   **Yes**   **No**

4. _____   Does he or she still stutter?   **Yes**   **No**

5. _____   Does he or she still stutter?   **Yes**   **No**

3. Is there a family history of stuttering on the **biological mother's** side of the family? (Please circle one.)

Yes   No   **Unknown**

4. If yes, please list all family members on the **biological mother's** side of the family who have **ever** stuttered. Please give their **relationship to the child** (e.g., child's uncle, aunt, grandfather, etc.).

1. _____   Does he or she still stutter?   **Yes**   **No**

2. _____   Does he or she still stutter?   **Yes**   **No**

3. _____   Does he or she still stutter?   **Yes**   **No**

4. _____   Does he or she still stutter?   **Yes**   **No**

5. _____   Does he or she still stutter?   **Yes**   **No**

3

Appendix 7.2

Modified Impact of Stuttering on Preschoolers and Parents (ISPP) Questionnaire

<u>Part I.</u>

1. Has stuttering ever caused any **changes in how easy it is for your child to talk** with other children?

   ☐ NO   YES

   ☐ Easier ☐ More difficult

2. Has stuttering ever caused any changes in your **child's self-confidence**?

   ☐ NO   YES

   Gain self-confidence ☐ Lose self-confidence

3. Has stuttering ever caused any changes in your child's **general talkativeness**?

   ☐ NO   YES

   ☐ More talkative ☐ Less talkative

4. Has stuttering ever caused any **changes in how much your child plays with other children**?

   ☐ NO   YES

   ☐ More   ☐ Less

5. Has stuttering ever caused any changes **in the way your child plays with other children**? *This question refers to a broad range of possible changes in the way children play. For example, a child may change from being more or less assertive, may use gestures to communicate in play, or may give up when he/she can't get or keep a playmate's attention.*

6.
   ☐ NO   ☐ YES   Please comment on the way your child's play has changed:

   _____
   _____
   _____
   _____

7. Has stuttering ever caused any **changes in your child's general mood**?

   ☐ NO   ☐ YES   Please comment on how your child's general mood has changed:

   _____
   _____
   _____
   _____

8. Has stuttering ever caused any **changes in your child's quality of life**?

   ☐ NO   ☐ YES   Please comment on the changes:

   _____
   _____
   _____
   _____

9. Has your child ever been **frustrated when stuttering**?

☐ NO ☐ YES

10. Has stuttering ever caused your child to become **withdrawn**?

☐ NO ☐ YES

If you think stuttering has affected your child in any way other than in the ways referred to above, please summarize.

_____
_____
_____

Part II.

11. Has your child ever been **teased** by other children because of his/her stuttering?

☐ NO ☐ YES   Please describe what children do or did when they tease(d):

_____
_____
_____
_____

12. Has stuttering ever caused a **change in how much children play with your child**?

☐ NO   YES

☐ More   ☐ Less

13. Has stuttering ever caused **a change in the way children play with your child**? *Again, this question refers to a broad range of possible changes in the way children play with your child. For example, playmates may become more empathetic and watch out for your child, they may not wait for your child to say what he/she wants to say, or they may become more "bossy" or directive.*

☐ NO   YES ☐   Please describe the change:

_____
_____
_____
_____

14. Have other **children ever reacted** in any other way to your child's stuttering?

☐ NO   YES ☐   Please describe how the children react(ed):

_____
_____
_____
_____

15. Is there **anything else** about how children react to your child or your child's stuttering that you wish to share?

_____
_____
_____

Part III.

16. Has your child's stuttering ever affected you emotionally?

_____

_____

_____

17. Has your child's stuttering ever affected how you communicate with your child?

_____

_____

_____

18. Have you ever not known what to do or say when your child was stuttering?

_____

_____

_____

19. Has your child's stuttering ever affected the relationship between you and your child in so far as it would be affected by a breakdown in communication?

_____

_____

_____

6

Appendix 7.3

Vanderbilt Responses to Your Child's Speech (VRYCS) Rating Scale

RESPONSES TO YOUR CHILD'S SPEECH

	Never	Rarely	Sometimes	Often	Always	Responses to Your Child's Speech Rating Scale In the past 2 months, how often did you:
1.	0	1	2	3	4	Slow down your speech.
2.	0	1	2	3	4	Become tense when your child was speaking.
3.	0	1	2	3	4	Fill in words for your child.
4.	0	1	2	3	4	Talk for your child.
5.	0	1	2	3	4	Say your child's words for him/her.
6.	0	1	2	3	4	Ask your child to think about what he/she is going to say.
7.	0	1	2	3	4	Ask your child to take a deep breath before speaking.
8.	0	1	2	3	4	Finish what your child was saying.
9.	0	1	2	3	4	Pause before responding to your child.
10.	0	1	2	3	4	Remain relaxed when your child was speaking.
11.	0	1	2	3	4	Let your child lead the conversation.
12.	0	1	2	3	4	Ask your child to slow down while talking.
13.	0	1	2	3	4	Use simpler language when your child was talking.
14.	0	1	2	3	4	Ask simple questions.
15.	0	1	2	3	4	Worry about your child's talking.
16.	0	1	2	3	4	Wait for your child to finish talking before you spoke.
17.	0	1	2	3	4	Praise what your child said.
18.	0	1	2	3	4	Tell your child to relax.

7

Appendix 7.4

Intelligibility in Context Scale (ICS)

(McLeod, Harrison, & McCormack, 2012)

Child's name:_____

Child's date of birth:_____ Male/Female:_____

Language(s) spoken:_____

Current date: _____ Child's age:_____

Person completing the ICS:_____

Relationship to child:_____

The following questions are about how much of your child's speech is understood by different people. Please think about your child's speech over the past month when answering each question. Circle one number for each question.

	Always	Usually	Sometimes	Rarely	Never
1. Do **you** understand your child[1]?	5	4	3	2	1
2. Do **immediate members of your family** understand your child?	5	4	3	2	1
3. Do **extended members of your family** understand your child?	5	4	3	2	1
4. Do your **child's friends** understand your child?	5	4	3	2	1
5. Do other **acquaintances** understand your child?	5	4	3	2	1
6. Do your **child's teachers** understand your child?	5	4	3	2	1
7. Do **strangers**[2] understand your child?	5	4	3	2	1
TOTAL SCORE =	/35				
AVERAGE TOTAL SCORE =	/5				

[1] This measure may be able to be adapted for adults' speech, by substituting *child* with *spouse*.
[2] The term *strangers* may be changed to *unfamiliar people*

This version of the *Intelligibility in Context Scale* can be copied.
Intelligibility in Context Scale is licensed under a Creative Commons Attribution-NonCommercial-NoDerivs 3.0 Unported License.

Further information: McLeod, S., Harrison, L. J., & McCormack, J. (2012). The Intelligibility in Context Scale: Validity and reliability of a subjective rating measure. *Journal of Speech, Language, and Hearing Research, 55*(2), 648-656. http://jslhr.asha.org/cgi/content/abstract/55/2/648

8

8 School-Age Children

Kenneth J. Logan and Hayley S. Arnold

Abstract

This chapter presents an overview of methods and strategies that are used in contemporary clinical practice when assessing stuttering in school-aged children. The chapter is designed to guide clinicians through an assessment process that takes into account the school-aged child's functioning, impairment, activity limitations, and participation restrictions, as well as personal and environmental factors that can influence communication performance. Application of assessment information to stuttering diagnosis, severity determination, and, if appropriate, treatment planning are discussed as well.

Keywords: stuttering, assessment, school-aged children, diagnosis, speech fluency

8.1 Introduction

In this chapter, we describe the processes and procedures used to assess stuttering in school-aged children. Assessment is the foundation of clinical practice. School-aged children typically are referred for assessment of stuttering when someone—usually a parent or a teacher—is concerned that stuttering may be present and limiting the child's spoken communication, academic performance, educational access, or social acceptance. The clinician's assessment goal is not only to diagnose a child's stuttering but also to determine how stuttering affects the child's communication functioning at home, in school, and in other settings, and more generally, to determine how it affects the child's quality of life and sense of well-being. After acquiring this information, the clinician works with the child, caregivers/parents (hereafter parents), and teachers to formulate a plan for what should happen next, including whether referrals to other professionals are warranted.

This chapter is organized into five main sections. First, we present a framework for planning and implementing assessments. Next, we describe an assessment protocol that provides clinicians with a comprehensive menu of assessment options, including tools and strategies for collecting background information and for obtaining informal and formal norm-referenced descriptions of fluency performance and its impact. Next, we discuss how to interpret assessment data for the purposes of diagnosing stuttering, determining its severity and impact on a child, and forming treatment recommendations. We then provide a case study of a school-age child who presents with stuttering and other concerns to help readers apply information from the chapter to assessment planning. We close the chapter with a discussion of future directions in the assessment of school-aged children who stutter.

8.2 A Framework for Assessing Stuttering in School-Aged Children

We organize stuttering assessment around the International Classification of Functioning and Disability, and Health (ICF),[1] which is a tool developed by the World Health Organization to provide health care professionals with a framework for classifying and describing the health-related functioning of people. When applied to people who stutter, the ICF offers a template for designing an assessment that is likely to yield a description of not only a person's fluency disorder but also how the fluency disorder fits into the broader context of a person's life.[2]

In the ICF framework, an individual's functioning is described in three main ways: (1) body structure and function (i.e., anatomical and physiological characteristics); (2) activities and activity limitations (i.e., daily activities, how they are performed, and performance difficulties that are demonstrated); and (3) participation and participation restrictions (i.e., the type and extent of engagement in daily activities, and the extent to which engagement is limited).

There are several key concepts that are essential for understanding the ICF framework and its application to children who stutter. The concept of *functioning* focuses on characteristics a child *has* and on what a child *does*, regardless of whether it is "typical" or not. Thus, it has a positive connotation. Functioning is contrasted with *disability*, which refers broadly to *impairment* in body structure or functioning, *limitations* in the ability to perform daily activities, and *restrictions* in the extent of participation in daily activities. Thus, *disability* refers to those aspects of functioning that are atypical or different from what people in the general population do. Both perspectives—functioning and disability—are important to examine during stuttering assessment as each provides unique information about a child. These concepts and several others from the ICF model are presented in ▶ Table 8.1. As shown, the table is organized around the two broad components of the ICF framework: (1) functioning and disability and (2) contextual factors; several more specific concepts are introduced and explained under each component. ▶ Table 8.1 also includes examples of *quantitative* (i.e., numerical, objective) and *qualitative* (i.e., impressionistic, subjective) measures that a clinician can obtain to gather information about a child's functioning and disability.

When assessing school-aged children who stutter, one main goal is to describe the child's current fluency performance and, in doing so, to identify evidence of fluency *impairment* (i.e., stuttering) as well as any concomitant communication disorders that may exist. The clinician then seeks to refine this description by determining how contextual factors affect the expression of a child's stuttering in daily life. As shown in ▶ Table 8.1, contextual factors include a mix of personal and environmental variables. Ideally, the clinician will collect information about home and school speaking situations, as well as other speaking situations that are important to the child and family (e.g., speech during an after-school sporting activity). This leads to the identification and description of situations with the most and least severe stuttering, the most and least participation, and so forth.

8.2.1 School-Age Children and Stuttering

There is little justification for taking a "wait-and-see" approach when deciding whether to assess concerns about stuttering in school-aged children. Stuttering onset typically occurs during the preschool years. Most school-aged children with stutter-like speech are likely to have been showing signs of the disorder for several years and, thus, are beyond the age at which unassisted recovery from stuttering typically occurs.[3,4,5,6,7] Onset of stuttered speech during the school years also is a concern, because an older-than-average age of stuttering onset is associated with an increased risk of persistent stuttering.[8,9] Consequently, when a school-aged child is referred for concerns about stuttering, the assessment should take place promptly, and if treatment is warranted, then it too should commence promptly.

Although it may seem counterintuitive, the length of time a child has stuttered does not strongly predict how much stuttering-related disfluency will be produced.[10] For example, some children exhibit a relatively high frequency of stuttering soon after the onset of stuttered speech appears, only to see it decline later. Other children show the inverse pattern, and still others exhibit relatively stable amounts of stuttered speech over time. The more important point is that stuttering severity consists of more than the number of stuttered syllables a child produces; as shown in ▶ Fig. 8.1, associated symptoms (e.g., extraneous physical movements and physically tense speech musculature) and coping and concealment strategies (e.g., word substitution and speech avoidance) are prominent components of the disorder in many older school-aged children, especially as compared to preschool and early school-aged children.[8,10] ▶ Fig. 8.1 also illustrates that increases in these stuttering-related behaviors coincide with increased self-awareness of stuttered speech as children age. These data are consistent with findings from other studies that show that the communication-related attitudes of children who stutter become increasingly less positive with age[11] and that their speech becomes increasingly effortful, as evidenced by the emergence of muscle tremor during speech in older children.[12] The relationships between children's speech disfluencies and the ways in which they respond to and cope with them are important to clarify during assessment.

Table 8.1 Application of the International Classification of Functioning, Disability, and Health (ICF) framework to the assessment of school-aged children who stutter

ICF components and description		Examples of corresponding assessment measures	
		Quantitative	Qualitative
Functioning and disability	*Functioning*: neuroanatomy/neurophysiology of speech-production system *Impairment* (disability): atypical speech functioning resulting from impaired speech production system; other areas of impairment (e.g., speech sound production)	Measures of stuttering-related disfluency	Child's descriptions of speaking experiences and stuttering-related symptoms/challenges
	Activities (functioning): daily speaking activities *Activity limitations* (disability): impairment that limits functioning in daily life; Speaking activities that feature atypical fluency performance	Measures of stuttering-related disfluency across speaking tasks/situations	Parent accounts of child's situational fluency performance
	Participation (functioning): extent of speaking engagement in various activities *Participation restrictions* (disability): atypical reductions in how often or how much a child speaks during various activities	Measures of verbal output (e.g., words spoken per activity, number of activities avoided per day)	Child's reports of situational avoidance or of saying less than desired
Contextual factors	*Personal*: client-specific factors that influence expression of stuttering	Measures of stuttering-related thoughts, beliefs, emotions	Parent/teacher descriptions of how stuttering affects child's quality of life
	Environmental: background factors (e.g., cultural factors, listener reactions to stuttering, access to speech-language pathology services) that influence expression of stuttering	Measures of listener behaviors such as verbal interruptions, disparaging comments about speech	Teacher reports of bullying; child reports on effects of listener behaviors on fluency

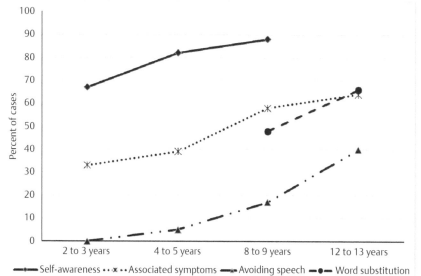

Fig. 8.1 Percent of children who stutter exhibiting various characteristics of stuttering behaviors. The three *dashed lines* illustrate how selected data from one study of the developmental progression of stuttering symptoms from early childhood through adolescence.[8] The *solid line* shows selected data from another study regarding self-awareness of stuttering in children who stutter.[9] (Percentages for self-awareness are approximate values that are based on a figure in the original publication).

8.2.2 An Assessment Protocol for School-Aged Children Who Stutter

In the context of fluency assessment, the term *protocol* refers to the procedures and practices that the clinician uses to collect information about an individual's communication functioning. With the school-aged population, an assessment protocol provides a format for answering relevant clinical questions about a child. A sample protocol for assessing school-aged children who stutter is presented in ▶ Fig. 8.2. As shown, the protocol in ▶ Fig. 8.2 has seven primary components. It may not be necessary to include all protocol components in every assessment. Rather, the clinician can adjust the protocol to fit the needs of individual children and/or accommodate time constraints. That said, we recommend that, as much as possible, clinicians use similar procedures from one case to the next. This approach provides clinicians with a standard context for evaluating children's stuttering, which will help the clinician build a mental database of how children who stutter typically perform and how their performance can vary. Clinicians are also likely to find that repeated administration of a core set of assessment tasks will increase the accuracy and efficiency of their assessments. ▶ Table 8.2 adds to the information in ▶ Fig. 8.2 by providing an overview of key questions to ask when assessing stuttering in school-aged children who stutter, as well as examples of specific procedures or tools the clinician can use when attempting to answer those questions.

▶ Fig. 8.3 offers details about specific analyses that a speech-language pathologist (SLP) can perform when assessing stuttering in a school-aged child. As shown there, a child's speech production can be measured in terms of its continuity, rate, rhythm, and effort. Each of these measures is relevant to understanding a child's fluency functioning. Analysis of continuity and rhythm yields information about the connectedness and prosody of speech, whereas analysis of rate yields information about the speed with which information is communicated, and analysis of effort yields information about the how hard a child "works" to produce spoken utterances. Analysis of these aspects of speech across the various activities in a child's life provides insight into the extent to which activity limitations and participation restrictions are present.[13]

Tools and Procedures for Collecting Background Information

Concepts presented in ▶ Table 8.2 and ▶ Fig. 8.3 are described in more detail in the following sections.

The Case History Form

The case history form is a tool that organizes information around questions pertaining to the child's functioning and experiences. Examples of case history forms and formats for stuttering assessments are available in various sources.[13,14,15] In many work settings, however, clinician-developed forms are used. Ideally, the clinician sends the case history form to the parents prior to the assessment so they can complete it thoughtfully and accurately. When stuttering is the presenting complaint, the case history form should include questions about age of stuttering onset, types of symptoms observed, changes in symptom presentation over time, the child's and others' reactions

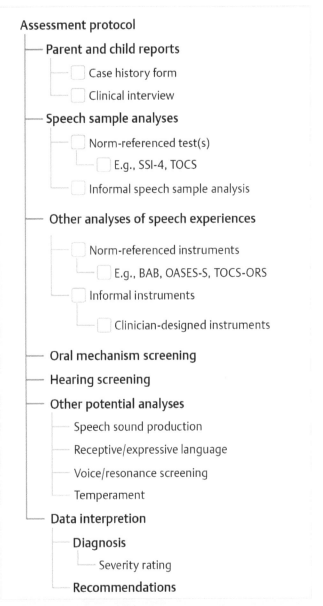

Fig. 8.2 A sample assessment protocol for use with school-aged children who stutter.

to stuttering, outcomes from previous assessments or therapy, family history of stuttering and other communication disorders, and so forth. Case history forms also commonly include questions about the child's developmental history, current and past performance in other aspects of communication and academics, emotional, behavioral, and attentional characteristics, as well as medical history and current health (e.g., illnesses, injuries, medications, general health). Case history forms also typically include questions about the child's family context and extracurricular activities and interests.

The Clinical Interview

The clinical interview is a clinician-directed discussion that is organized around questions and prompts pertaining to the child's past and current functioning and experiences. With the school-aged population, the clinician typically seeks to

Table 8.2 Key assessment questions and associated assessment instruments

Assessment question	Case history form	Clinical interview	SSI-4	TOCS	BAB	OASES-S	Informal speech sample analysis	Other formal and informal ratings and measures
Is stuttered speech present?	✓	✓	✓	✓	✓	✓	✓	✓
If so, how severely?	✓	✓	✓	✓	✓	✓	✓	✓
Which stuttering symptoms are present?	✓	✓	✓	✓	✓	✓	✓	✓
How does stuttering affect the child's communication in daily activities?	✓	✓	✓	✓	✓	✓	✓	✓
How does stuttering affect the child's participation in daily activities?	✓	✓	✓	✓	✓	✓	✓	✓
How do others respond to the child's stuttering?	✓	✓		✓	✓	✓		✓
Does the child exhibit self-limiting thoughts/emotions/beliefs?	✓	✓	✓	✓	✓	✓		✓
How does the child cope with or react to his or her stuttering?	✓	✓	✓	✓	✓	✓	✓	✓
Are there aspects of the environment that affect the child's fluency/communication functioning?	✓	✓	✓	✓				✓
Are there other aspects of communication that are a cause for concern?	✓	✓						✓
What does the parent/child hope to learn from the assessment?	✓	✓						

Abbreviations: SSI-4, Stuttering Severity Instrument, 4th edition; TOCS, Test of Childhood Stuttering; BAB, Behavior Assessment Battery; OASES-S, Overall Assessment of the Speaker's Experience of Stuttering, School-Age version.

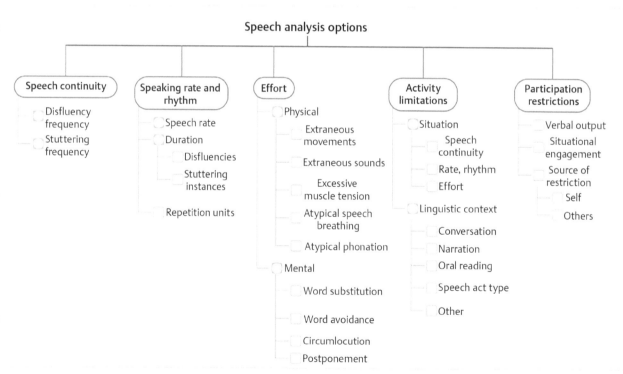

Fig. 8.3 Overview of options for analyzing informal speech samples.

interview both the child and parent(s), depending on factors such as parent accessibility, time constraints, and the child's willingness and ability to talk about their speaking experiences. The goal of the interview is to elicit a rich description of the child's past and current functioning with regard to the presenting complaint, medical history, academic history, and general developmental history, as well as the context within which the child lives (e.g., family structure, family members' history of communication disorders and responses to the child's fluency difficulties).

During the clinical interview, the SLP can follow up on information provided on the case history form and can explore topics that arise incidentally during the clinical interview. The SLP should attend to the emotional tone that parents and children use while describing their experiences, as this can provide insight into the degree or intensity of difficulties that the child has faced, as well as the parent's or child's comfort level with discussing stuttering and the parent's or child's level of enthusiasm about participating in intervention.

► Table 8.3 includes examples of questions and prompts that clinicians can present during a clinical interview to inquire about the child's stuttering-related experiences. The questions/prompts are phrased in two ways: one for use with parents and the other for use with children. Obviously, it is important to adjust the wording of these questions/prompts to fit the situation. Older school-aged children are likely to be better informants than younger ones; however, age is not a perfect predictor of how much information a child will provide or how accurate the information will be. Accordingly, we are hesitant to suggest a minimum age for conducting clinical interviews

with school-aged children. The questions/prompts in ► Table 8.3 can be expanded as needed to obtain information about topics such as family history of communication disorders, the family/household structure, and the child's developmental, medical, and educational histories.

As shown in ► Table 8.3, clinical interviews typically begin with an open-ended question about the parent's or child's chief concerns and, with parents, the primary reasons for seeking a speech-language evaluation. For example, with a mother who is concerned that her child might be stuttering, the SLP can ask her to describe or demonstrate the speech behaviors that are creating concern. As parents talk, the SLP listens for mention of stuttering symptoms, how the symptoms have changed over time, which parts of stuttering are most concerning, and which daily activities are most and least impacted by stuttering. When parents mention limitations in their child's communication participation, the clinician must try to separate aspects of a child's temperament, such as shyness or sensitivity, from communication avoidance that is associated with stuttering.

Table 8.3 Prompts for interviewing parents/caregivers and children about stuttering-related behavior and experiences

Interview prompts		
Information sought	Parents/caregivers	Children
Chief reason for seeking evaluation	What brings you here for the assessment today? • What have you observed? • What concerns you most? • When did you first become concerned? • Has your child's speech changed over time? How? • Has your level of concern changed over time? How?	Some children find talking is mostly easy to do and others find it is hard. Tell me about your speech and how you talk. • Is it easy or hard for you to talk? Tell me more. • Some kids get "stuck" while talking. Does this happen with you? How often? When? Tell me what happens. • Do you remember when you first started getting stuck/stuttering? Has it changed since then?
Activity limitations	Tell me how your child's stuttering affects different speaking situations. • Which situations are most/least difficult? Why? • To what extent does stuttering limit your child's communication in these situations?	Where/when is it easiest/hardest to talk? • What makes some kinds of talking hard to do? • Do you feel like you still get your message across even if your speech gets stuck when you're talking?
Participation restrictions	Does your child talk as often and as much as they would like when at home, school, or in community settings? • Does your child restrict the amount of talking because of speech difficulties? • Do others exclude your child from speaking situations because of speech difficulties?	Do you talk as often and as much as you would like? • Do you talk more in some places or situations than others? • Do you talk more to some people than others? • Do you ever not talk at all? • Do you ever say less than you would like to say? • What causes you to hold back from talking? • When/where do you do a lot of talking?
Environmental factors	How do people in your home, at school, and out in the community respond to your child's speech? • Are there aspects of the communication environment that are helpful to your child? Are there aspects that make speaking more difficult? • Have you or others tried to help when they stutter? Tell me more.	What do people do or say and how do they act when your speech is stuck/when you stutter? • Does anyone try to help you? Who tries to help? What do they do? • Are there things they do that help your speech? • Are there things they do that make speaking harder for you?
Attitudes, thoughts, feelings, and emotions about stuttering and communication	How does your child react when stuttering? • Do they show awareness of stuttering? • How do they act or feel when stuttering? • In which situations/settings do they seem most/least comfortable talking? What are you thinking/feeling when your child stutters? Has your child ever met anyone else who stutters?	Do you have times when you notice your speech is stuck? Tell me more. • What do you think when your speech is stuck/you stutter? How do you feel? • Overall, how do you feel about talking? Is it something you like or do not like to do? • Have you ever been around anyone else who stutters? Tell me what that was like.
Treatment and desired outcomes	Has your child ever had speech-language treatment? • How was that? What was the outcome? What are your hopes/dreams for your child? • What changes would you like to see in your child's communication/interactions with others? • What do you think would help your child most? • What would your child like to do better?	Have you ever met with a speech teacher like me before? • What was helpful/not helpful about that? Are there parts of your speech you want to change? • Tell me more. What would change? Talking more easily? Talking more often, in more places, or with more people? • What would you like to do 1 year from now with your talking that you are not doing now?

The SLP also attempts to elicit information about how the child and others react to the stuttering. Information about the child's awareness and concern about stuttering are obtained, along with information about how the child's speaking environment affects communication performance. The SLP listens for evidence of supportive environmental elements (e.g., speaking partners who wait for the child to finish a stuttered word, school-based accommodations for graded speaking assignments) and nonsupportive elements (e.g., speaking partners who interrupt stuttered speech or who offer unsolicited advice or assistance with stuttered speech). Synthesis of this information helps the clinician and family determine the extent to which environmental factors need to be addressed in a treatment program that follows the assessment.

Information about the child's family context such as the number of people in the household, number and age(s) of siblings, family routines, and schedules can provide insight into the types of communication demands the child encounters each day and the extent to which family members can support the goals of intervention.

Clinicians should also ask about family history of stuttering and other communication disorders. Although this information does not factor into the diagnosis of stuttering, it may help the clinician estimate the child's risk for persistent stuttering, as a positive family history of stuttering is a risk factor for persistence, particularly when the affected relative exhibits persistent stuttering.[15] (See ▶ Chapter 3 in this book for more about the genetic bases of stuttering.)

Clinical interviews also usually address the child's past assessment and treatment experiences. Such information helps the SLP put the present assessment into perspective and may shape any treatment recommendations that are made. In the cases where treatment is recommended following the evaluation, clinicians should collaborate with the child and the parents to shape both the treatment goals and approach, rather than to prescribe them to the family. The clinician can begin this process during the clinical interview by asking children who stutter and their parents what they hope to gain from the assessment and what goals they think they might want to work toward in any subsequent treatment. Children who stutter sometimes present with co-occurring disorders that affect other aspects of speech-language functioning as well as general academic performance[2] (see ▶ Chapter 4 and ▶ Chapter 13 for more information). For example, speech sound disorder and language disorder are two of the most common diagnoses that co-occur with stuttering in children, and social anxiety disorder has emerged as a relatively common co-occurring diagnosis in teens and adults who stutter.[21,22] Thus, the SLP needs to inquire about functioning in these domains to appropriately plan for assessment, and to consider them when designing treatment and making referrals (Box 8.1).

Box 8.1 Recommended Interviewing Practices

1. *Create a context for the interview.* Preface the clinical interview with a brief explanation of the goals for the assessment and the role of the interview in the assessment. The SLP should then ask the parent or child if they have any questions about the assessment, as well as what they hope to learn from it.

2. *Define terms that may be unfamiliar.* Clinicians should limit the use of professional jargon when interviewing parents and children. When professional terms (e.g., *disfluency*) are used, a brief, simple explanation should follow. Most parents and many school-aged children will be familiar with the term *stuttering*, so it is fine to use that word when discussing speech fluency performance. In the cases where a diagnosis of stuttering is uncertain or a child seems unfamiliar with the term, alternate wording should be used (e.g., "speech problem," "repeating a word," "getting stuck when talking").

3. *Begin each interview topic with an open-ended, neutrally worded question.* For example, when asking parents about their child's speech symptoms, it is preferable to ask *What have you observed about your child's speech?* rather than *Tell me about the problems your child experiences when talking.* The first prompt is worded neutrally and thus allows for the possibility that the child has had only positive experiences or a mix of both positive and negative speaking experiences. The SLP can follow up with questions that elicit details about whatever positive or negative experiences are mentioned in the initial response.

4. *Engage in active, empathetic listening.* When engaged in active listening, the clinician should occasionally make statements to assure the parent or child that they not only heard the content but also empathized with the accompanying thoughts and feelings.[16] Imagine a scenario where the mother of a child who stutters tells the clinician that she feels helpless and upset when her son stutters and this has led her to attempt to help him by talking for him. Although the mother's behavior is not a practice SLPs would recommend, the clinician nonetheless should refrain from correcting it during the interview. Doing so might lead the parent to feel guilty, which in turn would make it less likely that she will answer the remaining questions completely or honestly. Instead, it is preferable for the clinician to deliver an empathetic response such as, "It sounds like you've come up with something to do when your son has difficulty speaking. Yet, despite your efforts, you still feel overwhelmed and upset about what you should do."

5. *Prepare for how to respond to children who are reluctant to talk about their stuttering.* Some children may not be ready to talk openly about stuttering and the feelings and emotions associated with it, especially to a clinician they have just met. For many children who stutter, their fluency difficulties are a source of daily frustration and embarrassment. Over time, this can lead to emotions such as fear, anxiety, and shame, which can be of sufficient intensity to cause children to feel uncomfortable when discussing the behaviors, thoughts, feelings, and emotions that surround their stuttering. Such children may downplay the severity of their stuttering and the impact it has on their quality of life.

   One way to overcome a child's reluctance to share personal experiences with stuttering is to depersonalize the discussion. This can be done by asking the child questions about other children who stutter.[17,18] For example, the clinician can show the child informational materials featuring other children who stutter and then ask questions like "What do you think other kids who stutter feel when they are talking to friends?" As the child responds, the clinician can acknowledge and validate the content and feelings in the child's response, and then follow with questions like, "Do you ever feel that way when *you* are talking to friends?" If the child remains reluctant to talk, it is best not to press for an answer. The child's lack of responsiveness may provide the clinician with about as much information on how they feel about stuttering as a lengthy response would provide.

Informal Approaches to Assessing Fluency

SLPs have developed a variety of measures to describe speech fluency performance. Some of these measures are informal and can be used instead of or in addition to measures found on norm-referenced tests such as the ones described later in this chapter. Informal fluency analyses often are used with samples of connected speech that are elicited in conversational and narrative/monologue (e.g., storytelling) contexts. Informal measures are particularly useful when applied to speech samples that are elicited from beyond-clinic situations. The informal assessment data can be used to complement findings from norm-referenced tests and, in doing so, provide clinicians with a more complete understanding of the child's speech fluency. In the remainder of this section, several informal measures are described. It takes practice to implement some of the informal measures described below accurately, reliability, and efficiently. FluencyBank, listed in the Further Readings section at the end of this chapter, provides speech samples that can be used for practice with informal measures.

Speech Continuity Measures

Measurement of *speech continuity* is the most common type of informal fluency analysis. In the context of stuttering assessment, speech continuity is measured by determining the frequency with which various types of disfluency are produced. Methods for computing disfluency frequency are explained in Box 8.2.

Box 8.2 Speech Sample Elicitation Strategies

Informal speech sample analysis is usually conducted with either conversational or narrative speech (i.e., monologue, storytelling). Either type of sample is acceptable to use; however, conversation may offer a better representation of school-aged children's communication skills since that is the speaking context they primarily use to express their thoughts and ideas. Sample lengths of at least 300 to 600 syllables are recommended to obtain a valid representation of fluency performance.[2] With younger school-age children, conversational samples are best elicited in a play setting, using topics that pertain either to the ongoing activities or to other things that interest the child.

An alternative to play-based conversation is to use a text-free picture book such as Mercer Mayer's "Frog, Where Are You?"[22] or David Wiesner's "Flotsam"[23] as a stimulus for eliciting speech. The clinician guides the child through pages of the book, making remarks as needed to maintain conversation with the child. The setup for an activity like this is shown in ▶ Fig. 8.4a, b. The use of simple comments and open-ended questions and requests in combination with ample periods of silence usually is sufficient to elicit an adequate conversational sample. As shown in ▶ Fig. 8.4b, when obtaining a speech sample with children in the middle elementary grades and older, the clinician can identify topics beforehand that are familiar and of interest to the child, such as favorite games, books, extracurricular activities, hobbies, and pets, and then talk with the child about them. Topics that relate to a past or future event often elicit more speech than those that deal with immediately present objects or events.

Clinicians sometimes may find that a child does not stutter to the degree that the case history or clinical interview suggests. In such instances, the clinician can introduce mild forms of communicative pressure or stress during the speech sample. Examples of such clinician-administered strategies include breaking eye contact with the child as the child talks (see ▶ Fig. 8.4c, d for depictions of these strategies), increasing the pace by posing a series of questions in rapid succession, and increasing speech rate.

Measuring Frequency of Speech Disfluency

Speech disfluency frequency is a quantitative measure of speech continuity that captures the amount of speech disfluency a child produces in relation to the size of the speech sample. Data are reported as either "disfluencies per 100 syllables" or "disfluencies per 100 words." Although the two measures do not yield equivalent frequency scores, in most cases the discrepancy between them is unlikely to be great enough to affect decisions about stuttering diagnosis or severity.[24] We advise clinicians to select a base unit (i.e., syllables or words) and use it consistently.

Disfluency frequency measures can be based on typed or handwritten verbatim transcripts, but this approach can be very time-consuming. Unless a written transcript is needed for another purpose (e.g., to analyze a child's expressive language), it is preferable to use a coded form of transcription in lieu of a verbatim written representation. A grid for conducting a coded analysis of fluency is presented in ▶ Fig. 8.5. Each of the 100 cells in the grid corresponds to either a syllable or a word, depending on the clinician's preferred unit of analysis. Syllables or words that are said without disfluency are coded with a dash (i.e., "-"). Syllables or words produced with accompanying disfluency are described either generally (e.g., with the letter "D," for disfluent) or with a set of more specific codes that indicate the types of disfluency produced. When conducting a detailed analysis of speech disfluency, a clinician may report frequency scores for specific types of disfluency, such as the following:

- Part-word repetition (sounds, syllables, or part of words are repeated, e.g., *y-you*; *be-be-because*; *Washing-Washington*).
- Monosyllable word repetition (e.g., *She-she-she said it*).
- Multisyllable word repetition (e.g., *Josie-Josie-said it*).
- Phrase repetition (e.g., *After school, after school, I went to my aunt's house*).
- Audible sound prolongation (e.g., *Wwwe went to my aunt's house*).
- Inaudible sound prolongation or block (articulatory postures are fixed or held such that speech appears to be "blocked", e.g., *{holding the /b/ posture silently for 1 second}boy*).
- Interjection (e.g., *um, uh*).
- Revision (e.g., *She-he said it*).

As shown in ▶ Fig. 8.5, a total of 9 syllables were preceded by interjection (I), 13 featured either audibly prolonged (P) or inaudible, blocked (B) speech sounds, 7 syllables featured

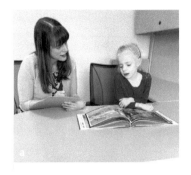
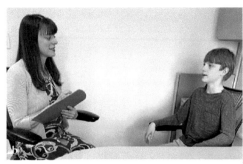
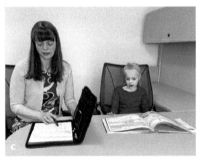
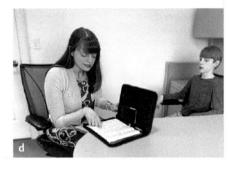

Fig. 8.4 Depiction of a speech-language pathologist eliciting speech samples for the purpose of conducting a disfluency analysis. (a) Elicitation of a speech sample with a 7-year-old child using a text-free picture book. (b) Elicitation of a speech sample with a 12-year-old child without visual stimuli. (c, d) The clinician intentionally breaking eye contact or shared eye gaze with the children in order to recreate communicative stress experienced in daily life.

P	Rv	I	Rv	Rv	Rv	Rv	Rv	P	Rv	Rv	P	Rv	R	Rv	B	Rv	Rv	P	Rv	Rv	Rv	B	Rv	R
Rv	Rv	R	Rv	Rv	B	Rv	Rv	Rv	I	Rv	B	Rv	Rv	Rv	I	Rv	Rv	I	Rv	Rv	Rv	Rv	P	Rv
I	Rv	Rv	R	Rv	Rv	Rv	Rv	P	Rv	Rv	Rv	P	Rv	Rv	Rv	Rv	Rv	P	Rv	I	Rv	Rv	Rv	Rv
R	Rv	Rv	I	I		Rv	R	Rv	Rv	I	Rv	Rv	Rv	Rv	B	Rv	R	Rv	Rv					

Cells represent:

☑ Syllables

☐ Words

coded: 95

Fig. 8.5 Example of a completed fluency analysis grid. B, blocked speech sound (inaudibly prolonged speech sound); I, interjection; P, audibly prolonged speech sound; R, part-word repetition (sound or syllable repetition); Rv, revised speech

part-word (sound or syllable) repetitions (R), and there was 1 instance of revision (Rv). The first six codes shown in row 1 in the analysis grid correspond to an utterance such as [Rrr] *ain is* [*um*] *in the forecast*, where the first syllable, *rain*, features prolongation of /r/ and the interjection *um* is assigned to the following syllable (i.e., the third syllable, *in*). A blank 300-syllable or word count sheet is provided in ► Chapter 7.

When using a syllable-based analysis, only one disfluency is counted per cell. For example, if a child began a syllable with a repetition of the initial consonant and then prolonged the vowel within the same syllable (e.g., *dog* → [*d-d-d-oooo*]*g*), the clinician could enter one code for sound/syllable repetition and one code for sound prolongation into the cell that corresponds to "dog." This would be counted as one disfluent syllable, with two codes used to describe the disfluency. Alternately, the clinician could simply code the syllable as containing one "complex" disfluency (in this case, a *disfluency cluster* that includes both repeated and prolonged speech. The clinician could use a unique code to show that a cluster of stutterlike disfluencies has occurred (e.g., CSLD).

After the coding is complete, disfluency frequency scores are computed for each disfluency type by dividing the number of each disfluency type by the number of coded syllables and then multiplying by 100. This yields the percentage of syllables with each type of disfluency. As shown in ► Fig. 8.5, if each cell represents one syllable, then a total of 95 syllables were coded. The frequency scores, expressed as "percent of syllables," for the four disfluency types observed in the sample are computed as follows:
- Interjection frequency: = (9/95) × 100 = 9.47%.
- Revision frequency: = (1/95) × 100 = 1.05%.
- Prolongation/block frequency: = (13/95) × 100 = 13.68%.
- Part-word repetition frequency = (7/95) × 100 = 7.37%.

Repeated speech sounds and syllables or prolonged/blocked speech sounds differentiate children who stutter from children with typical fluency. For this reason, clinicians often refer to them as "stutter-like disfluencies" (SLDs) and compute the combined frequency with which a speaker produces them. For example, in ► Fig. 8.5, there are 20 SLDs (13 prolongations/blocks and 7 sound/syllable repetitions) and 10 "other" (also

called "non-stutter-like" or "typical") disfluencies. Using the information from ▸ Fig. 8.5 as an example, the frequencies for these categories of disfluency are computed as follows:
• Frequency of SLDs = (20/95) × 100 = 21.05%.
• Frequency of other (non-stutter-like) disfluencies = (10/95) × 100 = 10.53%.

The frequency across all disfluency types is computed as follows:
• Overall frequency of disfluency (all types) = (30/95) × 100 = 31.58%.

Clinicians also commonly report the percentage of all disfluencies that are stutter-like. In this example, where 20 of the 30 disfluencies are stutter-like, this is computed as follows:
• Percent of total disfluencies that are stutterlike = (20/30) × 100 = 66.7%.

The analysis described earlier and shown in ▸ Fig. 8.5 is based on coding syllables. However, word-based analyses can also be used. Computation procedures are mostly the same as those used with a syllable-based analysis; however, for children who produce words that contain more than one instance of disfluency, the "percentage of words stuttered" metric will undercount the amount of disfluency produced (e.g., [mu-]multi[pli-]plication for "multiplication" is scored as one disfluent word, which misses the fact that the word contains two instances of disfluency). To account for this possibility, it is best not to report a word-based analysis as a percentage, but instead as "number of disfluencies per 100 words." Finally, it also is important to note that although disfluency is a common marker of stuttered speech, it is not the only marker of stuttered speech. For example, a word that sounds fluent may be judged as "stutterlike" if a speaker exhibits rhythmic finger tapping (a "physical concomitant" of stuttering) leading into the start of the word. In such instances, additional codes can be added to the clinician's disfluency analysis system to document the occurrence of such behavior. After continuity data are collected, they can be compared to the normative data in ▸ Table 8.4 for children who stutter and typically fluent peers.

Measures of Rate and Rhythm

SLPs may wish to supplement disfluency frequency measures with measures that capture the rate and rhythm of speech. Several options are available.

Measuring Speech Rate

Speech rate is computed by determining the number of syllables or words a speaker produces per second or per minute of speech.[26] To compute speech rate, the clinician first randomly selects at least 10 utterances from a recording of the child's conversational speech. The clinician then measures the duration of each utterance, including any disfluent speech and within-utterance pauses. Next, the clinician counts the number of syllables (or words) in each utterance, excluding any syllables that occur in disfluent portions of the utterance. For example, in the utterance [On-] on the table the first iteration of the word on is excluded from the count of the utterance's syllables, but it is included in the timing of the utterance duration. Syllable (or word) counts and durations are summed across utterances and then divided to yield the average speech rate for the set of sampled utterances.

In most cases, the more disfluency a child produces, the slower the speech rate will be. This is because disfluency consumes time that a child would otherwise spend producing fluent words to communicate. In one study of school-aged children's speech rates during conversation, narration, and sentence production tasks, children who stutter spoke significantly slower than children who did not stutter.[26] Across the three tasks, the mean speech rate for children who did not stutter was 172.87 syllables/min (SD = 30.50) and for children who stutter, it was 151.20 syllables/min (SD =30.6).

Speech rate is a potentially useful way to gauge a child's communicative competence. Not only does it provide information about the pace at which a child articulates, but it also provides information about the pace at which the child conveys information to others. Speech rate reductions that result from frequent disfluency may help explain research that shows poorer listener recall of auditorily presented information in presentation conditions that feature frequent stuttering compared to those with infrequent stuttering.[27] The reasons for this are not completely understood; however, slow, highly disfluent speech may tax a listener's working memory to a greater extent than minimally disfluent speech, thus making the speech more challenging and more effortful to process.

Disfluency Duration

Disfluency duration is another useful measure when assessing stuttered speech. Longer disfluencies disrupt speech rhythm

Table 8.4 Reference data for interpreting disfluency measures that are commonly computed as part of a speech sample analysis

Disfluency measure[a]	Scores indicative of a stuttering diagnosis[b]
Total disfluency frequency[c]	8 or greater (plus an SLD frequency of 2 or more)[53]
SLD frequency	3 or more per 100 syllables[32,53,54,55]
Percent of total disfluencies with SLD	More than 60% of all disfluencies are stutterlike[32,55]
M number of repetition units per SER[d]	More than 1.30 units per repetition and more than 33% of all SERs have >1 unit[31]

Abbreviation: SLD, stutterlike disfluency.
[a] See chapter section on Measuring Frequency of Speech Disfluency and ▸ Fig. 8.5 for computational procedures associated with each disfluency measure.
[b] Frequency refers to the number of disfluencies produced per 100 syllables or words.
[c] Superscript Arabic numerals indicate the supporting references for the scores.
[d] Short-element repetitions, which include repetitions of sounds, syllables, and one-syllable words.

and information flow to a greater extent than those of relatively brief duration. To compute the average duration of a child's speech disfluencies, the clinician randomly selects at least 10 speech disfluencies from a recording of a child's speech. The selected disfluencies should be limited to part-word or monosyllabic word repetitions, and prolonged or blocked sounds. Using a stopwatch, the clinician measures the interval between the start and end of the disfluency. For example, the italicized segments of the following utterances would be measured:

- *b-* bank (the unsuccessful attempt at advancing through the /b/ in "bank" is timed).
- *mmm*oney (the duration of the prolonged /m/ is timed).
- *t–*-alking (the duration of the blocked /t/ is timed).
- *at-* at night (the initial, unsuccessful attempt of "at" is timed).

To compute the average duration, the clinician sums the durations of each measured disfluency and then divides by the total number of disfluencies measured. Studies of preschool- to early-elementary-aged children who stutter show mean durations for SLDs to be in the range of 0.65 to 0.90 seconds.[28,29] In a study of teens and adults who stutter, minimum durations for instances of stuttering averaged 0.41 seconds and maximum durations averaged 4.32 seconds.[30]

Another approach to quantifying disfluency duration is to determine the mean number of *repetition units* in repetitions of sounds, syllables, or one-syllable words. For this measure, the clinician randomly selects at least 10 disfluencies from a sample of the child's speech. For each disfluency, the clinician counts the number of unsuccessful attempts the child makes at completing the syllable. For example, [g-] *go* features one unsuccessful attempt at saying the target *go*; thus, this repetition has one repetition unit. Similarly, the disfluency on the word *can* in the utterance "[*Can- Can- Can-*] *Can I go home*?" has three repetition units. The number of repetition units in each of the analyzed disfluencies is summed and divided by the total number of disfluencies analyzed, yielding the average number of repetition units per disfluency (Box 8.3).

Box 8.3 A Weighted Index of Stutterlike Disfluency

Ambrose and Yairi described the use of a *Weighted SLD Index* (WSI),[32] which is a composite measure of disfluency that can differentiate children who stutter from children who do not stutter. WSI is computed using the following formula:

[(frequency of short-element repetitions) × mean RUs per repetition] + (2 × frequency of dysrhythmic phonations).

As the formula shows, the index takes into account the frequency of two SLD categories: short-element repetitions (i.e., part-word and monosyllable repetitions) and "dysrhythmic phonation" (i.e., sound prolongations, blocks, breaks in vowel production). The repetitions are weighted by multiplying their frequency by the mean number of repetition units (RUs) per repetition. The dysrhythmic phonations are weighted by multiplying their frequency by a factor of 2.

In a study of preschool-aged children, Ambrose and Yairi reported that all 54 typically fluent children had WSI scores of ≤3.99, while all 90 children who were diagnosed as stuttering had WSI scores of ≥4.00.[32] Ambrose and Yairi suggested that WSI scores of 4.00 to 9.99 were indicative of mildly severe stuttering, 10.00 to 29.99 of moderately severe stuttering, and ≥30 of severe stuttering. Although the WSI seems to reliably differentiate preschool-aged children who stutter from those who do not, it has not, to our knowledge, been applied to school-aged children who stutter. Nonetheless, in school-aged children in whom a diagnosis is uncertain and the clinician lacks access to a standardized diagnostic test like the *Test of Childhood Stuttering* (TOCS),[14] the WSI measure may be useful for this purpose.

Measures of Speaking Effort

Speaking effort can be measured from two perspectives: physical effort and mental effort. Researchers have used various instrumental approaches to assess physical effort, including measures of muscle activation (i.e., electromyography) and physical force (e.g., strain gauges). Because these types of equipment are unavailable in many work settings, SLPs are more likely to implement informal tools such as rating scales (described in the following section) to assess physical effort. These types of clinician-designed data collection tools can be implemented to examine the extent to which extraneous movements are present during speech or immediately prior to speech initiation. This approach can also be used to assess the extent of extraneous sounds, excessive physical tension, atypical speech breathing, and atypical phonation during speech.

As shown in ▶ Fig. 8.1, children become increasingly aware of their stuttering as they age. Along with this, they become increasingly likely to respond to their stuttering with the use of self-devised stuttering management strategies that require substantial mental effort to implement. For example, children may use strategies such as word substitution and avoidance, as well as others like them (e.g., postponement/stalling strategies, pretending to think about or remember something) to conceal stuttering. Extensive use of any of these strategies requires near-continuous self-monitoring of one's speech, as the speaker scans upcoming speech for words that may be stuttered upon. SLPs can collect information about the amount or nature of mental effort a child expends by using self-designed checklists and rating scales. These instruments can be administered to children who stutter, parents, or teachers to obtain multiple perspectives on this aspect of stuttering. As will be discussed in the following section, there are also normed instruments with items or sections that address speaking effort and coping strategies for stuttering.

Informal Rating Scales

Informal rating scales are useful for evaluating many aspects of stuttered speech; however, most commonly, they are used to make global ratings of stuttering severity. Parents' and clinicians' severity ratings are especially useful because they

Circle the rating that goes with your impressions of the child's stuttering severity.

1	2	3	4	5	6	7	8	9
No stuttering	Very mild stuttering							Very severe stuttering

Fig. 8.6 Example of a 9-point rating scale that can be used for rating stuttering severity.

provide the clinician with information about children's stuttering in settings beyond the clinic.[33] Scores from these rating scales have been shown to be both reliable and highly correlated with SLPs' stuttering frequency and severity measures.[34,35] ▶ Fig. 8.6 contains an example of a 9-point rating scale that has text labels attached to some of the scale numbers. On the scale, a rating of 1 corresponds with typical speech, 2 corresponds with relatively mild stuttering, and 9 corresponds to very severe stuttering.

Examples of other aspects of stuttering that can be rated include stuttering frequency, disfluency duration, muscle tenseness, and speaking effort. Informal rating scales can also be adapted to assess the frequency and intensity of emotions such as fear and anxiety during speech, as well as speakers' level of satisfaction with their speech or success in managing stuttering. Ratings of speech naturalness are particularly helpful to use near the completion of a stuttering treatment program, especially when the intervention has heavily emphasized the use of controlled articulation rate to manage stuttered speech.[36] The clinician uses the rating to provide the child with feedback about the extent to which speech sounds "natural" (i.e., rate, prosody, and inflection sounds like a typical speaker). Naturalness ratings can also be used to describe a child's speech in various settings (e.g., during a specific speaker task, over the course of an entire day).

Norm-Referenced Tests of Speech Fluency

Norm-referenced tests that are used in the assessment of stuttering incorporate standard procedures for collecting and analyzing speech samples and they provide the clinician with standardized scores such as percentile ranks. These features allow clinicians to compare the performance of the child who is being assessed against a reference group (e.g., children who do stutter, children who stutter) and to evaluate changes in a child's stuttering over time.

Stuttering Severity Instrument, Fourth Edition

The *Stuttering Severity Instrument, Fourth Edition* (SSI-4)[20] is a norm-referenced test that clinicians use to rate the severity of a speaker's stuttering. The SSI-4 contains separate norms for preschool-aged, school-aged, and teens/adult-aged individuals who stutter. The stuttering severity rating on the SSI-4 is organized around a *speaking task* and, for children who read at a minimum of a third-grade level, a *reading task*. The *speaking task* on the SSI-4 uses pictures and verbal prompts to elicit speech samples in and outside of the clinic. After these samples are obtained, the clinician analyzes them to compute the percentage of stuttered syllables per task (see the section *Speech Continuity Measures*). The speech samples are also used to determine the average duration of the three longest instances of stuttering that occur. The child's stuttering frequency and duration measures are converted to weighted "task scores" using tables on the SSI-4

scoring form. The clinician also rates the child's speech for the presence of "physical concomitants" using four 6-point rating scales that capture the extent to which behaviors such as distracting sounds, facial grimaces, and extraneous head and extremity movements accompany instances of stuttering. The score from the physical concomitants scale is added to the weighted frequency and duration scores to yield a total score, which is then compared to SSI-4 norms to yield a percentile rank and a corresponding "severity equivalent" (i.e., a descriptive label such as "very mild," "mild," "moderate, and so forth).

The SSI-4 is normed only on speakers who stutter. Thus, the main use of the test is to compare the person who is being assessed to other people who stutter for the purpose of obtaining a severity rating of the person's stuttering. Because the SSI-4 is not normed on typical speakers, it is less useful for differentiating stuttering from typical disfluency. Nonetheless, the frequent presence of disfluencies that are characteristic of stuttering, lengthy disfluencies, and disfluencies that are accompanied by physical concomitants are usually sufficient to help a clinician decide independently whether a child should be classified as a person who stutters.

Test of Childhood Stuttering

The TOCS[21] is normed on 4- to 12-year-old children to diagnose stuttering and determine its severity. The TOCS has two norm-referenced assessment components: the *Speech Fluency Measure* and the *Observational Rating Scales* (ORS). The test also includes a third, optional section, *Supplemental Clinical Assessment Activities*, which contains materials and methods for conducting clinical interviews and informal quantitative analyses of speech fluency like those described previously in this chapter (i.e., disfluency frequency scores, disfluency duration scores, speech rate, stuttering frequency scores). Scales for rating speech naturalness and documenting the frequency with which various associated behaviors are provided as well.

The *Speech Fluency Measure* portion of the TOCS takes about 20 minutes to administer and features four types of talking tasks: rapid picture naming, sentence production, conversation, and narration. The ORS portion of the TOCS, completed by parents and teachers, includes two nine-item subscales, one that measures the extent to which stuttering symptoms are present in the child's speech and another that measures the consequences of stuttering (e.g., social and communicative penalties resulting from disfluency). The ORS, which provides the clinician with a norm-referenced measure of the child's speech fluency and consequences of stuttering in settings beyond the immediate testing environment, is further described in the norm-referenced assessment section later.

In contrast to the SSI-4, the TOCS is normed on both typical children and children who stutter. This makes it possible not only to obtain an estimate of stuttering severity but also to make statistical conclusions about the extent to which a child's speech fluency is like that of children in the general population. On the TOCS' *Speech Fluency Measure*, a child's performance on the speaking tasks is compared to both typical children (i.e., children without a diagnosis of stuttering) and children who stutter. These comparisons are based on the frequency with which children produce part-word repetitions, whole-word repetitions, and prolonged or blocked speech sounds (i.e., the disfluency types that are most characteristic of stuttering). Because children who do not stutter rarely produce repetitions of sounds, syllables, and words and prolonged/blocked speech sounds, an individual who produces even a modest number of these disfluencies on the test will drop outside of the normal range. Data from the ORS are used similarly. That is, comparisons between a child's rating scores and the test norms provide both diagnostic and severity information that is based on parent and teacher perspectives—individuals who interact with the child regularly outside of the assessment setting.

Norm-Referenced Scales of Stuttering Experiences

Behavior Assessment Battery for School-Aged Children Who Stutter

The *Behavior Assessment Battery for School-Aged Children who Stutter*[37] contains three stand-alone rating scales, each of which is normed. The first of these, the *Speech Situation Checklist* (SSC) consists of two 50-item self-rating scales. The essential content of the items on these two subscales is the same; however, on the *SSC–Emotional Reactions* version, children rate the extent to which they are afraid to talk in various situations. On the *SSC–Speech Disruption* version (SSC-SD), children rate the amount of "trouble" that they have with their speech in various situations. Examples of contexts that children rate on both subscales include talking with certain types of people (e.g., adults, same-age boys and girls), performing various speech acts (e.g., answering questions, making a class presentation), and talking in specific contexts (e.g., on the telephone, arguing with a friend). The SSC is normed on children with typical fluency (ages 6–13 years) and children who stutter (ages 6–15 years). The norms consist of mean scores for each age level and their associated standard deviations.

The second component of the *Behavior Assessment Battery for School-Aged Children who Stutter*, the *Behavior Checklist* (BCL), is also a self-rating instrument. It consists of 50 items that deal with specific stuttering-related behaviors. Children are asked to indicate via a yes/no response whether they do various behaviors "to help (their) sound or words come out without trouble." Examples include pressing the lips together, clicking the tongue, and tightening stomach muscles. Like the SSC, norms for the BCL consist of means and associated standard deviations, for each year from ages 6 through 13 years for children who do not stutter and 6 through 15 years for children who stutter.

The third component of the *Behavior Assessment Battery for School-Aged Children who Stutter*, the *Communication Attitude Test* (CAT) is also a self-rating instrument. Children indicate their agreement with 33 statements via true/false responses. Examples of test items include the following: "It is hard for me to talk to people" and "People worry about the way I talk." The norms for the CAT are structured like the norms for the SSC and

the BCL. There is a revised version of the CAT (*Children's Attitudes About Talking–Revised*, or CAT-R),[38] consisting of 32 items, many of which are worded similarly to items on the CAT. Norms for the CAT-R feature mean scores and associated standard deviations for each year from ages 7 through 11 for children who do not stutter and children who stutter.

Overall Assessment of the Speaker's Experience of Stuttering–Student Version

The *Overall Assessment of the Speaker's Experience of Stuttering–School-Age* version (OASES-S)[39] is a norm-referenced rating scale designed for use with 7- to 12-year-old children who stutter. It is designed to provide information about the impact of stuttering from the speaker's perspective. The OASES-S contains 60 items, which are organized into four sections: *General Information* (15 items), *Speaker's Reactions* (20 items), *Daily Communication* (15 items), and *Quality of Life* (10 items). Each item is accompanied by a 5-point rating scale. Children who stutter are asked to read each test item and then circle the number on the scale that corresponds to their perspective on the item's content.

In the *General Information* section, children rate test items such as the extent of their stuttering-related knowledge and feelings about speaking. In the *Speaker's Reactions* sections, children rate how often they experience various emotions when thinking about stuttering, how often their stuttered speech is accompanied by physical and avoidance behaviors, and the extent to which they agree with various statements about stuttering. In the *Daily Communication* section, children rate the degree of stuttering-related communication difficulties they experience in various speaking situations at school, home, and during social activities. In the *Quality of Life* section, they rate the extent to which stuttering adversely affects their life.

Test of Childhood Stuttering: Observational Rating Scales

As mentioned previously, the ORS portion of TOCS includes two nine-item subscales that parents and teachers complete to provide the SLP with information about the child's stuttering. Nine items are rated to indicate how frequently the child has exhibited the described stuttering behavior(s) during the previous 2 months. Six of the nine items pertain to disfluency characteristics that align with stuttering and the remaining three items pertain to the frequency with which the child's speech is disfluent in different settings. Alternately, on the *Disfluency-Related Consequences* section, parents and teachers rate the frequency with which the child exhibits physical movements, emotions, coping mechanisms, and social penalties because of stuttering. Findings from one recent study show that parents' ratings of their child on the TOCS-ORS align well with direct observations of the child's stuttering-related behavior made by experienced SLPs.[40]

Additional Areas for Assessment

Phonology and Language

A significant percentage of children who receive treatment for stuttering in school-based settings will also qualify for treatment of concomitant disorders that affect either speech sound production and/or receptive and expressive language.[13] Thus, during an assessment, the clinician should be alert for difficulty in these areas. In the cases where there is cause for concern, the SLP can select from a range of formal, norm-referenced tests and informal procedures to examine the child's functioning in greater detail.

Children who stutter—even those with typically developing speech and language—are more likely to stutter when saying utterances that are motorically or syntactically complex.[29,41] Clinicians can design speech tasks that feature varying degrees of motor complexity (e.g., a picture-naming task with one-, two-, and three-syllable target responses) or language complexity (e.g., a sentence imitation task with stimuli that differ in the syntactic difficulty). Such tasks can provide valuable information about how the child's fluency varies with speech and language complexity.

Another way of examining the relationship between fluency and language complexity is for the clinician to intentionally vary the types of utterances they use during conversation with the child. For example, a clinician's closed-ended requests for information are likely to elicit short, simple responses from the child (e.g., SLP: *What color is it?* → Child: *Red*), while statements and open-ended requests for information tend to elicit longer, more complex utterances (e.g., SLP: *I like turtles because they move slowly.* Child: *I like cheetahs because they are fast.* SLP: *Tell me about your birthday party.* Child: *It was really fun. First, we played games and then we opened presents. After that, we had cake*). Informal probes like these are straightforward to design and administer, and thus easy to embed in an assessment protocol. They can provide useful information about fluency variability with any type of case, even those for whom articulation and language functioning are not identified as areas of concern.

Stuttering occurs within the context of utterances that require phonological, syntactic, and semantic planning. SLPs should also consider the possibility that a child who is referred for stuttering assessment may, instead, be demonstrating signs of an undiagnosed language impairment. Several researchers have reported that children with language impairment produce revisions, interjections, long silent pauses, and even SLDs more frequently than children with typical language skills.[42,43,44] With such cases, the frequency of SLDs is usually not sufficient to warrant a diagnosis of stuttering. The presentation of this type of "borderline" disfluency profile may be a sign of language impairment rather than stuttering and thus might prompt the clinician to conduct a comprehensive language assessment.

Temperament

Temperament is a biological construct that accounts for individual differences in emotional, motor, and attentional reactivity, and the extent to which a child is capable of self-regulating these reactive components.[19] Some recent theories of stuttering include temperament as a key factor in both the onset and development of the disorder.[45,46] There are different views on whether temperament should be considered in assessment or treatment of stuttering in children.[47] One main argument for assessing temperament is that information about this aspect of a child's functioning may help in making decisions about stuttering therapy. For example, a treatment program that emphasizes parent corrective feedback to the child about their stuttering may not be the best choice for a child who reacts strongly to any sort of evaluation or correction. More broadly, it is best practice to adjust assessment or therapy procedures for children who are extremely shy, visibly uncomfortable in a clinical environment or with an unfamiliar adult, or who show concern about their own performance during an evaluation or in therapy (see ▶ Chapter 11 School-Age Children in this volume for descriptions of therapy approaches for stuttering in school-aged children). An opposing view is that presently, there is not enough evidence to support the routine assessment of a child's temperament as part of a stuttering evaluation or treatment.[47]

When a clinician plans to evaluate temperament as part of a broader assessment, several options are available for the school-aged population. The first is to informally collect information about the child's emotional, behavioral, and attentional characteristics through a case history form or clinical interview (▶ Table 8.2). Clinicians could ask about how the child responds to new situations/people, positive/exciting events, difficult tasks, losing a game, not getting one's way, and being corrected. Some of these situations often occur during the assessment, allowing the clinician to observe whether the child has strong reactions (e.g., withdrawal, expressions of anxiety) or difficulty coping with such reactions. A second option, available for younger school-aged children up to 8 years old, is to administer the *Children's Behavior Questionnaire–Very Short Form* (CBQ-VSF).[48] This formal, norm-referenced tool provides information about temperament. Children demonstrating behaviors indicative of strong reactions and low levels of regulation may not only benefit from stuttering treatment that gently introduces challenges but also strategies for regulating such reactions, especially if communication related.

Drawing Conclusions and Making Recommendations

Diagnosing Stuttering

Diagnosis of stuttering in the school-aged population generally is a straightforward process. For most children who are diagnosed with stuttering, the following three criteria will be met within a 300- to 600-syllable sample: (1) repetitions of sounds, syllables, or words and prolonged or blocked sounds (i.e., SLDs) on ≥3% of syllables; (2) the combined frequency of these disfluency types will constitute the majority of all disfluencies the child produces (i.e., >50%); and (3) one of these SLD types will be the most frequent disfluency type the child produces. ▶ Table 8.4 contains additional information about what is typical of children's fluency.

As children progress through the elementary school years, they tend to become increasingly aware of their disfluencies and can describe the experience of stuttering accurately and in detail. In fact, during the assessment, a school-aged child may be able to tell the clinician that they stutter. In these cases, the clinician's primary job is to determine the accuracy of the child's self-diagnosis and, when stuttering is present, describe its characteristics, severity, and impact on communication.

Occasionally, there are cases where the diagnosis of stuttering is unclear at the conclusion of the assessment. For example, a child's frequency of SLD may not be particularly high, and the child does not seem to be able to describe speaking experiences in detail. In the cases where the frequency of the child's stuttering is borderline, the clinician can look for other markers of stuttered speech, detailed in the previous section on informal measures, such as mean RUs, SLD duration, presence of behaviorally complex or clustered SLDs, or marked presence of physical concomitants during speech, to clarify the diagnosis.

In the cases where parents report that their child stutters at home but the child does not stutter during the standard assessment tasks administered in clinic, the clinician can use the communicative stressors discussed earlier in this chapter and other beyond-clinic speech samples (i.e., school-based speech sample) to see if the behaviors that are causing concern can be elicited. Alternately, the clinician can use normed parent- and teacher-based rating scales (e.g., the TOC-ORS) or data from clinical interviews to confirm that the child stutters. Parental concern about stuttering has been shown to be a reliable indicator of the presence of stuttering in children, so much so that it has been used as an inclusionary criterion for stuttering group classification in many research studies. Finally, a child's responses on self-rating measures that assess the severity and/or impact of stuttering on quality of life, participation, and so forth (e.g., OASES-S, Behavior Assessment Battery, CAT-R) can help the clinician arrive at a diagnosis by providing information about the extent to which stuttered speech adversely affects the child.

Determining Severity

Stuttering severity is a multidimensional construct. One approach to describing it is to quantify the extent to which SLDs and accompanying behaviors are observed and measured in the child's speech. Norm-referenced tests such as the SSI-4 and TOCS provide this type of quantitative measure of severity, as do normed self-rating scales like the SSC-SD and speech fluency measures obtained from samples of the child's speech. Although this information helps the clinician, child, and parent get a sense of how the child speaks, quantitative measures of speech fluency do not always accurately reflect the extent to which stuttering adversely impacts a child's day-to-day life. For example, a child might earn a rating of "mild" on the SSI-4, yet report experiencing moderate to severe participation restrictions and elevated anxiety in classroom situations that require speaking. In this case, a more thorough statement of severity, such as "mildly stuttered speech that has a moderate negative impact on communication and psychological well-being," is needed. The main point here is that the combination of speech-based measures of stuttering severity along with measures that capture the cognitive and emotional consequences of stuttering will yield the most valid severity rating and will better inform recommendations for therapy.

Making Recommendations

At the conclusion of an assessment, the clinician conveys assessment results and accompanying recommendations to the parent and, when applicable, the child. At this point, the therapeutic process commences. The clinician begins by sharing with the parent and child the most helpful things to do in the coming weeks and months. The presentation of recommendations at the end of the assessment provides an opportunity to educate parents and the child about stuttering and what can be done to

help the child reach their goals. Such education is important as research indicates that people are more likely to engage in helpful behaviors when they hold accurate beliefs about stuttering.[49]

Assessment recommendations for school-age children typically address the following issues:
- Is treatment recommended? If so,
  - Why is it necessary and what are the general goals?
  - What type and intensity of treatment is recommended, and who will be involved in the process?
  - Is the child's or family's participation in a stuttering support group recommended?
  - Are there other concerns related to stuttering that need to be addressed (e.g., bullying)?
  - Are there barriers to delivering treatment (e.g., transportation or scheduling problems)?
- If treatment for stuttering is not recommended:
  - Is assessment or treatment for other speech-language disorders needed?
  - Is a reassessment of the child's speech fluency needed in the future? If so, when?
  - What should the parent or child do if concerns about stuttering persist or worsen?
- Regardless of whether treatment is recommended:
  - Are referrals to other professionals warranted?

Treatment Eligibility Considerations in Public School Settings

The Individuals with Disabilities Education Act (IDEA), which is a federal law in the United States, indicates that public education should provide free and appropriate services to children with disabilities so that they are "prepared to lead productive and independent adult lives, to the maximum extent possible" (c5 Aii).[50] Considering the ways that untreated stuttering can adversely impact children's lives, addressing stuttering is consistent with the IDEA's aim. Relative to assessment, IDEA stipulates that the evaluation should "use a variety of assessment tools and strategies to gather relevant functional, developmental, and academic information, including information provided by the parent" (b2 A). The law also states that the local educational agency should "not use any single measure or assessment as the sole criterion for determining whether a child is a child with a disability or determining an appropriate educational program for the child" (b2 B). For this reason, clinicians in the United States who work in settings where qualification for services is linked to a disfluency frequency threshold can point to this stipulation in federal law (which supersedes local policies) as support for considering more than one type of assessment measure to determine whether a child qualifies for services.

As we have detailed in this chapter, a multidimensional approach to assessment is useful when evaluating school-aged children who stutter.[51] Such an approach is needed when the goal is to demonstrate that a child who is doing well *academically* may not be functioning well *educationally*. In the language of IDEA, the term "educational" has been interpreted as including learning in the domains of social, emotional, and interpersonal development. Thus, even though a student may be passing, or even excelling, grade-wise in their academic work, the child's stuttering still may negatively impact educational performance. For example, stuttering may result in the child being excluded by classmates from academic activities, and it may cause the child to withdraw from speaking situations, thereby limiting their ability to fully benefit from social, emotional, and interpersonal experiences that are central to public education.[52]

8.3 Case Scenario

The following case study of a school-aged child, "Jake," illustrates key concepts from this chapter. It includes information from the intake form completed by the parents and information from the clinical interviews with the parents and Jake. While reading the case description, notice what questions need to be addressed. After the case information is presented, you will be asked what should be included in the remaining components of the assessment.

8.3.1 Intake Information

Jake is an 8-year-old boy and a rising third grader at the time of his current assessment. His parents scheduled him for a 90-minute evaluation at a university speech-language-hearing clinic to address concerns that they had about his long-standing difficulties with stuttering.

8.3.2 Clinical Interview

In the clinical interview, the clinician began by asking the parents to describe their concerns about Jake's speech fluency. The parents indicated that they first noticed symptoms of stuttering—primarily repetitions of sounds and syllables—in Jake's speech when he was 4 years old, but stated the symptoms seemed to resolve within about 6 months. They stated that Jake began showing symptoms of stuttered speech again after starting first grade, but the stuttered speech was mainly limited to "stressful situations." Symptoms at the start of first grade included repeating word-initial sounds and syllables as well as prolonging and blocking on consonant sounds, sometimes for several seconds. The parents reported that at the midpoint of second grade (about 4 months prior to the third grade assessment), the frequency of Jake's stuttering increased significantly, was present in most situations, and consisted primarily of prolonged and blocked consonant sounds, which were sometimes accompanied by eyelid closing, "tense looking muscles," and facial grimacing. His parents stated that they and Jake became concerned about the changes in his stuttering, spurring them to schedule the present evaluation.

Jake's parents reported that, during the 6 months preceding the current assessment, he had become very aware of his stuttering and that, when he was unable to communicate, he sometimes sighed loudly, groaned, and said, "Never mind." They also reported that he occasionally reacted to his stuttering by running away to his bedroom. Overall, however, Jake's parents reported that he displayed appropriate social skills when interacting with peers and that he participated in most or all communication situations.

Related to family history, Jake's mother reported that her brother (Jake's uncle) stuttered noticeably from childhood through adolescence. Although the uncle's stuttering improved greatly by early adulthood, Jake's mother stated that

her brother still stutters in some situations and that he "avoids speaking in front of large groups." In addition, Jake's father reported that he had received services from an SLP as child because of difficulties with "pronouncing some of his speech sounds."

The parents reported no major concerns about Jake's development other than his stuttered speech and his sounding "a little less mature" than his classmates because he "says certain sounds wrong." Although the parents described Jake's overall academic abilities as "average to above average," they expressed concern about his reading comprehension, observing that he sometimes does not recall details about what he has read. They also indicated that in the past few months he "does not explain things as clearly" as he previously did.

When the clinician interviewed Jake about how he felt about his stuttering and his ability to communicate with others, he reported that he felt "great." However, when the clinician depersonalized the interview by asking how other children might feel when they stuttered in a conversation with friends, Jake reported they would feel upset and embarrassed.

8.3.3 Clinical Application Questions for the Case Study

1. Which questions from ▶ Table 8.2 did the intake and case history help to answer?
2. What questions remain after reading this case summary?
3. Based on the remaining questions, use ▶ Table 8.2 to develop an assessment battery.
4. After developing your assessment battery, check ▶ Table 8.1 to see that all components of the ICF model are being evaluated.

8.4 Future Directions

Although research has led to the development of useful tools for assessing stuttering in school-aged children, there is room for improving the accuracy, reliability, and efficiency of these clinical instruments and measures. We expect that, in the near future, advances in speech recognition technology will lead to widespread use of automated analyses of stuttered speech samples. Such analyses will be performed much faster and more reliably than today's manual analyses and should yield detailed information about not only stuttering-related disfluency but also other relevant aspects of communication performance such as speech rate, disfluency duration, and language functioning. In the absence of fully automated tools, current web-based tools, such as those associated with FluencyBank,[58] provide computer-based analyses that are created from clinician-entered transcripts and other learning tools for speech fluency and rate analysis.

It is also worth considering that although linguistic context and demand are included in most multifactorial models of stuttering, there is a lack of evidence for including formal language assessment, beyond a basic screening, as a standard component of a stuttering evaluation for school-aged children. Similarly, it is unknown whether routine formal assessment of temperament is necessary for this age group. Further research will help clinicians gain clarity on these issues.

8.5 Conclusion

Assessment is the bedrock of the clinical management of stuttering. Use of an assessment battery that is based on the WHO's ICF model helps clinicians develop a comprehensive understanding of a child's speech fluency by yielding information about factors necessary to diagnose stuttering, describe its severity and life impact, and weigh the need for treating it. Clinicians can develop a comprehensive understanding of children's stuttering by conducting a combination of formal and informal measures. Although the SLP assumes primary responsibility for planning and administering an assessment, school-aged children and their families should be involved in the process so that issues that are important to them are addressed. Their perspectives on stuttering will not only provide clinicians with information about stuttering severity but also foster the development of treatment plans that are aimed at improving not only children's speech fluency but also their communication effectiveness and general quality of life.

References

[1] World Health Organization. International Classification of Functioning, Disability, and Health: Short Version. Geneva: World Health Organization; 2001

[2] Yaruss JS, Quesal RW. Stuttering and the International Classification of Functioning, Disability, and Health: an update. J Commun Disord. 2004; 37(1):35–52

[3] Yairi E, Ambrose NG. Early childhood stuttering: for clinicians by clinicians. Austin, TX: Pro-ed; 2005

[4] Yairi E, Ambrose NG, Paden EP, Throneburg RN. Predictive factors of persistence and recovery: pathways of childhood stuttering. J Commun Disord. 1996; 29(1):51–77

[5] Yairi E, Ambrose NG. Early childhood stuttering I: persistency and recovery rates. J Speech Lang Hear Res. 1999; 42(5):1097–1112

[6] Andrews G. The epidemiology of stuttering. In: Curlee RF, Perkins WH, eds. Nature and treatment of stuttering: New directions. Boston, MA: College-Hill Press; 1984;1–12

[7] Sheehan JG, Martyn MM. Stuttering and its disappearance. J Speech Hear Res. 1970; 13(2):279–289

[8] Bloodstein O. The development of stuttering. I. Changes in nine basic features. J Speech Hear Disord. 1960; 25:219–237

[9] Boey RA, Van de Heyning PH, Wuyts FL, Heylen L, Stoop R, De Bodt MS. Awareness and reactions of young stuttering children aged 2–7 years old towards their speech disfluency. J Commun Disord. 2009; 42(5):334–346

[10] Pellowski MW, Conture EG. Characteristics of speech disfluency and stuttering behaviors in 3- and 4-year-old children. J Speech Lang Hear Res. 2002; 45(1):20–34

[11] Vanryckeghem M, Brutten GJ. The relationship between communication attitude and fluency failure of stuttering and nonstuttering children. J Fluency Disord. 1996; 21(2):109–118

[12] Kelly EM, Smith A, Goffman L. Orofacial muscle activity of children who stutter: a preliminary study. J Speech Hear Res. 1995; 38(5):1025–1036

[13] Logan KJ. Fluency Disorders. 2nd ed. San Diego, CA: Plural; 2022

[14] Gillam RB, Logan KJ, Pearson N. Test of childhood stuttering. Austin, TX: Pro-ed; 2014

[15] Yairi E, Seery C. Stuttering: foundations and clinical applications. 2nd ed. Boston, MA: Pearson; 2015

[16] Luterman DM. Counseling persons with communication disorders and their families. 3rd ed. Austin, TX: Pro-ed; 1996

[17] Kully DA, Langevin M, Lomheim H. Intensive treatment of stuttering in adolescents and adults. In: Conture EG, Curlee RF. eds. Stuttering and Related Disorders of Fluency. 3rd ed. New York, NY: Thieme Medical Publishers; 2007:213–232

[18] Logan KJ, Mullins MS, Jones KM. The depiction of stuttering in contemporary juvenile fiction: Implications for clinical practice. Psychol Sch. 2008; 45(7):609–626

[19] Rothbart MK. Becoming who we are: temperament and personality in development. New York, NY: Guilford Press; 2011

[20] Riley GD. Stuttering Severity Instrument-4th Edition (SSI-4). Austin, TX: Pro-ed; 2009

[21] Gillam RB, Logan KJ, Pearson NA. Test of childhood stuttering. Austin, TX: Pro-ed; 2009

[22] Mayer M. Frog, Where Are You? New York, NY: Dial Press; 1969

[23] Wiesner D. Flotsam. New York: Clarion Books; 2006

[24] Yaruss JS. Converting between word and syllable counts in children's conversational speech samples. J Fluency Disord. 2000; 25(4):305–316

[25] Brundage SB, Ratner NB. Measurement of stuttering frequency in children's speech. J Fluency Disord. 1989; 14(5):351–358

[26] Logan KJ, Byrd CT, Mazzocchi EM, Gillam RB. Speaking rate characteristics of elementary-school-aged children who do and do not stutter. J Commun Disord. 2011; 44(1):130–147

[27] Panico J, Healey EC. Influence of text type, topic familiarity, and stuttering frequency on listener recall, comprehension, and mental effort. J Speech Lang Hear Res. 2009; 52(2):534–546

[28] Zebrowski PM. Duration of the speech disfluencies of beginning stutterers. J Speech Hear Res. 1991; 34(3):483–491

[29] Logan KJ, Conture EG. Selected temporal, grammatical, and phonological characteristics of conversational utterances produced by children who stutter. J Speech Lang Hear Res. 1997; 40(1):107–120

[30] Johnson W, Colley WH. The relationship between frequency and duration of moments of stuttering. J Speech Hear Disord. 1945; 10(1):35

[31] Ambrose NG, Yairi E. The role of repetition units in the differential diagnosis of early childhood incipient stuttering. Am J Speech Lang Pathol. 1995; 4(3):82–88

[32] Ambrose NG, Yairi E. Normative disfluency data for early childhood stuttering. J Speech Lang Hear Res. 1999; 42(4):895–909

[33] Onslow M, Jones M, O'Brian S, et al. Comparison of percentage of syllables stuttered with parent-reported severity ratings as a primary outcome measure in clinical trials of early stuttering treatment. J Speech Lang Hear Res. 2018; 61(4):811–819

[34] Karimi H, O'Brian S, Onslow M, Jones M. Absolute and relative reliability of percentage of syllables stuttered and severity rating scales. J Speech Lang Hear Res. 2014; 57(4):1284–1295

[35] O'Brian S, Packman A, Onslow M, O'Brian N. Measurement of stuttering in adults: Comparison of stuttering-rate and severity-scaling methods. J Speech Lang Hear Res. 2004; 47(5):1081–1087

[36] Ingham RJ, Sato W, Finn P, Belknap H. The modification of speech naturalness during rhythmic stimulation treatment of stuttering. J Speech Lang Hear Res. 2001; 44(4):841–852

[37] Brutten GJ, Vanryckeghem M. Behavior Assessment Battery for School-age Children who Stutter. San Diego, CA: Plural; 2007

[38] De Nil LF, Brutten GJ. Speech-associated attitudes of stuttering and nonstuttering children. J Speech Hear Res. 1991; 34(1):60–66

[39] Yaruss JS, Coleman, CE, Quesal, RW. Overall Assessment of Speaker's Experience of Stuttering-School Age. McKinney, TX: Stuttering Therapy Resources; 2016

[40] Tumanova V, Choi D, Conture EG, Walden TA. Expressed parental concern regarding childhood stuttering and the Test of Childhood Stuttering. J Commun Disord. 2018; 72:86–96

[41] Byrd CT, Logan KJ, Gillam RB. Speech disfluency in school-age children's conversational and narrative discourse. Lang Speech Hear Serv Sch. 2012; 43(2):153–163

[42] Boscolo B, Ratner NB, Rescorla L. Fluency of school-aged children with a history of specific expressive language impairment: an exploratory study. Am J Speech Lang Pathol. 2002; 11(1):41–49

[43] Finneran DA, Leonard LB, Miller CA. Speech disruptions in the sentence formulation of school-age children with specific language impairment. Int J Lang Commun Disord. 2009; 44(3):271–286

[44] Guo LY, Tomblin JB, Samelson V. Speech disruptions in the narratives of English-speaking children with specific language impairment. J Speech Lang Hear Res. 2008; 51(3):722–738

[45] Conture EG, Walden TA, Arnold HS, Graham CG, Hartfield KN, Karrass J. Communication-emotional model of stuttering. In: Bernstein Ratner N, Tetnowski J, eds. Current Issues in Stuttering Research and Practice. Mahwah, NJ: Lawrence Erlbaum; 2006:17–46

[46] Smith A, Weber C. How stuttering develops: the multifactorial dynamic pathways theory. J Speech Lang Hear Res. 2017; 60(9):2483–2505

[47] Onslow M, Kelly EM. Temperament and early stuttering intervention: two perspectives. J Fluency Disord. 2020; 64:105765

[48] Putnam SP, Helbig AL, Gartstein MA, Rothbart MK, Leerkes E. Development and assessment of short and very short forms of the infant behavior questionnaire-revised. J Pers Assess. 2014; 96(4):445–458

[49] Arnold HS, Li J. Associations between beliefs about and reactions toward people who stutter. J Fluency Disord. 2016; 47:27–37

[50] US Department of Education. Individuals with Disabilities Education Act, 20 U.S.C. § 1400. 2004. Available at: https://uscode.house.gov/view.xhtml?path=/prelim@title20/chapter33&edition=prelim. Accessed June 10, 2020

[51] Olson ED, Bohlman P. IDEA '97 and children who stutter: evaluation and intervention that lead to successful, productive lives. Semin Speech Lang. 2002; 23(3):159–164

[52] Thomas JL. Decoding eligibility under the IDEA: Interpretations of "adversely affects educational performance". Campbell Law Rev. 2016; 38(1):73–107

[53] Tumanova V, Conture EG, Lambert EW, Walden TA. Speech disfluencies of preschool-age children who do and do not stutter. J Commun Disord. 2014; 49:25–41

[54] Boey RA, Wuyts FL, Van De Heyning PH, Heylen L, De Bodt MS. Characteristics of stuttering in Dutch-speaking individuals. Clin Linguist Phon. 2009; 23(4):241–254

[55] Yairi E. Disfluency characteristics of childhood stuttering. In: Curlee RF, Siegel, GM, eds. Nature and treatment of stuttering: New directions. 2nd ed. Boston, MA: Allen and Bacon; 1997;49–78

Further Readings

Bernstein Ratner N, Luckman CR, Baer M. FluencyBank Voices-CWS Corpus. Available at: https://fluency.talkbank.org/access/Voices-CWS.html

Blood GW, Blood IM. Long-term consequences of childhood bullying in adults who stutter: social anxiety, fear of negative evaluation, self-esteem, and satisfaction with life. J Fluency Disord. 2016; 50:72–84

Iverach L, Jones M, McLellan LF, et al. Prevalence of anxiety disorders among children who stutter. J Fluency Disord. 2016; 49:13–28

Smith A, Weber C. How stuttering develops: the multifactorial dynamic pathways theory. J Speech Lang Hear Res. 2017; 60(9):2483–2505

Yaruss JS, Quesal RW. Stuttering and the International Classification of Functioning, Disability, and Health: an update. J Commun Disord. 2004; 37(1):35–52

9 Adolescents and Adults

Eric S. Jackson and Anthony DiLollo

Abstract

The purpose of this chapter is to describe procedures for the assessment of stuttering in adults and adolescents, along with the rationale for our approach to evaluation. Although stuttering is conventionally considered to be primarily a disorder of speech or speech fluency, most of what we will discuss relates to key characteristics of stuttering other than observable speech (dis)fluency. This focus on under-the-surface features of stuttering is critical because, as we will detail, measuring surface behaviors alone does not provide a comprehensive picture of stuttering or its impact. In fact, relying on surface measures can greatly underestimate the magnitude of the stuttering problem. As such, for many teens and adults who stutter, focusing on the overt behaviors of stuttering becomes secondary in both the assessment and therapeutic processes. After a brief introduction, which describes the purposes of stuttering assessment for adolescents and adults, we will provide an outline of the essential components in the diagnostic process. Resources to assist clinicians in assessment will be discussed and examples, including a case study, will be provided. Our goal is for readers to understand the entirety of both the principles and procedures in the assessment process and how to implement them when working with adolescents and adults who stutter.

Keywords: stuttering, fluency disorder, assessment, variability, anticipation, adults who stutter, adolescents who stutter

---

> ### Clinical Note
>
> Some readers may take issue with the term "problem" when describing stuttering, as it may ultimately contribute to the stigmatization of stuttering. We use this term because if an individual comes to us for therapy, stuttering is likely a problem or challenge in their mind. Indeed, the purpose of therapy for all adolescents and adults who stutter is to reduce the magnitude of this problem rather than any individual feature of stuttering (e.g., number of disfluencies).

9.1 Introduction

9.1.1 Basic Assumptions

To begin, it is safe to say that there is no universal agreement about the best way to assess stuttering. The procedures discussed in this chapter are based on a number of assumptions about adolescents and adults who stutter, derived from a number of sources including, most importantly, people who stutter. These premises direct the diagnostic process and influence the choices we make for assessment, including the questions we ask, the procedures we use, and our interpretation of the findings.

The first, and arguably most important assumption is that adolescents and adults who stutter—hereafter referred to as "adults who stutter" or "people who stutter" because adolescents have more in common with adults who stutter than with children who stutter—have lived with the disorder for a decade or more (see ▶ Chapter 1 in this volume). Given the relatively long duration of stuttering, we can reasonably conclude that they are unlikely to completely recover.[1] In other words, they will experience at least *some* amount of stuttering for the rest of their lives, regardless of therapy. This first assumption leads to our second, which is that unless we discover during intake and evaluation that the person exhibits cluttering or neurogenic stuttering (see ▶ Chapter 16 in this volume), we assume that they began to stutter in early childhood (i.e., they exhibit "developmental" stuttering). For these reasons, the information in this chapter will focus primarily on the assessment of the disorder of stuttering that begins during the preschool years.

One's history with stuttering is likely to have led them to try various ways of dealing with the problem. These attempts can include speech-language or psychologically oriented therapy; advice from well-meaning (but often misinformed) relatives, teachers, and friends; information found in books, booklets, pamphlets, and on the Internet; or self-taught strategies.[2] Individual experiences with stuttering have likely impacted their educational, social, and vocational experiences.[3,4] Although not all of these things will be true for all people who stutter, at least some of them will be true for most people who stutter.

9.1.2 Client Expectations: A Word about Controlled Speech versus Spontaneous Fluency

Many clients come to us with the primary goal of being fluent, or not stuttering, and it is both reasonable and expected for speech-language pathologists (SLPs) to adhere to their wishes. Although the desire for increased fluency is easy to understand (why wouldn't someone want to talk without stuttering and without thinking about the mechanics of speech?), the clinician must discuss with the client what is realistic. Although learning to use different speaking strategies can increase the control that a speaker has over their speech mechanism, spontaneous or natural fluency may not be attainable, especially for people with long histories of stuttering, at least not all of the time. Rather, the goal is controlled fluency, or "less effortful stuttering," or "managed stuttering." That is, the speaker learns a different way of talking and stuttering, with less effort, and this is considered to be the optimal outcome of therapy.

It is important to appreciate that behavioral approaches such as stuttering modification and fluency shaping do not *directly* target increased spontaneous or natural fluency. As mentioned earlier, they focus on teaching the person how to either stutter more easily (i.e., with less physical tension or with shorter duration) or produce controlled speech. It is also essential to recognize that speech techniques used to intentionally change how one uses their articulatory and phonatory systems to produce speech are actually at odds with the automaticity that underlies spontaneous fluency. Increased automatic or spontaneous fluency can emerge when these new ways of talking and stuttering are consistently practiced over time. In this way, fluency should be considered a *distal*, not *immediate*, goal of therapy. All of this is to say that from the very beginning, it is the responsibility of the SLP to provide information about the nature of stuttering and stuttering therapy. It is not to limit goals in therapy for people who stutter. Rather, goals should be realistic and achievable. These early discussions are likely to include education about stuttering, improving attitudes about stuttering, changing one's self-concept as a person who stutters, stuttering with less effort, and increasing one's ability to say what they want to say regardless of the amount of stuttering.

9.1.3 Impact of Stuttering and What Needs to Change

An important goal of assessment is to help the person who stutters to expand their thinking about therapy goals beyond speech fluency. In our experience, when a client tells us that they want to be fluent, or they want to stop stuttering, what they often mean is that they want to speak without thinking about stuttering. In other words, they want to be spontaneously fluent. Most, if not all, of the stuttering clients we see will continue to stutter to some degree throughout their lives. And for many individuals who stutter, all it takes is one instance of stuttering in a situation that they deem is especially important or during which they do not want to stutter to experience the negative thoughts, emotions, or impact on their quality of life that were the very reasons they sought therapy in the first place. Therefore, our position is that the primary goal of an assessment should not be quantifying how much a person stutters, but rather how they are responding physically, psychologically, and emotionally to stuttering. Identifying these responses to stuttering will allow the SLP to develop an intervention plan specific to the individual that is focused on how stuttering is an obstacle or problem in the client's life.

9.2 A Clinical Definition of Stuttering

A working definition of the stuttering disorder is critical to assessment because it determines the variables we want to observe and measure as we undertake the diagnostic process. Our clinical definition reflects our view, described earlier in this chapter, that stuttering is a complex phenomenon comprised of a spectrum of features that range from unobservable to observable and that vary both within and across individuals who stutter. By the time a person who stutters reaches adolescence, they have undoubtedly experienced many social interactions in which their speech system has broken down—and they have had to learn to cope with or manage these situations. For example, how does one handle a situation in which they introduce themselves in a classroom and stutter when saying their name, and someone jokes that they "don't know their own name"? They may not care, or they may remember this mocking the next time they introduce themselves in a similar situation. What do they do? Do they ask the teacher if they can opt out of introducing themselves? Do they leave the room when it is

their turn so that they can avoid potential negative listener reactions? Or do they forge ahead, potentially flooded with anxiety until it is their turn to speak, and hope for the best? The point here is that as a result of a neurobiological condition that manifests itself intermittently (i.e., stuttering behavior), people who stutter are forced to make decisions that nonstuttering individuals do not have to make, particularly in reconciling their desire to speak with potential listener or environmental reactions. And this is what we, as SLPs, are assessing—the role that stuttering plays in shaping an individual's everyday experiences.

Historically, the biggest challenge clinicians have faced is finding ways to observe and quantify the unobservable or "under-the-surface" characteristics of stuttering. These include cognitive and affective or emotional constructs such as anticipation, avoidance, fear, shame, guilt, and others. Listeners hear and see surface disfluency and, as a result, this is what has typically been emphasized in assessment and therapy. The problem with this focus is that there can be a discrepancy between what is produced and seen on the surface and what is experienced beneath the surface. Thankfully, in recent years a growing body of research investigating these "unobservable" aspects of stuttering has led to a shift away from surface-centric approaches to assessment, and one area that has received a significant amount of attention due to its central role in how speakers respond to stuttering is *anticipation*.

9.3 Anticipation: Stuttering Below the Surface

Surface breaks in speech fluency do not always provide a reliable measure of a moment of stuttering. This is because children, teens, and adults who stutter frequently anticipate when they are about to stutter and can quickly engage in strategies to alter speech, such as avoiding or concealing, or using a speaking strategy.[5,6] Anticipation refers to the speaker's awareness that something has gone wrong during speech-language planning and that they will stutter overtly if they do not do something to alter the ongoing process of speech production (e.g., by avoiding or changing a word). ▶ Fig. 9.1 presents a conceptual timeline of the stuttering event for a single word.

Clinical Note

We currently do not have a good understanding of what goes "wrong" in the speech-language systems of people who stutter when they stutter. There are some data that suggest that this glitch is represented at a neural level, but we are far from understanding the neural processes that underlie stuttering events. However, we find that using the term glitch is helpful to the speaker because it indicates that something goes wrong prior to actually producing the word, and the speaker can learn to respond to this in a way that is helpful or adaptive to them. We are hopeful that the coming years will shine light on the neural and other processes that lead to the manifestation of overt stuttering events.

As shown in ▶ Fig. 9.1, the speaker first has intention to say a word. During the processes of speech-language planning, there

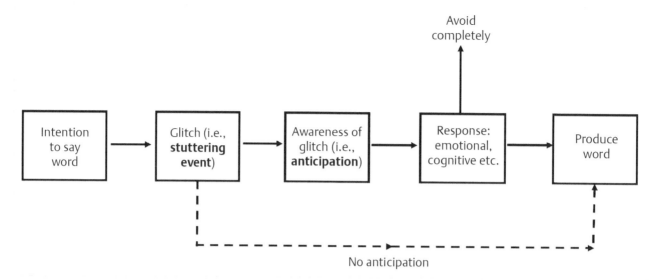

Fig. 9.1 Timeline of the stuttering event.

is some sort of "glitch"—something goes wrong in the speaker's speech-language system. The speaker then becomes aware that something has gone

wrong, and is faced with a decision regarding how to respond (e.g., stall, disguise, use a speaking strategy). The speaker then produces the word. In many cases, the speaker may choose to avoid the word, or speaking, completely, because the risk of stuttering overtly outweighs the benefit of saying what they want to say, at least at that moment. Also, there may be many instances in which the speaker is not aware that something has gone wrong, and therefore does not anticipate stuttering. This could happen due to the inherently rapid nature of speech (e.g., there is not enough time to become aware), or because the speaker is simply not paying attention to their speech. However, it is important to note that given enough time, people can predict (or anticipate) overt stuttering moments with a high degree of accuracy. As such, anticipation is a central feature of stuttering because the things that people who stutter do in reaction to, or to cope with, impending stuttering shape both their observable stuttering behaviors and their experience of stuttering in general. Thus, the client's anticipation of stuttering is the *problem* that SLPs should understand, explore, and identify.

Clinical Note

Dean Williams, an SLP, researcher, and person who stuttered, wrote a lot about the stutterer's perception that stuttering is something out of their control—that it just happens, they don't know why, and as a result, doing anything about it is difficult if not impossible. This is a very passive perspective of the problem—stuttering is going to happen and take me with it, and there's little I can do about it. Williams encouraged SLPs to help their clients develop a more active perspective of their problem (i.e., "...stuttering is something that I am doing"). Although the initial breakdown in speech is not under the speaker's control, how they respond to this breakdown certainly is, or at least speakers can learn how to increase their sense of control over how their stuttering physically manifests itself.[7]

Defining and measuring such unobservable stuttering characteristics as anticipation is challenging. Most of what we know about these under-the-surface experiences and coping strategies comes from people who stutter themselves. In particular, many people who stutter report that the intermittent and involuntary nature of stuttering—or at least their belief, feeling, or sense that stuttering is involuntary and "just happens"—leads to a variety of coping behaviors that may become the most detrimental feature of the problem.[8,9,10,11,12] For example, due to uncertainty about whether or when they will stutter, a speaker may choose not to approach a romantic partner or not ask for a raise at work due to a fear of stuttering. These situations are inherently challenging for many people, but for people who stutter, this challenge is compounded by the possibility of stuttering.

Clinical Note

The reader may be wondering how a stutterer can experience the ability to anticipate moments of stuttering with high accuracy, as well as the intermittency of stuttering (sometimes it happens and sometimes it doesn't). This is indeed a challenging problem for stutterers, and for those who work with stutterers. One way to think about this challenge is that intermittency, or variability, of stuttering is contextual—the social milieu is constantly changing and with these changes when and where a person stutters also changes. Thinking about the social milieu prior to being in a speaking situation, for example, can bring with it a looming sense of anticipatory anxiety that is not specific to certain words, but a more general anxiety about impending danger (i.e., stuttering). In contrast, people who stutter also have a shorter-term and more specific sense regarding which specific words will be stuttered, which typically occurs just prior or close to the actual production of that word.

One final note related to anticipation and other covert features of stuttering is the dissociation that people often experience between the overt speech behaviors of stuttering—the repetitions and prolongations of sounds, for example—and their covert coping strategies and cognitive or affective experiences. For example, there are some individuals who present, on the surface, with a mild stuttering problem (i.e., low frequency of observable stuttering), but report that stuttering has a significant adverse impact on the quality of their life. For other people who stutter, the opposite dissociation is true—a high frequency of observable stuttering yet a limited effect on their overall quality of life. The observation that severe stuttering on the surface does not always align with a negative life experience—and vice versa—is a strong indication for the need to examine these under-the-surface aspects of stuttering during the assessment process. As many have pointed out, there is much more to stuttering than meets the eye, particularly in adolescents and adults.[3,13,14]

9.4 Measuring the Unobservable and Observable: A Framework for Stuttering Assessment

As Yaruss[18,19] has pointed out (and describes in ▶ Chapter 11 of this text), the World Health Organization's *International Classification of Functioning, Disability, and Health* (ICF),[15] an updated version of the earlier *International Classification of Impairments, Disabilities, and Handicaps* (ICIDH),[16,17] provides an internationally recognized framework for assessing complex human conditions—developmental, neurotypical, or disordered. As such, it provides an appropriate structure for the assessment of stuttering (▶ Fig. 9.2).

The ICF takes into account the *experiences* of the individual with any complex health problem, not merely the overt manifestation of the condition. Furthermore, the ICF model implies that all people with a specific condition will not respond to it in the same way; rather, a variety of factors both within the individual and their environment play a role in one's lived experience of the problem. The ICF framework can be used to describe all aspects of an individual's health experience, including both normal and disordered functioning. Therefore, the ICF supports the consideration of a wide range of factors that might be relevant for any one person who stutters; that is, the factors that should be assessed during an evaluation (for a more detailed discussion of stuttering and the ICF, see Yaruss and Quesal[20]).

9.4.1 Impact of Stuttering

With the previous discussion in mind, we propose that the main purpose of the stuttering evaluation is to determine the *impact* of stuttering on the individual as opposed to the *amount* of stuttering a person exhibits. Teens and adults who stutter come to us for a variety of reasons. They may be having difficulties in school because they stutter. Stuttering may be impacting their ability to achieve success at work. They might be feeling held back socially because of stuttering. They may have had previous therapy that focused largely or solely on changes in surface fluency and, because they have been unable to maintain the level of fluency that they achieved during therapy, they feel like they are doing something wrong. They may feel guilty because they are not able to achieve the level of fluency with

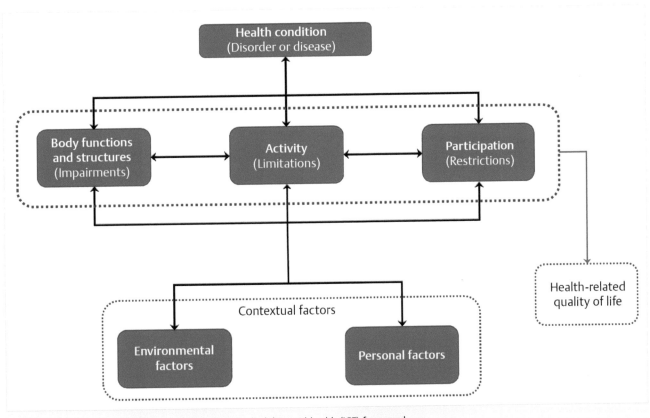

Fig. 9.2 The international classification of functioning, disability, and health (ICF) framework.

their teacher or boss that they can with their friend or spouse. These experiences lead them, and those around them, to believe that they can or should be able to control their stuttering "if they just tried harder." This, of course, is not true. Although a person who stutters may learn to be largely in control of how they respond to stuttering, they will have much less control over when and where stuttering occurs.

9.4.2 Variability Not Frequency of Stuttering

We suggest that the most useful way to consider the salience of disfluency to the overall impact of stuttering is to shift the focus away from the frequency and type of disfluency to the *intermittency* or *variability* of stuttering. The contextual variability of stuttering is a hallmark characteristic of the disorder (see ▸ Chapter 1 for a detailed discussion of the contextual variability of stuttering) and the feature that challenges clinicians who work with people who stutter, researchers who study stuttering, and, most importantly, people who stutter themselves. Typically, the intermittency of stuttering is confusing to the individual as well as to their family, friends, coworkers, and colleagues. People who stutter often ask us why they are fluent sometimes (e.g., speaking to a young child or pet) but not at other times (e.g., meeting a potential partner on whom you want to make a good impression). Imagine the confusion and distress experienced by people who stutter when they can produce the same speech sounds and articulatory gestures with relative ease in one situation, but with great difficulty in another, even immediately or a short time later. This aspect of stuttering presents individuals who stutter with an incredible challenge—navigating the "stuttering minefield." Responses from listeners to unexpected fluency breaks in the speech of people who stutter are challenging for both the speaker and the listener as well because these seemingly random interruptions are difficult to understand ("You weren't stuttering before…why are you stuttering now?"). Thus, an understanding (and acceptance) of the intermittency of stuttering is likely the most critical if one is to effectively assess (and ultimately treat) stuttering.

In the following sections, we describe a contemporary framework for assessing the covert and overt features of stuttering. We start with a useful way for clinicians to conceptualize the covert and overt features of stuttering in terms of the challenges they pose to both clients and the clinicians working with them. This conceptualization provides us with useful terminology that can help clinicians more clearly understand their role in helping clients cope with the complexities of their stuttering experience.

9.4.3 Reframing Overt and Covert Aspects of Stuttering: Technical and Adaptive Challenges

DiLollo and Neimeyer[21] described the ways in which concepts from adaptive leadership[22,23] map onto therapeutic processes in speech-language pathology. Of particular interest to us in this current chapter are the concepts of "adaptive" and "technical" challenges, as these provide clinicians with a way to more

clearly conceptualize the needs and challenges associated with the surface, speech-related aspects of their client's stuttering, while also considering the more covert, affective, and cognitive aspects of the problem, and the overall impact that stuttering has on the person's quality of life (▸ Fig. 9.3).

As described by Heifetz and Laurie,[22] *technical challenges* are those that can be clearly defined by an expert, and strategies for addressing these challenges are most effectively implemented through the application of expert knowledge. In the context of stuttering, technical challenges include surface behaviors, such as the types and duration of disfluencies, and accessory behaviors (see ▸ Chapter 1). The corresponding technical solutions are strategies to reduce or smooth out the overt stuttering behaviors (see ▸ Chapter 12 for a discussion of therapeutic strategies for modifying speech and stuttering).

In contrast, *adaptive challenges* involve the less observable aspects of problems. According to Heifetz and Laurie,[22] adaptive challenges are difficult to identify, typically have no clear, straightforward solution, and require changes in beliefs, lifestyle, and ways of thinking. For persons who stutter, adaptive challenges involve those cognitive and affective aspects of the disorder that impact the person's thinking, lifestyle, and self-image. Importantly, whereas technical challenges are typically addressed with a known solution, by someone other than the person facing the issue (e.g., a professional such as an SLP), adaptive challenges are addressed in more personal ways by the individual. In the case of people who stutter, a technical solution for altering speech production so as to move through speech in an easier way might address the immediate needs or expectations of the client to reduce the overt signs of stuttering. However, addressing the adaptive challenge of changing thinking and feeling is a process that, with the support of an SLP and an extended network of social supports, must be led by the person experiencing stuttering. In many cases, this involves moving away from the "stutterer" identity—that is, not thinking of oneself solely as a person who consistently struggles with speech, but rather as an individual who is many things and sometimes happens to stutter. In the case of the SLP, technical solutions involve the things that they can observe, including overt behavior, whereas adaptive solutions involve things that the SLP can learn to see more of.

Heifetz and colleagues[24] reported that one of the most common mistakes in leadership is a failure to recognize both adaptive and technical challenges in a situation, resulting in attempts to address the problem only from a technical perspective. As previously discussed, this is also a common mistake in the evaluation (and treatment) of stuttering, when clinicians focus only on counting and cataloging overt speech disfluencies as the measure of a client's stuttering. In such cases, the adaptive aspects of the stuttering problem are ignored or minimized—often because clinicians are unsure or uncomfortable with how to assess the intrinsic, less observable aspects experienced by the person who stutters and the ways in which they experience and cope with them. Fortunately, there are a number of relatively simple ways in which clinicians can assess the adaptive aspects of a client's stuttering, starting with a more person-focused approach to the diagnostic interview, followed later in the evaluation session or sessions by the use of tools such as attitude and self-efficacy scales, more comprehensive inventories such as the relevant form(s) of the *Overall Assessment of the Speaker's*

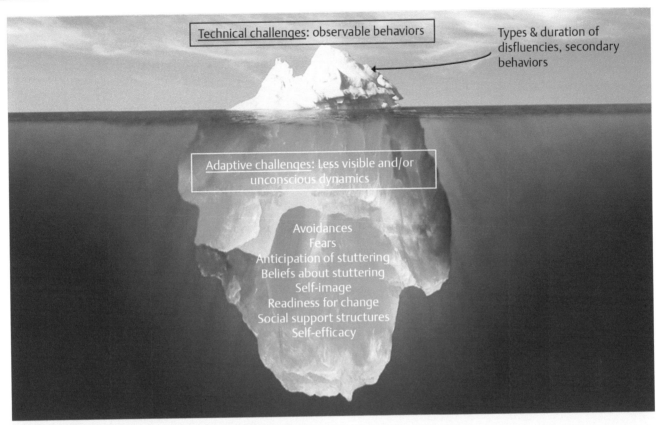

Fig. 9.3 Adaptive and technical challenges associated with stuttering.

Experience of Stuttering (OASES),[25] or other informal tools that ask clients to reflect on their experience of stuttering.

Although we have just contrasted technical and adaptive challenges, it is important to note that these are constructs that are created to allow us to more easily understand and examine complex processes like stuttering. In many ways, especially in the everyday lived experience of persons who stutter, technical and adaptive challenges are inextricably woven together. Thinking back to our earlier discussion of anticipation, the beginning of the stuttering event is first known by the speaker, and how the speaker responds to it is a very private experience—until they decide to show (or not show) their stuttering to the world. The manifestation of the behavior (i.e., the technical) is tightly linked to the person's response to stuttering, and reflects the adaptive experience of the breakdown. Therefore, the first step in an assessment of stuttering is to learn about the person to develop a foundation for understanding how they respond to intermittent interruptions in speech production.

In the following section, we provide an outline of the assessment process. A comprehensive evaluation will include a thorough assessment of both covert and overt (or adaptive and technical) features associated with the client's stuttering. We discuss the various components of an assessment, from the initial case history to the closing interview. Importantly, this section is only intended to provide the reader with a framework for assessment of an adult who stutters. Ultimately, the SLP will determine assessment techniques and protocols that they find most useful for a comprehensive assessment that is individualized for a specific client.

9.5 The Assessment Process

▶ Fig. 9.4 summarizes the basic evaluation procedures showing how they target aspects of the individual's stuttering along the continuum of "technical" to "adaptive" challenges.

It is critical to assess *both* technical and adaptive aspects of the clients' stuttering in order to gain a holistic understanding of how they might successfully manage stuttering. Importantly, however, it is not how *many* scales or tests you use that makes an assessment "comprehensive." Rather, it is how you *interpret* the information you obtain. That is, the ways in which the client responds informs us not only about their stuttering-related challenges but also where they are on their stuttering journey, and how ready and motivated they are to make a change. Consequently, all tests, scales, and other tools that are used with clients should be viewed as a *starting point* for gathering information, with the clinician not only discussing with the client his or her overall scores/outcomes but also asking about responses to specific items/questions that stand out as suggesting a strength or an area that is particularly challenging.

9.5.1 Case History

Ideally, the SLP should obtain case history information before conducting the assessment session. This information is often obtained by sending a case history questionnaire to the client. The case history provides us with a "mental snapshot" before we meet the client in person. Case history information typically includes things such as demographic information, therapy history, why the client

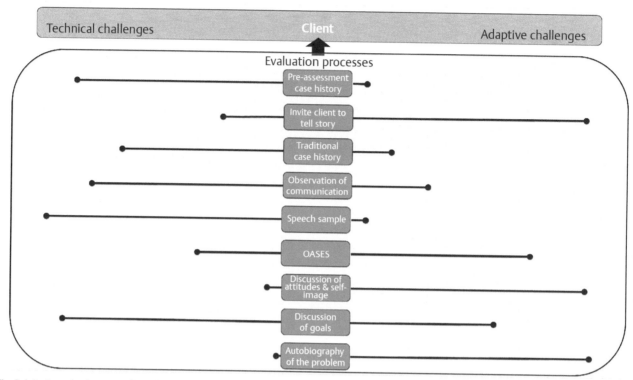

Fig. 9.4 Basic evaluation procedures for stuttering.

is interested in therapy at this particular time, whether the client is self-referred or was referred by someone else (e.g., an employer or teacher), and the impact that stuttering is having on the person. Appendix 9.1 includes a sample case history form.

9.5.2 Diagnostic Interview

At the beginning of the evaluation, we ask open-ended questions to allow the person who stutters to tell their story. Each story will be different. The goal, however, is to determine the ways in which stuttering impacts the individual's life and what we can do in therapy to help the client lessen the impact of stuttering on their life. Although there are general questions we can ask (Box 9.1), skilled SLPs will follow the client's lead during the assessment. As a result, each client's assessment will be different. Just like there are no "cookbook" treatments for stuttering, there is no "cookbook" approach to assessment. Box 9.1 presents guidelines for the key areas of focus during the diagnostic interview.

Box 9.1 Sample questions that may be asked during interview of an adult stutterer

- Why are you here today? Tell me about your speech problem.
- When did you first notice that stuttering was a problem?
- Has your speech changed since then? How?
- Is your speech better or worse at some times than others? Give me some examples.
- Do you have more trouble speaking in some situations than others? Do certain words or sounds give you more trouble than others? Are some people harder to talk to than others? Give me some examples.
- Do you avoid certain situations? Words? Sounds? Listeners? Give me some examples.
- Can you describe or show me what happens/what you do when you stutter?
- If you think you are going to have trouble saying a word or speaking in a particular situation, do you do anything to "help?" (Alternative: Do you use any "tricks" when you stutter?)
- Have you ever had speech therapy? When? Where? What did you do in therapy? Did it help? Why or why not?
- Do you have any idea why you stutter? Has anyone offered any suggestions, etc., regarding why you stutter?

- How has your life been affected by stuttering? How would your life be different if you didn't stutter?
- What would you like to get out of this evaluation? Are there any specific things that you are interested in or that I can do for you?
- Why have you decided to look for help now?
- When did you begin to stutter?
- Has it changed over the years?
- Does anybody you know stutter? Anybody in your family?
- What do you think caused your stuttering?
- Does your stuttering change from situation to situation?
- How would your life be different if you didn't stutter?
- Do you avoid certain speaking situations/words?
- Do you make decisions based on the fact that you (might) stutter?
- Have any of your relationships been affected by the fact that you stutter?
- What do you think other people think of your stuttering?
- Do you ever talk about stuttering with anybody?
- Do you have any questions for me?

Start with the Person not the Problem

When clients come to us for a stuttering evaluation, they typically expect us to ask a lot of questions, get samples of their speech, and maybe ask about attitudes. In other words, they expect us to be primarily focused on the overt characteristics of stuttering. Unfortunately, this approach remains anchored in the "technical" aspects of the client's problem and provides little to no accounting of the "adaptive" aspects of the problem. Given the need to explore both the technical and adaptive aspects of the client's stuttering, clinicians should plan their diagnostic interview in a way that first signals the client that we are interested in him or her as a *whole person* and not just his or her stuttering.

Inviting the Person to Tell Their Story

The importance of personal narratives in understanding and treating health problems has been widely discussed across health care settings.[26] Likewise, a number of authors have discussed the value of eliciting the client's "story" in the assessment and treatment of communication disorders in general,[21,27,28] and specifically for persons who stutter.[14,29,30] In the context of the evaluation of stuttering, the client's story includes all aspects of the person's life—who they are, how they see themselves, what they like and dislike, how they spend their time, etc.—and it is not restricted to "stuttering's story," which provides only a limited account of the person who is seeking help. Consequently, the first steps in a comprehensive evaluation for an adult who stutters are the following:

1. *Invite the person to tell his or her story.* Do this by saying something like, "Tell me about yourself" or "Tell me about your life."
2. *Listen.* The only questions that the clinician needs to ask at this time are to clarify something the client has said or to request more detail.

Starting an evaluation in this way enables the *client* to direct the initial content and provides the clinician with insights into what the client views as the most important aspects of his or her story. This is why it is important for the clinician to ask as few questions as possible at this time (something that is difficult for many SLPs!) because asking questions takes control of the story away from the client, focusing instead on what the clinician believes to be important.

9.5.3 Adaptive Measures

In addition to the interview, a number of measures are available to assess the less observable features of stuttering.

The Overall Assessment of the Speaker's Experience of Stuttering

OASES is available for both adults *(OASES-A)*[25] and teenagers between the ages of 13 and 17 years *(OASES-T)*.[25] Both the *OASES-A* and *OASES-T* include four sections: *General Information about Stuttering*, *Reactions*, *Functional Communication*, and *Quality of Life*. The *OASES-A* contains 100 items and the *OASES-T* has 80 items; the items on both forms require the client to rate the extent to which different aspects of stuttering impact a range of activities, responses, and goals (i.e., from "not at all" to "completely"). These ratings are used to derive an "impact score" for each of the four sections and an overall impact score that reflects the degree to which stuttering adversely impacts the speaker. As noted earlier, there is often a mismatch between the frequency and severity of surface disfluency and *OASES* scores; for example, some people who produce relatively few moments of overt stuttering experience a severely adverse impact of stuttering on their lives. The opposite can also be true (e.g., high frequency of stuttering with mild or moderately adverse impact).

The Stuttering Anticipation Scale

The Stuttering Anticipation Scale (SAS)[6] is a nonstandardized tool used to assess the extent to which individuals anticipate stuttering, as well as how they respond to anticipation. The *SAS* was developed as the result of a qualitative investigation of the ways in which adults who stutter respond to anticipation.[5] The data collected in the study provided one of the first glimpses into how people respond to the internal knowledge that they are about to stutter. The 25 most common responses to anticipation revealed in the study were used on a questionnaire that asks respondents to rate how often they anticipate stuttering in general, and the frequency with which they use a range of responses to the anticipation of stuttering. Sample items include the following: How often do you switch words when you know you are going to stutter? and How often do you stall when you know you are about to stutter? The *SAS* is a flexible tool such that it is not necessary for clients to complete all 25 questions, wording of questions can be altered to more closely reflect the speaker's background, and new questions can be added if the client indicates that they have responses to anticipation not included in the *SAS*.

The Modified Erickson Scale of Communication Attitudes

The Modified Erickson Scale of Communication Attitudes (S-24)[31] assesses attitudes about stuttering through 24 true/false questions (e.g., "I find it easy to talk with almost anyone"; "I find it very easy to look at my audience while speaking to a group").

Perceptions of Stuttering Inventory

Stuttering inventory[32] examines clients' self-rating of their degree of avoidance, struggle, and expectancy, whereas the *locus of control of behavior*[33] measures the ability of a person to take responsibility for maintaining new or desired behaviors. Although the aforementioned scales developed by researchers are readily available and empirically valid, individual clinicians can create their own rating scales to gain information about any aspect of stuttering that is relevant to any particular client (e.g., "How much do you avoid on a typical day?", "How hard is for you to speak on a typical day?", and "How representative is your current level of stuttering compared to what you experience on a normal day?").

Finally, DiLollo and Neimeyer[21] provide a number of activities, drawn from narrative therapy, that can facilitate the client's expression of the adaptive challenges of stuttering. For example, they describe having the client write an "autobiography of the problem" in which the person who stutters writes from the perspective of stuttering, describing its relationship with the client, what it wants from the client, and how it gets its way with the client. Such creative writing activities help externalize the problem and have been shown to help develop new and alternative insights into the impact of problems such as stuttering, and to foster potential ways of dealing with the effects of the problem.[21] For example, writing about a time when stuttering was very difficult, but from the perspective of stuttering, can help the adult and teen who stutters to take a step back and view their stuttering in a different, more objective way, opening up discussion about how they might resist stuttering's negative influence on their life and well-being.

9.5.4 Technical Measures

Following the client's telling of his or her story, the clinician can ask questions about the history and course of the client's stuttering with reference to the broader story that the client has just shared, thereby placing this information in a context that is specific and unique to that particular client.

Throughout the interview, we have been "sampling" the person's speech, in the sense that we have been observing the client's overt stuttering behaviors as they tell their story. Throughout our discussion with them, we are developing a sense of how the client stutters—how often, what types, and any accessory or associated behaviors accompanying their stuttering. We record the session, not necessarily to go back and analyze the frequency, type, and duration of stuttering (although we may do that if needed) but to review what the client said so that we are clear about what they have told us. In some cases, measures of surface disfluency (e.g., frequency or severity) may be asked for by other professionals, agencies, or third-party reimbursors. Our position is that these measures are most useful when they reflect *how* an individual stutters more than *how much* the individual stutters. Our clinical experience has shown that when clinicians consider the frequency of stuttering alone as a measure of progress, they often fail to notice important qualitative changes in speaking behavior that take place during therapy. For example, a client may enter therapy using tense pauses or abrupt and physically tense speech onset as their primary way of stuttering. Treatment may focus on teaching an easier, more physically relaxed approach to speaking, or being more open about stuttering (i.e., approaching stuttering, stuttering openly without avoiding or attempting to hide it; see ▶ Chapter 12). As the person begins to use these strategies, the result is a change from tense pauses to more forward-moving or "easier" disfluencies in the form of sound or word repetitions and smooth initiation of speech. In such a case, it is likely that the overall disfluency count would actually show an *increase* in stuttering as therapy progressed, at least in the beginning stages of therapy, even though the client's speech is becoming less effortful. This is likely due to two things. First, the person may feel more comfortable "letting stuttering out" without avoiding or hiding it. Second, the individual may be changing from a physically tense and static articulatory posture (i.e., holding articulators still, ceasing airflow and phonation) toward one that is characterized by movement across all the subsystems of speech production. For these reasons, it is more helpful to describe the *type* and *severity,* rather than the *number* of disfluencies. Related measures that describe what the person is doing when they stutter also include duration of audible/inaudible prolongations and pauses, and the number of iterations or repeated units in a sound or word repetition.

A major concern with speech sampling is that it is heavily influenced by the variability of stuttering. As we previously discussed, for people who stutter speech fluency is quite unstable from situation to situation and from time to time.[34,35] Even the tried-and-true "conversation, reading, monologue" samples that have been the standard for many years provide unreliable "data" upon which to make clinical decisions in that they are obtained at a single point of time in a single context.

In addition to sampling specific characteristics of the person's overt stuttering, we administer the *Stuttering Severity Instrument, Fourth Edition (SSI-4),*[36] probably the most well-known of all stuttering assessment tools. The *SSI-4* focuses exclusively on what we have described as the *technical aspects* of stuttering. It includes three sections that allow the clinician to assess the frequency, duration, and physical concomitants of stuttering. Stuttering *frequency* is determined by calculating the percentage of syllables stuttered in samples of at least 150 syllables. *Duration* of stuttering is measured by averaging the three longest stuttering events. Finally, the physical concomitant score is determined using a 6-point Likert scale (from most to least severe) to rate *distracting sounds, facial grimaces, head movements,* and *movements of extremities.* The speech samples that are elicited for analysis include a reading passage and two spontaneous conversations. The authors suggest collecting these data in different contexts (e.g., on a phone call, conversation with another speaker). Scores from the frequency, duration, and physical concomitant sections are converted to an overall severity rating score.

9.5.5 Closing Interview

Following the assessment, we share our preliminary findings with the client. These observations most likely include measures of the impact of stuttering on the client's overall quality of life, as well as stuttering severity in terms of how the individual physically responds to stuttering (i.e., surface behaviors, responses to anticipation). We want to make sure that we address the initial concerns that the client described at the beginning of the session to make sure those have been addressed. After describing our understanding of the client's concerns and perspectives, and our own interpretation of what we have observed during the evaluation, we open the discussion to possible options for treatment. We answer any questions the client has about the potential avenues for therapy, and, if needed, we explain the similarities and differences between various intervention approaches (see ▶ Chapter 12 for description of treatment for teens and adults). We also provide resources such as pamphlets, articles, videos, and support-group opportunities that are offered by such organizations as the *Stuttering Foundation,* the *National Stuttering Association,* and *FRIENDS* (the national association of young people who stutter). Finally, we refer the client and/or family for further assessment by other professionals (e.g., mental health professional, neurologist, otolaryngologist, educational psychologist) if we observe concomitant issues, or if we think the client's stuttering is not developmental in nature (e.g., secondary to physical or psychological trauma or illness, cerebral vascular accident [CVA], or drug use), or if the fluency problem seems to be related to something other than stuttering.

In the following section, we present a case study demonstrating one way to use the procedures and tools described in the previous sections to conduct an assessment of a young adult who stutters.

9.6 Case Study

Bernie is a 23-year-old man who contacted the clinic about receiving therapy for stuttering, which he has reportedly been struggling with since childhood. In response to questions posed on a case history form, Bernie stated that he has had many years of therapy. His primary reason for seeking therapy at this point in time is that he wants to "be able to do [his] upcoming interviews." Bernie says his stuttering has "never been so bad."

During the initial interview, we first want to get to know Bernie—we want him to tell his story. Consequently, we invite Bernie to tell us about himself, being careful to emphasize that we are interested in *his* story, not stuttering's story of *him*. Bernie starts by saying, "Well, I started stuttering when I was around 4, I think, but the first time I really remember stuttering was on the first day of school, when I tried to say my name. I remember kids laughing at me." As Bernie pauses, we take the opportunity to reorient his story by pointing out that what he just told us was the start of "Stuttering's" story of him. We ask Bernie if he can tell us "his" story by putting Stuttering's story aside for a moment and just focusing on what Bernie likes, thinks, wants, and dreams about. This approach helps us to establish two things: (1) that we are interested in Bernie as a whole person and not just his stuttering and (2) that Bernie indeed does have a story that is independent of stuttering and that stuttering does not have to be the dominant feature in his life.

As a part of this initial conversation, we not only learn about Bernie and his story but we also build empathy and trust—often referred to as "rapport"—so that Bernie might be willing to share personal details that may be difficult, but which will ultimately provide a comprehensive picture of his stuttering experience. We accomplish this by engaging with Bernie using active listening skills and our demonstration to Bernie that we are interested in him as a whole person, and not just his stuttering. Active listening can be achieved by maintaining eye contact and neutral facial expressions, relaxed posture, offering affirmative responses such as head nodding, short phrases or syllables/words (e.g., "I see," or "uh huh," or "I understand"), and, most importantly, not talking! During this conversation, we learn that getting a good job, maintaining close relationships with family and friends, sports, and staying healthy and active are all important to Bernie. Through some follow-up questions, we find out that Bernie is in business school and is very proud of his accomplishments, being named to the Chancellor's Honor Roll every semester that he has been in college. Bernie shows real excitement and engagement when he talks about his studies and it becomes increasingly clear that his excellence in his field is an important aspect of his identity. At the same time, Bernie confided that he is terrified about several interviews coming up for summer internships. He is afraid that, because of his stuttering, he might not perform well in the interviews and

this would be devastating for his career plans. Knowing this information about Bernie provides us with an initial understanding of his thinking, and suggests that he is motivated to make some change. Such readiness will serve him well as he embarks on the journey to change both *how* he stutters and how he *responds* to stuttering (i.e., if that's what he wants to do!).

Although we are not focusing on Bernie's speech patterns at this point, we do note that he seems to enjoy communicating except for those times when he stutters (e.g., he consistently looks down when he overtly stutters). In addition, he tends to "back up" when he experiences stuttering (e.g., restarts utterances, uses filler words). These initial behavioral observations will prime us to pay attention to how Bernie physically responds to stuttering throughout the assessment.

We then ask Bernie questions specifically related to his stuttering, helping us to focus primarily on the *technical* aspects of his problem while still listening for additional information about the *adaptive* challenges posed by stuttering (e.g., avoidances, emotional responses, etc.). Bernie tells us that he has received "a lot" of speech therapy throughout his life, "though none of it has been helpful," because he's "still stuttering." This statement suggests that Bernie is very focused on the technical aspects of stuttering, or what listeners can observe when he stutters. We take this as an opportunity to explore his goals for this assessment and possible therapy. Specifically, what does Bernie hope will come from this evaluation? What would a successful therapy look like for him? We ask him about his history with stuttering: When did it start? How has it changed over the years? Does it change in different contexts? This last question deals with variability—for example, is it easy to speak with certain individuals (family/friends) and hard to speak to people he doesn't know? Bernie tells us that situations like interviews are the most challenging for him, which is an indicator that his main motivation for coming to therapy may be due to the stress caused by his upcoming interviews. This is a common feeling for young adults about to begin their "professional" life, possibly develop serious relationships, etc. When asked why he thinks these contexts are most difficult, Bernie replies that he does not know, indicating a lack of awareness, or at least that structured attention has not been paid to stuttering. We also ask Bernie how stuttering impacts his life and whether he makes life decisions based on stuttering. He indicates that he thinks stuttering has forced him to become a more thoughtful and patient person. He also reports that stuttering often dictates who he decides to talk to (e.g., "...there have been many women who I haven't approached due to the possibility of stuttering"). These responses indicate that Bernie feels that at times his stuttering negatively impacts his life/participation, and also that he is able to see the positive impact that stuttering can have.

Throughout the interview, we noticed that Bernie avoided eye contact (e.g., looked down) and to our trained eyes and ears, appeared to use avoidance behaviors (e.g., word switching, circumlocution) during moments of stuttering. These behaviors indicated that Bernie has developed numerous "tricks" to attempt to escape the moment of stuttering, and also that there may be fear, shame, and embarrassment associated with stuttering for Bernie. When asked if he knew why he used these behaviors, Bernie said, "I don't really know...sometimes I know I'm gonna stutter and I just want to get through it as fast as possible." This statement prompted us to use the *SAS* as a tool to explore more about how Bernie responds to the sense or feeling that he is going to stutter (i.e., anticipation). Of interest is that completing the *SAS* helped increase Bernie's awareness of these behaviors; he stated that "...I never really thought of how many things I do to try not to stutter." Finally, it is important to note that when we see and hear evidence of avoidance strategies, we always follow up with the client to check the accuracy of our observations. And, as previously stated, we also use the client's responses to relevant items on the *SAS* and *OASES* to corroborate our impression that they are using overt/covert avoidance strategies.

Given Bernie's responses, we decided to ask him to write an "autobiography of stuttering"[21] to further explore his relationship with stuttering. Box 9.2 shows Bernie's autobiography of stuttering, reflecting a complex relationship that includes stuttering's dominant role in decision-making, some positive aspects of stuttering's influence, and how stuttering casts doubt on Bernie's ability to stand up to it.

Box 9.2 Stuttering's Autobiography, as written by "Bernie"

I have always been with Bernie. I was there as he spoke his first words, even if no one else knew it at the time. Eventually, other people started to notice me. Bernie didn't seem to care at first. But then I started to make things hard for him. His friends at school sometimes made fun of him because of me and he became scared of talking. That is me! I did that to Bernie! I started to get more and more control of him and I liked it! By the time Bernie was in high school, I was in complete control. I told him when he could talk, who he could talk to, and even when and where he could go. I even stopped him from dating for a long time!

Despite this, I think Bernie actually likes me! I have made him more aware of others who struggle with a problem. I force him to be more thoughtful about everything—partly because he has to consider me in every decision that he makes. But he is a more kind and patient person because of me!! I also protect him. I am his excuse for not succeeding. I can keep him safe from failure and rejection. With me, he doesn't have to push himself or try to be someone that he is not!

Of course, despite this, Bernie has tried to fight me. He has had lots of people try to help him fight me, too. But they all failed! I am too strong! Or, maybe, Bernie is too weak? He likes to think that he is smart and good at things, but he has never been smart enough to beat me! He can try all he likes, but he will never be rid of me! I will always be in charge and telling him what to do. I will even destroy his chance of getting a good internship and making a good career. I don't care if he fails, because, if he fails, then I win! He will have to come crawling back to me and let me have my way. We can stay safe in our bubble. Once Bernie accepts this, I have won and he will always be mine!

After Bernie read the autobiography to us (and provided us with a written copy), we talked with him about what he learned from the experience. He told us that it was really hard for him to go back and read what he had written—that it made

him question if he really can "beat stuttering." As a part of this conversation, we asked Bernie if he could think of times that he had "stood up to" stuttering. We noted the examples that Bernie provided and asked him, "How were you able to do that, if stuttering is really too strong for you?" In this way, we plant a seed that there might be an alternative to Bernie's story of stuttering being too strong for him to overcome.

We video recorded our conversation with Bernie so that we could conduct our speech analysis after the interview. This allowed us to focus completely on interacting with Bernie, as opposed to splitting our attention between interacting with Bernie and recording speech behaviors. If video recording is not possible, the clinician will need to be flexible and find a way to take notes during the evaluation without sending a message to their client that they are uninterested. It was observed that most of Bernie's overt stuttering consisted of blocks with significant tension and eye blinking. That is, Bernie appeared to use significant physical effort in trying to "fight" through stuttering moments. In addition, he relied on starter phrases (e.g., "uh," "um," "ya know"), which we interpreted as his attempts to get through stuttering events and avoid overt stuttering. Importantly, while significant physical effort and avoidance strategies were observed, the overall frequency of Bernie's stuttering was limited (more below, perhaps due to his use of avoidance strategies). When asked, Bernie indicated that he felt "tight" during stuttering, but that he was not aware where in his body he felt this tightness. After receiving permission from Bernie to ask him about stuttering events during the evaluation, following a stuttered disruption we asked, "What did you do right before you stuttered...and what were you thinking?," and Bernie identified both his physical and cognitive responses (i.e., "...my throat tightened and I got that feeling, you know, I knew I was gonna stutter on that word and didn't really want to..."). This demonstrates that given prompts, Bernie is very aware of his responses and reactions to stuttering.

Regarding formal testing, we administered both the *OASES* and the *SSI-4*. Bernie received a total impact rating of "*moderate to severe*" on the *OASES*, indicating that stuttering has a moderate to severe adverse impact on Bernie's life. For the SSI-4, we used the interview during the evaluation to obtain a 500-word spontaneous speech sample, and asked Bernie to orally read a passage to obtain an additional speech sample. Based on these two samples (conversation with the clinician during the interview and oral reading) along with the *physical concomitants* score, Bernie received a *mild* severity rating. As discussed previously, the discrepancy between the *OASES* (moderate to severe) and SSI-4 (mild) scores further reflects the importance of focusing on harder-to-observe aspects of Bernie's stuttering. In addition to using the ratings from the *OASES* and *SSI-4*, Bernie's responses to individual items on the *OASES* were reviewed with him, targeting items that he rated particularly high or low and asking him to elaborate further on why he responded in that way. For example, Bernie indicated that he "strongly agreed" with the OASES item, "If I did not stutter, I would be better able to achieve my goals in life." We then asked Bernie, "Why do you think you would be better able to achieve your goals if you didn't stutter?" This provided us with a greater depth of understanding of Bernie's stuttering, how it impacts his daily life, and how he reacts to it in various contexts.

Bernie was self-referred, and appeared to be motivated to start making changes related to how he experienced stuttering. Bernie was seeking therapy during a challenging time in his life, as he was about to begin interviewing for potential summer internships. He reported a long history of stuttering, and also a long history of trying to conceal his stuttering and negative emotions surrounding stuttering (e.g., anxiety, shame, embarrassment). Bernie indicated that he had allowed stuttering to make major life decisions for him (e.g., not speaking to certain individuals that he wanted to out of a fear of stuttering). The cognitive and emotional responses to stuttering, as well as decisions Bernie allowed stuttering to make for him, reflected adaptive challenges, which were also reflected in the OASES score and the autobiography of stuttering. Bernie also exhibited an engrained pattern of responding to his stuttering with tensing and pushing, as well as relying on well-practiced strategies or "tricks" to get through stuttering moments (e.g., switching words, starter phrases). These visible physical characteristics reflected additional technical challenges.

Given Bernie's experiences, background, and motivation, he appeared to be a good candidate to begin therapy. The initial focus in therapy was to explore with Bernie how stuttering was impacting his life, and what decisions Bernie was making because of stuttering. Through motivational interviewing (see ► Chapter 12), we helped Bernie to begin to figure out why he responded to stuttering in the ways that he did—an important first step in therapy. Results from the evaluation suggested that Bernie would benefit from openly talking about stuttering and also working to desensitize to stuttering through, for example, pseudostuttering, education, and stuttering openly. We discussed our impressions with Bernie, and also provided him with information about resources to explore on his own (e.g., The National Stuttering Association (NSA), FRIENDS: The National Association of Young People Who Stutter, The Stuttering Association for the Young (SAY), StutterTalk podcast). Finally, we asked Bernie if he had any specific ideas about potential therapy, and we discussed possible treatment approaches with him.

9.7 Conclusion

A comprehensive assessment of stuttering in adolescents and adults requires the SLP to determine not only how *much* a person stutters but also, more importantly, *how* they stutter and the extent to which stuttering adversely impacts their life. This is because measures of overt stuttering, particularly frequency, are prone to misrepresent the extent of the individual's stuttering problem—primarily because of the variability of stuttering and the individual's ability to anticipate stuttering events. This is not to say that overt features should be ignored. In fact, the covert features of stuttering mediate overt features, such that how an individual responds to the possibility of stuttering shapes how stuttering overtly manifests itself. In this chapter, we presented a framework for thinking about and developing an assessment that appropriately balances attention paid to covert and overt features of stuttering in adolescents and adults. We then applied this framework to a case study and included some initial thoughts about the direction of therapy.

9.8 Definitions

Under-the-surface features of stuttering: The characteristics of stuttering that are not easily observed by others.
Over-the-surface features of stuttering: The characteristics of stuttering that are easily observed by others.
Spontaneous fluency: Fluency that occurs automatically or without conscious thought of speech or the speaking process.
Controlled fluency: Fluency that is produced with intentional use of speaking strategies or techniques.
Anticipation: The sense that upcoming speech will be stuttered if the utterance is attempted as initially planned.
Avoidance: Making a decision to conceal or disguise overt stuttering behaviors.
Fear: The result of being unable to anticipate the consequences of stuttering or anticipating negative consequences of stuttering.
Shame: The sense that "I am fundamentally flawed or broken."
Guilt: The feeling of having done something wrong or presenting one's self in a way that is inconsistent with one's identity.
Stuttering variability: The inconsistency with which stuttering events occur, in large part, if not entirely, due to contextual factors.
Whole person: Viewing the person beyond the problem. This includes interests, likes/dislikes, hopes, fears, relationships, careers, etc. The focus of inquiry here is the person separate from the problem.

References

[1] Yairi E, Ambrose NG. Early Childhood Stuttering for Clinicians by Clinicians. Austin, TX: Pro-Ed; 2005

[2] Finn P, Howard R, Kubala R. Unassisted recovery from stuttering: self-perceptions of current speech behavior, attitudes, and feelings. J Fluency Disord. 2005; 30(4):281–305

[3] McClure JA, Yaruss JS. Stuttering survey suggests success of attitude-changing treatment. ASHA Lead. 2003; 8(9):3–19

[4] Yaruss JS, Quesal RW, Reeves L, et al. Speech treatment and support group experiences of people who participate in the National Stuttering Association. J Fluency Disord. 2002; 27(2):115–133, quiz 133–134

[5] Jackson ES, Yaruss JS, Quesal RW, Terranova V, Whalen DH. Responses of adults who stutter to the anticipation of stuttering. J Fluency Disord. 2015; 45:38–51

[6] Jackson ES, Gerlach H, Rodgers NH, Zebrowski PM. My client knows that he's about to stutter: how can we address stuttering anticipation during therapy with young people who stutter? Semin Speech Lang. 2018; 39 5:356–370

[7] Williams DE. A point of view about stuttering. J Speech Hear Disord. 1957;22(3):390–397

[8] Tichenor S, Yaruss JS. A phenomenological analysis of the experience of stuttering. Am J Speech Lang Pathol. 2018; 27 3S:1180–1194

[9] Tichenor SE, Yaruss JS. Stuttering as defined by adults who stutter. J Speech Lang Hear Res. 2019; 62(12):4356–4369

[10] Plexico LW, Manning WH, Levitt H. Coping responses by adults who stutter: part I. Protecting the self and others. J Fluency Disord. 2009; 34(2):87–107

[11] Plexico L, Manning WH, Levitt H. Coping responses by adults who stutter: part II. Approaching the problem and achieving agency. J Fluency Disord. 2009; 34(2):108–126

[12] Constantino CD, Eichorn N, Buder EH, Beck JG, Manning WH. The speaker's experience of stuttering: measuring spontaneity. J Speech Lang Hear Res. 2020; 63(4):983–1001

[13] Murphy WP. A preliminary look at shame, guilt, and stuttering. In: Bernstein-Ratner N, Healey C, eds. Stuttering Research and Practice: Bridging the Gap. Mahwah, NJ: Lawrence Erlbaum Associates; 1999:131–143

[14] Manning WH, DiLollo A. Clinical decision-making in fluency disorders. San Diego, CA: Plural Publishing; 2017

[15] World Health Organization. International Classification of Functioning, Disability and Health. Geneva: World Health Organization; 2001

[16] World Health Organization. International Classification of Impairments, Disabilities, and Handicaps: A Manual of Classification Relating to the Consequences of Disease, Published in Accordance with Resolution WHA29. 35 of the Twenty-Ninth World Health Assembly, May 1976. Geneva: World Health Organization; 1980

[17] World Health Organization. International classification of impairments, disabilities, and handicaps. Wkly Epidemiol Rec. 1993; 68(15):101–103

[18] Yaruss JS. Describing the consequences of disorders: stuttering and the international classification of impairments, disabilities, and handicaps. J Speech Lang Hear Res. 1998; 41(2):249–257

[19] Yaruss JS. Evaluating treatment outcomes for adults who stutter. J Commun Disord. 2001; 34(1–2):163–182

[20] Yaruss JS, Quesal RW. Stuttering and the International Classification of Functioning, Disability, and Health: an update. J Commun Disord. 2004; 37 (1):35–52

[21] DiLollo A, Neimeyer RA. Counseling in speech-language pathology and audiology: reconstructing personal narratives. San Diego, CA: Plural Publishing; 2014

[22] Heifetz RA, Laurie DL. The work of leadership. Harv Bus Rev. 2001; 79(11)

[23] Heifetz RA, Linsky M. A survival guide for leaders. Harv Bus Rev. 2002; 80(6): 65–74, 152

[24] Heifetz R, Grashow A, Linsky M. Leadership in a (permanent) crisis. Harv Bus Rev. 2009; 87(7–8):62–69, 153

[25] Yaruss JS, Quesal RW. OASES: Overall Assessment of the Speaker's Experience of Stuttering. Minneapolis, MN: Pearson; 2016

[26] Charon R. The patient-physician relationship. Narrative medicine: a model for empathy, reflection, profession, and trust. JAMA. 2001; 286(15):1897–1902

[27] Shadden BB, Hagstrom F. The role of narrative in the life participation approach to aphasia. Top Lang Disord. 2007; 27(4):324–338

[28] Hinckley JJ. Telling the story of stroke when it's hard to talk. Top Lang Disord. 2015; 35(3):258–266

[29] DiLollo A, Neimeyer RA, Manning WH. A personal construct psychology view of relapse: indications for a narrative therapy component to stuttering treatment. J Fluency Disord. 2002; 27(1):19–40, quiz 41–42

[30] Leahy MM, O'Dwyer M, Ryan F. Witnessing stories: definitional ceremonies in narrative therapy with adults who stutter. J Fluency Disord. 2012; 37(4): 234–241

[31] Andrews G, Cutler J. Stuttering therapy: the relation between changes in symptom level and attitudes. J Speech Hear Disord. 1974; 39(3):312–319

[32] Woolf G. The assessment of stuttering as struggle, avoidance, and expectancy. Br J Disord Commun. 1967; 2(2):158–171

[33] Craig AR, Franklin JA, Andrews G. A scale to measure locus of control of behaviour. Br J Med Psychol. 1984; 57(Pt 2):173–180

[34] Constantino CD, Leslie P, Quesal RW, Yaruss JS. A preliminary investigation of daily variability of stuttering in adults. J Commun Disord. 2016; 60: 39–50

[35] Tichenor SE, Yaruss JS. Variability of stuttering: behavior and impact. Am J Speech Lang Pathol. 2021; 30(1):75–88

[36] Riley GD. SSI-4 Stuttering Severity Instrument. Austin, TX: Pro-Ed, Inc.; 2009

Further Readings

Behrman A. Facilitating behavioral change in voice therapy: the relevance of motivational interviewing. Am J Speech Lang Pathol. 2006; 15(3):215–225

Cheasman C, Everard R, Simpson S, eds. Stammering therapy from the Inside. New perspectives on working with young people and adults. Guildford, UK: J&R Press; 2013

Fraser M. Self-therapy for the stutterer. The Stuttering Foundation; 2002

Nippold MA. When a school-age child stutters, let's focus on the primary problem. Lang Speech Hear Serv Sch. 2012; 43(4):549–551

Perkins WH. What is stuttering? J Speech Hear Disord. 1990; 55(3):370–382, discussion 394–397

Peter R, Reitzes D, eds. Stuttering: Inspiring stories and Professional Wisdom. Chapel Hill, NC: StutterTalk; 2012

Quesal RW. Empathy: perhaps the most important E in EBP. Semin Speech Lang. 2010; 31(4):217–226

Stuttering Foundation of America. Advice to those who stutter (No. 9). Stuttering Foundation of America: 1998

Williams D. The genius of Dean Williams. Stuttering Foundation of America; 2004

Williams DE. A point of view about stuttering. J Speech Hear Disord. 1957; 22(3): 390–397

Yaruss JS, Coleman CE, Quesal RW. Stuttering in school-age children: a comprehensive approach to treatment. Lang Speech Hear Serv Sch. 2012; 43(4): 536–548

Zebrowski PM, Arenas RM. The "Iowa Way" revisited. J Fluency Disord. 2011; 36(3): 144–157

Appendix 9.1 Sample Case History Form for Adult Stutterers

Case History (Oral): Adult

Date: _____

Name: _____

Age: _____

Date of Birth: _____

Gender: M/F _____

Preferred Pronouns: _____

Person filling out form and relationship to client: _____

Phone number: _____

E-mail: _____

Reason for referral

Why are you interested in stuttering assessment or therapy?

_____

Speech and language development

Is English your first language? Do you speak other languages? If so, which?

_____

When did you start talking? Babbling? First word? Combine words?

_____

Have you ever had any speech, language, or communication problems?

_____

Did you ever receive services/therapy for speech or language? If so, when?

_____

Other development

Have you ever been diagnosed with any sort of neurological, learning, hearing, or psychological problem?

_____

If yes, have you had therapy for any problem (other than stuttering)? Have you had any major illnesses/surgeries?

_____

Family history

Does anyone in your family have (or have they had) speech or language problems? Other problems?

_____

Stuttering

When did you start stuttering? Do you remember, or did someone tell you?

_____

Has your stuttering always been the same?

_____

Have you ever had therapy for stuttering? If so, when/how long? What did you do in therapy?

_____

Are there things you do to manage or change your speech?

_____

How severe would other people rate your stuttering? (1 = not severe at all; 5 = extremely severe)

_____

Overall, how severe would you rate your own stuttering? (1 = not severe at all; 5 = extremely severe)

_____

Overall, how much does stuttering impact your life? (1 = not at all; 5 = a tremendous amount).

_____

Section IV

Treatment of Stuttering

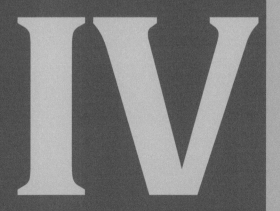

10 Preschool-Age Children

Marie-Christine Franken, Sharon Millard, and Anna Hearne

Abstract

The purpose of this chapter is to describe the factors that contribute to decisions about stuttering therapy for young children, specifically whether treatment is both warranted and recommended, and to describe three treatment approaches that may be adopted. Readers will be provided with a global overview of the motivating theory, principles, and methods of the *Palin Parent–Child Interaction Therapy, the Lidcombe Program, and Restart-Demands and Capacities Model-based treatment*, the treatment approaches that presently have the highest levels of research evidence to support their implementation by trained therapists. It should be recognized, however, that as empirical evidence emerges, there are likely to be additional therapy approaches that may prove equally or indeed more efficacious as those discussed in this chapter. These approaches are intended to be delivered by qualified clinicians. Across the globe, a range of titles and terms are used to refer to such clinicians including speech and language therapist, speech and language pathologist, and logopedist, among others. Throughout this chapter, we will use the term speech and language therapist (SLT) and therapist to refer to these professionals, for the purposes of consistency.

Keywords: stuttering, fluency disorders, preschool, children, therapy, treatment, intervention

10.1 Introduction

Compared to the long history of stuttering therapy with adults, intervention with young children is in its infancy. While there are now at least three evidence based interventions with young children (Palin Parent-Child Interaction Therapy,[1] the Lidcombe Program,[2] and Restart-DCM treatment[3]), because up to 80% of stuttering resolves without intervention,[4] and with little evidence of the effectiveness of treatment, there was a strong argument for waiting until such unassisted recovery was unlikely. Further, the "influential diagnosogenic theory that assigned the cause of stuttering to parents' attitudes toward a child's speech"[5] led clinicians to advise parents to ignore stuttering, with treatment often begun if the child was still stuttering during the school years. However, such advice did not lead to a reduction in stuttering prevalence and as evidence emerged that early intervention with young children is efficacious, this perspective changed.

Presently, early intervention for young children who stutter has become standard practice, although there is still discussion about when treatment should begin. In the 1980s, Starkweather and colleagues advocated prevention and early intervention as soon as possible after stuttering onset, arguing that doing so would reduce the chances of a persistent problem.[6,7] In contrast, Yairi and colleagues advised that treatment should be delayed while actively monitoring the course of the child's stuttering for 9 to 12 months.[5,8] This recommendation was based on their findings that the stuttering severity of children who recovered from stuttering was significantly lower in the final quarter of the first year compared to that observed shortly after onset. This was not the case for children whose stuttering would persist. Importantly though, these authors suggested that such a monitoring phase should be shortened or even skipped entirely if danger signs (risk factors for persistent stuttering) are apparent.

There have been a number of longitudinal studies that have sought to identify the factors that differentiate children at greater risk of persistent stuttering from those whose risk is small.[9,10,11,12,13,14,15,16,17,18,19,20] Evidence for the role of factors such as child language ability, socioeconomic status, maternal education, and stuttering severity is somewhat inconsistent and inconclusive. While that is the case, a recent meta-analysis combined the outcomes of 11 studies and identified the following clinical characteristics to be associated with higher risk of stuttering persistence: being male, being older at stuttering onset, a family history of stuttering, higher stuttering frequency, lower speech sound accuracy, and lower expressive and receptive language skills.[21] Discussing these predictors with parents can facilitate the decision-making process when considered in the context of the child's and parents' needs and wishes. It is important that these risk factors be interpreted as probabilities and not absolutes, and the following limitations should be considered so that the clinician may interpret and apply the findings appropriately:

- There are inconsistencies across studies with respect to which factors are considered predictive of outcome, likely reflecting the complex nature of childhood stuttering, limitations of sample size, and methodological differences across studies.
- It is not known if and how the findings from the nonclinical populations studied (e.g., children who stutter but who do not present at clinics) generalize to the clinical group of children who receive therapy for stuttering.
- Group findings cannot be reliably or validly applied to individuals. It is not possible to make a judgment about whether that specific child is going to continue to stutter or whether stuttering will resolve based on trends in the population as a whole.
- The relative or cumulative risk of individual factors is not known, and neither is the degree to which particular factors might protect the child from developing persistent stuttering.
- For those children who continue to stutter, the early experiences of stuttering and responses to it (by both parents and child) will influence the behavior, experience, and impact of stuttering in the long-term. Further, early childhood experiences and family stressors can have long-term implications for overall mental health and well-being.[22] As clinicians, we have an opportunity to support the development of positive stuttering management skills and attitudes, with the aim of reducing the potential long-term consequences of living with stuttering.
- Even though the majority of children may resolve stuttering without intervention 2 to 3 years after the problem first emerges, the experience at the time of onset is often upsetting, alarming, and anxiety provoking (both for the child and his or her parents). At the very least, if we as therapists can reduce these negative consequences, we should.[23]

There is no evidence that the factors identified to be either risk or protective for persistent stuttering are the same as those which predict therapy outcome. In fact, in a recent study examining the effectiveness of Palin Parent–Child Interaction (PCI) Therapy, the authors did not find these factors to be relevant to treatment outcome.[24] Given these limitations, in practice there has been a move away from trying to determine whether or not an individual child is likely to resolve stuttering without intervention as the main criterion informing the decision for therapy. Rather, the experience of stuttering and the impact that it has on both the child and parents holds greater significance with regard to whether therapy is warranted. Presently, an assessment of all children who have started to stutter is recommended, regardless of the risk factor profile. Those who believe that all stuttering experiences have potential to harm the young child will recommend no delay of starting treatment.[1,25] Alternately, as the majority of children will recover without treatment, others will recommend actively monitoring the child's stuttering until 9 to 12 months after stuttering onset, when the child and parents are not very concerned and there is no serious risk profile.[5] The nature and extent of this monitoring will vary according to the standards and availability of local services. Besides, the dynamic and fluctuating nature of stuttering over time means that its impact, and therefore the need for therapy, is also subject to change. That said, once therapy is indicated, the clinician has a choice of evidence-based interventions that may be utilized. The three approaches described below represent those with the strongest evidence, those that are used internationally, and those for which structured training for therapists has been developed. In the following sections, the principles, methods, and empirical evidence for each approach are described.

10.2 Therapy Approaches for Preschool Children Who Stutter

10.2.1 Palin Parent–Child Interaction Therapy

Palin Parent–Child Interaction Therapy (*Palin PCI*) is a therapy approach developed over many years at the Michael Palin Centre for Stammering in London, United Kingdom. The authors refer to *Palin PCI* as an approach, rather than a program, to reflect the flexible nature of its design and implementation. The intention is that each family will experience a similar overall structure of sessions, while the content can be adapted to the child's and family's individual needs. Therapist training is required before *Palin PCI* should be undertaken, and while the main elements of the approach are described here, the reader is directed to the second edition of the therapy manual for further detail regarding the theoretical underpinnings, principles, and methods of the approach, and the existing evidence base.[1]

Palin *PCI* is based on the understanding of stuttering as a multifactorial disorder (see ▶ Chapter 1 and ▶ Chapter 2),[26] with some children born with the neurophysiological predisposition to stutter.[27,28] This genetic predisposition interacts with physiological, linguistic, psychological, and environmental factors, which influence the moments of stuttering that are produced, along with the chronicity, experience, and impact of the

disorder on the child. These factors are discussed in detail in previous chapters and presented in ▶ Fig. 10.1.

At the center of the model is the child who is born with the predisposition to stutter, and the psychological, physiological, and environmental factors that will influence its expression. The stuttering itself and the speech motor system required for the production of fluent speech are incorporated into the bottom left corner of the triangle. At the top of the triangle are the child's speech, language, and communication skills. These will interact with neurophysiological vulnerability to stutter, making it easier or harder for the child to communicate. The child's other communications skills (e.g., appropriate eye contact and turn taking) can further enhance or reduce their ability to communicate or may indeed be affected by stuttering. At the bottom right of the triangle in ▶ Fig. 10.1 are the child's temperament and cognitive skills. These will also interact with moments of stuttering and influence the child's emotional and behavioral responses and reactions, as well as the development of their emotional well-being.

As shown in ▶ Fig. 10.1, the circles around the outside represent the child's communicative environment, which, in the case of the preschool child, is by and large the parents. Childcare and educational contexts may also be involved, but the primary caregivers will have the greatest and most consistent influence on the child, both in the short and long-term. *Palin PCI* is built on the evidence that parents:

- do not cause stuttering.
- can make changes in their interaction style that support the child's speech fluency and communication skills.
- have the skills and capacity they need to make effective change but may lack the knowledge and confidence to do so.

The aims of *Palin PCI* are the following:
- To help each child become a confident and competent communicator, whether or not they continue to stutter.
- To reduce the impact of stuttering on the child and parents.
- To enhance the child's fluency.
- To increase the parents' and the child's knowledge about stuttering and confidence to manage it.

Evidence Base for the Palin PCI Approach

In order to evaluate the parents' perspectives of change in their child's stuttering and related reactions, Millard and Davis developed the *Palin Parent Rating Scales*,[29] a standardized measure that can be used with the parents of any child who stutters, and any therapy program. To begin, they conducted a Delphi study to identify what parents viewed as desirable outcomes from therapy, yielding a series of statements that reflected what was most important to the majority of the participants. A psychometric evaluation of the resulting questionnaire revealed that it measures three distinct components:
- Factor 1: the impact stuttering has on the child.
- Factor 2: the severity of stuttering and its impact on the parents.
- Factor 3: parents' knowledge about stuttering and confidence in managing it.

A summary of the evidence base for Palin PCI is presented in ▶ Table 10.1. Briefly, both efficacy[30,31] and effectiveness studies[24]

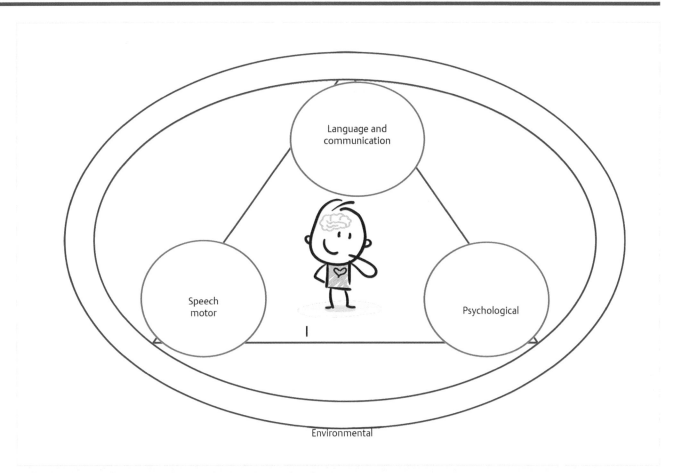

Fig. 10.1 The Palin Parent–Child Interaction Model. Image provided courtesy of Michael Palin Centre 2019.

Table 10.1 The evidence base for Palin Parent–Child Interaction (PCI), Lidcombe Program (LP), and Restart-Demands and Capacities Model (Restart-DCM): main publications and findings

Study	Design	Participants	Outcome measures	Main findings
Millard et al[30]	Replicated single-subject studies	6 children aged 3.3–4.10 y >12 mo since onset	Stuttering frequency (speech samples recorded at home)	• 4/6 significantly reduced stuttering frequency during phase B with both parents and indirect components only • 1 child reduced stuttering frequency during phase B with one parent • 2 children who did not reduce stuttering frequency with both parents during phase B received direct therapy components
Millard et al[31]	Replicated single-subject studies	6 children who received Palin PCI 4 waiting list controls >12 mo since onset	Stuttering frequency (speech samples recorded at home) Palin PRS	• All 6 children who received Palin PCI significantly reduced stuttering frequency of the period of the trial • Parents reported reduced impact on child and themselves; increased knowledge and confidence in managing stuttering • 3/4 children in no intervention condition did not demonstrate improvement over time
Millard et al[24]	Clinical outcome study with data collected at four points over 1 y	n = 55 Age: 30–84 mo	Stuttering frequency Palin PRS KiddyCAT	• Significant improvement in all outcome variables, maintained for 1 y posttreatment onset • Parents' view of the impact of stuttering on the child (F1 PRS) and the severity of the stutter and impact on the parents (F2) predicted parents' knowledge and confidence (F3) • Stuttering frequency did not predict F3 pretherapy but did posttherapy • "More successful" group had a greater proportion of children who had a persistent family history and girls, and proportionally fewer children with advanced language skills

Table 10.1 (*Continued*) The evidence base for Palin Parent–Child Interaction (PCI), Lidcombe Program (LP), and Restart-Demands and Capacities Model (Restart-DCM): main publications and findings

Study	Design	Participants	Outcome measures	Main findings
Jones et al[32]	Randomized controlled trial (RCT)	• *n* = 54 children • Age: 3–6 y • 29 in LP arm • 25 in control arm • Stuttering above 2% SS	• %SS in three different speaking situations before randomization and at 3, 6, and 9 mo after randomization	• Highly significant difference (*p* = 0.003) at 9 mo • Mean %SS after 9 mo • LP: 1.5%SS • Control: 3.9%SS
Jones et al[33]	Retrospective clinical audit	• *n* = 261 • age: 3–6 y	• %SS • Age • Sex • Period from onset to treatment • Treatment time	• Longer treatment time related to more severe stuttering • Age and sex were not significant • A short delay in commencing treatment did not increase treatment time for preschoolers
Bonelli et al[34]	Single group study	• 9 children from outcome studies by Onslow et al[47]	• % syllables disfluent • Articulation rate • Interturn speaker latency • Mean length of utterance • Development sentence score • Number of different words • Requests for clarification • Requests for information	• Despite clear reductions in stuttering, no changes in child or parent speech rate, interspeaker turn latencies or pragmatic functioning • Possibility that treatment results in decreased language functioning ruled out
Bridgman et al[35]	RCT	• *N* = 49 children • Age: 3.0–5.11 y	• %SS at 9 months post randomization • Number of consultations	• Webcam delivery of LP achieved similarly efficacious results
Goodhue et al[36]	Qualitative study	• 16 mothers	• Semi-structured interviews about their experiences with the LP	• Themes from the interviews including practicalities of implementing the treatment, positive aspects, emotions and obstacles
Franken et al[37]	RCT	• *n* = 30 children • aged <6.0 y • Stuttering above 3% SS • Time since onset >6 mo • 15 in DCM arm, 15 in LP arm	• % SS (speech samples recorded at home) • Parent and clinician severity ratings	• 12 weeks post treatment onset, the stuttering frequencies and severity ratings significantly decreased for both treatment groups. No differences between groups were found. Parents of children in both groups were cooperative in many respects, and there were no differences between them on scales that measured their satisfaction with the two treatments • For LP treatment, the means decreased from 7.2% (SD = 2.0) to 3.7% (SD = 2.1). For DCM treatment, the means decreased from 7.9% (SD = 7.1) to 3.1% (SD = 2.1)

de Sonneville-Koedoot et al[38]	RCT	• *n* = 199 children
		• aged 3.0–6.3 y
		• Stuttering above 3% SS
		• Time since onset >6 mo
		• 100 in Restart-DCM arm, 99 in LP arm
			• Percentage of nonstuttering children at 18 mo
			• %SS; Parent Severity
			• Ratings
			• Health-related quality of life
			• Emotional and behavioral problems (CBCL)
			• KiddyCat
				• Percentage of non- (or minimally) stuttering children at 18 months:
				  76.5% for LP
				  76.5% for LP
				  76.5% for LP71.4% for Restart-DCM
				• Mean %SS after 18 mo:
				  1.2% (SD: 2.1) for LP
				  1.5% (SD: 2.1) for Restart-DCM
				• At 18 mo post onset treatment, no differences between Restart-DCM and the LP were significant
				• At 3 mo post onset treatment, children treated by LP showed a greater decline in %SS

de Sonneville-Koedoot et al[39]	RCT	• *n* = 199 children • aged: 3.0–6.3 y • Stuttering above 3% SS • Time since onset >6 mo • 100 in Restart-DCM arm, 99 in LP arm	• Number needed to treat, • Health-related Quality of • Life (EQ-VAS and HUI3) at 3, 6, 12, and 18 mo, V-QALYs, direct and indirect costs	• The economic analysis showed that at 18 mo, the V-QALYs of LP was slightly higher (0.018; 95% CI: 0.008–0.027) with a small effect size (Cohen's *d* = 0.17). Besides, mean costs for the LP group were significantly higher compared to the Restart-DCM group (€3199 vs. €3032), again with a small effect size (Cohen's *d* = 0.14) • The results indicated a high probability that the LP (in the NL: the new treatment) is cost-effective compared to Restart-DCM treatment (in the NL: the standard) given a threshold for willingness to pay of €20,000 per QALY

Abbreviations: CI, confidence interval; EQ-VAS, EuroQol-visual analogue scales; KiddyCAT, Communication Attitude Test for Preschool and Kindergarten Children Who Stutter; PRS, Parent Rating Scale; SD, standard deviation; V-QALYs, Value-based quality adjusted life years.

demonstrate that *Palin PCI* reduces the negative impact of stuttering on the child, increases the child's fluency, reduces parental anxiety, and help parents to feel more confident and knowledgeable in how to support their child. These positive outcomes reflect the specific aims of the program.

Essential Pieces

Initial Assessment

The assessment process is considered to be the foundation of the *Palin PCI* approach. It is comprehensive and thorough. Through this engagement and joint understanding, the parents and therapist identify priorities for therapy and begin to establish the therapeutic alliance that is crucial for successful therapy outcome.[40]

When parents contact a therapist, it is because they are worried and are seeking support. In the first instance, the therapist will provide the parents with information about stuttering such as incidence, prevalence, and the factors that put the child at risk of persistence,[41] without making predictions about whether or not an individual child is likely to experience unassisted recovery. It is important, however, to note that a decision

about whether to offer therapy is not based on these risk-of-persistence factors; rather, it is made on the basis of whether the stuttering is having an impact on the child or parents. Having heard the information about stuttering, some parents will choose to wait for a few months to "see how it goes." Other parents continue to express concern and wish to have help, in which case a full assessment is offered. Parental concern is evidence that the child's stuttering is having an impact on the family.

The assessment process reflects the multifactorial nature of stuttering. The aim is to identify specific physiological, linguistic, environmental, and emotional factors that are supporting the child's communication and fluency as well as those that are making communication more challenging. Using a range of formal and informal methods (such as those described in ▶ Chapter 7 of this volume, alongside parent and child interviews[1]), the therapist explores the perspectives of the child and their parents/guardians (in *Palin PCI*, both parents who live in the home with the child are involved).

Once the assessment is completed, the therapist explains the findings from both the child assessment and parent case history to the parents. ▶ Fig. 10.2 provides an example of how the

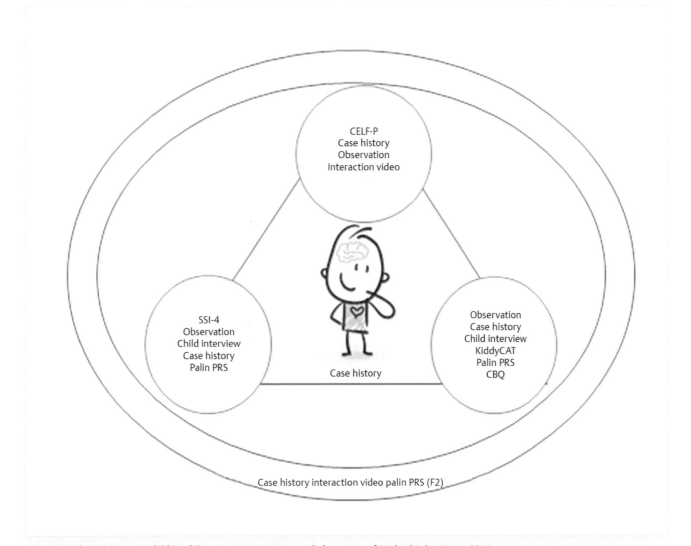

Fig. 10.2 The Palin Parent–Child Model Assessment. Image provided courtesy of Michael Palin Centre 2019.

assessments and the findings map onto the *Palin PCI* model shown in ▸ Fig. 10.1.

Using ▸ Fig. 10.1 as a reference and visual aid, the therapist explains that stuttering is complex and there are some factors that make it easier for the child to communicate and be more fluent, and some that make it harder for children who stutter to talk easily, using the information from the assessment to highlight the relevant factors for the individual child so that the parents understand the nature of their child's stuttering, what they are already doing that is helpful, and how therapy might support this further.

There is a very particular style adopted by the *Palin PCI* therapist. *Palin PCI* seeks to help parents to build on their knowledge and develop their skills in a way that will empower them, reduce their worries, and give them confidence to support the child in the long-term. Strategies employed in *Solution-Focused Brief Therapy* (SFBT)[42] counseling have had a significant influence on the approach over recent years. SFBT assumes that people have the resources they need to manage their problems and it is the role of the therapist to help them identify those skills and strategies that are helpful. As such, within *Palin PCI* there is an assumption that parents will already have ways to support their child and those may be built upon, so teaching, instructing, correcting, and modeling are not required. The therapist shapes the conversations with parents in a way that helps them to explore their hopes and expectations from therapy, while also assisting them to focus attention on "what is going well" and notice "small steps in the right direction." Working within this framework, the *Palin PCI* therapist focuses on asking, not telling; finding, not showing; and encouraging attention to what is positive.

Therapy Structure

Therapy is delivered through six, once-weekly clinic sessions, which last approximately 1 hour. The parents who live with the child (including those who have a parenting role, such as stepparents or guardians) attend all therapy sessions. At the end of the six clinic sessions, the parents continue to implement the strategies they have learned at home for an additional 6-week period and provide feedback each week to the therapist. At the end of this so-called home consolidation period, the child's progress is reviewed and decisions about further therapy are made.

The focus of the initial session is to help the parents explore their "best hopes" with the therapist using the questions described in *SFBT* methods[42] as a way to elicit their hopes, expectations, and priorities for therapy. In this first session, the clinician introduces the structure of the program and observes a PCI session that provides the basis for goal selection. This is accomplished in the following ways:

- The family is introduced to the concept of "*Special Time.*" This is a 5-minute playtime that each parent will have with the child between three and five times per week. The child selects the toy/game and the parent's role is to play with them, focusing on what the child says, not on how they are saying it. Books, sports, and screen activities should be avoided during *Special Time* because the PCI is reduced/ different in these times. *Special Time* provides the time at home for parents to practice what they have learned

(i.e., interaction targets, described in the following pages) through the remainder of the program.

A video recording is made of each parent playing with the child. The recording provides the therapist with insight into the child's communication skills in a more familiar speaking context, and is used in therapy for the parents to identify a communication strategy to pay attention to in therapy. The content and focus of the remaining sessions are dependent on the strengths and needs identified in the assessment and the hopes and expectations expressed by the parents in session 1.

Therapy Strategies

Based on observations made during the assessment, the parent interview, and the video-recorded play session therapy includes three sets of strategies: interaction, family, and child strategies.

Interaction Strategies

Palin PCI does not assume that parents are doing something "wrong" or that they differ from other parents, but that there are features of the way in which they interact with their child that make it easier or harder for the child to communicate or speak fluently. There is also an understanding that because they are worried, behaviors/interactions may become distorted. For instance, in their attempt to reduce pressure on the child and to try to stop them from experiencing stuttering, parents may talk for the child, interrupt, or take lengthy conversational turns. Simply put, it is natural for our interaction to be influenced by our emotional state.

Interaction strategies are chosen during the parents' observation of the recorded interaction with their child (typically in session 2). The therapist asks each parent to identify "what are you doing that is helpful for your child's communication?" or "how are you helping your child's stuttering?" The parents are then asked to identify something they could do more of, or do differently that would further support their child's communication. The parent is asked to think about what they already know that helps their child (e.g., letting the child finish their thought, giving them time to respond), and the rationale for any change they would like to make ("why would that be helpful?"; "what difference would that make for your child?"). This helps the parents to be explicit about the reasoning behind any change they are proposing, making them specific and achievable. The parents then practice these in *Special Time* at home, keeping a record of what they did and the results they observed.

Parents typically focus on two to three Interaction Strategies over the 6-week period. Each week, they make a new recording of their interaction with the child in the clinic and use that to reflect on the target-specific changes they have been working on. Watching the recording gives the parents feedback about the changes they are making and to consider whether they will add a new strategy or not. Interaction strategies that are typically identified by parents are listed in ▸ Table 10.2.

Family Strategies

One or two *Family Strategies* might also be introduced within the first six sessions of therapy. These will have been identified during the assessment as additional strategies to help the parents

Table 10.2 Interaction, family and child strategies that might be included in an individual therapy program of Palin Parent–Child Interaction (PCI) theory

Parent interaction strategies	Family strategies	Child strategies
Following the child's lead during play and/or conversation	Being open about stuttering and using language that does not refer to stuttering in negative terms	Being open and talking about stuttering
Giving the child time to respond or finish what they want to say	Building confidence—recognizing strengths, reinforcing effort, using praise to maximum effect, and noticing what is going well	Desensitization about stuttering
Increasing pausing between turns	Turn taking during family conversations and activities to promote	Understanding and managing thoughts and emotions
Reducing their rate of speech to match that of the child	Dealing with feelings—encouraging openness about feelings and managing strong reactions	Speaking more slowly
Eye contact—using eye contact to maintain attention or demonstrate listening	Tiredness—encouraging and supporting good sleep hygiene and routine	Increasing pausing
Language—using shorter sentences; using less complex language to match that of the child	High standards—helping children to learn how to accept what is "good enough," coping with disappointment, building resilience, learning how to be kind to yourself	Being more concise
Questions and comments—getting a balance between comments and questions thinking about whether the questions are at the appropriate level for the child to respond easily	Behavior management—promoting consistency, predictability, clear boundaries, learning to accept responsibility for your actions, helping parents not to fear that they will make the stammer worse because they reprimand the child	Language or phonology therapy

and the child cope with stuttering in a more positive and proactive way. For example, parents of children who stutter often describe a loss of confidence in how to support their child and may treat the child differently because they stutter. Because stuttering is a multifactorial disorder, the child's development and interaction with their environment will affect how they respond, react, and manage their stuttering in the short and long-term. A child who is confident to talk, who is aware of their emotions and able to regulate them and their behaviors, who is resilient, has good problem-solving skills, is independent, and secure is more likely to speak without struggle and cope with their stuttering in the long-term. *Family Strategies* that might be included in a *Palin PCI* program can be seen in ▶ Table 10.2.

Child Strategies

For the majority of children, successful implementation of *Interaction* and *Family Strategies* reduces concerns about the child's stuttering. They support the child's speech fluency by helping parents to have realistic demands and expectations for behavior change while setting up practice sessions and building confidence through reinforcement. If the child or parents continue to be concerned about stuttering or if the child is showing evidence of developing unhelpful strategies for coping with stuttering (e.g., increased struggle or avoiding words), then further therapy may include more direct *Child Strategies*. These require the child to become more actively involved in therapy by learning more about speech and communication and developing their own helpful cognitive strategies for responding to stuttering. The number of additional sessions depends on the strategy required and the child's progress, but typically three to four additional sessions would be offered.

▶ Fig. 10.3 shows how the *Interaction, Family*, and *Child Strategies* work together to target the areas of need. Throughout the therapy process, it is the therapist's role to help the parents to notice the strengths in these areas as well as areas that can be developed. The therapist does this using the solution-focused style of questioning, and throughout the process, parents are asked to keep a record of "what I am pleased to notice."

Follow-up and Monitoring

At the end of the initial 6-week in-clinic therapy phase, there is a 6-week consolidation phase when parents continue with Special Times and their strategies. During that time, they provide the SLT with feedback about those tasks and at the end of that period, the child's progress is reassessed. The parent's and child's view of stuttering is considered (e.g., *Palin PRS*, observation and conversation with the parents and child). If the child is showing increased confidence to communicate, stuttering is reducing, and the parents are feeling more confident in their skills to support their child, the family is encouraged to continue to implement the strategies at home. The process of change continues over time, so the child's progress is monitored over a 1-year period using the measures.

10.2.2 The Lidcombe Program

Evidence Base for the Lidcombe Program

The LP is a parent-delivered treatment for early stuttering. It was developed in Australia in the 1990s and has grown in its use across the globe, including (but not limited to) the United Kingdom, European countries such as the Netherlands, Germany, France, and Belgium, the Middle East, South Africa, Singapore, Japan, Hong Kong, New Zealand, the United States, and Canada.

The theoretical underpinnings of the LP are behavioral, in that the child's stuttering is targeted directly, with the aim of reducing it. These behavioral roots come from research in the 1970s showing that stuttering in preschool children can be reduced through operant principles—primarily contingent consequences (e.g., verbal feedback following a moment or instance of stuttering or fluent, stutter-free speech).[43,44] This research provided the basis for development of the *LP*, and parental verbal feedback for both stutter-free speech and stuttering has always been the core of the essential components of the treatment.

There is a significant amount of research evidence, including randomized controlled trial (RCT) evidence and long-term follow-up data to attest to the LP's efficacy and effectiveness

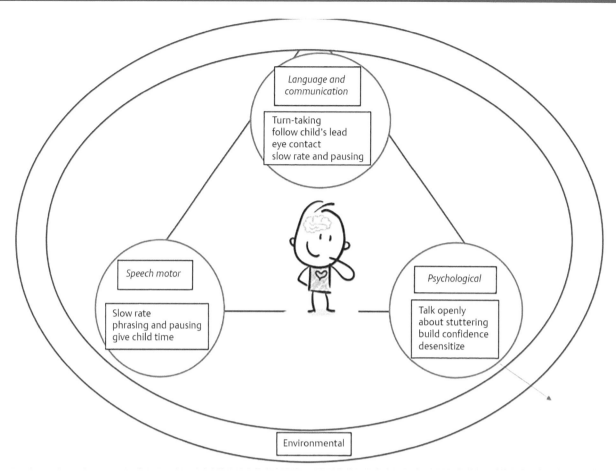

Fig. 10.3 The Palin Parent–Child Model Therapy Strategies.

(► Table 10.1). Research has shown that the treatment can be successfully implemented in community clinics, and across a variety of languages and a range of service delivery models including telehealth and group format (see ► Table 10.1). Readers are also encouraged to consult Mark Onslow's electronic textbook that contains an extensive summary of research relating to the LP.[45]

Essential Pieces

Initial Assessment

The LP does not prescribe a particular assessment process or standardized tools but is based on detailed discussion and direct observation of the child's stuttering (see ► Chapter 7 of this text for details of the assessment process for preschool children who stutter). The assessment marks the beginning of the collaborative process between the parent and the clinician and involves both giving and gathering information.

Therapy Structure

As shown in ► Fig. 10.4, the *LP* consists of two stages with distinct goals:
- *Stage 1*: achievement of zero or near zero levels of stuttering.
- *Stage 2*: maintenance of zero or near zero levels of stuttering in the long-term.

In *stage 1*, weekly appointments are scheduled during which the clinician works with the parent to individualize the treatment so that it can be effectively carried out in the family's everyday life. This individualization occurs by integrating the clinician's understanding of both the *LP* and stuttering in general, with the parents' knowledge of their child and family. In *stage 2*, once zero or near zero levels of stuttering have been achieved, a maintenance program begins. Treatment at home is withdrawn slowly and the frequency of appointments with the clinician reduces while zero or near zero levels of stuttering are maintained. Should the child's stuttering reemerge, parents increase treatment again until zero or near zero levels are reached and treatment can be withdrawn again.

During the weekly visits to the clinician in stage 1 of the LP, parents are taught how to conduct the essential components that make up the treatment:
- measurement of stuttering severity.
- practice sessions at home.
- feedback for stutter-free and stuttered speech.

Treatment involves all these components; however, the way each component is carried out is not rigidly defined and will differ from family to family. It is the clinician's responsibility to work with individual parents to ensure individualization for successful treatment. Each of these components and their individualization is explained below.

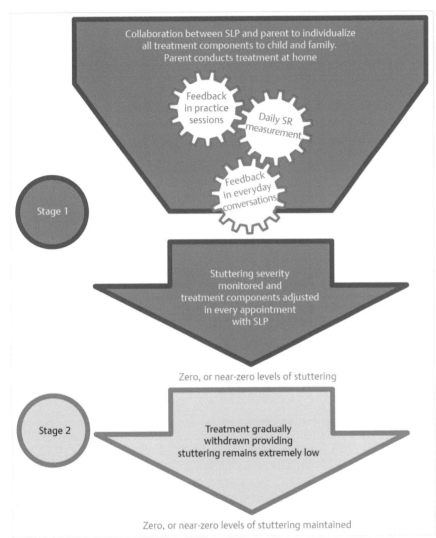

Fig. 10.4 The Lidcombe Program (SLP, speech-language pathologist, SR, Severity Rating).

Collaboration between SLP and parent to individualize all treatment components to child and family. Parent conducts treatment at home

Feedback in practice sessions

Daily SR measurement

Feedback in everyday conversations

Stage 1

Stuttering severity monitored and treatment components adjusted in every appointment with SLP

Zero, or near-zero levels of stuttering

Stage 2

Treatment gradually withdrawn providing stuttering remains extremely low

Zero, or near-zero levels of stuttering maintained

Measurement of stuttering in the *LP* is accomplished using a 0 to 9 rating scale, where 0 = *no stuttering*, 1 = *extremely mild stuttering*, and 9 = *extremely severe stuttering*. This tool is called the *Severity Rating (SR) scale* and evidence has shown that both parents and clinician can use it reliably with minimal training.[46,47,48] Reliability in using the SR scale is established by the parent and the clinician listening to several minutes of the child's speech and agreeing on a rating with no more than one scale value difference. This reliability is checked at every appointment with the same procedure. Throughout treatment, the SR scale provides a measurement tool to track progress or identify a lack of it. It is also used as a neutral and reliable way of communicating about changes in the child's stuttering severity, for example, instead of the parent saying the stuttering "was terrible on the weekend," they can say "the stuttering was a 7 on the weekend." Consistent use of the SRs is an essential part of the treatment. The trends they show are an important consideration in problem-solving and for any treatment decisions throughout treatment. As with all components of the *LP*, this measurement tool is used flexibly. Parents are asked to rate their child's speech in everyday conversations on a daily basis and plot this on the LP SR graph (see LP SR chart in Appendix 10.1). The ways in which parents carry out these

daily SRs are negotiated to suit the family's routine and/or the child's pattern of stuttering. For example, some parents graph one SR for the entire day, while other parents might elect to rate only the conversation at the dinner table, as this is a time they focus on their child's speech. Another example would be that some children typically stutter more in the evening than in the morning, hence one rating does not capture this trend appropriately and parents can graph two ratings, one for the morning and one for the evening. During appointments with the clinician, the trends in the daily ratings from home serve as the basis for decisions about how to maintain the progress being made or how to remediate a lack of progress. In either case, the type and number of practice sessions and the type and amount of feedback are discussed and evaluated by the clinician and parent in decisions about how to proceed.

Toward the end of stage 1, the SRs are used to identify when the child's stuttering is low enough to enter stage 2 of the *LP*. Once daily SRs show a pattern of minimal stuttering (mainly 0 with some ratings of 1) for a period of 3 weeks, stage 2 of the treatment commences. During stage 2, the parent and the SLT continue to use the daily SRs to identify any signs of relapse and adjust therapy accordingly.

Practice sessions are another essential component of the *LP*. Like measurement, practice sessions are a daily part of the treatment in stage 1. During a practice session, which typically lasts around 15 minutes, the parent selects an activity and carries on a conversation that facilitates mostly stutter free (e.g., an SR of 0 or 1). Although it is essential that parents conduct practice sessions with their children at home, exactly how they do them depends on many factors including the child's interests, their stuttering severity, and the family's routine.

The process of finding the best way for the parent and child to engage in practice sessions begins during the first appointment where the clinician provides a model. Following on from this, the clinician and the parent discuss and experiment with various activities to identify those that are not only engaging and fun for the child but also stimulate the kind of conversation that is mostly stutter free. This is a balancing act, in that the conversation should be as "simple as necessary" and at the same time "as complex as possible" while eliciting mostly stutter-free speech. To accomplish this, parents are taught communication strategies that reduce the length and complexity of their child's speech, but only to the extent that is necessary to achieve very low stuttering during the practice sessions. The conversation should not be too restricted. Every practice session provides an opportunity to see how long and complex the child's sentences can be while still remaining mostly stutter free. When the practice sessions are balanced in this way, they ensure the best context for the parent to give feedback and the child to practice stutter-free speech. This is an essential skill for the parent to learn and therefore is carefully explained and modeled by the clinician.

Different activities are selected not only on the basis of the child's interests but also at a complexity level that is matched to their current level of stuttering. As an example, a matching game typically elicits much simpler language from the child than a free-play activity, so it is best suited for children whose stuttering is more frequent and severe. For example, at the beginning of stage 1, a parent of a child with a significant level of stuttering likely needs to select simple activities such as a matching game or a coloring activity to stimulate conversation that is in the here and now (rather than focused on imagination or memory), and encourages utterances that are shorter and less complex than might be customary for the child. Another parent whose child is stuttering moderately may begin with practice sessions in the context of picture books, allowing conversation that is still in the here and now, but likely contains longer sentences than would be the case in a matching game. In the middle of stage 1, the stuttering severity of both these children might have reduced to the extent that the parents can select a pretend play activity with dolls or cars that allows for some conversation with long sentences about abstract topics in the child's imagination and memory. Finally, toward the end of stage 1, both these children's speech might be mainly stutter free and their parents can conduct practice sessions within ordinary conversation without needing to manipulate the activity or their child's language.

During every appointment with the clinician, the parent demonstrates the type of practice session they have conducted at home during the previous week. It is the clinician's role to provide feedback to the parent and demonstrate any changes in the practice sessions that might be needed to suit changes in the child's SRs, or any successes or difficulties the parent encountered in the previous week. Common issues that require problem-solving during appointments with the clinician include the following: keeping the conversation as simple as necessary and as complex as possible while stimulating mostly stutter-free speech from the child; finding varied activities that are fun as well as suitable for generating the appropriate level of conversation for a practice session; and finding time to conduct the practice sessions and occupying siblings while doing practice sessions.

This process of demonstration, experimentation, and problem-solving provides the basis for the clinician's recommendation for the coming week. It also ensures that the parent feels confident about being able to practice at home in ways that are fun and enable their child to speak at an optimum level (i.e., simple as necessary and as complex as possible) with mostly stutter-free speech. When parents are able to conduct practice sessions this way, it provides the best context for the parent to give feedback—the third essential component of the *LP*.

Therapy Strategies

The primary strategy used in LP is parent-administered feedback that is mainly given not only for stutter-free speech but also for stuttering. The following general principles apply for any feedback in the *LP*:

- Feedback for stutter-free speech is always introduced before feedback for stuttering.
- Feedback is given in practice sessions first and then in everyday conversations.
- Feedback for stutter-free speech is more frequent than feedback for stuttering.
- Feedback is embedded into the conversation and not intrusive or intensive.
- The child and the parent must be comfortable with all feedback given.

Although these general principles apply, each is individually adjusted. For example, although feedback for stutter-free speech is always introduced first, there are no hard and fast rules for when feedback for stuttering is introduced. It might be in the first few weeks or much later. Further, parents initially only provide feedback during the 15-minute practice sessions; however, there are no rigid guidelines for when feedback is introduced in everyday conversations. It might be introduced when the parents are noticing some stutter-free speech in everyday conversation and are accurately providing feedback in practice sessions. In addition, although feedback for stutter-free speech is always more frequent than feedback for stuttering, exactly how much of each is provided depends on how the child and their stuttering responds—it might be a dozen in each practice session, but it can also be fewer or many more. The child and the parent must be comfortable with all the feedback that is given.

As shown in ▶ Fig. 10.5, there are three types of feedback for stutter-free speech: *acknowledgment*, *praise*, and *request for self-evaluation*. These three types of feedback enable the parent to tailor their responses to their own and their child' style. For example, some children and parents prefer very enthusiastic praise or request for self-evaluation that can be considered

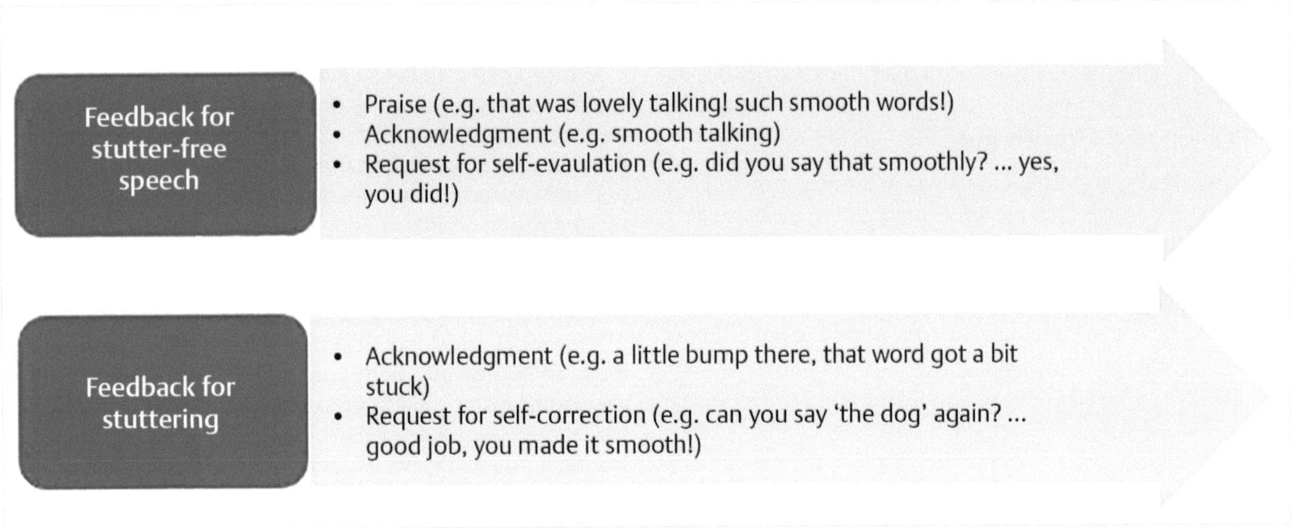

Fig. 10.5 Feedback for stutter-free speech and stuttering in the Lidcombe Program.

"double praise," for example, the parent asking "was that smooth?" and the child saying "yes" and the parent following up with "yes it was, well done!" Other parents' and children's styles are more suited to very low-key acknowledgment, such as the parent simply saying "smooth" to provide feedback. In any case, the feedback must feel (to the parent) and sound (to the child) sincere. If the child does not like the way the feedback sounds, it must be adjusted until a style of feedback that suits the child is found. Also, just as the wording and type of feedback is determined individually, so is the frequency of feedback. Although it should be given consistently throughout the practice session, it should be neither intrusive nor intensive. That is, feedback is "sprinkled" through the 15-minute practice session conversation and does not detract from the content of the conversation.

Feedback for stuttering is introduced once the parent is accurately providing feedback for stutter free-speech and both parent and child are comfortable with the feedback during the 15-minute practice sessions at home. Providing the child feedback after moments of stuttering can often occur as quickly as in the first few weeks, but it may also take several months. At first, as is the case with feedback for stutter-free speech, feedback for stuttering is only introduced during the 15-minute practice sessions. As shown in ▶ Fig. 10.5, there are two types of feedback for stuttering, *acknowledgment* and *request for self-correction*. Both are delivered in a neutral tone and are in no way punitive. In fact quite the opposite; a request for self-correction is delivered in a way that is helpful and gives the child the maximum chance of responding with a stutter-free utterance. The parent is taught to be specific and only ask the child to repeat the stuttered word or words, not the whole utterance. For example, if the child says "I I I like the ones with the chocolate sprinkles", the parent might respond, "So yummy!! Can you say 'I like' again?" If the correction is successful in that the child produces the stuttered word or words fluently, it is followed with praise, for example, "you made it smooth, well done! I like the chocolate sprinkles too!" and the conversation continues seamlessly. If it is not successful and the child responds with a stuttered word, the response is acknowledged but a second request for

self-correction is not provided, and once again, the conversation continues seamlessly. It is very important to ensure that the child is comfortable with this kind of feedback, as it has the potential to be perceived negatively. If the child is even slightly uncomfortable when asked to self-correct, this type of feedback is deferred, or left out altogether. It is not essential that it is used in the *LP*.

Once the parent and child are comfortable with giving and receiving feedback in the practice sessions and the parent is noticing some entirely stutter-free utterances in everyday conversations, the clinician teaches the parents how to give feedback in everyday conversations. As with feedback during the practice sessions, this feedback is individualized with respect to its wording, enthusiasm, and frequency across the day.

Collaboration between the clinician and parent is essential to individualized application of the *LP*. Although the clinician has expert knowledge in stuttering and it is their role to demonstrate and explain the components of the approach to the parent. It is not until this knowledge is synthesized with the parent's knowledge of their child, their family, and their child's stuttering that treatment can be successful. Collaboration in decision-making about how to conduct the treatment ensures that it is done not only correctly but also in a way that is possible within their family's individual circumstances and characteristics. Open discussion and experimentation with procedures occur during every appointment, for example, deciding the best times for practice sessions, selection of materials (e.g., books, toys), and checking with parents to ensure their comfort with the wording of reinforcement, for example, "I've just praised by saying 'fantastic smooth words,' do you think that would feel ok for you and Sam?" or "We're seeing SRs of mainly 4 s and that's with about 5 praises in everyday conversation; I think it might be good to do a few more. What would be another situation you would hear some stutter-free speech in that you could praise?" and so forth. Such problem-solving conversations support the parents' confidence and foster empowerment in their ability to manage not only successes but also the difficulties with treatment at home. Clinicians aim to develop a shared sense of responsibility for the treatment with the parent, so that the parent does not feel their role in the treatment weighing heavily on them. Creating this atmosphere of collaboration and sharing of responsibility is one of the foundations of the *LP*.

Follow-up and Monitoring

Once the child's stuttering has shown a pattern of mainly 0 s and some 1 s on the SR scale for 3 consecutive weeks, stage 2 of the *LP* commences. This stage of treatment consists of follow-up and monitoring, designed to prevent relapse and typically lasts around 12 months. If the child's SRs continue to be mainly 0 s and some 1 s, and the parent is aware of how to address any increases, the feedback in practice sessions and everyday conversations are gradually and systematically reduced. If relapse occurs, the feedback is increased or reinstated until the zero or near zero levels of stuttering are reached once more.

In practical terms, this means that appointments with the clinician are scheduled increasingly further apart: two times 2, 4, then 8, and finally 16 weeks apart. Parent collection of the SRs continues throughout stage 2; however, it is also reduced in frequency. Once appointments with the clinician are 8 weeks apart or more, parents are asked to monitor regularly and to comment on any increase in the child's stuttering, but only collect SRs for 2 weeks prior to an appointment. Practice sessions have usually ceased toward the end of stage 1, as the child's speech is mainly stutter free in everyday conversations. If they are still occurring, they are faded out in the early part of stage 2. Finally, assuming stuttering remains at a very low level, the feedback that the parents give in everyday conversations is reduced gradually from the amount that was being conducted daily in stage 1, to almost no feedback except occasional praise toward the end of stage 2.

10.2.3 Restart-Demands and Capacities Model Based Treatment

Evidence Base for Restart-DCM

Beginning in the 1970s, clinicians and researchers in stuttering began to develop treatment approaches for preschool stuttering based on the idea that "fluency breaks down when environmental and/or self-imposed demands exceed the organism's motoric, linguistic, emotional or cognitive capacities for responding."[49] This notion was formalized in the *Demands and Capacities Model (DCM)* of intervention developed for preschoolers and their parents.[6,7,50] This model assumes that stuttering arises when a child attempts speech performance beyond his or her actual capacities (skills and abilities) for fluent speech. It is viewed as a consequence of a mismatch between task demands, and the capacities that the child brings to the task at that moment in time. Demands for fluency will naturally increase as a child gets older; for example, listeners expect a quicker and more complete answer to a question from a 5-year-old than from a 3-year-old. In most cases, these increasing demands will be successfully met because the child's capacities for fluent speech mature as a function of time. In fact, it has been speculated that the synchronous development of both language and speech motor skills and performance with age may partly explain the high proportion of unassisted or natural recovery from stuttering in young

children (see ▶ Chapter 1 for a more detailed discussion of unassisted or natural recovery).

Although research has shown that some children who stutter exhibit relative weaknesses or dissociations in their capacities for fluency,[9,13,18,19,51,52,53,54,55,56] the *DCM model* assumes no deficits. That is, a child's capacities for fluency across all four domains—speech motor, linguistic, emotional, and cognitive—may be within normal or even above normal limits.[49] The latter may be especially true for linguistic capacities,[19,56] in that precocious language will place a high (internal) demand on a child's (typically or poorly) developing speech motor system.

The central premise of *DCM treatment* is that *decreasing* communicative demands, both internal and external to the child, can promote the child's speech fluency.[57,58,59,60] For example, parents' explicit acknowledgment of the child's difficulties with talking during moments when the child is clearly experiencing difficulty ("That was hard, wasn't it?" or "Learning to talk can sometimes be hard") will decrease the emotional demands on both. ▶ Fig. 10.6 illustrates *DCM's* assumption that stuttering results when the speech motor, linguistic, emotional, and cognitive demands (internal and external) placed on the child for fluent speech exceed the child's capacities in one, more, or all of these domains at that moment in time.

Results of early DCM therapy have been reported by its developers.[7,61] Later, the effectiveness of (Restart-)DCM was investigated in two studies in the Netherlands, both comparing (Restart-)DCM-based treatment—the standard treatment approach in the Netherlands—with the LP (▶ Table 10.1). Analyzing the long-term outcome data of the RESTART study is currently in progress.

Essential Pieces

Initial Assessment

A multifactorial assessment to identify the child's capacities for fluent speech production, and the communication demands placed on them, is an indispensable part of the *Restart-DCM* approach. In addition to the assessment domains specified in ▶ Table 7.3 in ▶ Chapter 7 of this book, Restart-DCM assessment also includes an assessment of the child's speech motor skills: the accuracy, smooth flow, and rate of speech motor movements.[62] In addition, a parent-child interaction (PCI) is analyzed[3] Appendix 10.2 A teacher's questionnaire covering the questions in ▶ Table 7.2 is optional.

The PCI analysis, which is specific to *Restart-DCM*, serves as the initial assessment activity. In this activity, the parents and the child are invited to engage about 7 minutes in free play, and preferably also about 7 minutes in a developmentally appropriate structured activity (e.g., working on a puzzle together) "just as they would do at home." This PCI sample is video recorded and analyzed using the *PCI Form* (Appendix 10.1).[3] This analysis includes observing and scoring specific parent and child conversation behaviors such as interspeaker pause time; number, type, and tone of parental questions; and parent's reactions to the child's stuttering (verbal and nonverbal).

All assessment data collected are analyzed and used to formulate hypotheses in preparation for a parent conference. Which demands appear to cause communicative pressure for the child? What capacities appear limited or poorly matched to demands at this moment in time? Which factors appear to be

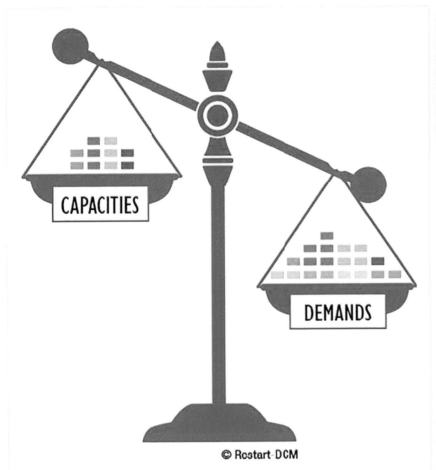

Fig. 10.6 Restart-DCM graphic depicting demands for fluent speech outweighing the child's capacities for fluent speech. Demands and capacities include motor (*light blue*), linguistic (*orange*), emotional (*yellow*), and cognitive (*dark blue*). On the demands side of the scale, lighter shades of one color express *internal* demands, whereas darker shades express *external* demands.

impacting the favorable balance between demands and capacities in an undesirable way? An example of how assessment data is used to develop treatment aims is provided (Appendix 10.2).

During the parent conference, the child's parents are asked to describe their idea or "theory" about what caused the child's stuttering. Often parents express feelings of guilt and worry about their child's stuttering, and the clinician should listen deeply so that they feel comfortable expressing their beliefs.[63] Reviewing the child's assessment data and explaining to parents how the identified capacities and demands fit within the Restart-DCM approach, the clinician can draw a plain scale and note a few "weights": salient examples of demands and capacities, and how well or poorly they are matched at this moment in time. For example, the child's asynchronous language development would be an example of capacity and the parent's speech rate would be an example of a demand, and so forth. *Special Times* and a logbook are introduced, which are considered to be the bridge to starting treatment. The parents are instructed to use the logbook to record the length and content of each *Special Time*, including when and what demands and capacities tools were practiced and the results, specific observations of the child's and parent's behavior, and questions for the clinician. Observations recorded in the logbook are guided by a series of questions that include the following: What did you do? For how long? How did it go? What was the result? How did you experience the "special time"? What did you notice about your child?

Therapy Structure

Treatment is delivered through once-weekly clinic sessions, which last approximately 1 hour, with one parent attending. After every fourth clinician–parent–child session, conferences with both parents (without the child) are scheduled. It is preferable to address parent concerns or difficulties without the child being present.

▶ Fig. 10.7 shows the key elements of *Restart-DCM* as the steps of a staircase to emphasize that each step in the process builds on the previous step.

As depicted in ▶ Fig. 10.7, *Restart-DCM* includes three discriminant treatment phases:

- *Phase I*: In the initial phase, therapy focuses on *lowering demands* by teaching the parents tools to facilitate a better match with the child's current capacities for fluency. Parents learn to change their interaction style, first during treatment sessions in the clinic, then at home during *Special Times*. Gradually, parents start to change their interaction behavior also in everyday situations. First, the relevant motoric demands, as identified in the assessment, are addressed, followed by linguistic, emotional, and, finally, cognitive demands. Besides changes in interaction style, parents also make changes in daily life to reduce demands placed on the child. For example, parents may *plan activities* to improve the predictability of events for the child and to adapt it to the child's temperament. Many children only need this the first

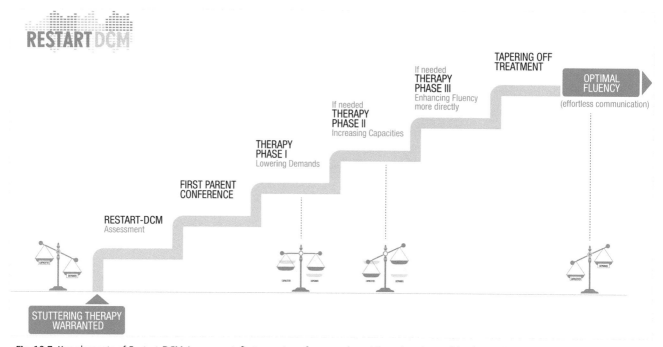

Fig. 10.7 Key elements of Restart-DCM Assessment: first parent conference, phase I (lowering demands), phase II (increasing the child's capacities), phase III (enhancing fluency more directly), tapering off treatment.

phase of Restart-DCM treatment (lowering relevant demands for fluency) to achieve normally fluent speech. If so, all behavioral adjustments gradually become normalized and treatment will be tapered off (▶ Fig. 10.7). Only if the child's level of fluency has not reached acceptable levels (i.e., more than occasional repetitions with one iteration) once relevant demands have been addressed, *phase II* of the program—*increasing capacities*—is added.

- *Phase II*: During this second phase, the clinician (in the clinic) and the parents (in the clinic and at home) maintain the achieved level of reduced communicative demands on the child, and treatment proceeds with training of relevant capacities for fluency. When the capacities of the child mature and improve enough to withstand communicative demands in everyday speaking situations, treatment will be tapered off.
- *Phase III*: In the final phase of the program, enhancing fluency more directly is initiated, but only if the child is still exhibiting unacceptable disfluency after lowering demands and increasing capacities.

In summary, a typical treatment session may include the following: the clinician observes the PCI and the child's fluency, reads the parents' notes in the logbook from the past week, debriefs about how parent–child Special Times/practice sessions went, reviews how treatment was implemented during the past week, and demonstrates, discusses, and models changes in procedures for the coming week. During the session, the parent takes notes and practices new strategies. Finally, a plan for the coming week and time allotted for discussion and problem-solving is provided.

Therapy Strategies

Phase I of the program, *lowering demands*, begins with *the motor domain* and targets decreasing the demands observed during the assessment. The most common demand on the child's speech motor system is a parental speech or articulation rate, which is much faster than the child's rate in conversation. Parents are trained to use an articulation rate that is comparable to the child's rate when they are speaking fluently, typically about three syllables per second for a 3- to 4-year-old. This reduction in parent speaking rate typically feels "abnormal" to them; indeed, while slower than the natural adult speech rate of about five syllables per second, it is a *temporary* adjustment intended to restore a favorable demands/capacities balance for the child. Another way to reduce the demands within the motor domain is by teaching parents to extend the breaks they take between the child's own conversations and their own conversations, and arranging turn taking.

Decreasing demands on the child in the *linguistic domain* includes training parents to ask fewer questions of their child in conversation and using more declarative and redundant language instead. Within the *emotional domain*, parents may be taught to respond helpfully when the child stutters, but only when the child shows signs of increased emotional reactivity or distress (e.g., "Saying that word was hard, wasn't it?"). In addition, providing the child with words to express emotions in daily situations can help the child to regulate strong emotional reactions in the moment (e.g., "You feel angry because you think it is unfair that you have to go to bed now"). This type of response can help reduce the child's level of emotionality, but only if the parent's tone of voice is empathetic and sincere. Once the parent has used wording to convey that they have heard and seen the child, they can proceed with a direction or explanation (e.g., "Four-year-old boys need good sleep so that they will be ready for the next day. Off we go"). This two-step model of responding to the child's emotion followed by providing language models and explanations was specifically developed for Restart-DCM treatment (Appendix 10.2),[3] and can be very helpful; however, only if the parent–child relationship is positive; otherwise, parents may sound hostile or punitive to the child. In addition, in the cases where the child is especially sensitive to his stuttering, parents can model easy, typical disfluencies for the child. Occasional modeling of normal disfluencies for the child, such as "Clean, clean up your toys" or "Clean up your, eh, toys," may decrease demands by lowering the child's internal (and high) "fluency standard." Finally, in the *cognitive domain*, parents can be taught to *show the child* how to respond in a specific situation rather than demanding speech; for example, modeling the sentence "Thank you for the slice of sausage, sir" as opposed to "What do you say?"

It is essential to remember that any changes in communication that are proposed to parents are always first modeled by the clinician, and then practiced with the parent during a treatment session before they start using them at home. Only after the parent feels comfortable using these strategies, and the clinician thinks they have sufficiently mastered the relevant behaviors (e.g., dealing with the child's frustration after losing a game), are they ready to practice at home. As an example, a mother who sought treatment for her 3-year-old son shared that she sometimes had cried in bed at night, feeling very guilty, because she could not manage to slow her speaking rate on her own, recommended to do so by a former clinician. For most parents, changing habitual communicative patterns is hard, so in Restart-DCM, we consider modeling and practicing essential to the success of the approach. In general, building a respectful, honest, and supportive working alliance with the parent is considered crucial: at home, the parent delivers the treatment and the clinician guides the parent to do this effectively and safely.

Phase II of the program, *increasing capacities*, also firstly targets the *speech motor domain*. If shown to be relevant from results of the assessment, the child's speech motor skills will be targeted.[62,64,65] The therapist will model sequences of nonsense words such as /zipe/ and /mitapo/ (14 levels of difficulty), and children are invited to repeat these syllable sets accurately, smoothly, and coarticulated. Speech motor training starts at a very slow rate (1 syllable/s), then slow (2 syllables/s), and then a normal rate (3 syllables/s), and with varying stress patterns and intonation. Nonsense syllable sets are followed by sequencing real words,[66] and are paired with other activities such as coloring and dancing, gradually generalizing these movements to spontaneous speech to stimulate automaticity. If the parents are able to successfully engage in these so-called "speech gym" activities with their child at home, two times a day for about 5 minutes and speech fluency does not normalize, training capacities in the relevant *language domain*, including phonology, will be added. For example, if the assessment results indicate that strengthening receptive or expressive language capacities would benefit the child's speech fluency, or in case of a language dissociation (e.g., a lower word knowledge as compared to other language capacities), then language intervention would be appropriate to reduce this imbalance. If the

child's speech fluency is still not normalized after relevant speech motor and language capacity training, and assessment results and observation indicate that *emotional factors* appear to contribute to more (severe) stuttering, increasing the child's capacities in the *emotional domain* can be targeted. Specific and more direct exercises to desensitize the child to stuttering (i.e., decreasing the child's reactivity to stuttering) may be relevant. Those children who stutter more in situations where they become easily and quickly upset or excited, or who withdraw quickly and regulate slowly, may benefit from direct activities to improve awareness of their emotions, and their emotional reactivity and improve self-regulation skills. For example, the therapist may first model for the child that losing a game can be hard and can make you angry (reactivity), but that you can still continue the game (regulate), which is more important. Then, the therapist will try to engage the child in the exercise. It goes without saying that directly teaching self-regulation strategies is always adapted to the child's maturity level. Finally, in the *cognitive domain*, the child can engage, for example, in activities to learn how to take turns during verbal interactions, if this is still a situation that seems to elicit more stuttering.

Phase III of the *Restart-DCM* program, *enhancing fluency more directly*, is initiated if the child's level of disfluency is still too high after lowering relevant demands and training relevant capacities. Phase III involves teaching the child how to modify instances of stuttering. For example, while playing games appropriate for the child's developmental level, examples of how to change stuttered speech in a playful way will be shown to the child. For example, contrasting an *easy* repetition with a *tense* prolongation, or comparing and contrasting *large* articulation movements (e.g., mouth more open, lips more rounded) with *small* articulation movements (e.g., mouth a little bit open, lips hardly rounding). All clinician modeling and practicing occurs in a playful manner, modeling an attitude of tolerance for stuttering and while the child is invited to participate. At home, parents replicate these strategies and games to ensure that the child experiences normal (dis)fluency and spontaneously starts to employ other, easier ways of speaking as a result of these experiences. The balance between demands and capacities continues to fulfill the pivotal role in treatment.

Follow-up and Monitoring

Over the course of treatment, the clinician periodically measures the child's stuttering severity (using the Stuttering Severity Instrument, Fourth Edition [SSI-4]),[67] and both the parent and clinician periodically rate the child's fluency on a qualitative 8-point scale,[8] where 0 = normal fluency, no stuttering, 1 = borderline fluency, 2 = mild stuttering, and 8 = very severe stuttering.[9] Parents also repeatedly (e.g., every 3 months) rate the impact of stuttering on the child (see ▶ Chapter 7). When the child exhibits normal speech fluency for several weeks, home treatment sessions will be gradually terminated, parental use of lowering demands in daily conversation with their child will become gradually normalized, and treatment sessions will be gradually tapered off. At the termination of therapy, parents should feel skilled in lowering communicative demand, so they will be able to respond to a relapse of stuttering immediately by lowering demands.

10.3 Discussion

With each of the approaches described in this chapter, there will be children who continue to stutter. One of the roles of the therapist is to ensure that intervention does not reinforce negative views of stuttering in either the child or their parents. In the case that early intervention does not achieve fluent speech, both parent and child may experience a sense of failure and a negative view of therapy. If these results are not discussed with sensitivity and care, there is a danger that the pursuit of fluency can give the child (and parents) an unintended message that stuttering is undesirable, something to be fixed, avoided, or hidden. If we reinforce the belief that the stuttering must be stopped no matter what, we run the risk of encouraging avoidance, shame, and guilt about stuttering, and strengthening a belief that a happy life is impossible when you stutter. Therapy for stuttering in the early years is the beginning of a process of tolerance and acceptance of difference, more in keeping with current attitudes and views regarding diversity in other walks of life. Supporting effective and confident communication, participation in daily activities, and the child's ability to reach their potential are the ultimate aim, whether or not they continue to stutter.

In some countries, a monitoring phase precedes the beginning of early intervention.[5] The length of this monitoring period depends on the presence of risk factors described in the introduction, and the impact stuttering has on the parents and child. Often, there will be good reasons to recommend immediate therapy, even in the cases where time since onset is only 3 months.

Given the options available, the clinician will need to decide which of the available treatments will be offered to an individual child and family. The similarities and differences between Palin PCI, *LP*, and *Restart-DCM* are shown in ▶ Fig. 10.8, and careful comparison of each when considered in the context of the child's and family's needs will facilitate decision-making. Importantly, recent research suggests that while all three treatments are effective, there is not one approach that yields a better outcome than another.[38]

As discussed throughout this chapter, parent preferences are considered, and should be a fundamental to shared decision-making. Parent preferences may be influenced by their own experiences of therapy, cultural norms, values, priorities, learning styles, or the child's temperament. In reality, however, the choice of treatment used may be heavily influenced by factors such as the needs and opportunities for postgraduate training of clinicians in the region, and the skills, background, and theoretical perspectives of graduate instructors and experienced colleagues. The approach of choice will be further influenced by the treatment setting (school, private practice, university clinic) and travel distances. Finally, there may be higher political or institutional directives within a service delivery model or insurance policy that restrict the family's and therapist's choice. Ultimately, what is important is for the therapist to seek the necessary training to reliably and validly deliver one or more of these approaches, and seek continuing education as caseloads demand.

In some circumstances, it is possible for individual clinicians to offer a choice of intervention, but this tends to be limited to more specialist therapy contexts (i.e., centers dedicated to stuttering and stuttering therapy), or in certain countries such as the Netherlands and the United States. If a clinician is unable to offer a choice, parents should be educated about the different approaches and provided support in accessing those elsewhere if they choose. In sum, it is most important for the therapist to be trained in the approach they use, the therapy is individualized to meet the family's needs, and that the impact of the intervention is monitored and jointly reviewed at regular periods.

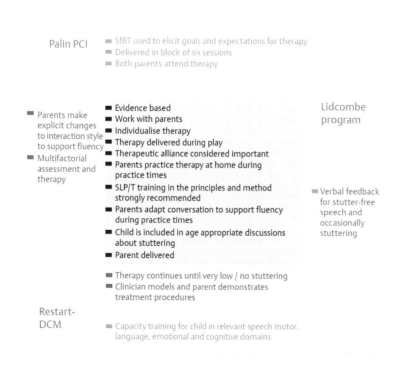

Fig. 10.8 Similarities (*dark center panel*) and differences (*light borders*) among Restart-DCM, Palin Parent–Child Interaction (PCI), and the Lidcombe Program.

Palin PCI
- SfBT used to elicit goals and expectations for therapy
- Delivered in block of six sessions
- Both parents attend therapy

- Parents make explicit changes to interaction style to support fluency
- Multifactorial assessment and therapy

- Evidence based
- Work with parents
- Individualise therapy
- Therapy delivered during play
- Therapeutic alliance considered important
- Parents practice therapy at home during practice times
- SLP/T training in the principles and method strongly recommended
- Parents adapt conversation to support fluency during practice times
- Child is included in age appropriate discussions about stuttering
- Parent delivered

- Therapy continues until very low / no stuttering
- Clinician models and parent demonstrates treatment procedures

Lidcombe program

- Verbal feedback for stutter-free speech and occasionally stuttering

Restart-DCM
- Capacity training for child in relevant speech motor, language, emotional and cognitive domains

10.4 Conclusions and Future Directions

At the Oxford Fluency Conference in 2014, it was recognized that fluency is not the only outcome for therapy and not necessarily the most important one. *Satisfaction with communication in everyday situations* was proposed as the primary outcome for stuttering therapy.[68] Unfortunately, research following up on this is still very limited.[69]

Further research into the mechanisms of change and critical components of therapy is required. In this respect, research into the LP is more advanced, with the researchers investigating the contribution of treatment components.[70,71] Research should also investigate the effectiveness of treatment components such as "lowering speech motor demands" or "increasing speech motor capacities." More information about what features of the LP, Restart-DCM, and Palin PCI are the *mechanisms of action* would help refine and enhance the methods and potentially increase treatment adherence and fidelity.[72] Although therapies have several commonalities (which might explain why they have comparable outcomes), and most treatments appear to work for most families and children, there is unlikely to be a "one-size-fits-all" intervention.[23] Understanding more about the variability in responses to intervention, the factors that influence that, will help improve the recommendations for which therapy might be more or less suitable for which child. Further, the efficiency of treatments needs to be compared. For example, *Palin PCI* and *Restart-DCM* are both indirect approaches, but *Palin PCI* takes only six sessions and one follow-up session, whereas *Restart-DCM* treatment has a mean of 20 sessions over the first 18 months from treatment onset.[39]

Last but not least, as we learn more about the genetic underpinnings and the neurophysiological mechanisms of stuttering, we hope that more targeted and effective therapies will be developed. Therefore, although we have support for our current methods, research into novel interventions should continue.

References

[1] Kelman E, Nicholas A. Palin Parent-Child Interaction Therapy for Early Childhood Stammering. Abingdon, UK: Routledge; 2020

[2] Onslow M, Webber M, Harrison E, et al. The Lidcombe Program treatment guide. 2020. Available at: https://www.uts.edu.au/research-and-teaching/our-research/australianstuttering-research-centre/asrc-resources/resources

[3] Franken, MC, Laroes, E. RESTART-DCM Method (2021). Revised edition. Available at: https://restartdcm.nl/wp-content/uploads/2021/05/RestartDCM-Method-2021_online.pdf

[4] Andrews G, Harris M. The Syndrome of Stuttering. London, England: Heinemann; 1964

[5] Yairi E, Seery CH. Stuttering: Foundations and Clinical Applications. 2nd ed. Boston, MA: Pearson; 2015

[6] Starkweather CW, Gottwald SR. The demands and capacities model II: clinical applications. J Fluency Disord. 1990; 15(3):143–157

[7] Starkweather CW, Ridener Gottwald S, Halfond MM. Stuttering prevention: a clinical method. Englewood Cliffs: Prentice Hall; 1990

[8] Yairi E, Ambrose NG. Early Childhood Stuttering for Clinicians by Clinicians. Austin, TX: Pro-Ed; 2005

[9] Yairi E, Ambrose NG. Early childhood stuttering I: persistency and recovery rates. J Speech Lang Hear Res. 1999; 42(5):1097–1112

[10] Kloth S, Janssen P, Kraaimaat F, Brutten GJ. Child and mother variables in the development of stuttering among high-risk children: a longitudinal study. J Fluency Disord. 1998; 23(4):217–230

[11] Rommel D, Häge A, Johannsen HS, Schulze H. Linguistic aspects of stuttering in childhood. In: Hulstijn W, Peters HFM, Van Lieshout PHHM, eds. Speech Production: Motor Control, Brain Research and Fluency Disorders. Amsterdam: Elsevier Science Publishers; 1997:603–610

[12] Kefalianos E, Onslow M, Packman A, et al. The history of stuttering by 7 years of age: follow-up of a prospective community cohort. J Speech Lang Hear Res. 2017; 60(10):2828–2839

[13] Ambrose NG, Yairi E, Loucks TM, Seery CH, Throneburg R. Relation of motor, linguistic and temperament factors in epidemiologic subtypes of persistent and recovered stuttering: Initial findings. J Fluency Disord. 2015; 45:12–26

[14] Häge A. Cognitive and linguistic abilities in young children: are they able to predict the further development of stuttering. Sprache Stimme Gehor. 2001; 25(1):20–24

[15] Hollister J, Van Horne AO, Zebrowski P. The relationship between grammatical development and disfluencies in preschool children who stutter and those who recover. Am J Speech Lang Pathol. 2017; 26(1):44–56

[16] Leech KA, Bernstein Ratner N, Brown B, Weber CM. Preliminary evidence that growth in productive language differentiates childhood stuttering persistence and recovery. J Speech Lang Hear Res. 2017; 60(11):3097–3109

[17] Spencer C, Weber-Fox C. Preschool speech articulation and nonword repetition abilities may help predict eventual recovery or persistence of stuttering. J Fluency Disord. 2014; 41:32–46

[18] Usler E, Smith A, Weber C. A lag in speech motor coordination during sentence production is associated with stuttering persistence in young children. J Speech Lang Hear Res. 2017; 60(1):51–61

[19] Watkins RV. Language abilities of young children who stutter. In: Yairi E, Ambrose N, eds. Early Childhood Stuttering: for Clinicians by Clinicians. Austin, TX: Pro-Ed; 2005:235–252

[20] Erdemir A, Walden TA, Jefferson CM, Choi D, Jones RM. The effect of emotion on articulation rate in persistence and recovery of childhood stuttering. J Fluency Disord. 2018; 56:1–17

[21] Singer CM, Hessling A, Kelly EM, Singer L, Jones RM. Clinical characteristics associated with stuttering persistence: a meta-analysis. J Speech Lang Hear Res. 2020; 63(9):2995–3018

[22] Essex MJ, Kraemer HC, Armstrong JM, et al. Exploring risk factors for the emergence of children's mental health problems. Arch Gen Psychiatry. 2006; 63(11):1246–1256

[23] Bernstein Ratner N. Selecting treatments and monitoring outcomes: the circle of evidence-based practice and client-centered care in treating a preschool child who stutters. Lang Speech Hear Serv Sch. 2018; 49(1): 13–22

[24] Millard SK, Zebrowski P, Kelman E. Palin Parent-Child Interaction therapy: the bigger picture. Am J Speech Lang Pathol. 2018; 27 3S:1211–1223

[25] Onslow M, Kelly EM. Temperament and early stuttering intervention: two perspectives. J Fluency Disord. 2020; 64:105765

[26] Smith A, Weber C. How stuttering develops: the multifactorial dynamic pathways theory. J Speech Lang Hear Res. 2017; 60(9):2483–2505

[27] Kraft SJ, Yairi E. Genetic bases of stuttering: the state of the art, 2011. Folia Phoniatr Logop. 2012; 64(1):34–47

[28] Chang SE. Research updates in neuroimaging studies of children who stutter. Semin Speech Lang. 2014; 35(2):67–79

[29] Millard SK, Davis S. Palin Parent Rating Scales. Available at: https://www.palinprs.org.uk/secure/pprs_connect.php

[30] Millard SK, Nicholas A, Cook FM. Is parent-child interaction therapy effective in reducing stuttering? J Speech Lang Hear Res. 2008; 51(3):636–650

[31] Millard SK, Edwards S, Cook FM. Parent-child interaction therapy: adding to the evidence. Int J Speech Lang Pathol. 2009; 11(1):61–76

[32] Jones M, Onslow M, Packman A, et al. Randomised controlled trial of the Lidcombe programme of early stuttering intervention. BMJ. 2005; 331(7518): 659–661

[33] Jones M, Onslow M, Harrison E, Packman A. Treating stuttering in young children: predicting treatment time in the Lidcombe program. J Speech Lang Hear Res. 2000; 43(6):1440–1450

[34] Bonelli P, Dixon M, Bernstein Ratner N, Onslow M. Child and parent speech and language following the Lidcombe programme of early stuttering intervention. Clin Linguist Phon. 2000; 14(6):427–446

[35] Bridgman K, Onslow M, O'Brian S, Jones M, Block S. Lidcombe program webcam treatment for early stuttering: a randomized controlled trial. J Speech Lang Hear Res. 2016; 59(5):932–939

[36] Goodhue R, Onslow M, Quine S, O'Brian S, Hearne A. The Lidcombe program of early stuttering intervention: mothers' experiences. J Fluency Disord. 2010; 35(1):70–84

[37] Franken MC, Kielstra-Van der Schalk CJ, Boelens H. Experimental treatment of early stuttering: a preliminary study. J Fluency Disord. 2005; 30(3):189–199

[38] de Sonneville-Koedoot C, Stolk E, Rietveld T, Franken MC. Direct versus indirect treatment for preschool children who stutter: the RESTART randomized trial. PLoS One. 2015; 10(7):e0133758

[39] de Sonneville-Koedoot C, Bouwmans C, Franken MC, Stolk E. Economic evaluation of stuttering treatment in preschool children: the RESTART-study. J Commun Disord. 2015; 58:106–118

[40] Wampold BE. How important are the common factors in psychotherapy? An update. World Psychiatry. 2015; 14(3):270–277

[41] Yairi E, Ambrose N. Epidemiology of stuttering: 21st century advances. J Fluency Disord. 2013; 38(2):66–87

[42] De Shazer S. Keys to solution in Brief Therapy. New York, NY: Norton; 1985

[43] Martin RR, Kuhl P, Haroldson S. An experimental treatment with two preschool stuttering children. J Speech Hear Res. 1972; 15(4):743–752

[44] Reed CG, Godden AL. An experimental treatment using verbal punishment with two preschool stutterers. J Fluency Disord. 1977; 2(3):225–233

[45] Onslow M. Stuttering and Its Treatment: Eleven Lectures. 2020. Available at: https://www.uts.edu.au/research-and-teaching/our-research/australian-stuttering-researchcentre/asrc-resources/resources

[46] Eve CL, Onslow M, Andrews C, Adams R. Clinical measurement of early stuttering severity: the reliability of a 10-point scale. Aust J Hum Commun Disord. 1995; 23(2):26–39

[47] Onslow M, Andrews C, Costa L. Parental severity scaling of early stuttered speech: four case studies. Aust J Hum Commun Disord. 1990; 18(1):47–61

[48] Onslow M, Harrison E, Jones M, Packman A. Beyond-clinic speech measures during the Lidcombe Program of early stuttering intervention. ACQ Speech Pathology Australia. 2002; 4:82–85

[49] Adams MR. The demands and capacities model I: theoretical elaborations. J Fluency Disord. 1990; 15(3):135–141

[50] Starkweather CW. Fluency and Stuttering. Englewood Cliffs, NJ: Prentice-Hall Inc; 1987

[51] Anderson JD, Pellowski MW, Conture EG. Childhood stuttering and dissociations across linguistic domains. J Fluency Disord. 2005; 30(3):219–253

[52] Bauerly KR, Gottwald SR. The dynamic relationship of sentence complexity, childhood stuttering, and grammatical development. Contemp Issues Commun Sci Disord. 2009; 36(Spring):14–25

[53] Coulter CE, Anderson JD, Conture EG. Childhood stuttering and dissociations across linguistic domains: a replication and extension. J Fluency Disord. 2009; 34(4):257–278

[54] MacPherson MK, Smith A. Influences of sentence length and syntactic complexity on the speech motor control of children who stutter. J Speech Lang Hear Res. 2013; 56(1):89–102

[55] Usler E, Weber-Fox C. Neurodevelopment for syntactic processing distinguishes childhood stuttering recovery versus persistence. J Neurodev Disord. 2015; 7(1):4

[56] Watts A, Eadie P, Block S, Mensah F, Reilly S. Language ability of children with and without a history of stuttering: a longitudinal cohort study. Int J Speech Lang Pathol. 2015; 17(1):86–95

[57] LaSalle LR. Slow speech rate effects on stuttering preschoolers with disordered phonology. Clin Linguist Phon. 2015; 29(5):354–377

[58] Ryan BP. A longitudinal study of articulation, language, rate, and fluency of 22 preschool children who stutter. J Fluency Disord. 2001; 26:107–127

[59] Sawyer J, Matteson C, Ou H, Nagase T. The effects of parent-focused slow relaxed speech intervention on articulation rate, response time latency, and fluency in preschool children who stutter. J Speech Lang Hear Res. 2017; 60 (4):794–809

[60] Stephenson-Opsal D, Bernstein Ratner N. Maternal speech rate modification and childhood stuttering. J Fluency Disord. 1988; 13(1):49–56

[61] Gottwald SR, Starkweather CW. Stuttering prevention and early intervention: a multiprocess approach. In: Onslow M, Packman A, eds. The Handbook of Early Stuttering Intervention. San Diego, CA: Singular Publishing Group, Inc.; 1999:53–82

[62] Riley J, Riley G. Oral Motor Assessment and Treatment. Improving Syllable Production. Austin, Texas: Pro-ed; 1985

[63] Luterman D. Sharpening counselling Skills (DVD). Memphis, TN: Stuttering Foundation of America

[64] Riley J, Riley G. Speech motor training. In: Onslow M, Packman A, eds. The Handbook of Early Stuttering Intervention. San Diego, CA: Singular Publishing Group; 1999:139–158

[65] Riley GD, Ingham JC. Acoustic duration changes associated with two types of treatment for children who stutter. J Speech Lang Hear Res. 2000; 43(4):965–978

[66] Daly DA, Riley J, Riley G. Speech Motor Exercises: Applying Motor Learning Principles to Stuttering and Apraxia. Austin, TX: Pro-ed; 2000

[67] Riley GD. SSI-4: Stuttering Severity Instrument - Fourth edition; examiners' manual. 4th ed. Austin, TX: Pro-Ed; 2009

[68] Karimi H, O'Brian S, Sommer M, et al. The Croatia protocol: Improving clinical trials of stuttering treatment. Paper presented at the 10th Oxford Dysfluency Conference, Oxford, UK, July 17–20, 2014

[69] Karimi H, Onslow M, Jones M, et al. The Satisfaction with Communication in Everyday Speaking Situations (SCESS) scale: an overarching outcome measure of treatment effect. J Fluency Disord. 2018; 58:77–85

[70] Donaghy M, Harrison E, O'Brian S, et al. An investigation of the role of parental request for self-correction of stuttering in the Lidcombe Program. Int J Speech Lang Pathol. 2015; 17(5):511–517

[71] Donaghy M, O'Brian S, Onslow M, Lowe R, Jones M, Menzies RG. Verbal contingencies in the Lidcombe Program: a noninferiority trial. J Speech Lang Hear Res. 2020; 63(10):3419–3431

[72] Bernstein Ratner N. Evidence-based practice in stuttering: some questions to consider. J Fluency Disord. 2005; 30(3):163–188

Appendix 10.1

STUTTERING SEVERITY RATING SCALE

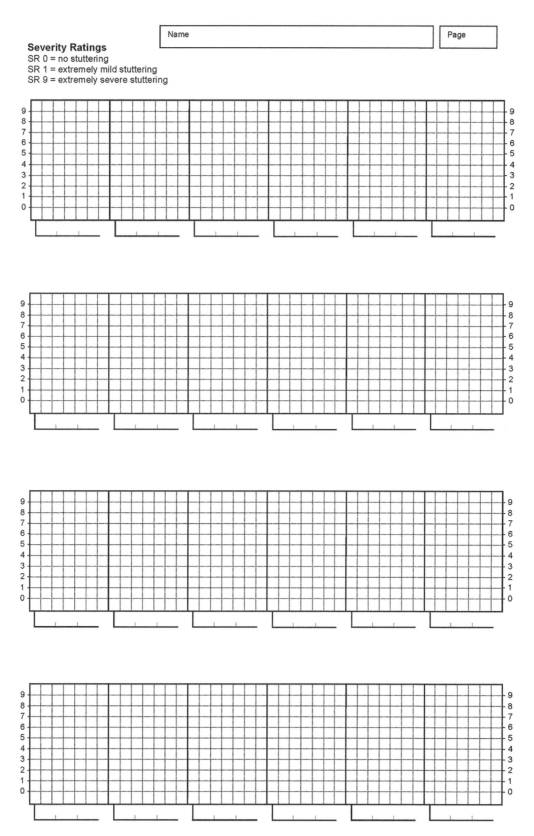

Severity Ratings
SR 0 = no stuttering
SR 1 = extremely mild stuttering
SR 9 = extremely severe stuttering

Name

Page

Appendix 10.2

SUMMARY OF RESTART-DCM ASSESSMENT OF CASE JILL

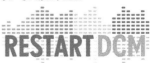

CASE __JILL_____ DATE_____ THERAPIST _____		
CASE DESCRIPTION BASED ON ANAMNESTIC INTERVIEW		
Personal information	Name:	Jill
	Age:	3 years 7 months
	Gender:	female
	Family:	Father (F), Mother (M), sister (9 years) and Jill
	Parental occupation:	F = finance controller, M = pedagogical assistant
	School/level:	Pre-school
Child's history – in general	Motor development:	Average – quick
	Illnesses:	Just regular colds
	Hearing:	Good
	Treatment (any):	None
	Physical complaints:	None
Child's history -- specific	First words:	at age 11 months
	Course:	Average, but exceptionally large vocabulary since early language development
	Age at onset:	2 years 11 months
	Possible cause(s):	Wants to tell so much; exciting times (Christmas holiday, skiing for the first time)
	Course stuttering following onset:	Sudden onset of severe stuttering; after 3 weeks recovery for a few weeks, then relapse with mild to severe stuttering with ups & downs.
	Family history:	None
	Current severity:	Severe stuttering Parents increasingly worried – VAS 7 (1-10 scale)
	Stable / variable pattern:	Ups & downs but never a day normal fluency
	Environmental factors:	More fluent while playing, more stuttering while telling story's
	Previous speech Therapy: (re. stuttering or other speech-language problems)	Parents contacted speech therapist 8 weeks after onset. She advised parents to tell Jill to slow down her speech and talk like a snail. This has not improved fluency
	Other significant information:	None
ASSESSMENT FINDINGS		
Stuttering	Description of stuttering, types of dysfluencies:	Mostly sound and part-word repetitions (multiple), prolongations sometimes with pitch rise (occasionally), blocks (more and more)
	Stuttering Severity Instrument Score:	Score ___25_____ = very mild / mild / **moderate** / severe / very severe

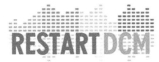

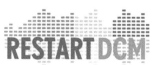

ASSESSMENT DATA: *DEMANDS*			
Test results, questionnaires, standardized observations, etc.			
Motor domain	Language domain	Emotional domain	Cognitive domain
- turns overlap - short interaction times - Jill 3.5 syll/sec - M 5.5 syll/sec	- M uses complex lexicon - M corrects J's lexicon - both often take long turns - M reads books at older sister's level	- teacher expects flexibility and adaptation - M does not know how to address J's *stubborn* behavior/temper tantrums, tries to calm Jill down (suspects she feels insecure) by telling her that she can feel safe and can talk about it	- M is offering complex concepts answering Jill's questions - M approaches Jill on the same level as her 9 years old sister

ASSESSMENT DATA: *CAPACITIES*			
Test results, questionnaires, standardized observations, etc.			
Motor domain (M)	Language domain (L)	Emotional domain (E)	Cognitive domain (C)
Speech Motor Assessment (OMAS) Jill refuses to cooperate. When invited to imitate /pe/, she is silent and stares at the floor. She ignores both her parents and the therapist Speech sound production: age appr.	*Receptive Language* Score : +1,4 SD *Expressive Language:* * Word production Score: - 0,4 SD * *Sentence production:* Score: - 0.7 SD *Peabody Picture Vocabulary test* + 1,4 SD	- difficulty adapting to change - seems rigid, stubborn - highly emotional when not being able to perform as sister can (temper tantrums) - whole body is tense while experiencing blocks, turns side-ways - Kiddy Cat: same response as taking the OMAS	- very precise - perfectionistic - mistakes are failures - highly competitive in regards to older sister - eager to learn - talks with great detail, looking for precise wording

TREATMENT PLAN		
Treatment Goals	Lowering (internal and external) Demands:	M: reducing articulation rate; Increasing interaction times L: matching turns of parents and Jill; parents using age appropriate lexicon E: prepare Jill for change, visualising daily routines in schedule; Communicating with Lowered Emotional Demands: two steps [3, App 5] C: offer more age appropriate concepts
	Increasing Child's Capacities:	M: retesting showed adequate OMAS score – Speech Motor Training not required L: Improving expressive language skills, more phrasing; being able to limit talking E-C: learning to cope with change, mistakes, not being able to do some things, stuttering

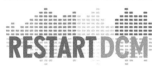

11 School-Age Children

J. Scott Yaruss, Craig Coleman, Janet Beilby, and Caryn Herring

Abstract

This chapter describes strategies for helping school-age children who stutter (i.e., children between the ages of 6 and 12 years) learn how to navigate the impact of stuttering on their communication and their lives as a whole. The treatment process is presented as a comprehensive approach that must be considered within the context of overall communication functioning; the overarching goal of therapy is to ensure that the child is able to speak freely and effectively, regardless of whether or not moments of stuttering are produced in the flow of speech. Because numerous approaches to stuttering therapy for school-age children have been described in the literature, we will provide readers with an overview of the general therapy process and its various components. In doing so, readers will learn how to identify relevant aspects of therapy for different children who stutter and how to select from and adapt available treatment options to meet the needs of each individual child. A set of targeted case examples, rather than a single, detailed case study, is used to demonstrate the steps in the clinical decision-making process so that readers can apply the general concepts underlying stuttering therapy to individual children.

Keywords: stuttering, treatment, therapy, intervention, school-age, speech fluency

11.1 Introduction

Working with school-age children who stutter offers speech-language pathologists (SLPs) countless challenges and opportunities. The challenges arise because the school-age years bring new uncertainties for children as they learn to navigate greater independence and responsibility in their speech and in their lives as a whole. The opportunities arise because there is much that SLPs can do, while working collaboratively with children, caregivers, and others, to reduce the impact of stuttering and to minimize the likelihood that the child will experience negative consequences associated with stuttering. The overarching principle guiding our approach to treatment for school-age children who stutter is that "stuttering is more than just stuttering."[1] This means that the experience of stuttering for the child involves more than just the production of stuttered speech disfluencies. Accordingly, therapy for stuttering must address more than the child's observable stuttering behaviors. In this chapter, we talk about how to address the entirety of the stuttering experience, including issues related to speech fluency as well as the ways the child, family/caregivers, and others react to stuttering, the ways in which stuttering might affect the child's ability to communicate effectively, and the impact that stuttering might have on the child's overall quality of life.

This chapter is organized as follows. We begin by highlighting the importance of diagnostic data to ensure that clinical decision-making is based on an appropriate foundation of evidence. We then discuss some of the reasons that working with school-age children who stutter is unique, emphasizing the challenges and opportunities mentioned earlier. We then move on to the details of treatment, starting with the primary goals of therapy for school-age children who stutter. To ensure that treatment is comprehensive in nature,[2] we base our goal-selection process on the World Health Organization's *International Classification of Functioning, Disability, and Health* (ICF),[3] a standard framework that is used around the world for categorizing all aspects of human health experience. Within the context of the ICF, we then describe various treatment options that can be used for each unique child who stutters and their caregivers. Following this, we illustrate how the process can unfold by sharing a set of case examples, highlighting how our treatment decisions are affected by particular characteristics of the child and caregivers. We then discuss two specific aspects of the therapy process that can greatly affect outcomes: the development of the therapeutic alliance and the clinician's demonstration of empathy. Finally, we end with some brief thoughts about the future of stuttering therapy for this age group, as we affirm that clinicians can make a positive difference in the lives of school-age children who stutter and their families. Our orientation to treating children who stutter is optimistic, and we hope that, by the time you finish with this chapter, you will agree.

11.2 The Importance of Assessment

This is a chapter on treatment, but before we can begin to discuss how to plan therapy, we must first ensure that we have appropriate assessment data. The components of a comprehensive stuttering assessment for school-age are described in ▶ Chapter 8, and we emphasize that one should never predetermine what a child needs in therapy based solely on the knowledge that "the child stutters." Put simply, different children who stutter need different therapy, and the only way to know what that therapy should be is to first have adequate information about the unique needs of each child and family. The best way to obtain this knowledge is through a comprehensive assessment process that involves more than just measuring stuttering frequency or severity.[4] Importantly, research has shown that the speakers' experience of stuttering is not solely determined by the amount, nature, or severity of stuttering that the speakers may produce.[5] For example, some children may stutter frequently yet experience minimal adverse impact resulting from their stuttering. On the other hand, some may stutter infrequently (at least as determined by listeners) yet experience significant negative impact.[6] Therefore, we must assess more than just observable stuttering behavior.

As described in ▶ Chapter 8 (see also ▶ Table 11.1), a comprehensive evaluation of a school-age child who stutters should include information about how the child and the people in the child's environment (friends, peers, teachers, family members, and other caregivers) react to and cope with stuttering. This includes details about how stuttering is affecting the child (often referred to as "adverse impact" or "impact on quality of life") and the child's interactions with others, as well as reports from the child and other relevant individuals

Table 11.1 Key aspects of a comprehensive assessment of school-age stuttering

Assessment activity	Sample data to be collected
Interview with the parents/caregivers	• Child's history of stuttering, speech and language development, and general development • Caregivers' knowledge and perceptions about stuttering • Caregivers' observations about the child's stuttering across situations • Caregivers' goals for therapy
Interview with the child	• Child's knowledge and perceptions about stuttering • Child's goals for therapy
Observation and assessment of child's speech in different speaking situations	• Measures of observable speech fluency and stuttering (e.g., frequency, duration, types of disfluencies, and severity of stuttering)
Observation and assessment of other aspects of child's experience of stuttering	• Child's affective, behavioral, and cognitive reactions to stuttering • Difficulties the child experiences when communicating in key situations (e.g., at home, at school, in social settings) • Impact of stuttering on the child's overall quality of life

in the child's life. Some of this information can be gathered through standardized assessments, though clinicians will also find it valuable to conduct detailed interviews with the child, the caregivers, and other relevant individuals who know and interact with the child. Going forward in this chapter, we assume that a comprehensive evaluation has already been conducted and that the clinician and family have decided that therapy is both warranted and recommended.

11.3 General Considerations for Working with School-Age Children

"Growing up is hard, and I'm trying not to do it."

–10-year-old child

Children who continue to stutter beyond the preschool years face several challenges that SLPs must be prepared to address. Put simply, school-age children who stutter are different from preschool children who stutter: they are more likely to continue stuttering,[7,8,9] and they are more at risk of experiencing negative reactions,[10,11,12] both from themselves and from others. Moreover, school-age children have unique psychosocial, affective, and behavioral developmental patterns that are distinct from those of younger children—and also from those of adolescents.

11.3.1 School-Age Children Who Stutter Are Still Growing

Although school-age children are often referred to as "big kids," they sometimes want to do "little kid" things, as well. As they move away from younger childhood and toward adolescence, school-age children may want to show increasing independence from their caregivers. Simultaneously, they also show increasing dependence on their peers for social, emotional, and academic development and validation.[13] School-age children are not only growing physically but also developing more complicated notions about their sense of self and their personal identity. Simultaneously, they are expanding their awareness of their future roles in society and relationship with others. Moreover, a growing body of research has shown that school-age children's temperament is likely to affect their experiences with stuttering over time.[14,15]

Developmentally, school-age children are at an age of instability, exploration, and self-focus; they are in a stage of being "in between," sandwiched between two more clearly identifiable age groups. For these reasons, school-age children often experience confused and confusing feelings about stuttering. It is critically important that we demonstrate unconditional positive regard for the child, their thoughts, and their emotions. We will return to the notion of providing support to our clients when we discuss empathy and the "therapeutic alliance" toward the end of this chapter. For now, we want to highlight the value of supporting school-age children through the unique position they find themselves in: not yet fully independent, but still expected to take on more responsibility and initiative every day—even in areas in which they may still feel the need for greater support. Dealing with the challenges presented by stuttering may be one of those areas. Children benefit when they know that we are there to help them even as they work to find their own way.

As you can see, it is necessary for SLPs to adapt their treatment to the unique developmental stage of school-age children. This means that we need to be aware of the rapid changes in development, learning, and preferred activities that children experience during this period (▶ Table 11.2). For example, like preschool-age children, children aged 6 to 7 years enjoy many different activities, including gross motor activities, such as riding bicycles and jumping rope; they generally like to be occupied and kept busy during treatment sessions. At the same time, they may also be able to engage in repeated practice activities in order to improve their skills and abilities. By the age of 8 or 9 years, children are becoming more proficient in their abilities; they can care for themselves more effectively, and they can employ finer motor skills, such as using tools, sewing, and drawing. Still, they like to play, and an important aspect of play at this age is learning to interact and socialize with others. During the school-age years, children tend to move from playing alone to having multiple friends and social groups. Friendships become more important across these years, but school-age children are generally still connected to their caregivers and like being part of a family unit. Generally, by the age of 10 to 12 years, children's interests move toward competition-based games; they may enjoy participating in clubs and groups, thereby highlighting the even greater role of social interaction. By this age, children are lively contributors to conversations, and they usually enjoy engaging with and talk-

Table 11.2 Sample activities appropriate for age and developmental stage

Age (y)	Executive functioning skill developing	Example activities
6–9	• Cognitive flexibility • Working memory • Decision-making	• Hearts and other card games • Opposites • Matching • Fantasy play/imagination
	• Monitoring	• Hide and seek • Tag
	• Self-monitoring • Working memory • Attention	• Dancing
	• Focused practice	• Jump rope
9–12	• Cognitive flexibility • Working memory	• Hearts and other card games • Sudoku • Crossword puzzles • Fantasy play
	• Decision-making • Monitoring • Time pressure	• Spit and other more competitive card games • Team sports
	• Planning • Anticipating possible outcomes	• Chess • Puzzles
	• Focused practice	• Jump rope
	• Selective attention • Self-monitoring • Coordination of working memory with attention, cognitive flexibility, and inhibition	• Playing a musical instrument • Singing in rounds

Table 11.3 Ways that stuttering might affect school-age children differently from preschoolers

- Increasing awareness of stuttering
- Increasing discomfort with the sensation of being stuck
- Increasing concern about other people noticing stuttering
- Increasing fear about other people's reactions to stuttering
- Increasing reliance on the opinions and feedback of other people
- Increasing value placed on talking and social interaction
- Increasing concern by parents and caregivers about the child's stuttering

ing to others. Talking plays an increasingly important role in the child's life, and this has particular relevance for understanding the impact of stuttering—and the role of the SLP in helping children who stutter. ▶ Table 11.3 summarizes some of the ways in which stuttering might affect school-age children differently from the way it affects preschool-age children.

11.3.2 Stuttering Affects School-Age Children Differently from Preschool Children

One of the key ways in which stuttering can affect school-age children is in their social interactions with others. Social competence, or skilled communication in social behavior, plays a substantial role in children's social development. The fact that stuttering can interfere with communication may have consequences for the child's participation in social discourse.[12] For example, social banter is one tool that young people may use to both test out and forge friendships. Knowing good jokes and being able to tell them, as well as using popular slang words and terminology, matters at this age; school-age children want to be able to interact with potential friends in an easy and effortless way, but stuttering can hamper their ability to do this. School-age children who stutter may also experience bullying and other negative reactions from their peers.[16,17] The result can be diminished opportunity for social interaction, increased

isolation, and greater adverse impact on the child's quality of life as a result of stuttering. All of these consequences reflect the unique challenges faced by school-age children who stutter, and so they must be carefully considered in a comprehensive plan of treatment.[18]

Another way in which stuttering affects school-age child differently than younger children is the basic fact that they have been stuttering for a longer period of time—and, the older they get, the more time they have spent stuttering.[13] They may not remember a time when they did not stutter, and this has consequences for their still-developing self-concept and self-identity. For example, children may see themselves only or primarily as a person who stutters, and ignore the other important roles they have, and other characteristics they possess. Moreover, the growing demands placed on school-age children for increasingly adultlike social, communicative, and academic competence may exacerbate concerns about speaking, stuttering, and communicating.[19]

11.3.3 School-Age Children Are Not Adolescents or Adults

Just as school-age children are different from preschool children, they are also different from adolescents and adults.[20] They are still developing their self-awareness skills and their ability to manage their behavior. Crucially, they may not be able to demonstrate the same level of commitment to change or independence as adolescents and adults. This has important consequences for therapy, affecting everything from goal selection to how sessions are structured and the nature of practice assignments. At the same time, the school-age years present numerous opportunities for children to develop healthy attitudes and learn ways of responding to stuttering that reduce the likelihood of later concerns with self-esteem and self-confidence. This, in turn, can minimize the adverse impact of stuttering on quality of life, something that is commonly experienced by adolescents and adults who stutter. If children can learn at an early age that what they say is valued—even if it is produced disfluently[21]—then this can go a long way toward diminishing the adverse impact of stuttering that they might otherwise experience later in life.

11.3.4 Stuttering Also Affects School-Age Children's Caregivers Differently

Another way in which treating school-age children who stutter differs from treating younger children who stutter is seen in the responses of caregivers. As parents and others begin to recognize that their child did not "grow out" of stuttering at an earlier age, they may worry more about how stuttering might affect their child's life.[22,23] For example, they may raise concerns about the potential effects of bullying, and they may wonder about whether or how stuttering will affect the child's later school performance, employment opportunities, and overall success in life. This concern can lead to an even greater sense of urgency for their child to make progress both in and out of treatment. In response to this increased worry about the impact of stuttering on the child's future, caregivers often become concerned that their child is not practicing enough or focusing enough on their speech. This can result in parents placing greater pressure on the child's communication, whether intentionally or unintentionally.[24] Teachers, too, may experience increasing concern about how to respond to a child's stuttering at school, and this can compound the difficulties that children experience, in and out of the classroom.[25,26]

The child's continued stuttering can also have an impact on the caregivers themselves,[27] as they continue to worry about the role that they may have played in their child's development—and lack of recovery from stuttering. They may have understandable fears about how to help their children cope with stuttering as they grow, and this can increase the impact of stuttering on the entire family. Thus, the experiences and hopes of caregivers must also be considered in treatment for children who stutter.[23] The discussions that SLPs have with caregivers of school-age children are going to be different from those they have with the caregivers of children in the preschool years. Accounting for the needs of caregivers is another reason that effective therapy for school-age children who stutter should be broad based, addressing not only the child's speech fluency but also their overall experience of stuttering, as well as the experiences and the reactions of those in the child's environment.

11.4 Comprehensive Treatment for School-Age Children Who Stutter

Readers will likely identify a consistent theme that runs throughout many of the chapters in this book: stuttering treatment should not focus only on observable stuttering behaviors. Although there may be differences of opinion about the specific nature and cause(s) of stuttering or about the specific form that assessment and treatment should take,[2,28] we believe that it is fair to say that there is general consensus across theorists and clinicians alike about the fact that stuttering is a complex condition that involves many different aspects of a person's life.

11.4.1 A Framework for Understanding Stuttering

Accounting for the various aspects of the experience of stuttering can be confusing, even for clinicians and researchers who specialize in stuttering and its treatment. To make the complexities of stuttering assessment and therapy easier to understand, we find it helpful to use a widely accepted framework for describing human health experience in general. In this chapter (as in ▶ Chapter 8), we use the ICF. This framework is used in the field of speech-language pathology in general, in part because it forms the core of our scope of practice,[29] and in part because it highlights the ways in which different aspects of the experience of communication issue can relate to one another.

The general structure of the ICF is described in ▶ Chapter 8, so we will not go into specifics here. Put simply, the ICF describes the overall experience of behavioral and health disorders in terms of two primary interacting components: (1) body function and structure and (2) activities and participation. Interacting with both of these components is (3) personal and environmental context. First, the *body function and structure* component includes all of the major structures and functions of the human body, along with the ways in which people can experience *impairments* in those body structures and functions. Second, *activities and participation* include the various activities that people might wish to engage in as they participate in their lives, as well as the limitations or restrictions on either that may be associated with the impairment. Finally, the ways a person's experience of a condition or disorder such as stuttering can be affected by their own *personal* reactions to the situations they face, as well as the reactions of those in their *environment*. These key components of the ICF and their application to stuttering in school-age children are summarized in ▶ Table 11.4.

Table 11.4 Key components of the World Health Organization's International Classification of Functioning, Disability, and Health[3,30]

ICF component (and potential difficulty)	Definition	Relevance to stuttering[30]
Body function and structure *(impairment)*	• Body structure: all the physical parts of the human body (anatomy) • Body function: the ways in which structures work (physiology)	• Sensation of being stuck, losing control, or being unable to move forward when speaking that may lead to observable speech disruptions
Activities and participation *(activity limitations and participation restrictions)*	• Activities: what people want to be able to do in their lives (e.g., activities of daily living) • Participation: ways in which people want to engage in their lives	• Activities: reading aloud in class, asking or answering questions, talking to friends (limitations reflect difficulties with these activities) • Participation: socializing with others, achieving educational goals (Restrictions reflect difficulty with these aspects of participation)
Personal and environmental context	• Personal context: individual's affective, behavioral, and cognitive reactions • Environmental context: reactions of other people	• Affective: fear and anxiety, embarrassment, shame, frustration • Behavioral: avoidance, tension or struggle behaviors, observable speech disruptions • Cognitive: low self-esteem or self-confidence • Environmental: negative comments by others, bullying by peers

Applying the ICF framework to stuttering assumes that the *impairment* in body function for people who stutter reflects underlying differences in the various linguistic, motoric, temperamental processes[31] that arise from genetic[32] and neurological[33] differences commonly seen in people who stutter. This fundamental impairment ultimately results in what might be termed the primary symptom of stuttering as experienced by people who stutter,[30] that is, the sensation of being "stuck" when trying to speak. Adults who stutter describe this sensation as a "loss of control,"[34] or a moment in which they know what they want to say but are unable to say it. This sensation can lead the speaker to exhibit and experience various *reactions* that can be described as affective (feelings), behavioral (actions), or cognitive (thoughts). Common affective reactions include feelings of embarrassment, shame, frustration, and anxiety.[35] Common behavioral reactions include disruptions in speech fluency (i.e., speech disfluencies), physical tension or struggle,[36] and avoidance or escape behaviors.[37] Common cognitive reactions include lower self-esteem or self-confidence,[38] a reduced sense of self-efficacy,[39] or self-stigma.[40] People in the speaker's *environment* can also react, for example, by cutting the speaker off, finishing sentences, or bullying the speaker, and this, in turn, can increase the individual's own negative reactions to their stuttering.[41,42] The sensation of being stuck, combined with the internal and external negative reactions, can lead to *limitations* in daily activities such as introducing oneself, joining in conversations, telling a joke, and reading aloud or asking questions in class. If a child experiences difficulties in these daily activities, then this might contribute to broader *restrictions* in the child's ability or willingness participate in the educational setting or in learning to socialize with others.

The ICF model is helpful when working with school-age children who stutter because it allows clinicians to view stuttering in the larger context of the child's everyday experiences. In this way, it reduces the likelihood that clinicians will focus primarily or only on surface-level characteristics (i.e., speech fluency) and intentionally or inadvertently ignore the child's thoughts and feelings—and the role they play in both the experience of stuttering. In the next portion of this chapter, we will demonstrate how the ICF can support the development of a comprehensive set of treatment goals that address the entire experience of stuttering for the school-age child.

11.4.2 Selecting Appropriate Treatment Goals

As we have noted, treatment for school-age children who stutter should be tailored to the needs of each individual child and family. Even so, there are commonalities[43] in treatment goals and procedures that are relevant across children and their families, even as the specific procedures used for achieving these goals need to be individualized. We present these general goals below following the structure of the ICF, then we provide more specific details about how to implement them later in the chapter. (A summary of sample goal areas as reflected by the ICF framework is shown in ▶ Table 11.5.)

Impairment

According to people who stutter,[30] the fundamental core or underlying experience of the moment of stuttering involves a sensation of being stuck or of losing control of the speech mechanism. It is this sensation of being unable to move forward that is believed to lead to the disruptions in speech that are characterized as "stuttered" or "stutterlike" disfluencies. Thus, a common goal for stuttering therapy is to help speakers learn to identify and navigate through the sensation of feeling or being stuck.[1] The different therapeutic strategies for doing this can result in an overall reduction in the frequency of stuttering as well as qualitative changes in the form that stuttering takes (e.g., a reduction in the perceived severity of stuttering). Examples of goals that address this aspect of stuttering center on so-called speech modification or speech restructuring strategies[44,45] that seek to enhance fluency, as well as so-called stuttering modification strategies[46,47] that seek to help people stutter with less physical tension or struggle, so that stuttering moments are less disruptive to ongoing communication. (Note that these aspects of therapy can also be seen as relating to the child's reactions, covered in the next section. Although we often think about the components of the ICF model in fairly independent terms, it is necessary to recognize that they are in fact interacting and overlapping.[3]) A brief comparison of speech modification and stuttering modification strategies is shown in ▶ Table 11.6.

Child's Reactions

As one might imagine, the experience or sensation of being stuck or of losing control is not pleasant. In reaction, children who stutter may tense their muscles when speaking or avoid talking altogether as they attempt to cope with the underlying disruption in speech planning[36] or difficulty in producing speech smoothly (behavioral reactions). At the same time, they may feel embarrassed, anxious, or upset about the resulting disruption in fluency (affective reactions) and, over time, they might come to believe that they cannot communicate effectively (cognitive reactions).

Table 11.5 Summary of key treatment areas in terms of the International Classification of Functioning, Disability, and Health (ICF) model

ICF component	Sample goal areas
Impairment	• Help children learn to handle the sensation of feeling stuck to reduce the frequency of observable stuttering behavior using speech modification and stuttering modification strategies
Child's reactions	• Reduce the child's embarrassment, fear, shame, or other negative affective and cognitive reactions to stuttering • Reduce avoidance, tension, and other negative behavioral reactions
Environment's reactions	• Educate people in the environment so that they understand stuttering and are less likely to react negatively to it
Activity limitations and participation restrictions	• Ensure that children are speaking in all desired situations and engaging fully in social and educational interactions

Table 11.6 Speech modification compared to stuttering modification

	Speech modification	Stuttering modification
Overarching goal	• Reduction in frequency and severity of observable stuttering behavior	• Reduction in physical tension and struggle during moments of stuttering
Implementation schedule	• All (or nearly all) speech is modified to prevent moments of stuttering from occurring	• Only moments of stuttering are modified; nonstuttered speech is not modified
Sample treatment strategies	• Easy onset • Pausing and phrasing • Light articulatory contacts	• Cancellation • Pullout • Voluntary stuttering

A substantial literature from the field of psychology has described methods for helping people understand and ultimately change these types of affective, behavioral, and cognitive reactions[48,49] to a wide range of issues. These so-called cognitive therapy approaches have direct relevance to the treatment of school-age children who stutter, and in recent years several authors have described ways to use cognitive methods in stuttering therapy. These include cognitive behavioral therapy,[50] acceptance and commitment therapy,[51,52,53] and mindfulness[54] approaches, and there is a growing literature on the use of these types of cognitive therapy approaches in helping children who stutter (and their families) come to terms with stuttering so that it causes less adverse impact in their lives. For example, Murphy and colleagues have described how to use cognitive restructuring (a common cognitive therapy strategy) to "de-awfulize" stuttering so that children can learn to respond less negatively to moments of stuttering.[55,56] This helps children learn to tolerate the discomfort of stuttering rather than trying to run from or avoid it. As children become desensitized to moments of stuttering, and as they learn to cope with the sensation of loss of control, they can communicate more easily and more effectively.

Environment/Reactions

Children experience a wide variety of communication environments, and there can be notable differences in how other people in their family and community react to stuttering. As a result, children need to learn how to navigate their communication experiences at home, at school, in social settings, at community-based events, and in many other potential situations (e.g., sports, band, dance, on the school bus, etc.). Unfortunately, children who stutter often find themselves in an environment that does not understand stuttering.[1] Parents and other caregivers, teachers, peers, and even SLPs may harbor misperceptions and misunderstandings about stuttering and stuttering therapy. Given these challenges, children need therapeutic support as they learn to advocate for themselves, to educate the people around them about stuttering, and to respond appropriately and effectively to challenging situations such as bullying.[56,57]

Activity Limitations and Participation Restrictions

The challenges associated with stuttering can result in a situation where children are less willing or able to (1) perform daily activities associated with speaking and (2) participate fully in communication situations. Goals related to reducing these activity limitations and participation restrictions are the culmination of all of the general goals described earlier: helping children

respond differently to the sensation of being stuck (thereby changing their speech fluency or stuttering), helping children reduce their negative reactions to stuttering so they are less concerned about speaking differently from other people, and creating an environment that is supportive of their communication differences. Put simply, it is easier for children who stutter to perform daily activities related to speaking and to participate more fully in social interaction when they can speak and communicate more easily, think and feel less negatively about themselves and their stuttering, and have an environment that understands and accepts them. SLPs can further support reductions in adverse impact due to stuttering by specifically helping children learn to fully engage in daily activities involving speaking and to participate in social interaction, for example, by intentionally entering feared situations that they might otherwise have avoided and by being open about stuttering so that they are not held back by a fear of being "found out" as a person who stutters.

11.4.3 Focusing on Communication Rather than Speech Fluency as a Primary Outcome

As should by now be apparent, the goals of therapy for school-age children will likely involve a mix of improving communication attitudes, increasing the child's and caregivers' understanding about stuttering, fostering the child's sense of empowerment and self-acceptance, *and* making changes in speech production that enhance overt fluency and minimize the severity of stuttering behaviors. Still, it is important to recognize that children (and their families) often come to therapy with one goal in mind: to increase the child's fluency. As we work to create meaningful goals for each individual child, we need to understand *why* the family (and perhaps the child) sought therapy in the first place. More than likely, fluency is only part of a bigger picture. When we dig deeper into motivations for therapy, we often find a broader desire for the child to be able to *communicate* more easily and more effectively. The true goal is not just for the child to be fluent when speaking but also for the child to be able to say what they want to say without being held back.[20] Likewise, the wider motivation for therapy is often the desire for the child to succeed in school, in their career, and in their life as a whole, regardless of whether or not they stutter. Put differently, the caregivers' sincere wish for therapy is that it will help their child to be "okay"—even if they continue to stutter.[1]

"I just want him to be okay."

–Parent of a school-age child who stutters

The caregivers' and child's genuine thoughts about therapy and what they hope it will accomplish can often be more thoroughly unpacked in the early stages of the therapy process. For example, children may share that they wish that they could raise their hand in class or order for themselves at a restaurant, or they may reveal that they want to be able to tell a joke or a story to their friends.[58] These are concrete, real-world changes that would make a positive impact on the child's life. Importantly, these are changes that can be accomplished *regardless* of whether the child speaks fluently. Likewise, caregivers may report that they want their child to feel good about themselves and to succeed at school. At first, they may think that the only way to accomplish this goal is for the child to "be fluent." As they learn more about stuttering and communication as a whole, they often come to realize that this goal can be achieved *even if the child continues to stutter in some fashion.* SLPs should not be lulled into focusing only on fluency simply because this is what children and families think they want; a deeper conversation and exploration of the child's and family's true motivations for pursuing therapy may reveal *why* they seek fluency. By taking a broader perspective, clinicians may be able to help their young clients and their caregivers come to understand that their ultimate goals can be accomplished regardless of whether or how much the child continues to stutter.

In fact, one of the easiest ways for clinicians, children, and caregivers alike to ensure holistic treatment is to look past the observable stuttering behaviors altogether. This might seem counterintuitive, given that the child and family may believe that they are seeking treatment in order to help their child achieve fluency. Still, as we have stated, focusing only on fluency is not enough—and, in fact, it might be detrimental to achieving the most impactful goals of therapy. Research has shown that having a primary goal of "speaking fluently" can actually be associated with an *increased* adverse impact of stuttering on a person's life.[37] Moreover, although overt disfluencies are often the most noticeable and seemingly relevant aspect of stuttering for listeners, this may not be the case for speakers who stutter themselves. It is critically important for SLPs to understand—and ultimately treat—stuttering as it is experienced by the speaker who stutters.[37] As we discussed earlier, this means addressing the ways a child *feels* and *thinks* about stuttering while ensuring that they can *communicate effectively* so that stuttering does not interfere with their ability to live a full and fulfilling life.

Here is another way of looking at the goals of stuttering therapy: We want children to feel better about themselves and their communication than they did before they met us. From a listener's perspective, this might mean that overt stuttering behaviors have changed. From the children's perspective, however, this means that they can better tolerate the moment of stuttering and the sensation of the loss of control, that they can communicate more easily and more effectively, that they can speak with a greater sense of spontaneity[59] and comfort, that they can engage in social interaction with increased confidence and satisfaction, and that stuttering no longer has a negative impact on their life. Any and all of these potential therapy outcomes constitute success, both in the grand scheme and in daily interaction. To achieve these goals, clinicians need to become facilitators who enable children to expand their choices, to reduce their emotional reactivity, and to improve their overall resilience,[60,61] thereby leading to a better long-term quality of life. The clinical practices that SLPs employ in the service of these goals must be flexible enough to allow for differences in children's skills, interests, and characteristics— and therein lie the challenges and the joys of working with school-age children who stutter and their families.

11.4.4 The Importance of Practice-Based Evidence

As any student in any field knows all too well, there is a difference between how something is presented in a textbook and how it is realized in real life. This is certainly the case when it comes to stuttering therapy. What we present in this chapter reflects the combined experience of advanced clinicians and researchers who have dedicated their lives to the study of stuttering assessment and treatment. We recognize that our experience allows us to adapt treatment to the individual needs of our clients seemingly effortlessly, but we do not come by this ability by magic or without thought. Instead, we continuously adapt and develop our clinical decision-making based on the best-available evidence from the ever-expanding research literature and our growing clinical experience. On a day-to-day basis, however, what allows us to make our decisions about how to proceed in therapy with our clients who stutter is the *data* that we collect in an ongoing fashion. This is particularly important as we seek to uphold and adhere to the principles of *evidence-based practice* (EBP), as is the expectation and obligation of all SLPs.[62,63,64] Certainly, one key aspect of EBP is the published literature.[65] Another key aspect, however, is the *practice-based evidence* (PBE) that each clinician collects with each client and family with whom they work as we move through the therapy process.[66] That is, SLPs must evaluate the relationship between what is addressed within therapy and the child's performance and experiences in the real world. This is particularly important when it comes to treating school-age children who stutter, for the existing evidence base in the published literature is sorely lacking.[28,62] Put simply, we need more research on the treatment of school-age children who stutter; this is a point on which even those who approach stuttering from different philosophical perspectives agree.[2,28]

To compensate for the lack of empirical evidence, it becomes particularly important for clinicians to *collect their own data* in order to evaluate the appropriateness and effectiveness of the treatment that they provide to school-age children who stutter and their families. Of course, ongoing data collection is always important for supporting clinical decision-making; in the case of school-age stuttering, however, it is even more crucial. Therefore, as we discuss treatment options in the next section, we also discuss methods for documenting the changes that clients might experience, so that we can keep our focus on ensuring that treatment is moving in the right direction—that is, helping school-age children communicate more easily and more effectively and minimizing the burden that stuttering might cause in their lives.

11.5 Sample Treatment Goals, Procedures, and Activities for School-Age Children Who Stutter

Given the material covered thus far as background and foundation, we now turn to specific treatment procedures and activities for individual school-age children who stutter and their families. Again, we emphasize that these procedures and activities will not all be necessary for all children and families. Different children will likely have different needs and priorities for what treatment should emphasize, both for the child and for the family as a whole. For example, some children will come to treatment with much higher levels of resilience than others[61]; these children may need less work on self-advocacy before moving to other areas of treatment. Other children may come to therapy with higher levels of embarrassment or shame; these children may need considerably more work on self-acceptance before moving on to other areas of treatment. It is incumbent upon the SLP to select appropriate therapy components based on the individual needs of their clients and to apply them in the order that is appropriate for each person; here, we seek to present a broad menu of options that may be considered and selected as necessary, based on a careful review of the literature, the child's and caregivers' needs, and the clinician's perceptions and experience. As before, we organize these options in terms of the ICF model to ensure that we address the entirety of the stuttering experience. (Note: Because the specific format and language required for treatment goals differ depending upon the institution or location, we have not presented these goals in a format that might meet the requirements of an Individualized Educational Plan [IEP] for a particular school district in the United States. Instead, the goals that we present below are worded generally, so that they can easily be adapted to different formats and requirements.)

11.5.1 Sample Goals, Procedures, and Activities: Stuttering Impairment

Helping children change the way they cope with the underlying sensation of being stuck involves helping them understand what they are doing during the moment of stuttering itself.[67,68] This begins with helping the child to build a strong foundational understanding of their speech mechanism (e.g., the "speech machine"[1]) and the ways they use it when speaking—and when stuttering.[20] A specific goal for this aspect of therapy might be, "The child will demonstrate knowledge of the parts of the body involved in producing speech." Sample procedures include teaching the child how we use the respiratory, phonatory, and articulatory systems alone and together to produce speech. For example, the clinician and child might talk about the speech mechanism, draw pictures of the parts of the body involved in producing speech, identify moments of "fake" stuttering in the speech of the clinician, and, ultimately, in the child's own speech. Relevant data might include evaluations of the child's ability to describe the speech mechanism to others and to relate the occurrence of physical tension to specific physiological systems.

Increasing awareness of stuttering in this way is an excellent first step that can help children to "stay present" during a moment of loss of control so that later in therapy, they can learn how to make changes in their stuttering behavior in real

time. Thus, another specific goal for this aspect of therapy might be, "The child will demonstrate the ability to identify a moment of stuttering in their own speech." Sample procedures might involve tallying activities, in which a child counts their moments of stuttering. This is a powerful way to build behavioral or physical awareness of stuttering, whether this awareness occurs before, during, or after the moment of speech disruption. Tallying activities can be as simple as asking a child to make a mark on a piece of paper when they feel stuck while talking; doing so in and of itself supports ongoing data collection and reflection. Importantly, such activities must *not* be done in a punitive fashion. The purpose of identifying moments of stuttering is not so that the child must "fix" their speech or recognize that they have made a "mistake"; we do not wish to send the message that "more stuttering is bad" or "less stuttering is good." Instead, the goal of these types of activities is to help children better understand and "tune in" to what they are doing when they talk. We want them to be able to experience stuttering during these exercises, so that they can learn more about stuttering. This helps build their self-monitoring skills; these exercises also help them to learn to tolerate the moment of stuttering and to experience stuttering without negative judgment from themselves or us. Rather than viewing stuttering as something to suppress or hide or feel bad about, children are being praised for their ability to "catch" or be aware of moments of stuttering. Once the child has an increased awareness of when they are stuttering, we can guide them toward staying present *during* a moment of stuttering. These lessons will be crucial for later work in which they learn to modify moments of stuttering if and when they choose to do so.

Another common goal for helping children learn to cope with the sensation of being stuck is to help them learn to hold on to, or stay in, a moment of stuttering while they are producing it. Thus, a goal might be, "The child will demonstrate the ability to 'freeze' while producing a moment of stuttering and remain in it." At first, this may seem counterintuitive, in that it is reasonable to assume that our goal is to help children move through moments of stuttering more easily. This is certainly true—we do teach the child how to move through stuttering moments efficiently. Before they can do that, however, they need to develop the self-monitoring skills to "catch" a moment of stuttering in real time. The ability to catch a moment of stuttering "on the fly" helps the child to develop the presence of mind to be able to make changes in stuttering. Staying with a moment of stuttering in real time also helps the child to tolerate stuttering enough that they do not feel compelled to rush through or run from the sensation of being stuck. We can accomplish this goal through "speech detective" or "catch me" games,[1] in which we "play around" with stuttering to help children learn more about what they do with their speech mechanisms during stuttering. Relevant data include tallies of the number of moments of stuttering that the child is able to catch and the speed with which they catch them (i.e., before, after, or during production).

▶ Table 11.7 lists sample goals and activities for addressing this aspect of treatment. Importantly, these activities also support the child's ability and willingness to stutter more freely and openly, and this, too, helps them learn to respond more easily to the sensation of being stuck. Rather than trying to hide, avoid, or mask stuttering, they can allow themselves to "let stuttering out" more easily. The resulting speech behavior—that is, speech that may be disrupted but does not contain

Table 11.7 Samples goals, activities, and data: Impairment

Goal	Sample activity to address goal	Examples of data collection
The child will demonstrate knowledge of the parts of the body involved in producing speech by creating a speech machine drawing	• Talk about the speech mechanism, draw pictures of the parts of the body involved in producing speech	• Create a speech machine • Describe the speech mechanism to others • Relate physical tension to specific physiological systems
The child will demonstrate the ability to identify a moment of stuttering in their own speech by tallying 10 moments of stuttering	• Tallying activities, in which a child counts their moments of stuttering	• Number of times a child marks on a piece of paper that they feel "stuck" while talking
The child will demonstrate the ability to "freeze" while producing a moment of stuttering and remain in it 10 times	• "Speech detective" or "catch me" games,[1] in which we "play around" with stuttering to help children learn more about what they do with their speech mechanisms during stuttering	• Number of times the child is able to freeze in a moment a stuttering • Child's ability to describe feelings and physical sensations during a moment of stuttering

tension or struggle behaviors—might be called "easier stuttering." As the child is able to tolerate the sensation of being stuck, they

becp,e able to stutter more openly, with less avoidance behaviors. Ultimately, this can lead to more forward-flowing speech.

Spotlight: Targeting Stuttering Impairment

Most, if not all, school-age children who stutter can benefit from work related to increasing their understanding of the moment of stuttering and the ways in which they respond to the underlying sensation of being stuck or of losing control. Thus, this is a component of therapy that we use for nearly all school-age children with whom we work. In particular, we often find that school-age children who stutter have not received sufficient support in learning about stuttering, even if they have previously been in therapy. When we talk with clinicians who are facing challenges in stuttering therapy, we often find that one of the key reasons is that they have not spent sufficient time building a foundation for the child's understanding of speaking and stuttering.

Consider the common situation of a school-age child who stutters whose prior testing and assessment have revealed low awareness of stuttering—although the child certainly knows that they stutter, they do not necessarily understand what they are doing during the moment of stuttering, and they cannot always identify stuttering in their speech. Therefore, an appropriate (and necessary) focus of therapy is to help them understand the parts of the body involved in producing speech (brain, lungs, larynx, and articulators)—presented at whatever level of complexity is appropriate for the child's age and cognitive development. This is followed by a detailed exploration of what they do with their speech mechanism when they are speaking fluently and what they do with their speech mechanism when they are stuttering. The more they learn about the moment of stuttering and how their speech mechanism is involved, the better prepared they will be for later work on changing the moment of stuttering (so-called stuttering modification techniques[46,47]). Children at this age and stage of therapy also benefit from "catch-me" and "speech detective" activities,[1] in which they explore the physical and cognitive/emotional sensations of being stuck and the surface speech disruptions that may result as they attempt to cope with their difficulty in producing speech in that moment.

11.5.2 Sample Goals, Procedures, and Activities: Child's Reactions to Stuttering

"Be yourself; everyone else is already taken."

–Oscar Wilde

The reactions that children may have toward their stuttered speech and the impact that it has on their quality of life has been investigated in several studies.[10,11,12] A principal finding from this work is that school-aged children who stutter experience negative reactions to their stuttering. This is not surprising, of course, but it is still important to recognize that such negative reactions to stuttering are often reflected in magnified affective, behavioral, and cognitive reactions to their speaking ability and difficulty, as well as significantly compromised communication in daily situations. More specifically, research has shown that the experience of stuttering for school-age children may involve elevated anxiety, interpersonal stress, and even social phobia.[6,15,35,69,70] These responses are compounded by the variable nature of stuttering,[71,72] which leads children to stutter more in some situations or at some times than in other situations or at other times. The uncertainty about stuttering

can be extremely frustrating for children who stutter,[73] and can lead them to struggle even more. Importantly, even children who do not stutter show some degree of negative reaction to their speaking ability.[12] Thus, the goals of therapy addressing negative reactions to stuttering do not need to seek an outcome of "zero negative reactions" in order to be successful. Helping a child achieve more neutral reactions to stuttering and speaking is a reasonable outcome, provided those reactions do not interfere with communication.

Thus, a common and important aspect of therapy for school-age children who stutter involves reducing negative emotions; this is often accomplished through desensitization and other cognitive therapy approaches that are designed to help the child become more comfortable with stuttering[2,55] (▸ Table 11.8). Desensitization, or the process of reducing negative thoughts and feelings through gradual exposure, is a key part of the treatment process, as it helps the child to be able to stutter more freely, to reduce avoidance of stuttering, and to minimize the fear of stuttering. A relevant goal might be, "The child will demonstrate reduced negative reactions to moments of stuttering." Common procedures for achieving this goal include exposure therapy, in which children learn—gradually—to allow stuttering in their speech while they systematically reduce their negative

Table 11.8 Sample goals, activities, and data: child's reactions to stuttering

Goal	Sample activity to address goal	Examples of data collection
The child will demonstrate reduced negative reactions to moments of stuttering	• Stutter openly by producing naturally occurring stuttering in a supportive environment (e.g., in the therapy room with us) • Voluntarily stutter to directly experience the behaviors and reactions associated with stuttering	• Number of times the child stutters openly or voluntarily stutters • Child self-reports about their feelings about stuttering • Standard tests and assessments related to their reactions of stuttering
The child will demonstrate reduced physical tension during moments of stuttering	• Produce speech at different tension levels with the aid of a 1–10 scale (1 being the most relaxed and 10 being the most struggled)	• Self-ratings or clinician ratings of the degree of tension
The child will attend a stuttering support group	• Research stuttering support organization with the child • Watch some videos of other people who stutter	• Self-reports about feelings related to meeting other people who stutter • Confirmation of attendance at a meeting (either virtual or face-to-face) • Number of times the child participates at a meeting

reactions. Children can learn to feel more comfortable stuttering by allowing naturally occurring stuttering to occur in a supportive environment (e.g., in the therapy room with us, while we encourage them to know that it is okay to stutter) or by using "voluntary" stuttering or "pseudostuttering" in order to directly experience the behaviors and reactions associated with stuttering—without the sensation of being stuck.[74,75,76] Relevant data may include children's self-reports about their feelings about stuttering, the number of times they were able to stutter openly or voluntarily along with the situations in which they were able to accomplish this, as well as results from standard tests and assessments of their reactions to their stuttering.[58,77]

As children learn to stutter with less fear and other negative responses, this leads to greater acceptance.[55] Acceptance in and of itself can help to reduce the adverse impact of stuttering overall. It can also help to reduce the physical struggle often associated with stuttering as the child learns not to wrestle with the sensation of being stuck. To achieve this, clinicians can build on the previously described foundational activities that help the child to increase their understanding and awareness of when and how they stutter. We like to explore pseudostuttering with more physical tension and then with less physical tension to help our students learn that they *can* make changes to how they stutter. These changes will require a significant amount of practice, but they provide a necessary foundation for later use of stuttering modification[46,47] strategies, if indicated

for a particular child. Speech modification strategies,[44] designed to reduce tension and struggle, can also be taught to reduce the behavioral reactions to the sensation of being stuck when speaking. Practicing these specific physical changes to the moment of stuttering (e.g., reducing muscular tension and moving forward in the utterance) can help the child to stutter more easily and with less physical tension.[46] Here, a relevant goal might be, "The child will demonstrate reduced physical tension during moments of stuttering," with ongoing data reflecting self-ratings or clinician ratings of the degree of tension.

As noted earlier, cognitive behavioral therapy strategies, including acceptance and commitment approaches and mindfulness-related procedures,[78] are also useful for helping children learn how to respond differently to difficulties in planning and producing speech.

Regardless of how much speech modification or stuttering modification is targeted in therapy, or experienced by the child, the most important goal is to help children learn that it is okay to stutter and to be a person who stutters. The more that children can learn and internalize that message, the easier it will be for them to cope with the fact that at times their speech will be different from the speech of their peers. And, when children believe that it is okay to stutter, they will come to recognize that *they* are okay—that they are not doing anything wrong when they stutter and that they should not judge themselves negatively because they sometimes do not produce speech fluently.

Spotlight: Targeting Child's Reactions to Stuttering

A common case scenario is the child whose stuttering is elevated (more frequent or physical tense moments of stuttering) in the classroom or when reading aloud in front of peers. Unfortunately, this increased difficulty is experienced in exactly those situations in which the child really wants to be able to talk easily (e.g., in front of peers). Therefore, an important component of therapy in such situations is to help students learn that "it is okay to stutter"—even in those situations where they wish that they could be fluent! SLPs typically experience this when school-age children express concern that they cannot participate in class the way other children can (e.g., they feel that they cannot ask or answer a question or read aloud like their peers can), or they cannot tell a joke like their friends can,[58] or they are afraid to speak lest they—or others—react negatively to their stuttering. Our job in such instances is not only to help them learn ways of coping with the sensation of being stuck, as described earlier, but also to help them learn to reduce their negative reactions to stuttering. The therapy builds upon prior work focused on educating children about speaking and stuttering, as described earlier, so that we can help children learn to tolerate—and ultimately accept—the moment of stuttering as something that sometimes happens when they are talking. Through exposure and desensitization therapy (teaching the child to use purposeful stuttering to become less fearful of it and helping them stutter in a way that may feel more comfortable for them), we help students learn to accept stuttering (affective reactions), to become less likely to avoid situations in which they might stutter (behavioral reactions), and to become less likely to judge themselves negatively or harshly because they stutter (cognitive reactions). As children learn that they are okay even though—and even when—they stutter, they become better able to cope with the difficult situations they face, and this ultimately helps them to improve their overall communication and to reduce the adverse impact of stuttering on their lives.

11.5.3 Sample Goals, Procedures, and Activities: Environment's Reactions to Stuttering

Educating the people in the child's environment about stuttering is a fundamental step in creating a supportive atmosphere (▶ Table 11.9). Importantly, the work that we do with caregivers, other family members, teachers, and peers has a bidirectional impact: the more we help the people in the child's environment to cope effectively with the child's stuttering and their own worries, the more it helps the child to do the same. This, in turn, helps the family and other important people in the child's life to feel less worried about stuttering and their child. One of our most fundamental goals when working with people in the child's environment is ensuring that they understand the nature of stuttering. For a child in the school-age years, this means helping parents and others to understand that, in all likelihood, the child will continue to stutter, in some fashion, throughout their life. It also means educating the child's support system that the adverse impact of stuttering may be greater in later childhood than in the preschool years. That means that the child is likely to need emotional support, not only from the SLP but also from the parents, other family members, teachers, and peers, and that the need for this support is likely to increase over time.

Depending upon the setting in which they work, clinicians may face challenges in working with parents, caregivers, or other family members. In the school environment in the United States, for example, clinicians might have relatively little contact with families—and even if they do, they may not have the time needed to guide caregivers through their own journey of stuttering acceptance. Therefore, much of the work in developing a supportive environment for the child may need to be done *through* the child rather than directly with the family. For example, helping children to increase their openness about stuttering will teach them how to discuss stuttering with their families and others in their environment. A goal might be, "The child will discuss basic facts about stuttering with family members, teachers, and peers." As children develop their expertise about stuttering in general and about their own stuttering in specific, they also develop the confidence they need for teaching others about their communication differences. This experience can be tremendously empowering for children in and of itself.

Similarly, engaging in self-disclosure activities,[79,80,81] in which children learn to openly acknowledge their stuttering, can help further reduce shame while simultaneously educating others about stuttering. For example, "The child will acknowledge their stuttering openly when talking to a friend" is an example of a therapy goal that targets self-disclosure. Of course, doing this can be quite challenging, especially if a child has previously worked hard to hide or avoid stuttering. Accordingly, we always begin such activities in a safe space (e.g., with us in the therapy room) before practicing with others. We then guide children through a hierarchy from easier to harder situations in which they can self-disclose (e.g., talking with a parent first and then, when ready, talking to a teacher), in order to provide support and foster generalization of skills to increasingly real-world situations.[82] Such activities help children learn to be proactive in dealing with stuttering while simultaneously giving them control over whether and when they tell others about their stuttering. The child's disclosure can also foster discussions about the nature of stuttering, thereby removing much of the "mystery" surrounding stuttering. This can ultimately lead to increased community awareness about stuttering and about people who stutter.

"Self-disclosure is easy! I'm just telling people the truth about me."
–Child who stutters

Indeed, we routinely work on how children can talk openly about stuttering, so that their peers, teachers, and caregivers will learn from them that stuttering is just a characteristic of how they talk and not something to be embarrassed about or ashamed of. We model different ways of talking about stuttering, we role-play responses to the comments of other children,[81] and we practice how to describe stuttering to others (e.g., "sometimes when I talk, I repeat sounds or words" or, even more simply, "I stutter"). Certainly, attaining the ability to talk about stuttering in an accepting fashion builds on a foundation of understanding (impairment) and acceptance (reactions) of stuttering, and comes with diligent practice.

In order to foster ongoing education about both the nature and treatment of stuttering for people in the child's environment,

Table 11.9 Sample goals, activities, and data: environment's reactions to stuttering

Goal	Sample activity to address goal	Examples of data collection
The child will discuss basic facts about stuttering with family members, teachers, and peers	• Research facts about stuttering • Compile a list of facts about stuttering • Practice explaining facts and answering questions	• Number of people the child educates
The child will acknowledge their stuttering openly when talking to a friend	• Brainstorm ways to self-disclose • Practice self-disclosure using role-play within therapy	• Number of self-disclosure scripts • Number of times the child self-discloses
The child will demonstrate appropriate responses to negative comments made by others	• Brainstorm possible responses • Role-play possible responses • Practice how to describe stuttering to others (e.g., "sometimes when I talk, I repeat sounds or words" or, even more simply, "I stutter")	• Number of times the child appropriately responds during role-play • Number of times the child appropriately responds to negative comments
The child will educate people in his life about the nature and treatment of stuttering	• Research facts about stuttering • Compile a list of facts about stuttering • Practice explaining facts and answering questions • Practice giving presentation within therapy • Give presentations to their class or other social groups	• Number of other people educated about stuttering

we encourage regular discussions between the child and care-givers about stuttering in general, and about the specific goals that a child is addressing at the time, both in and out of therapy. Children may give very brief presentations containing factual information related to stuttering (e.g., the prevalence of stutter-ing, the fact that more boys than girls stutter, etc.). This may be done first with family members, as the child may not yet be ready to talk about stuttering outside the comfort of home. Later, the child may be ready to give presentations about stuttering to their class or other social groups.[56] Children can vary the complexity of their presentations, for example, by describing basic facts about stuttering early in the therapy process and exploring theories of stuttering onset or therapy strategies later in therapy, as their knowledge and understanding develops. In addition, children may feel that it is helpful to discuss the impact of stuttering on their everyday life and communication, rather than just basic facts about stuttering. Child-delivered presentations[56] about stuttering are an effective way to educate other people about stuttering while also having the benefit of reducing the stigma associated with stuttering.

One common and troubling aspect of the environmental reactions to stuttering that we wish to highlight in particular is bullying.[83] Bullying is particularly problematic for children who stutter, not only because it increases the difficulty they experi-ence with communication but also because it can increase social isolation. Social isolation in and of itself is a significant risk factor for greater adverse impact from stuttering.[56] Helping children cope effectively with bullying includes educating them about stuttering and bullying, reducing their negative reactions to their own stuttering, and helping them learn to respond effectively and appropriately to the negative comments and behaviors of others.[57] Teaching such self-advocacy skills supports the child's development of self-esteem and self-acceptance. Goals for this aspect of therapy might include, "The child will demon-strate appropriate responses to negative comments made by others." The identification of appropriate responses can be a key focus of therapy,[56] and the data collected in and out of sessions could include the child's and the clinician's observations of how the child handled such difficult situations.

Importantly, not all environmental responses to a child's stut-tering should be viewed as negative. For example, a growing body of research shows that participation in support groups can help reduce a child's negative reaction to stuttering by providing a supportive network of people who understand and accept stuttering.[84,85] It is important to note that support groups are not the same as treatment groups. Although both types of groups have their place in the treatment process, treat-ment groups are often used as a means to target specific goals that the child may be working toward in therapy, but they are practicing within a group setting. Support groups, on the other hand, are not as likely to have specific speech-related goals attached to them. Instead, they offer opportunities for the child to speak freely about stuttering with others who may be at similar or different places in the treatment process (or not in treatment at all). Although SLPs can help facilitate the process of self-acceptance for the child who stutters, belonging to a community of children who stutter, in which they can safely share their thoughts, feelings, and experiences, is a powerful way to reduce isolation while normalizing the experience of stuttering. (Note that such activities can appropriately be viewed as involving both *environmental* reactions and *personal* reactions, as they cross domains in the ICF model.)

As with much of the literature in the field, the majority of research on the impact of support/self-help groups has focused on adults who stutter.[37,86,87,88,89,90] Still, a growing literature demonstrates the value of stuttering support and self-help activities and experiences for children, including participation in stuttering support groups and camps.[84,85,91,92,93] Support groups can also offer parents the opportunity to meet and talk with other parents who have faced similar issues in raising a child who stutters. This can be empowering for both groups, and it can help reduce the feeling of isolation. Another benefit of support groups is that they may be utilized even after formal treatment ends as a way for the child to continue working on generalization and maintenance of skills learned in therapy. Thus, we routinely introduce children and their families to the various support/self-help organizations for people who stutter. We are fortunate to have several organizations dedicated to the needs of children who stutter and their families. In the United States, this includes the National Stuttering Association (www.WeStutter.org), Friends: The National Association of Young People Who Stutter (www.FriendsWhoStutter.org), SAY: The Stuttering Association for the Young (www.SAY.org), and the Stuttering Foundation (www.StutteringHelp.org). Worldwide, there are many other organizations focused on helping those who are affected by stuttering; a comprehensive list is offered by the International Stuttering Association (www.isastutter.org). As children participate in stuttering support and self-help activities, they gain the opportunity to meet other children who stutter. Spending time with children who share their experiences helps them see that they are not alone in facing their stuttering, and this in and of itself can be a powerful lesson.[88] Support groups that include parents, caregivers, and families also help the important people in the child's life to see people who are living their lives successfully despite—or even because of—the fact that they stutter. This helps foster a sense of hope and optimism about their child's future. Support/self-help organizations give people who stutter the opportunity to speak freely in a safe space, and they provide them a place to be themselves, regardless of whether or how much they stutter. Although people who participate in support or self-help groups benefit in varying ways, one common outcome is the overall reduction in the adverse impact on the quality of life attributed to stuttering.[84,86,85,87,94] It is no exaggeration to say that we have seen children and care-givers experience life-changing growth during a single weekend at a conference hosted by a support organization; ongoing par-ticipation can bring even greater gains. Put simply, we strive to connect every child and family with whom we work with a stut-tering support organizations in one fashion or another,[89] and we are always gratified by the results.

"If you stutter, you're not alone."
–Motto of the National Stuttering Association

"If you stutter, you have friends."
–Motto of Friends: The National Association of Young People Who Stutter

---

Spotlight: Targeting Environment Reactions to the Child's Stuttering

A common situation we face with respect to the environment's reactions to stuttering is the situation in which a parent is actually more concerned about stuttering than the child is. There are many reasons for this; one key factor is the parents' ability to look toward the future and envision the problems that the child *might* experience as a result of stuttering. Not all of the feared outcomes are likely to come to pass, though it is understandable for parents to worry about the potential consequences of stuttering and to try to take steps to reduce the likelihood that their worst fears will come true. Therefore, we often find it important to educate parents about the experiences that people who stutter do actually have in their lives. This process has typically already started by the time a child reaches the school-age years; education of parents is an important component in many approaches to early childhood stuttering therapy. Still, the role of the parents—and the information that they need to know—changes as the child enters the school-age years. It is crucial for parents to receive updated information about stuttering so that they will be prepared to support their children through the many changes that they face. It is also crucial for parents to come to terms with the fact that their child stutters so that they are less likely to put inappropriate pressure on their child to speak fluently all the time when that can be quite difficult for children to do. Thus, parents will need to understand that the goals of therapy involve more than just increasing speech fluency, so it is important for clinicians to provide necessary background information to parents, in person during therapy sessions or via handouts and other materials. Another excellent way to accomplish this goal is to connect parents with adults who stutter, so that the parents can see that it *is* possible for their child to continue stuttering yet still live a good and fulfilling life. Seeing adults who stutter who are successfully pursuing and achieving their life goals can help reduce parents' fears about the future. Yet another way to educate parents is to encourage children to share their own thoughts about stuttering with their parents so that the parents can come to understand what stuttering is *really* like—not just what they fear it might be like. Of course, this does lead to parents hearing about the negative experiences that their children might have, but fostering open lines of communication in this way gives parents the opportunity to provide support and encouragement to their children, and this connection can have remarkable benefits for the child and parents alike. Working together, parents and children can come to understand that stuttering does not have to have a negative impact on the child's life and that there is much that they can do together.

11.5.4 Sample Goals, Procedures, and Activities: Activity Limitations and Participation Restrictions

The sensation of being stuck when speaking, the emotional and cognitive discomfort that accompanies that feeling, the physical reactions and avoidance that result from that feeling, and the environmental reactions to speech disruptions all combine to cause the child who stutters to experience adverse impact in the form of activity limitations and participation restrictions involving communication. Moreover, the negative emotions and cognitive reactions to stuttering experienced by young people have been shown to directly impact their participation in social events, their development of friendships, their school success, and ultimately their future career choices.[10,11,35,95] Therefore, an appropriately broad conceptualization of the impact of stuttering (and an appropriately broad approach to stuttering therapy) should address surface behaviors along with the intertwined consequences for the child's overall quality of life.

One of the most important ways to achieve this goal is to ensure that treatment activities are designed to promote generalization to real-world settings as early as possible.[82] This means that clinicians must not create goals that are geared only toward improving fluency or attitudes or communication in the clinical setting. Instead, goals must be comprehensive and

target all aspects of the experience of stuttering in all of the various communication contexts where the child interacts. Examples are shown in ▸ Table 11.10. Note that generalization should not only be targeted at the end of the therapy process; it must also be integrated throughout intervention. Only by addressing generalization right from the beginning of therapy will clinicians be able to help their clients expand their success beyond the therapy setting. Further, it is only by expanding success beyond the therapy setting that children who stutter can overcome the potential activity limitations and participation restrictions that are so commonly a part of the experience of stuttering. Goals should be written to target objectives outside of the therapy room as quickly as possible. Examples of ways generalization can be targeted include teaching peers about stuttering at school, ordering food at a restaurant while stuttering on purpose, and making a phone call while using speech or stuttering modification.

A particularly important aspect of overcoming activity limitations and participation restrictions associated with stuttering is the reduction of sound, word, or situational avoidance. The reasons that children engage in avoidance are particularly important for clinicians to understand. Generally, children avoid stuttering because they are embarrassed by it or afraid of it. They may be afraid not only of the discomfort associated with the moment of being stuck but also of the reactions of parents, teachers, and

Table 11.10 Sample goals, activities, and data: activity limitations and participation restrictions

Goal	Sample activity to address goal	Examples of data collection
The child will engage in activities and situations that are presently avoided	• Create a hierarchy of feared situations • Start at bottom of hierarchy (easiest situation) and slowly engage in the environment. Talking about the situation, role-playing the situation, or even entering the situation may be the first steps before the child actively participates • Examples of hierarchies might be working toward raising hand in class, ordering at a restaurant, or talking on the phone	• Lists of small steps within hierarchy • Tally when the child enters the situations • Tally when child meets each level of the hierarchy

peers who may respond negatively to stuttering. Reducing avoidance, in all its forms, can help children to increase their ability to perform daily activities and participate fully in life. A sample goal for reducing avoidance might be, "The child will engage in activities and situations that are presently avoided," and data collection can involve lists of the situations themselves and tallies of the child's success in facing those situations. It is important to note that the child's fluency in these situations is irrelevant; the goals are to *enter* and *participate in* an activity or situation, regardless of whether or how much the child stutters when doing so. The more that we can help children understand the negative consequences of avoidance, the more they will come to understand the value of speaking when they want to speak, rather than selecting whether, when, or how much to speak based on their fear of stuttering or its sequelae.

Another important way for SLPs to reduce the overall adverse impact of stuttering on children's lives is to maintain contact with them over the long term in order to monitor progress and make adjustments as the child faces new situations over time. One of the biggest mistakes we can make in stuttering treatment is to assume a definitive endpoint to the clinical interaction. This expectation on the part of the SLP or the child and family is problematic in a number of ways. First, discharging the child from therapy without developing a comprehensive monitoring plan can lead children who stutter and their caregivers to assume that treatment is over forever and will no longer be needed at any time in the child's life. If (and when) this turns out not to be the case, the situation might be viewed as "relapse."[96,97] The term "relapse" itself is associated with negative stigma, and it may lead children and their families to feel that the child (or the clinician) has failed in some fashion, even though this is not the case. The clinician should create the expectation for children and their caregivers that stuttering and its consequences may require some type of intervention at various points across the lifespan. For example, SLPs may work with children who do very well in therapy in the school-age years and no longer require formal treatment services. When these same children approach high school, however, they move on to more challenging communication situations that are very different from those they successfully navigated in middle school. They may also need to discuss specific situations such as job interviews, class presentations in front of peers, and talking with people they find attractive. Additional therapy or support may be necessary to help them deal with these situations; this is perfectly normal. For reasons such as these, children who stutter and their families should maintain some connection with a clinician, a trusted friend, or a support/self-help organization to gain the encouragement they might need in coping with their stuttering—and ensuring minimal adverse impact—throughout their lives. One way of achieving this is through regular "check-ins" with the clinician, perhaps consisting of brief phone calls, online video check-ins, or e-mails. The main goal of maintaining these relationships is for children to understand that support and help are available if they ever need further treatment or advice—and, if they do they have not failed or done anything wrong; it is simply the nature of dealing with a chronic condition such as stuttering.

Spotlight: Targeting Activity Limitations and Participation Restrictions

When children come to us exhibiting behavior patterns that involve avoidance, we immediately recognize that we will need to engage in treatment goals and activities focused on helping them overcome their fears so that they speak freely and openly in any situation. Some particularly common situations in which children are likely to avoid speaking involve asking or answering questions in class or reading aloud. The result of these behavior patterns is reduced participation in the academic setting. Children who are reluctant to participate in class may be worried about how their peers will react to stuttering; they may also be worried about how much effort may be required on their part to say what they want to say. To address these concerns, we talk directly with our clients about their underlying reactions toward stuttering. We seek to and determine the level at which they feel comfortable participating in class, and then we seek to increase that level through gentle and carefully paced guidance toward greater participation. Note that in some cases, children may not be ready to participate in class at all. They may first need significant work in addressing underlying reactions toward stuttering. When we all agree that they are ready to move toward participating more fully in class, we discuss goals for how often and in what context they will volunteer to participate in class. Structuring therapy in this way can help reduce the children's fears that they will be called upon before they are ready to participate. Thus, children can go into class knowing what their goals are, knowing how they will work to accomplish their goals, and knowing that they will not be put in overly distressing situations while they are still working toward easier and fuller participation in their educational settings. Note that we must also involve and engage classroom teachers in the therapy process when we establish these types of goals. This will allow them to react appropriately and to provide feedback to the clinician, caregivers, and even the child about how the plan is proceeding.

Another common situation in which school-age children who stutter may experience limitations in their daily activities and reduced participation is in everyday social situations. Indeed, as children move through the school-age years and toward adolescence, a large part of their social time may be spent with friends at malls, restaurants, or other establishments. In such settings, "placing an order" is an obligatory part of their conversational speech. People who stutter often report that not being able to order their own food is a frustrating experience,[58] and people may even resort to ordering something other than what they actually want. This can feel self-defeating, as the child may come to belief that stuttering must necessarily prevent them from getting what they want, not just at a restaurant but also in life as a whole. Thus, one of the more empowering activities we can have for children who stutter is to help them order their own food or ask questions when they are out in public. This can initially be addressed in therapy sessions as SLPs guide their students through the process of practicing ordering food from menus, asking questions related to a menu, and role-playing various scenarios that might occur in the real world. As children begin to feel more comfortable with the tasks—and, in particular, as they become more comfortable *stuttering* during these tasks—then the activities can be transferred out to the real world, where the clinician and clients can practice ordering food together, either in person or over the phone. In doing this, we want to be sure not to overwhelm the child by moving to real-world situations too quickly; therefore, we typically practice such activities gradually, moving up a hierarchy from easier to harder situations that take us from the therapy room to the real world. An example of a hierarchy for ordering food is shown in ▶ Table 11.11. (Note that following a hierarchy is also a great way to practice self-disclosure and pseudostuttering, as well as speech modification and stuttering modification strategies, as appropriate for each individual child.)

Table 11.11 Sample hierarchy for ordering food at a restaurant

Step	Task
1	Within therapy: research favorite restaurant online and looking over the menu
2	Practice ordering food from the menu with the clinician
3	Practice asking questions related to the menu
4	Role-play the ordering food situation within therapy
5	Practice self-disclosure, open stuttering, voluntary stuttering, or other modification strategies, as appropriate for each child
6	Observe while the clinician orders at restaurant (while voluntary stuttering)
7	Voluntarily stutter while at restaurant
8	Order food at a restaurant with support from clinician
End goal	Order food at a restaurant independently

11.6 Discussion

In this chapter, we sought to provide a general overview of important considerations in planning and implementing comprehensive therapy for school-age children who stutter. Throughout, we emphasized the importance of individualizing therapy to the needs of each specific child and family. Of course, we cannot cover all possible situations or outcomes in a single chapter, especially given our emphasis on the fact that "one size does not fit all" in stuttering therapy.[98] Still, as we bring this chapter to a close, we wish to address two additional considerations—the value of an empathetic clinician and the value of the therapeutic alliance—that significantly affect clinical decision-making and application with this population.

Building an effective working relationship with children who stutter is at the core of successful therapy. Effective clinicians are those who are professional and confident, and who display an understanding of the nature and treatment of stuttering.[99] Effective clinicians are also passionate and committed; they have a belief in the therapeutic process, and they express faith in the child's (and family's) ability to change. In addition to being empathetic,[100] effective clinicians are honest and able to relate to their clients on both personal and professional levels.[99]

One way that clinicians can express empathy is by showing respect for children as autonomous individuals—that is, as people who have meaningful agency in their own life decisions, commensurate with their age, development, and experience. This means collaborating with them in developing and individualizing therapy goals. Successful collaboration results from deep listening, asking meaningful questions, and providing validation. We must also be prepared to provide a safety net for school-age children who may be hurting as they come to terms with their differences. Although school-age children may be more adept at managing their wants and needs compared to younger children, they are still just developing. The respect that we show them, the belief that we express in their abilities, and the validation that we offer them are all invaluable for supporting their ability to cope effectively with stuttering.

The *therapeutic alliance* is the foundation of successful therapy.[101,102,103] It is a cooperative working relationship between the client and the clinician—a partnership that reflects the trust that the clinician and child will reach an agreement

about the goals of therapy and share an understanding of the processes to achieve these goals. Collaboration begins early in therapy as clinicians adjust their therapy methods to suit the needs and capacities of each individual client. The perspectives on these early needs in therapy do not have to match, and it is important not to be judgmental or defensive but to be open and direct the client and clinician work together to negotiate the therapeutic goals. Routinely checking on the child's and caregivers' perspectives is an important way to establish a strong alliance and increase positive outcomes.[101]

11.7 Future Directions

"Cupcakes are muffins that believed in miracles."
–Zen Buddhist quotation

As new data about stuttering emerge, we will need to continue examining our treatment practices. In particular, we must increase our understanding of the ways in which individual differences, as well as individual experiences in and out of therapy, may relate to stuttering treatment outcomes. As a field, we have achieved a strong consensus that stuttering treatment should be comprehensive;[2] we are still learning about the ways in which therapy can be better *individualized*. We must also work to ensure that all SLPs have adequate training and continuing education opportunities to understand how to address stuttering in a comprehensive manner. And we must continue to develop means of evaluating the changes that children make in therapy across a range of objectives (e.g., measuring success not just in terms of changes in observable stuttering behavior but also in terms of the other aspects of therapy, such as reductions in negative reactions, increases in functional communication, and improvements in quality of life).[58] Although our field has made and continues to make great strides in improving our understanding, assessment, and treatment of stuttering, we still have work to do.

11.8 Conclusion

Stuttering treatment for school-age children should focus on the entire experience of stuttering, addressing the unique needs of individual children and their families. Common components of therapy can be described in terms of the WHO's ICF model, meaning that therapy should address several related but distinct components. Aspects of therapy related to the *impairment* include strategies to help the child manage the experience of being stuck or of losing control when talking, so that they can move forward in speaking. Aspects of therapy related to the *child's affective, behavioral, and cognitive reactions* relate to helping children understand—and, ultimately change—the way they react to the sensation of being stuck, so that they can feel less embarrassed or ashamed of stuttering, are less likely to avoid moments of stuttering, can judge themselves less negatively, and, generally, can come to accept their stuttering. Aspects of therapy relating to the *environment's* reactions to stuttering involve educating parents and other caregivers, teachers, and peers about stuttering so they are less likely to react negatively. Doing so creates a supportive environment of individuals who understand and accept the child's stuttering. Finally, aspects of therapy designed to reduce *activity limitations* and *participation restrictions* are focused on ensuring that children say what they want to say without holding back, enter situations that they might otherwise find challenging, and engage fully in their lives.

When a child can recognize that stuttering is merely a characteristic of how they talk (and not the defining characteristic of their whole being), they can live their lives to the fullest without being held back or burdened by it. As clinicians, we can facilitate a child's journey toward improved communication and self-acceptance. We find this to be an extremely rewarding path for our young clients, their caregivers, and ourselves. We hope that you will also come to find this sense of satisfaction and accomplishment as you learn to help school-age children who stutter and their families.

11.9 Definitions

Affective reactions: The emotions that a person might feel in response to stuttering, such as embarrassment, fear, shame, anxiety, or frustration.

Behavioral reactions: The actions that one might take in response to the sense of being stuck or losing control, such as overt disfluencies, tension or struggle during moments of stuttering, or avoidance behaviors in an attempt to reduce the occurrence of stuttering.

Cognitive reactions: The thoughts that people might have about stuttering or themselves, such as low self-esteem or reduced self-confidence.

Desensitization: The process of reducing people's negative reactions through gradual exposure to the feared behavior or experience.

International Classification of Functioning, Disability and Health (ICF): A framework developed by the World Health Organization for describing human health experience.

Speech modification: Therapy strategies focused on changing the way a person speaks in order to facilitate the production of more perceptibly fluent speech.

Stuttering modification: Therapy strategies focused on changing the way a person stutters in order to reduce the observable severity of individual moments of stuttering.

Support/self-help organization: A group comprised primarily of individuals who share common differences or experiences that is focused on reducing the burden of living with those differences or experiences.

References

[1] Reardon-Reeves NA, Yaruss JS. School-age stuttering therapy: a practical guide. McKinney, TX: Stuttering Therapy Resources, Inc.; 2013

[2] Yaruss JS, Coleman CE, Quesal RW. Stuttering in school-age children: a comprehensive approach to treatment. Lang Speech Hear Serv Sch. 2012; 43 (4):536–548

[3] World Health Organization. The International Classification of Functioning, Disability, and Health (ICF). Geneva, Switzerland: World Health Organization; 2001

[4] Brundage SB, Ratner NB, Boyle MP, Eggers K, Everard R, Franken MC et al. Consensus guidelines for the assessments of individuals who stutter across the lifespan. American journal of speech-language pathology. 2021 Nov;30(6):2379–2393

[5] Yaruss JS, Quesal RW. Overall Assessment of the Speaker's Experience of Stuttering (OASES): documenting multiple outcomes in stuttering treatment. J Fluency Disord. 2006; 31(2):90–115

[6] Mulcahy K, Hennessey N, Beilby J, Byrnes M. Social anxiety and the severity and typography of stuttering in adolescents. J Fluency Disord. 2008; 33(4): 306–319

[7] Yairi E, Ambrose NG. Early Childhood Stuttering: For Clinicians by Clinicians. Austin, TX: Pro-Ed; 2005

[8] Andrews G, Harris M. The Syndrome of Stuttering. London, UK: Heinemann; 1964

[9] Månsson H. Childhood stuttering: incidence and development. J Fluency Disord. 2000; 25(1):47–57

[10] Rocha M, Rato JR, Yaruss JS. The impact of stuttering on Portuguese school-age children as measured by the OASES-S. Speech Lang Hear. 2021; 24(1): 38–47

[11] Chun RYS, Mendes CD, Yaruss JS, Quesal RW. The impact of stuttering on quality of life of children and adolescents. Pró-Fono Rev Atualização Científica. 2010; 22(4):567–570

[12] Beilby JM, Byrnes ML, Yaruss JS. the impact of a stuttering disorder on western australian children and adolescents. Perspect Fluen Fluen Disord. 2012; 22(2):51–62

[13] Conture EG, Guitar BE. Evaluating efficacy of treatment of stuttering: school-age children. J Fluency Disord. 1993; 18(2–3):253–287

[14] Eggers K, Millard S, Kelman E. Temperament and the impact of stuttering in children aged 8–14 years. J Speech Lang Hear Res. 2021; 64(2):417–432

[15] Rocha MSMS, Yaruss JSS, Rato JRJR. Temperament, executive functioning, and anxiety in school-age children who stutter. Front Psychol. 2019; 10: 2244

[16] Davis S, Howell P, Cooke F. Sociodynamic relationships between children who stutter and their non-stuttering classmates. J Child Psychol Psychiatry. 2002; 43(7):939–947

[17] Blood GW, Blood IM. Preliminary study of self-reported experience of physical aggression and bullying of boys who stutter: relation to increased anxiety. Percept Mot Skills. 2007; 104(3, Pt 2) s uppl:1060–1066

[18] Hughes CD, Mahanna-Boden S. Results from a stuttering clinic for school-age children who stutter: a pilot study using a comprehensive approach. Perspect ASHA Spec Interest Groups. 2017; 2(4):54–65

[19] Coleman C, Yaruss JS. A comprehensive view of stuttering: implications for assessment and treatment. Perspect Sch Issues. 2014; 15(2):75–80

[20] Conture EG. Stuttering: its nature, diagnosis, and treatment. Boston, MA: Allyn & Bacon; 2001

[21] Yaruss JS, Reardon-Reeves NA. Early childhood stuttering therapy: a practical guide. McKinney, TX: Stuttering Therapy Resources, Inc.; 2017

[22] Rocha M, Yaruss JS, Rato JRR. Stuttering impact: a shared perception for parents and children? Folia Phoniatr Logop. 2020; 72(6):478–486

[23] Millard SK, Davis S. The Palin Parent Rating Scales: parents' perspectives of childhood stuttering and its impact. J Speech Lang Hear Res. 2016; 59(5): 950–963

[24] Reeves NA, Yaruss JS. School-age stuttering: information and support for parents. McKinney, TX: Stuttering Therapy Resources, Inc.; 2019

[25] Irani F, Gabel R, Hughes S, Swartz ER, Palasik ST. Role entrapment of people who stutter reported by K-12 teachers. Contemp Issues Commun Sci Disord. 2009; 36:48–56

[26] Arnold HS, Li J. Associations between beliefs about and reactions toward people who stutter. J Fluency Disord. 2016; 47:27–37

[27] Beilby J. Psychosocial impact of living with a stuttering disorder: knowing is not enough. Semin Speech Lang. 2014; 35(2):132–143

[28] Nippold MA. Stuttering in school-age children: a call for treatment research. Lang Speech Hear Serv Sch. 2011; 42(2):99–101

[29] ASHA. Scope of Practice in Speech-Language Pathology. 2016. Available at: www.asha.org/policy

[30] Tichenor SE, Yaruss JS. Stuttering as defined by adults who stutter. J Speech Lang Hear Res. 2019; 62(12):4356–4369

[31] Smith A, Weber C. How stuttering develops: the multifactorial dynamic pathways theory. J Speech Lang Hear Res. 2017; 60(9):2483–2505

[32] Kraft SJ, Yairi E. Genetic bases of stuttering: the state of the art, 2011. Folia Phoniatr Logop. 2012; 64(1):34–47

[33] Craig-McQuaide A, Akram H, Zrinzo L, Tripoliti E. A review of brain circuitries involved in stuttering. Front Hum Neurosci. 2014; 8:884

[34] Perkins WH. What is stuttering? J Speech Hear Disord. 1990; 55(3):370–382, discussion 394–397

[35] Iverach L, Jones M, McLellan LF, et al. Prevalence of anxiety disorders among children who stutter. J Fluency Disord. 2016; 49:13–28

[36] Tichenor S, Leslie P, Shaiman S, Yaruss JS. Speaker and observer perceptions of physical tension during stuttering. Folia Phoniatr Logop. 2017; 69(4): 180–189

[37] Tichenor SE, Yaruss JSS. group experiences and individual differences in stuttering. J Speech Lang Hear Res. 2019; 62(12):4335–4350

[38] De Nardo T, Gabel RM, Tetnowski JA, Swartz ER. Self-acceptance of stuttering: a preliminary study. J Commun Disord. 2016; 60:27–38

[39] Ornstein AF, Manning WH. Self-efficacy scaling by adult stutterers. J Commun Disord. 1985; 18(4):313–320

[40] Boyle MP. Enacted stigma and felt stigma experienced by adults who stutter. J Commun Disord. 2018; 73:50–61

[41] Blood GW, Blood IM. Long-term consequences of childhood bullying in adults who stutter: social anxiety, fear of negative evaluation, self-esteem, and satisfaction with life. J Fluency Disord. 2016; 50:72–84

[42] Hugh-Jones S, Smith PK. Self-reports of short- and long-term effects of bullying on children who stammer. Br J Educ Psychol. 1999; 69(Pt 2): 141–158

[43] Wampold BE, Imel ZE. The great psychotherapy debate: the evidence for what makes psychotherapy work. 2nd ed. London: Taylor & Francis; 2015

[44] Bothe AK. Speech modification approaches to stuttering treatment in schools. Semin Speech Lang. 2002; 23(3):181–186

[45] Blomgren M. Behavioral treatments for children and adults who stutter: a review. Psychol Res Behav Manag. 2013; 6:9–19

[46] Williams DF, Dugan PM. Administering stuttering modification therapy in school settings. Semin Speech Lang. 2002; 23(3):187–194

[47] Van Riper C. The treatment of stuttering. 2nd ed. Englewood Cliffs, NJ: Prentice-Hall; 1973

[48] Beck AT. Cognitive therapy and the emotional disorders. New York, NY: International Universities Press; 1976

[49] Ellis A. Rational psychotherapy and individual psychology. J Individ Psychol. 1957; 13:38–44

[50] Kelman E, Wheeler S. Cognitive behaviour therapy with children who stutter. Procedia Soc Behav Sci. 2015; 193:165–174

[51] Sønsterud H, Halvorsen MS, Feragen KB, Kirmess M, Ward D. What works for whom? Multidimensional individualized stuttering therapy (MIST). J Commun Disord. 2020; 88:106052

[52] Beilby JM, Byrnes ML. Acceptance and commitment therapy for people who stutter. Perspect Fluen Fluen Disord. 2012; 22(1):34–46

[53] Palasik S, Hannan J. The clinical applications of acceptance and commitment therapy with clients who stutter. Perspect Fluen Fluen Disord. 2013; 23(2): 54–69

[54] Boyle MP. Mindfulness training in stuttering therapy: a tutorial for speech-language pathologists. J Fluency Disord. 2011; 36(2):122–129

[55] Murphy WP, Yaruss JS, Quesal RW. Enhancing treatment for school-age children who stutter I. Reducing negative reactions through desensitization and cognitive restructuring. J Fluency Disord. 2007; 32(2):121–138

[56] Murphy WP, Quesal RW, Reardon-Reeves NA, Yaruss JS. Minimizing bullying for children who stutter. McKinney, TX: Stuttering Therapy Resources, Inc.; 2013

[57] Yaruss JS, Reeves N, Herring C. How speech-language pathologists can minimize bullying of children who stutter. Semin Speech Lang. 2018; 39(4): 342–355

[58] Yaruss JS, Quesal RW. Overall Assessment of the Speaker's Experience of Stuttering (OASES). McKinney, TX: Stuttering Therapy Resources, Inc.; 2016

[59] Constantino CD, Eichorn N, Buder EH, Beck JG, Manning WH. The speaker's experience of stuttering: measuring spontaneity. J Speech Lang Hear Res. 2020; 63(4):983–1001

[60] Plexico LW, Erath S, Shores H, Burrus E. Self-acceptance, resilience, coping and satisfaction of life in people who stutter. J Fluency Disord. 2019; 59(59): 52–63

[61] Caughter S, Crofts V. Nurturing a resilient mindset in school-aged children who stutter. Am J Speech Lang Pathol. 2018; 27 3S:1111–1123

[62] Yaruss JS, Pelczarski K. Evidence-based practice for school-age stuttering: Balancing existing research with clinical practice. EBP Briefs. 2007; 2(4):1–8

[63] Bernstein Ratner N. Evidence-based practice in stuttering: some questions to consider. J Fluency Disord. 2005; 30(3):163–188

[64] Greenwell T, Walsh B. Evidence-based practice in speech-language pathology: where are we now? Am J Speech Lang Pathol. 2021; 30(1):186–198

[65] Bothe AK. Evidence-based treatment of stuttering: V. The art of clinical practice and the future of clinical research. J Fluency Disord. 2003; 28(3): 247–257, quiz 257–258

[66] Langevin M, Kully D. Evidence-based treatment of stuttering: III. Evidence-based practice in a clinical setting. J Fluency Disord. 2003; 28(3):219–235, quiz 235–236

[67] Zebrowski PM, Arenas RM. The "Iowa Way" revisited. J Fluency Disord. 2011; 36(3):144–157

[68] Quesal RW, Yaruss JS. Historical perspectives on stuttering treatment: Dean Williams. Contemp Issues Commun Sci Disord. 2000; 27:178–187

[69] Craig A, Hancock K, Tran Y, Craig M. Anxiety levels in people who stutter: a randomized population study. J Speech Lang Hear Res. 2003; 46(5):1197–1206

[70] Messenger M, Packman A, Onslow M, Menzies R, O'Brian S. Children and adolescents who stutter: further investigation of anxiety. J Fluency Disord. 2015; 46:15–23

[71] Constantino CD, Leslie P, Quesal RW, Yaruss JS. A preliminary investigation of daily variability of stuttering in adults. J Commun Disord. 2016; 60:39–50

[72] Gerlach H, Subramanian A, Wislar E. Stuttering and its invisibility: why does my classmate only stutter sometimes? Front Young Minds. 2020; 7:153

[73] Tichenor SE, Yaruss JS. Variability of stuttering: behavior and impact. Am J Speech Lang Pathol. 2021; 30(1):75–88

[74] Grossman HL. Voluntary stuttering: a mixed-methods investigation. Diss Abstr Int Sect B Sci Eng. 2009; 70(1-B):244

[75] Byrd CT, Gkalitsiou Z, Donaher J, Stergiou E. The client's perspective on voluntary stuttering. Am J Speech Lang Pathol. 2016; 25(3):290–305

[76] Yaruss JS. Evaluating and treating school-aged children who stutter. Semin Speech Lang. 2010; 31(4):262–271

[77] Vanryckeghem M, Brutten GJ. Behavior Assessment Battery. San Diego, CA: Plural Publishing; 2018

[78] Harley J. The role of attention in therapy for children and adolescents who stutter: cognitive behavioral therapy and mindfulness-based interventions. Am J Speech Lang Pathol. 2018; 27 3S:1139–1151

[79] Boyle MP, Milewski KM, Beita-Ell C. Disclosure of stuttering and quality of life in people who stutter. J Fluency Disord. 2018; 58:1–10

[80] Byrd CT, McGill M, Gkalitsiou Z, Cappellini C. The effects of self-disclosure on male and female perceptions of individuals who stutter. Am J Speech Lang Pathol. 2017; 26(1):69–80

[81] Murphy WP, Yaruss JS, Quesal RW. Enhancing treatment for school-age children who stutter II. Reducing bullying through role-playing and self-disclosure. J Fluency Disord. 2007; 32(2):139–162

[82] Yaruss JS, Reardon NA. Fostering generalization and maintenance in school settings. Semin Speech Lang. 2003; 24(1):33–40

[83] Hughes S. Bullying: what speech-language pathologists should know. Lang Speech Hear Serv Sch. 2014; 45(1):3–13

[84] Gerlach H, Hollister J, Caggiano L, Zebrowski PM. The utility of stuttering support organization conventions for young people who stutter. J Fluency Disord. 2019; 62:105724

[85] Herring C, Millager RA, Yaruss JS. Outcomes Following Participation in a Support-Based Summer Camp for Children Who Stutter. Lang Speech Hear Serv Sch. 2022;53(1):17–29

[86] Trichon M. Self-help conferences for people who stutter: an interpretive phenomenological analysis [dissertation]. Lafayette, LA: University of Louisiana; 2010

[87] Trichon M, Tetnowski J. Self-help conferences for people who stutter: a qualitative investigation. J Fluency Disord. 2011; 36(4):290–295

[88] Yaruss JS, Quesal RW, Murphy B. National Stuttering Association members' opinions about stuttering treatment. J Fluency Disord. 2002; 27(3):227–241, quiz 241–242, III

[89] Yaruss JS, Quesal RW, Reeves L. Self-help and mutual aid groups as an adjunct to stuttering therapy. In: Conture EG, Curlee RF, eds. Stuttering and Related Disorders of Fluency. 3rd ed. New York, NY: Thieme Medical Publishers, Inc.; 2007:256–276

[90] Borkman T. Understanding Self-Help/Mutual Aid: Experiential Learning in the Commons. New Brunswick, NJ: Rutgers University Press; 1999

[91] Byrd CT, Gkalitsiou Z, Werle D, Coalson GA. Exploring the effectiveness of an intensive treatment program for school-age children who stutter, camp dream. speak. live: a follow-up study. Semin Speech Lang. 2018; 39(5):458–468

[92] Byrd C, Chmela K, Coleman C, Kelly E, Reichhardt R, Irano F. An introduction to camps for children who stutter: what they are and how they can help. Perspect ASHA Spec Interes Groups SIG 4. 2016; 1(4):55–69

[93] Byrd C, Hampton E, McGill M, Gkalitsiou Z. Participation in camp dream speak live: affective and cognitive outcomes for children who stutter. J Speech Pathol Ther. 2016; 01(03):116

[94] Yaruss JS, Quesal RW, Reeves L, et al. Speech treatment and support group experiences of people who participate in the National Stuttering Association. J Fluency Disord. 2002; 27(2):115–133, quiz 133–134

[95] Yaruss JS, Pelczarski KM, Quesal RW. Comprehensive treatment for school-age children who stutter: treating the entire disorder. In: Guitar B, McCauley, Rebecca J, eds. Treatment of Stuttering: Conventional and

Controversial Interventions. Baltimore, MD: Lippincott Williams & Wilkins; 2010:215–244

[96] Tichenor SE, Yaruss JS. Recovery and relapse: perspectives from adults who stutter. J Speech Lang Hear Res. 2020; 63(7):2162–2176

[97] Craig A. Relapse following treatment for stuttering: a critical review and correlative data. J Fluency Disord. 1998; 23(1):1–30

[98] Yaruss JS. One size does not fit all: special topics in stuttering therapy. Semin Speech Lang. 2003; 24(1):3–6

[99] Millard SK, Cook FM. Working with young children who stutter: raising our game. Semin Speech Lang. 2010; 31(4):250–261

[100] Quesal RW. Empathy: perhaps the most important E in EBP. Semin Speech Lang. 2010; 31(4):217–226

[101] Plexico LW, Manning WH, DiLollo A. Client perceptions of effective and ineffective therapeutic alliances during treatment for stuttering. J Fluency Disord. 2010; 35(4):333–354

[102] Sønsterud H, Kirmess M, Howells K, Ward D, Feragen KB, Halvorsen MS. The working alliance in stuttering treatment: a neglected variable? Int J Lang Commun Disord. 2019; 54(4):606–619

[103] Manning WH. Evidence of clinically significant change: the therapeutic alliance and the possibilities of outcomes-informed care. Semin Speech Lang. 2010; 31(4):207–216

Further Readings

Cooke K, Millard SK. The most important therapy outcomes for school-aged children who stutter: an exploratory study. Am J Speech Lang Pathol. 2018; 27 3S:1152–1163

Conture EG, Guitar BE. Evaluating efficacy of treatment of stuttering: school-age children. J Fluency Disord. 1993; 18(2–3):253–287

Healey EC, Scott LA. Strategies for treating elementary school-age children who stutter: an integrative approach. Lang Speech Hear Serv Sch. 1995; 26: 151–161

Murphy WP, Quesal RW, Reardon-Reeves NA, Yaruss JS. Minimizing bullying for children who stutter. McKinney, TX: Stuttering Therapy Resources, Inc.; 2013

Murphy WP, Yaruss JS, Quesal RW. Enhancing treatment for school-age children who stutter II. Reducing bullying through role-playing and self-disclosure. J Fluency Disord. 2007; 32(2):139–162

Murphy WP, Yaruss JS, Quesal RW. Enhancing treatment for school-age children who stutter I. Reducing negative reactions through desensitization and cognitive restructuring. J Fluency Disord. 2007; 32(2):121–138

Reardon-Reeves NA, Yaruss JS. School-age stuttering therapy: a practical guide. McKinney, TX: Stuttering Therapy Resources, Inc.; 2013

Tichenor SE, Yaruss JS. Stuttering as defined by adults who stutter. J Speech Lang Hear Res. 2019; 62(12):4356–4369

Yaruss JS. Evaluating and treating school-aged children who stutter. Semin Speech Lang. 2010; 31(4):262–271

Yaruss JS, Coleman CE, Quesal RW. Stuttering in school-age children: a comprehensive approach to treatment. Lang Speech Hear Serv Sch. 2012; 43(4): 536–548

Yaruss JS, Quesal RW. Stuttering and the International Classification of Functioning, Disability, and Health: an update. J Commun Disord. 2004; 37(1):35–52

Yaruss JS, Reardon NA. Fostering generalization and maintenance in school settings. Semin Speech Lang. 2003; 24(1):33–40

12 Adolescents and Adults

Patricia M. Zebrowski, Naomi Rodgers, and Hope Gerlach-Houck

Abstract

The purpose of this chapter is to provide clinicians with a framework for working with their teen and adult clients in designing and implementing stuttering therapy. Our guiding principles for working with people who stutter have been inspired by the work of researchers and practitioners in communication sciences and disorders, counseling psychology, and health psychology. We propose that stuttering therapy and its outcomes require us to consider (1) how important speech and stuttering modifications, thoughts and feelings about stuttering, and avoidance strategies are to the client and (2) how ready clients are to change any or all of these components of the stuttering experience. With this in mind, we offer strategies for helping your clients make decisions about what they *want* and *can* do about stuttering, ways you can assist them in achieving these goals, and case examples of the therapy process.

Keywords: stuttering, fluency disorder, therapy, adults, adolescents

12.1 Introduction

As you learned in ▸ Chapter 1, developmental stuttering first emerges between 2 and 4 years of age. For approximately 75% of young children who begin stuttering, the core speech behaviors of stuttering—sound/syllable repetitions and prolonged sounds—decrease measurably over the next 36 months, with most children recovering within 12 to 24 months post onset. This means that teenagers and adults who present with developmental stuttering (i.e., stuttering that first began in early childhood) represent 25%, or the minority, of all cases. What do these numbers mean for the treatment of stuttering in adolescents and adults, the subject of this chapter? First, they indicate that teens and adults who stutter are, in some ways, not representative of the group of people with developmental stuttering, in that the majority experience unassisted (i.e., little or no treatment) recovery. That is, there is a unique set of risk factors that lead to the persistence of stuttering in these 25%. We understand developmental stuttering to be the result of a complex interaction of multiple risk factors (see ▸ Chapter 1), and that none of the candidate risk factors (i.e., genetics, speech motor skills, etc.) are necessary or sufficient for stuttering to emerge. These two facts—that teens and adults who stutter are a relatively small subgroup of the stuttering population and that the stuttering "recipe" is different and possibly unique for any given individual—lead to the conclusion that (1) the principles underlying intervention for persistent stuttering are largely different from those for young children and (2) treatment should be tailored to the person's individual situation and needs. This second point relates to the ways in which the "age" of the stuttering problem (along with, but likely more important than, the age of the person who stutters) shapes the experience of stuttering for teens and adults who stutter, often profoundly. That is, the more time that has passed since stuttering onset, the more

opportunities the person has had to experience and internalize both social and personal reactions to stuttering. For many teenagers and adults who stutter, these reactions tend to be negative, leading to an array of chronic and unhelpful behaviors, thoughts, and feelings.[1] It is this constellation of negative reactions (e.g., visible and physical tension and struggle while speaking and stuttering; avoidance of specific words, sounds, or situations, and verbal interactions in general; and negative thoughts and feelings about communication and self) that are necessarily the focus of stuttering therapy. That is, the *way* the person stutters or interferes with talking[2] and the habitual way they react to stuttering and its social and emotional consequences are the larger obstacles to well-being than the speech disfluencies themselves.

This chapter is organized into three distinct, yet interrelated, topics. First, we will describe two lines of research that have converged to reveal key cognitive processes underlying intentional behavior change. As mentioned earlier, we use this work and associated theoretical bases as a framework for making decisions about therapy goals and clinical approaches for teenagers and adults who stutter. Next, we present a series of related measures and dialogue methods that are rooted in one of these theories—*Stages of Change*—and discuss their use in determining *how* ready a client is to make a positive change to stuttering, *what* they are willing and able to address in both the present and future, and how *confident* they are that they can continue working on those new behaviors in the face of challenges or setbacks. We propose that this multidimensional framework should be used in the first step of therapy, as it forms the basis for intervention goals and approaches that are matched to the client's readiness to use them. Previous and emerging research supports the view that tailoring intervention in this way increases the likelihood of a positive, durable outcome. Finally, we discuss approaches for teaching clients how to engage in behaviors that lead to success in living with stuttering: learning to modify speech and stuttering, addressing negative thoughts and feelings, and increasing approach behaviors by talking without avoiding words or situations.

12.2 What Needs To Be Changed about Stuttering and Who Decides?

The field of speech-language pathology emerged from a collaboration of researchers and clinicians in multiple disciplines, including but not limited to education, physics, neurology, and psychology. This cross-disciplinary origin remains a key strength of our field. At the same time, it can pose challenges for students who must take coursework in a wide array of subject areas! Because we are therapists, we have been particularly influenced by research and practice in both counseling and health psychology to help us understand how best to facilitate behavioral and cognitive change in our clients. In the past 20 years or so, speech-language pathologists have learned more and more from psychology about the essential ingredients of successful therapy, and how to help clients choose personally meaningful goals. These two pieces of the therapy experience are the touchstones of the work we do.

12.3 What Contributes to Treatment Outcomes?

12.3.1 The Common Factors

For several years, researchers in counseling psychology have compared the efficacy of treatment approaches for mood disorders. The purpose of these meta-analyses has been to determine which treatment approach or set of techniques leads to the best outcomes and, therefore, represents the best approach. To the surprise of many investigators and replicated across several meta-analyses, results showed that (1) therapy for different mood disorders is better than no therapy and (2) one approach does not lead to a significantly better outcome than another. These findings have been consistent regardless of disorder (e.g., anxiety, depression, posttraumatic stress disorder, etc.).[3,4] How can one interpret these results and how might they apply to stuttering? A likely explanation is that while specific therapy techniques differ among treatment approaches, there is a set of commonalities across them that contribute *more* than technique to a good outcome in therapy. Researchers in psychology have labeled these the *common factors* in therapy and argue that each must be addressed if therapy is to be successful. Although stuttering is *not* a mood disorder, these findings are relevant to stuttering, a disorder that impacts a speaker's cognitive, emotional, and social well-being. We will more clearly connect the common factors and stuttering therapy shortly.

What are the common factors that contribute to successful therapy outcomes? Both researchers and therapists have identified four such factors: (1) the specific treatment approach and related techniques that are used, (2) what the client and their environment contributes to therapy, (3) the collaboration or alliance between the client and the clinician, and (4) both the client's and clinician's optimism in the client's ability to change and the clinician's ability to facilitate that change. The first one (treatment approach) is *specific* in that it is unique to different clinicians working with their individual clients; the rest, however, are factors that *cut across all therapy contexts* (thus, referred to as *common factors*), regardless of the specific approach and strategies used to target behavior change. In fact, some researchers have argued that these three factors, common across all therapy approaches both together and even separately, contribute the more to treatment outcomes than the specific techniques used.[5] This helps us to explain a common observation in clinical practice: although therapy approaches yield good outcomes overall for a population of clients, there is a large degree of variability in outcomes across individuals. ▶ Table 12.1 provides a description of the common factors.

What is the relevance of common factors to stuttering therapy? We continue to develop a solid evidence base that therapy "works" while also investigating the efficacy of different approaches for various disorders. In more recent years, however, researchers in speech-language pathology have been able to replicate findings from the psychotherapy literature. To a limited extent, meta-analyses have shown that therapy is better than no therapy across different speech and language disorders (e.g., child language disorders, aphasia, stuttering, etc.),[7,8] but that no single approach or therapy technique results in a significantly better outcome. Some researchers in stuttering have delved deeper to show that people who stutter believe that common factors, such as the *therapeutic alliance*, are essential to successful treatment outcomes.[9,10]

In summary, previous and emerging research in both psychotherapy and speech-language pathology points convincingly to

Table 12.1 The common factors in psychotherapy and their proportional contribution to treatment outcomes[6,61,62]

Extratherapeutic change (40%)	
The skills, abilities, constitutional factors, and environmental features that the client brings to therapy	• Age and gender • Educational and employment history • Support systems • Physical and mental health • Financial resources • Cognitive abilities • Readiness to make changes[61]
Therapeutic alliance (30%)	
The working relationship between the client and clinician	• Clinician empathy, warmth, and listening skills • Clinician and client communication skills • Shared decision-making • Client willingness to take risk • Client confidence in clinician's expertise and understanding of the client's experience
Expectancy (15%)	
Client and clinician belief that change can happen	• Confidence in the validity of the therapeutic approach • Client understanding of rationale for therapeutic strategies • Clinician and client confidence in overall plan and ability to sustain efforts when it is difficult
Technique (15%)	
The strategies and activities that comprise the therapy approach	• Strength of empirical and practice-based evidence • Goodness of fit between client and techniques • Clinician training and skill in teaching strategies

the need for clinicians to understand the importance of factors *beyond the technique* itself to treatment outcomes. We believe that this is also true for stuttering intervention.

12.3.2 Spotlight on the Client's Contribution to Therapy Outcomes: Stages of Change

Recall that the attributes of the client and what they bring to the therapeutic context are one of the common factors in treatment outcome. There are numerous characteristics of individual clients and their environments that either facilitate or hinder progress in treatment. One factor that has received considerable attention by behavioral health and counseling psychologists is the client's *readiness* to make a change toward a healthier physical or emotional state. In many studies across a wide variety of clinical populations, researchers have shown that a key factor in the outcomes of behavioral intervention is the goodness of fit between the therapy techniques used and the individual's *readiness* to use them.[11] The central idea is that one's readiness to engage in therapy is aligned with a specific *stage of change* (SOC) within a series of five temporally linked stages.[12] These five stages, and the shifts in thinking that facilitate movement across them, are at the heart of the *Transtheoretical Model* (TTM), or *SOC* model of intentional behavior change.[13] ▶ Fig. 12.1 shows the stages of change and a description of each.

Each of the five stages of change depicted in ▶ Fig. 12.1 represents an individual's cognitive state at a particular point in time. The current stage a person is in depends on two cognitive processes: (1) how important they personally find the pros and cons of making a change and (2) their level of confidence in their ability to stay on the path toward change when it is difficult. These processes are referred to as *decisional balance* and *situational self-efficacy*, respectively, and have been shown to predict where an individual is in the process of change.

Decisional balance is a dynamic process of internal conflict resolution that occurs when a person weighs the gains (pros) and losses (cons) of making a behavioral change. Shifts in decisional balance predict which SOC the person is in, as well as their movement across stages of readiness.[14,15] As one moves from Precontemplation toward Action, the number and importance of the benefits (i.e., the "good things") of making a change increase, while the number and importance of the losses (i.e., the "not-so-good things") of making that change decrease. As the balance tips in favor of the pros (i.e., the client places more importance on the pros than the cons), the client finds themselves closer and closer to being ready to engage in new behaviors. For example, a person who is in Action likely perceives that there are several pros related to making a change to stuttering (e.g., feeling calmer or more confident when speaking) and that these pros are more important to them than the fewer number of associated cons (e.g., time and financial commitment). In contrast, a person who is in Precontemplation may perceive that there are more cons to making a change to stuttering than pros and that these cons are important enough to dissuade them from making a change.

Situational self-efficacy is also a dynamic cognitive process. The confidence a person has in their ability to use a new behavior in challenging situations and remain engaged in behavior change after "failure" is susceptible to change. Similar to decisional balance, situational self-efficacy predicts where a person is in their readiness to change; people in earlier stages tend to have lower levels of situational self-efficacy, while people in later stages tend to have higher levels.[16,17] Whereas someone who is in Action may feel moderately confident that they can maintain their new behavior when faced with challenges, someone who is in Precontemplation would likely not feel as confident.

In summary, we propose that a client's readiness to make a positive change to stuttering (i.e., their SOC) is a key "common factor" in determining the goals of stuttering therapy. The client's thoughts and beliefs about what needs to change and

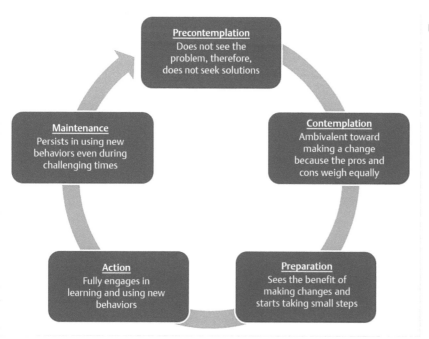

Fig. 12.1 The five stages of change.

how personally important it is for them to make those changes are powerful contributors to treatment outcomes. Your role as a clinician is to collaborate with the person who stutters to make sure that the approach and techniques used in therapy are matched with their readiness to use them.

12.4 Getting Started: A Stage-Based Framework for Therapy Planning

In the sections that follow, we describe a stage-based hybrid approach. Inspired by the *Stages of Change* model we just discussed, we offer a framework that guides adults and teens who stutter to make decisions about what they want to change about stuttering, and how to go about it. This approach, sequential in nature, begins with completing *readiness scales* that focus the client's attention on what they want to change about stuttering and how personally important it is to them. Their point of view, which is uncovered by completing these scales, is explored more deeply through *motivational interviewing*, a dialogic method that clarifies and strengthens the client's personal motivation for doing something helpful about stuttering. Finally, the information gained from both the scales and motivational interview guides the selection of therapy goals, and techniques are chosen that match the client's readiness to learn and use them.

12.4.1 Creating the Therapy Plan: Deciding What is Helpful

Both the *Common Factors* and *Stages of Change* models support the importance of starting therapy by helping the client decide what they want to be different about stuttering. Obviously the most straightforward way to do this is to ask and doing so will hopefully lead to fruitful discussions. Our clinical experience suggests that more often than not, the client's default answer is that they want to talk more fluently or stop stuttering; obviously, this makes sense and is valid. Just as often, however, the clinician can dig a little deeper to uncover less obvious and more nuanced ideas that the client has about what they want to be different about stuttering. These may include an overall wish to feel better about stuttering and talking, or to not worry so much about stuttering. The person may also want to be able to talk to friends or family members about stuttering or to talk freely without avoiding. These thoughts and desires are often below the surface and, in some cases, the client may even be unaware of them or how important they are to their overall quality of life. Because stuttering is multidimensional in its onset and development, choosing to focus solely on one dimension (e.g., speech modification) without exploring the meaning the client attaches to it may lead to therapy goals that are not well matched to the client's readiness to address them.

The process of deciding what needs to change about stuttering requires the client and clinician to collaboratively unpack the client's thoughts and beliefs about what is personally important and how change can occur. Our own work with adolescents and adults who stutter, and the previously described SOC research with other clinical populations, serves as the foundation for choosing the focus of therapy.

What are You Ready to Do?

In our own recent work,[18,19] we have shown that the *Stages of Change* model is a good fit for the population of adolescents and young adults who stutter. As a part of that process, we asked teens who stutter and speech-language pathologists who identified as stuttering specialists: "If someone was making a positive change to their stuttering, what would they be doing?" We carefully analyzed the content of these interviews and discovered there were common themes that ran through them. Using qualitative analysis methods,[20] we determined three global themes, or collection of behaviors, that reflect successful management of stuttering:

- Learn and use speech strategies or techniques for speaking more fluently and/or stuttering with less tension and struggle.
- Change negative thoughts and feelings about stuttering.
- Approach talking with less avoidance of words, sounds, or situations.

We used this three-part definition of stuttering management to create an *SOC* readiness scale for teenagers and young adults who stutter, using their responses to distinguish among the five different stages of change.[11,21] As seen in ▶ Fig. 12.2, our SOC scale first instructs the person who stutters to read the definition as a *whole* (i.e., think about all three "ingredients" necessary to successfully manage stuttering) and choose from one of five stages of readiness to address the holistic, three-pronged approach to managing stuttering. The five choices consisted of the following: (1) I am not thinking about doing any of these things in the next 6 months (reflecting the Precontemplation stage), (2) I am thinking about doing one or more of these things in the next 6 months (Contemplation), (3) I am planning to do one or more of these things in the next month (Preparation), (4) I have been doing one or more of these things for at least 6 months (Action), or (5) I have been doing one or more of these things for more than 6 months (Maintenance).

Next, the person is asked to consider their readiness to address each of the three behaviors *alone* and choose one of the five stages described earlier for modifying speech, changing thoughts and feelings, and reducing avoidance. In this way, we can see whether they are in a similar, or different, SOC across the three ingredients for making a positive change to stuttering. And in fact, we did find that individuals can be in different stages of change for various aspects of stuttering management when we received almost 200 completed scales from adolescents and young adults who stutter. For example, although a client may be in Action for modifying speech (indicating that they are currently working on it), they may be in Precontemplation for changing attitudes and reducing avoidance.[19]

How Important is Doing It?

As previously described, the pros and cons of making any sort of change, and the importance one assigns to each, are a central determinant of readiness to change. Put simply, people are more ready to embark on the change process when they believe that there are more *good* than *not-so-good* things about making change, and the good things are relatively important to them. That said, as part of our investigation of change readiness in people who stutter, we wanted to identify the pros and cons of making a positive change to stuttering according to teens who

Stages of Change

The best way for someone who stutters to do something to help with stuttering is to:

1. Learn and use strategies for speaking more fluently and/or stuttering with less tension and struggle;
2. Change negative thoughts and feelings about stuttering; and
3. Approach talking with less avoidance of sounds, words, or situations.

It's important to pay attention to all three of these things because just focusing on one is not enough to make long-lasting changes. For any of these things to become automatic, you will need help and regular practice for up to one year or more.

Thinking about the three things above **all together** (learning and using speech strategies, changing negative thoughts, and speaking without avoiding), how ready are you **right now** to do something about your stuttering?

Place a check mark in the box next to the sentence that best describes you **right now.**

	I am <u>not</u> thinking about doing any of these things in the next 6 months.
	I am thinking about doing one or more of these things in the next 6 months.
	I am planning to do one or more of these things in the next month.
	I have been doing one or more of these things for LESS than 6 months.
	I have been doing one or more of these things for MORE than 6 months.

Thinking of these three things separately, one by one:

1. How ready are you **right now** to get help to <u>learn and use speech techniques for speaking more fluently or stuttering with less tension and struggle</u>?

	I am <u>not</u> thinking about doing this in the next 6 months.
	I am thinking about doing this in the next 6 months.
	I am planning to do this in the next month.
	I have been doing this for LESS than 6 months.
	I have been doing this for MORE than 6 months.

2. How ready are you **right now** to <u>change your negative thoughts and feelings about stuttering</u>?

	I am <u>not</u> thinking about doing this in the next 6 months.
	I am thinking about doing this in the next 6 months.
	I am planning to do this in the next month.
	I have been doing this for LESS than 6 months.
	I have been doing this for MORE than 6 months.

3. How ready are you **right now** <u>to say what you want to say without avoiding sounds, words, or situations</u>?

	I am <u>not</u> thinking about doing this in the next 6 months.
	I am thinking about doing this in the next 6 months.
	I am planning to do this in the next month.
	I have been doing this for LESS than 6 months.
	I have been doing this for MORE than 6 months.

Fig. 12.2 The Stages of Change scale for stuttering.

stutter and stuttering specialists. Our analysis revealed eight pros and eight cons that were reliable predictors of a young person's readiness to change stuttering. ▶ Fig. 12.3 shows the resulting *Decisional Balance* scale containing these essential pros and cons. The pros (i.e., the good things about making a positive change to stuttering) include such things as "you would feel better about yourself" and "you would feel calmer." The cons, or not-so-good things, include "you would be disappointed in yourself if you change the way you speak just to make other people happy" and "you might not be able to change the way you speak." Respondents were asked to judge how important each of the pros and cons were to them when considering making a change to their stuttering. When we dug further into what they reported, we saw that in fact, there was a relationship between the number and importance of the pros and cons and SOC: teens who stutter who placed higher value on the pros of making a change were more likely to be in the action and maintenance stages. Why is this important? Until we can unpack these relationships in more detail, at the very least our observations support the idea that regardless of one's readiness to make a positive change to stuttering, an individual's beliefs regarding what is good and not so good about making this change provide therapists and clients with important insight for choosing therapy goals. Identifying therapy goals the client is ready to address maximizes the likelihood they will experience success.

How Confident Are You That You Can Do It?

In addition to uncovering a person's beliefs about the good and not-so-good aspects of changing the overt or covert aspects of stuttering, it is important to have a sense of how confident the person is in their ability to stay on the path of change when it is difficult to do so. We asked young people who stutter and a group of stuttering specialists to tell us the situations that make it hard to continue to make the three-pronged changes in stuttering. Using the same methods that we employed to create the two previously discussed measures of change readiness, we uncovered a core set of nonoverlapping situations that comprised our *Self-Efficacy* scale. As shown in ▶ Fig. 12.4, the scale contained 11 situations that make it challenging to "stay the course" or continue implementing positive changes to stuttering, including "you are telling a story" and "you are afraid you are going to stutter." Our large national sample of teens who stutter rated how confident they felt managing stuttering in each of these situations.

Pros and Cons About Making a Change to Stuttering

Please rate how important each of the following statements is to you when you think about making a change to your stuttering. pick a number on a scale from 1 to 5 where:

1 = Not important at all
2 = A little important
3 = Moderately important
4 = Very important
5 = Extremely important

When thinking about making a change in your stuttering, how important is it to you if....

	Not important				Extremely important
You would feel better about yourself?	1	2	3	4	5
You wouldn't feel like yourself if you stuttered differently?	1	2	3	4	5
You would talk more?	1	2	3	4	5
You wouldn't feel like stuttering runs your life?	1	2	3	4	5
You might hot be able to change the way you speak?	1	2	3	4	5
You would feel a sense of accomplishment?	1	2	3	4	5
Other people would disapprove of you trying to change the way you speak?	1	2	3	4	5
You would worry less about talking?	1	2	3	4	5
You could just be yourself?	1	2	3	4	5
Your speech would sound and feel weird and unnatural to you?	1	2	3	4	5
Your may miss out on other activities to spend time working on your stuttering?	1	2	3	4	5
You would feel calmer?	1	2	3	4	5
People would treat you just like any other person?	1	2	3	4	5
You would be disappointed in yourself if you change the way you speak just to make other people happy?	1	2	3	4	5
Your speech would sound weird and unnatural to other people?	1	2	3	4	5
You would lose part of who you are if you stuttered differently?	1	2	3	4	5

Fig. 12.3 The Decisional Balance scale for stuttering.

In summary, the information that a client shares through these three interdependent measures of readiness (SOC, Decisional Balance, and Self-Efficacy) can lay the foundation for treatment. By gaining insight into what the client is the closest to being ready to do about stuttering, how important it is to them to do it, and how confident they are that they can stick with the process, the clinician can help the client select therapy goals and tools that are a good match for their ability to learn and use them. Further, the process of working with the client to uncover their beliefs about what can help and what they feel ready to do is at the core of a strong therapeutic alliance.[10]

Filling in the Missing Pieces: The Motivational Interview

The client's responses on the three readiness scales set the stage for the focus of stuttering therapy and the approaches and techniques that will be used. Specifically, the client's

Confidence

Please rate how sure you are that you can make a positive change to stuttering when you find yourself in each of the following situations. pick a number on a scale from 1 to 5 where:

1 = Not at all sure
2 = A little sure
3 = Moderately sure
4 = Very sure
5 = Extremely sure

How sure are you that you can do something about stuttering when...

	Not at all sure				Extremely sure
You are talking in front of a group of people.	1	2	3	4	5
You are talking to a teacher or boss.	1	2	3	4	5
You are ordering at a restaurant.	1	2	3	4	5
You are being interviewed for a job.	1	2	3	4	5
You are telling a story.	1	2	3	4	5
You are meeting new people.	1	2	3	4	5
You are introducing yourself.	1	2	3	4	5
It's a hard talking day.	1	2	3	4	5
You are feeling stressed out.	1	2	3	4	5
You are calling someone on the phone.	1	2	3	4	5
You are afraid you are going to stutter?	1	2	3	4	5

Fig. 12.4 The Self-Efficacy scale for stuttering.

self-judgment of their readiness to engage in changing any or all the behaviors, thoughts/feelings, and responses to stuttering, along with their ratings of how personally important that change is, and how confident they are in doing so can help broadly determine what the client is ready and able to take on in therapy. The scales do not, and cannot, be a substitute for deeper conversations that reveal the unique thoughts and beliefs that either inhibit or facilitate change for an individual. A powerful method for revealing a client's specific thoughts and feelings about change is the motivational interview, described by William Miller and Stephen Rollnick[22] and written about extensively since the concept first emerged. Motivational interviewing involves a dialogue between the clinician and client to elicit "change talk" from a client, or information about what the client wants to change and how they can do it.[23] A comprehensive discussion of the theory and practices of motivational interviewing is beyond the scope of this chapter. The format helps strengthen the person's understanding of the gap between what they *are doing* and what they *want to do*. The therapist

then helps the client to recognize what they already *know* and *do* that can help them to make those changes they desire.

The basic ingredients in a motivational interview can be described by the acronym *DARN*, which stands for *desire, ability, reason*, and *need*. As such, the clinician engages the client in conversation that helps uncover the specifics about what the person wants to do, what they think they can do, why it is important to them, and why they think they need to do it. What is important to understand about a motivational interview is that these discussions are prompted by both direct and indirect questions and prompts from the clinician. It is also important to listen to and value what the client says, rather than inform or persuade.[24] For example, to reveal the client's *desires* (what they want to change), the clinician can ask directly, by asking "What do you want to do about stuttering?" or indirectly, by asking "What would you like to be different about stuttering?" or "Sometimes people have a theory or an idea about what can help them make a positive change to stuttering. What do you think you could do that would be helpful here?"

As an example of how a motivational interview can clarify a client's readiness to change, imagine that the clinician administers the *SOC*, *Decisional Balance*, and *Self-Efficacy* scales (▶ Fig. 12.2, ▶ Fig. 12.3, ▶ Fig. 12.4) to a teenager who stutters. The client's responses indicate that they are in the Action stage for learning and using strategies for changing speech and/or stuttering, in *Contemplation* for changing thoughts and feelings, and in Precontemplation for talking without avoiding. Using the client responses on the three scales as starting point, the clinician can dig deeper into the client's desire (D), perceived ability and confidence in making changes (A), the reasons these changes are more or less personally important and why (R), and the urgency, now and in the future, for making changes (N). Sample questions for each component of the motivational interview (i.e., DARN) are shown in ▶ Table 12.2.

Administering and discussing the SOC, *Decisional Balance*, and *Self-Efficacy* scales, and conducting the motivational interview are key to developing a shared understanding of the client's thoughts and feelings regarding change. As such, these practices form the foundation of a collaborative plan for therapy. We structure the articulation of this plan with Behrman's example of a "change plan" format.[23] Specifically, with clinician support, the client decides the following:

- The changes I want to make are....
- The steps I plan to take in changing are....
- The ways other people (clinician, family members, coworkers, friends) can help me are....

- I will know that my plan is working if...Some things that could interfere with my plan are....
- What I will do if the plan is not working....

In summary, helping the client explore and consider the usefulness of their thoughts and beliefs about doing something about stuttering is time well spent. In addition to sharing the responsibility for the direction of therapy, these conversations strengthen the therapeutic alliance in that they convey to the client that their viewpoints are honored and that their journey through treatment is a collaborative partnership with you.

12.4.2 Implementing the Therapy Plan: Learning the Things that Help

Therapy goals and approaches are chosen when the client and clinician come to a consensus about which of the three ingredients for successful stuttering management the client is either ready (i.e., Action) or close to ready (i.e., *Preparation*; ▶ Fig. 12.2) to learn. For example, some clients may be *contemplating* doing something to change the way they talk soon (i.e., learn and use speech strategies or techniques for speaking more fluently and/or stuttering with less tension and struggle), but are not ready to approach feared words and speaking situations without avoidance (Precontemplation). In fact, as we have discovered from our own work that it is not unusual for teens and adults who stutter

Table 12.2 Motivational interview components (i.e., DARN) and related questions

Desire (D)	
What the client wants to change about stuttering	• Is there a way you would like to think differently about stuttering? • What ideas do you have about how to do this? • How has stuttering affected your life (1, not at all; 10, it affects me every day)? • What would need to happen for you to move that number closer to "1"? • If in 3 mo or so you said "Wow, things are much better!", what would you be doing differently, or what would be changed about yourself? • How would others know that something has changed? • How can I help you in this process?
Ability (A)	
The client's thoughts about their ability to make desired changes to stuttering	• How might you go about changing (behavior, thoughts, self-confidence)? • Which of the changes you'd like to make seem most possible? • If you woke up tomorrow feeling confident about your ability to make the changes in stuttering that are important to you, what would you be doing or have done? • What might you do to increase your confidence?
Reason (R)	
The reasons the client wants to make changes to stuttering	• What are the good and not-so-good things about changing something about stuttering (i.e., pros and cons)? • Can you imagine a situation *right now* where changing something about stuttering would make things better for you? • What might those changes be, and how important are they to you *right now*? • What is the best that can happen if you start to work toward change? What is the worst? What is most likely?
Need (N)	
The client's view about the importance of changing something about stuttering, for both the present and the future	• How urgent does the need to make changes to stuttering seem to you *right now* (1, not at all; 10, extremely urgent)? • Do other people in your life think it is urgent for you to change something about stuttering? Who? How urgent (1–10)? • Is it important for you to make changes to stuttering for these people? • How will your life be different 1 y from now, or 5 y from now, if you *don't* make changes to stuttering? How different will it be if you *do*?

to be at different stages of change for the three components of successful stuttering management (see ▸ Fig. 12.2).

The following sections are organized by the three components of successful stuttering management that people who stutter and stuttering specialists endorse: (1) learn and use speech and stuttering modification strategies to make talking easier, (2) change how they think and feel about stuttering, and (3) increase approach behaviors by not avoiding words, sounds, or situations. For each component, we will describe general therapeutic approaches and specific techniques that are appropriate for individuals who are either preparing or ready to make a change as revealed through the *SOC* scale. In addition, we will discuss ways in which the clinician can integrate the client's beliefs about the pros and cons of making a change and their confidence in "staying the course" to guide the focus of therapy. ▸ Table 12.3, ▸ Table 12.4, ▸ Table 12.5 provide summaries of different approaches for the three components of successful stuttering management.

12.5 Selecting Therapy Approaches: Learn to Speak More Fluently or Stutter More Easily

If the client is ready to focus on speech production in therapy, or is close to doing so, there are three established approaches that have been developed to teach people who stutter how to either speak more fluently or stutter with less physical tension and struggle. These approaches can help in different ways and

have different levels of support for their efficacy. The first approach has been referred to as the *Normal Talking Process*, the second is referred to as *Speak More Fluently* (commonly known as fluency shaping), and the third as *Stutter More Easily* (commonly known as stuttering modification). ▸ Table 12.3 provides additional information about each of these approaches.

12.5.1 Normal Talking Process

This approach was developed by Dean Williams, a researcher/clinician and a person who stuttered himself. Williams was heavily influenced by his own experiences with stuttering, and by Wendell Johnson, his mentor at the University of Iowa. Like Johnson, Williams took a "strength-based" approach to the successful management of stuttering. Simply put, he argued that instead of working toward eliminating stuttering or replacing it with a different way of talking, a person who stutters should focus on what they already know how to do. In other words, they should pay attention to their spontaneously fluent speech and "do more of it." On its face, this perspective seems both obvious and overly simplistic, but in that lies much of its appeal. The clinician guides the client toward an understanding of how speech is produced and, more importantly, what it *feels* like to use the speech mechanism in different ways, including fluent and disfluent speech. This exploration leads the client to develop a physical awareness of what they *do* to speak fluently and what they *are doing with the same system* to interfere with fluency, or "forward-moving speech."[2,25,26] At the same time, the clinician helps the client identify their emotional reactions

Table 12.3 Strategies or techniques for speaking more fluently and/or stuttering with less tension and struggle

Therapy approach	Description	Examples of therapy techniques	Helpful for...
Normal talking process	Increases physical awareness of how we produce spontaneous fluency, and how we interfere with this process, resulting in speech disfluency	• Experiment with manipulating the five physiological parameters (airflow, voicing, movement, timing, and tension) to speak in different ways; • Increase physical awareness of fluent and disfluent speech and how to change between the two; • Decrease emotional arousal in moments of stuttering;	• Clients who have limited behavioral awareness of what talking *feels like*; • As a foundation for teaching strategies to increase *controlled fluency* and *easier stuttering*; • Young teens; • Beginning desensitization work

Speak more fluently (fluency shaping)	Client changes entire speaking pattern to produce controlled, stutter-free speech	• Slow rate through:
		  - Phrasing and pausing
		  - Prolonged vowels and/or syllables
		  - Longer turn-switching pauses
		• Decreased muscle tension through:
		  - Slow, relaxed onset of phonation
		  - Light or physically relaxed articulatory contact
			• Clients for whom fluency is highly important;
			• Clients with very severe stuttering who want to experience forward-moving speech;
			• Clients who can "shape" controlled fluency to *feel* and *sound* natural (to themselves and others);
			• Clients who can *navigate through* or *cope with* negative thoughts and emotions, or who approach talking without avoidance

Stutter more easily (stuttering modification)	Client identifies and changes moments of stuttering in real time, resulting in stuttered disruptions that are less frequent, shorter in duration, and less physically tense or struggled. May also result in fewer associated behaviors	• A sequence of strategies that include:
		  - Identifying an instance of stuttering in real time, **then**
		  - Staying in the stuttering moment (holding and tolerating), **then**
		  - Easing or pulling out by moving forward into the next sound or syllable with ease, **or**
		  - Cancellation by saying the word again using an easy onset or light contact immediately after the stuttered disruption
			• Clients with a high degree of emotional reactivity to stuttering;
			• Clients who frequently avoid sounds, words, or situations;
			• Clients who produce a high frequency of inaudible sound prolongations or disfluencies characterized by long periods of phonatory cessation;
			• Clients who do not want to change the entirety of their speech pattern through controlled fluency

Table 12.4 Strategies or approaches for changing negative thoughts and feelings about stuttering

Therapy approach	Description	Examples of therapy techniques	Helpful for...
Listening and valuing	• Clinician elicits the client's thoughts and feelings through intentional use of specific questions/prompts; • Clinician listens to and validates client's views about and reactions to stuttering, as opposed to informing or persuading client what to do about it	• Clinician uses questions/prompts to reveal thoughts and feelings and to deepen client–clinician relationship. These include: – Providing information – Open-ended questions – Affirming statements – Reframing statements – Affect response – Sharing self	• All clients and their families; • Diagnostic evaluations; • Beginning stages of therapy
Cognitive behavioral therapy (CBT)	• Clinician helps the client to identify and challenge their cognitive distortions (irrational thoughts that lead to negative emotion and behavior); • Comprised of 10 basic principles that guide the therapy process: formulating the problem in cognitive terms, strong therapeutic relationship, client's active participation, focusing on the problem, focusing on the present, teaching the client to become their own therapist, time-limited, structured sessions, identifying and responding to dysfunctional thoughts/beliefs, using a variety of techniques to change thinking/mood/behavior	• Client keeps a journal to record "thinking traps" or in-the-moment, automatic thoughts (quickly surfacing thoughts that are unrelated to logic or reason) about stuttering and related issues, and the emotions that immediately follow; • Journal entries are used as a platform for reframing these "thinking traps" into more neutral cognitions and emotions, and problem-solving more helpful responses	• Clients who present with "all-or-nothing" thinking, or for whom stuttering has a significant adverse impact on quality of life; • Clients with a high degree of emotional reactivity and a relatively limited ability to regulate emotional responses; • Clients who express a desire to change negative stuttering-related thoughts
Mindfulness	• Client is taught to intentionally and nonjudgmentally attend to internal and external experiences in the present moment	• Noticing but not evaluating thoughts, allowing them to pass while refocusing attention on an external point of focus, often the breath (inhaling and exhaling); • Discussing and practicing ways to "respond" rather than "react" to unhelpful thoughts	• Client reports preoccupation with unhelpful stuttering-related thoughts; • Client wants to devote less cognitive effort and attention to stuttering
Acceptance and commitment therapy (ACT)	• Clinician helps client to recognize and use personal values to inspire, motivate, and guide their behaviors while accepting painful and uncomfortable aspects of stuttering that they cannot change; • Comprised of six core processes that can guide the therapy process: self as context, defusion, acceptance, mindfulness, values, and committed action	• Distinguishing subjective thoughts from objective facts (defusion); • Values assessment to identify and clarify the client's values that then inform the goal-setting process (values)	• Clients who place a high value on communication and relationships and their importance to quality of life
Narrative therapy	• Client explores the ways in which their life is shaped by the stories they tell about themselves, and that others tell about them	• Clinician helps client to write their stuttering "story" to identify and reconstruct dominant themes that are not self-serving; • Externalizing stuttering in conversations and in writing by giving it a name and framing it as something separate from the person	• Clients who view stuttering as a major negative influence in their lives; • Clients who express feelings of guilt or shame about stuttering and being a person who stutters
Solution-focused brief therapy (SFBT)	• Clinician helps client to recognize their strengths and innate capacity for change, and to take small steps toward realizing their "preferred future"	• Clinician poses the "miracle question" to guide shared decision-making with the client: "If you woke up tomorrow, and a miracle happened so that you no longer stutter, what would be different?"; What would be the first signs that the miracle occurred?"; • Client uses a 10-point scale to rate "where they are now" and "where would be good enough" on their path to achieving their goals	• Client has difficulty recognizing and acknowledging their strengths, or helpful steps they have already taken to do something about stuttering
Self-help and support organizations	• Client participates in virtual or face-to-face group events aimed at providing social and emotional support for people who stutter	• Client engages in informal group discussions or activities with other individuals who stutter to gain perspective and to increase awareness of different ways to live with stuttering in a positive way; • Opportunities for volunteering or mentorship serve as positive coping mechanism	• Clients who report feelings of isolation or of being an outsider; • Clients who are in Contemplation or Preparation stages; • Clients who report that they have never met another person who stutters

Table 12.5 Strategies for approaching talking with less avoidance

Therapy approach	Description	Examples of therapy techniques	Helpful for...
Avoidance Reduction Therapy for Stuttering (ARTS)	Client learns to reduce struggle, confront fear, and deal with shame related to stuttering	• Clinician helps the client identify the helpful and unhelpful things they do in attempts to manage stuttering; • Clinician helps client develop a "fear hierarchy" of increasingly challenging social interactions. The client then intentionally engages in "open stuttering" (i.e., speaking freely, without the use of speech or stuttering modification strategies) in situations along the hierarchy, from least to most difficult	• Clients who report the use of multiple avoidance behaviors in attempts to keep from stuttering; • Clients with a high degree of emotional reactivity and a relatively limited ability to regulate emotional responses; • Desensitization; • Resilience training
Pseudostuttering	Client voluntarily produces simulated or imitated moments of stuttering, as realistically as possible	• Clinician models pseudostuttering and encourages clients to pseudostutter in various real-world contexts to promote desensitization (e.g., on the phone, at work)	• Clients who demonstrate high levels of emotional and physiological reactivity during moments of stuttering; • Clients who demonstrate high level of concern or worry about listener reactions to stuttering; • Desensitization
Self-disclosure	Client shares that they are a person who stutters with others, either before or during interactions	• Clinician helps client to develop and role-play a variety of verbal disclosure statements; • Clinician and client debrief following disclosure activities, using CBT strategies; • Exploring other ways to be "open" about stuttering (e.g., posting about stuttering on social media, wearing stuttering-related clothing, discussing stuttering with others)	• Clients who demonstrate high level of concern or worry about listener reactions to stuttering; • Clients who wish to inform others about their stuttering or reduce shame associated with being a person who stutters

and responses to moments of speech disruption. The goal is to recognize the emotional response to a moment of stuttering as *a feeling* that can be separate from the physical behaviors required to speak. In this way, the person learns that they can use and attend to the "normal" speaking process, even when strong emotions are present.

What does this approach look like in practice? To begin, the clinician provides the client with a clear and easily understood description of the speech mechanism and how we use it. This naturally involves both visual and written information about the anatomy of the subsystems involved (i.e., respiration, phonation, articulation), their various structures, and how we temporally coordinate the behaviors associated with each to produce *spontaneous* fluency (as opposed to *controlled* fluency, discussed further below). Although the client learns broadly about anatomy, they spend more time unpacking the physiology of speech production by experimenting with the manipulation of a set of five behaviors or "parameters"[2] that comprise speech production: *airflow, movement, timing, tension,* and *voicing*. First, the person is guided toward a physical awareness of how they are using these processes when they speak easily or in a forward-moving fashion. That is, what are they doing with *airflow* (continuous), *movement* (continually moving articulators from point to point), *timing* (of airflow and voicing with articulator movement), *tension* (of speech muscles), and *voicing* (on or off)? At the same time, the client is encouraged to manipulate these same processes to disrupt the forward flow of speech. For example, the clinician can instruct the client to stop their airflow while counting to 10 or place their tongue behind their upper teeth while saying /t/ in the word "two" and leave it there for too long (i.e., timing) or press it hard against their teeth by using too much muscle tension (i.e., tension). In this way, the person who stutters is learning the relationship

between what they physically *do* and how these behaviors underlie both fluent and disfluent speech. In Williams' own words[2]:

"With an increased awareness of behavior during the normal talking process, (the person who stutters) can begin to compare what they do to interfere with talking with what they can do to facilitate it. This provides the framework for constructive behavior change. They practice interfering on each speech parameter and then changing what they are doing to normal functioning on the parameter. Following this, they can practice on interfering on combinations of speech parameters (e.g. voicing and movement) and then change to normal talking behavior. As they practice in different speaking situations, they learn that they can be in charge of what they are doing. This reduces or eliminates most of the fears of stuttering."

In summary, the *Normal Talking* process emphasizes the importance of understanding and feeling the way one talks in general—both fluently and disfluently—as the primary mechanism for speech change. There are two main caveats offered here. One is that this approach is relatively unknown by practitioners in the field. The second is the lack of research support for its efficacy or effectiveness. These two important points are undoubtedly linked to the fact that Williams and his students published relatively little about how to implement the approach, and the desired outcomes of the approach are not clearly defined (i.e., increased spontaneous fluency, acceptance of stuttering, decreased emotional reactivity, or all of these?). That said, there is widespread acknowledgment that an emphasis on behavioral awareness of how we talk, both fluently and disfluently, is foundational to learning how to *change* the way one speaks, suggesting a role for this approach in the beginning stages of therapy for speech modification.

12.5.2 Speak More Fluently

This approach is commonly known as fluency shaping, but it also includes techniques called smooth speech, prolonged speech, or speech restructuring.[27,28,29,30] Some clinicians have even developed their own idiosyncratic titles for this approach such as "superfluency"[31] or "easy, relaxed approach, smooth movement."[32] Despite the variety of names of this approach, they all share the same primary goal: teach the client strategies that lead to *controlled fluency*, or speech that is *stutter free*. Intervention programs rooted in the major tenets of the speak more fluently approach are widely used around the world and are backed by relatively strong empirical support for reducing the frequency of stuttering, in some cases reporting minimal to no stuttering posttreatment. That is, when individuals who stutter use the techniques associated with this approach, they can produce greater amounts of fluent speech (controlled or spontaneous) at least in the short-term (up to 1 year posttherapy).

In practice, the techniques that yield stutter-free speech target *time*, *tension*, or both.[33] With regard to speech *timing*, the main goal is to teach the client how to reduce the overall rate of speech in conversation. To be sure, it is not the case that people who stutter speak at an atypically fast rate, but rather that slowing down facilitates smoother within- and between-word transitions, and thus, fluent speech. As shown in ▶ Table 12.3, speech techniques that lead to a reduced speaking rate include phrasing and pausing, prolonged syllables, and slow and smooth initiation of speech (particularly at the initiation of utterances). Techniques that target muscle *tension* and facilitate a more physically relaxed speaking mode include light articulatory contact, slow and smooth speech initiation, and physically relaxed or "easy" onset of phonation.

When a person who stutters uses these strategies correctly, the result is *controlled fluency*. As previously mentioned, this is not to be confused with *spontaneous fluency*, which is the fluent speech that an individual automatically produces without attending to *how* they are speaking and, thus, *without intentional use of strategies or techniques*. This distinction is important for clinicians who are using this approach with their clients in that it is essential to reinforce *what is being taught*, which in this case is controlled fluency. The contextual variability of stuttering (see ▶ Chapter 1) almost guarantees that over the course of therapy, people who stutter will produce increased amounts of spontaneous fluency within the session. Although this is important to note—if the goal is fluency—it is not what is being taught. The clinician should focus both teaching (through modeling and verbal instruction) and feedback on controlled fluency, perhaps noticing and commenting on the client's increased spontaneous fluency but not necessarily praising it (e.g., "I just noticed a lot of effortless fluency" instead of "I just noticed a lot of great fluency. Nice work!").

An additional point to note about controlled fluency relates to the client's perceptions of naturalness and spontaneity, and the extent to which this new way of talking impacts both. Studies have shown that while the use of strategies to reduce speech rate and decrease muscular tension yields fluent speech, individuals using them report that their speech sounds, and more importantly *feels*, unnatural. Further, controlled fluency requires a relatively high degree of attentional focus until it becomes automatic, resulting in diminished spontaneity of communication. These experiences undoubtedly interfere with the long-term use of any technique that results in the person changing the entirety of their speech pattern such that they don't "feel like themselves."[34] It is essential, therefore, that the clinician teach the client to self-rate how *natural* their controlled fluency feels to them, how *comfortable* they are in intentionally using it in any situation, and how to adjust the use of techniques to increase both automaticity and spontaneity.

12.5.3 Stutter More Easily

This approach, also referred to as *Stutter More Fluently* or *Stuttering Modification*, employs a set of techniques that teach the client how to intentionally change the moment of stuttering in real time. By reducing muscle tension and sustaining airflow, voicing, and articulator movement while producing a moment of stuttering, the person can essentially change a long, physically tense moment of stuttering into a shorter, smoother, and therefore more "acceptable" form of stuttered disruption.[35,36,37] Simply put, the person "catches" a moment of stuttering, sustains it (or "holds on") until they are able to reduce muscle tension and/or initiate airflow, voicing, and movement (or "loosen up"), and smoothly transitions into the following sound, syllable, or word.

The most significant difference between the *Speak More Fluently* and *Stutter More Easily* approaches is that the first requires the client to change the entirety of their speech pattern to replace stuttering with controlled fluency, while the goal of the second is to modify only moments of stuttering. In addition to a focus on identifying and changing moments of stuttering, a goal of the *Stutter More Easily* approach is to *desensitize* the person to stuttering and, in doing so, reduce feelings of distress and help them to more readily approach speaking. Specifically, these techniques provide multiple opportunities for the client to confront stuttering both physically and cognitively, gradually reducing the negative reactivity and fear that can exacerbate the behaviors of stuttering.

The strategies that characterize *Stutter More Easily* and can lead to both changes in stuttering and reduced fear are presented in ▶ Table 12.3. They are typically taught in sequence as they build upon each other. For example, accurate and rapid *Identification* of individual moments of stuttering by the client as they are produced precedes modification of these instances. Changing any behavior, including stuttering, requires the individual to know *when* and *how* they produce it. Once the client is behaviorally, or physically, aware of when they stutter and how they are using their speech mechanism in those moments, they are ready to begin the process of modification. First, by *Holding and Tolerating* an instance of stuttering, the individual learns to "stay in" the moment rather than pushing through or recoiling. At these times, the individual who stutters is typically filled with emotional awareness and in a vacuum of behavioral (or physical) awareness.[38] Holding on to the moment of stuttering, just staying with it, allows the client to experience the associated fear, panic, and out-of-control feeling in a safe and accepting space, which is the essence of exposure therapy. With time, repeated opportunities to hold and tolerate stuttered disruptions allow these negative reactions to subside and in doing so, the client can attend to the physical feeling of stuttering—what they are doing with airflow, voicing, and articulators in that moment. In short, holding and tolerating facilitates a decrease in emotional awareness and an increase in physical awareness, which is a necessary skill for making behavioral change. Once the client can identify and sustain (hold) instances of stuttering, they can learn to *Pullout* by intentionally decreasing muscle tension, initiating airflow and voicing, and smoothly transitioning into the next sound, syllable, or word. In the cases where the client is not ready or able to identify and sustain actual moments of stuttering, they can produce imitated or simulated stuttered disruptions, also known as *voluntary stuttering* or *pseudostuttering*. Holding on to and pulling out of moments of pseudostuttering may not be as confrontational as during moments of authentic stuttering; nevertheless, doing so provides the client a close approximation of what they do when they stutter. In addition, through pseudostuttering or mimicking stuttering "on purpose," the client can practice holding and tolerating and pulling or easing out of instances of stuttering. It is important to note that pseudostuttering still requires skill at identification and training in behavioral awareness; that is, for the client to simulate moments of stuttering, they will need to know, on a physical level, how to use their speech mechanism to disrupt the forward flow of speech.

12.5.4 Summary

When the clinician and the client work together to determine what the client wants to change about stuttering and why, it is frequently the case that the individual decides that they are ready to learn ways to change speech or stuttering to make talking easier. In these cases, there are three primary approaches that can help. The first is the *Normal Talking Process*, which helps the client to attend to what they do physically to speak both fluently and disfluently. The focus is on increasing spontaneous, or automatic, fluency by comparing the physical feeling of fluent and disfluent speech. Through a process of experimentation with the various parameters required for speaking—airflow, voicing, movement, tension, and timing—the client learns how we vary muscle tension and coordinate respiratory, phonatory, and articulatory movements to speak. By paying attention to the physical feeling associated with spontaneous fluency (something that people who stutter produce most of the time when they speak), they can make adjustments when they begin to interfere with this process and return to "home base," or easy, forward-moving speech. The second approach to changing talking discussed in this section is *Speak More Fluently*, a method for teaching the client to change the entirety of their speech pattern. The goal is to use a set of techniques that lead to controlled fluency, or stutter-free speech. These strategies focus primarily on changing speech timing (e.g., rate reduction) and tension (e.g., easy onset of phonation, light articulatory contacts). Whereas the *Normal Talking Process* leverages awareness of spontaneous fluency to increase normally fluent speech, *Speak More Fluency* approaches focus on teaching ways to make overall changes in speech production that, when used properly, result in the elimination of overt stuttering through controlled fluency. The third approach, *Stutter More Easily*, differs significantly from the first two in that the focus is on the moment of stuttering, not fluency. In practice, the client is taught to identify, sustain, and ease out of moments

of stuttering. Here the goal is so-called acceptable stuttering, or moments of stuttering that are shorter, more physically relaxed, and less struggled—possibly accompanied by fewer associated or secondary behaviors (i.e., eye blinks, head movements).

Each of these approaches can be helpful and should be presented to the client as options. Although the client is the one who decides what they would like to change about the way they talk, there are some general rules of thumb, based on our experience, that the clinician should consider. First, we have found that regardless of what the client wants to do—learn to use controlled fluency, change moments of stuttering, or both—a good foundation for speech change is to begin therapy with instruction in the *Normal Talking Process*. Following the principles of this approach, the clinician helps the client to increase their physical awareness of talking easily and interfering with this process. In focusing directly on talking as something the client *is doing*, rather than something that is happening *to* them, the long process of desensitization and the decrease of emotional reactivity to stuttering begins. Second, for clients for whom fluency is highly important overall, or those for whom it is important to be *dependably* fluent in specific situations, *Speak More Fluently* approaches can be the most appropriate. In addition, we have found that for clients presenting with a high frequency of stuttering accompanied by physical struggle and associated behaviors, beginning therapy by teaching techniques to elicit controlled fluency can relatively quickly allow them to communicate more efficiently (i.e., produce more words per minute) and provide a boost of confidence that change is possible. Of course, for these individuals, it is also often the case that *Stutter More Easily* strategies are also desirable as they help desensitize to and promote behavioral awareness during moments of stuttering. Finally, for those clients who produce relatively mild stuttering (i.e., low-frequency disfluencies, short duration, few to no associated behaviors), the *Normal Talking Process* can be most helpful in that it highlights skills that the client already possesses (relatively large amounts of spontaneous fluency) by strengthening their behavioral awareness of what they do when they talk easily. This can lay a strong foundation for the client to figure out ways to ease out of moments of stuttering "on the fly," which is a skill subsumed under the *Stutter More Easily* approach.

In closing, it must also be said that many people who stutter, and their clinicians, begin therapy by experimenting with an integrated approach, that is, trying out strategies from all approaches so that (1) they can become physically aware of what they do when they talk, (2) they can be *intentionally* fluent at times of their choosing, and (3) they know how to and feel confident that they can change moments of stuttering, *in real time*, when they choose. After the client experiments with the strategies that either yield controlled fluency or easier stuttering, they can make decisions about which they prefer to focus on in therapy.

12.6 Selecting Therapy Approaches: Changing Thoughts and Feelings

As described in several places in this chapter, and throughout this book, people living with stuttering often experience negative thoughts, attitudes, and feelings about stuttering, communication, and themselves. There is a rich literature base showing that these thoughts and emotions develop over time as people who stutter experience the personal, academic, vocational, and social consequences of stuttering, as well as the stigma and self-stigma associated with being a person who stutters.[39,40] Clinicians working with teenagers and adults who stutter must be prepared to help clients express the thoughts and emotions they experience that cause distress and, in many cases, drive much of their behavior. Undoubtedly, when a person who stutters gains a measure of autonomy over the way they speak—by using controlled fluency or modifying instances of stuttering—their positive thoughts and feelings often increase as well. However, this is not always the case. A comprehensive approach to the treatment of stuttering must include the cognitive and affective pieces of the problem that, for many, represent the most significant challenges.

Here we can revisit the discussion at the beginning of this chapter, namely, the importance of learning from related disciplines. Nowhere is this more critical than when deciding how to help a person who stutters change their thoughts and feelings about stuttering. This is an essential consideration in stuttering therapy, and is within the scope of practice for speech-language pathologists. In recent years, several researchers and clinicians in the field of stuttering have described ways in which established approaches in counseling psychology can be used in therapy. When the person who stutters is ready to confront and change the way they cope with stuttering, the clinician must have a working knowledge of how to get started on the journey. In the subsections that follow, we will provide brief summaries of the more widely used and promising approaches from counseling psychology and psychotherapy, along with additional resources for further study. A summary of the major principles underlying each approach, along with additional resources for more in-depth study, is provided in ▶ Table 12.4.

12.6.1 Listening and Valuing

In his seminal text on counseling in communication disorders, Luterman[24] asserts that the key to helping people to understand and act on what they need to feel better is for the clinician to *listen* and *value* what the individual reveals in conversation. What this means in practice is that the clinician engages the client in a dialogue, using a variety of different counseling responses to help them express and reflect upon their thoughts and feelings without providing a diagnosis of "what is wrong" or suggestions for how it can be "fixed." The role of the clinician is to select the response that will guide the client toward opening up and revealing their point of view. These responses are also strategic in that they invite varying levels of intimacy between the client and the clinician, and thus can strengthen (or keep neutral) the relationship between the two. For example, if a client says, "I'm embarrassed that I haven't been successful in therapy in the past," the clinician can respond with *information* about the types of stuttering therapies that are available and might also *persuade* the client to explore a specific program. Luterman refers to this as a *content* response, which essentially requires little or no follow-up from the client while keeping the relationship superficial. On the other hand, the clinician may say something as simple as "Tell me what makes you say that," an *open-ended question* that in some ways encourages the client to reveal what they have seen, heard, or

experienced that makes them believe they have failed and feel embarrassed. Of critical importance here is that the clinician does not offer an opinion on what the client thinks or how they feel. By bringing thoughts and emotions out into the open, by saying them out loud, and exploring them with another person, the client and clinician can unpack them together. Ultimately, it is up to the client to understand themselves in a way that helps them change the way they cope with stuttering and its consequences, both in their thoughts and in their emotions.

12.6.2 Cognitive Behavioral Therapy

This long-standing and widely used approach has been the bread and butter of counseling psychologists and psychotherapists for many years. In her excellent book, Judith Beck[41] describes cognitive behavioral therapy (CBT) as a process of understanding the perception of events and experiences that have led to the client's behaviors and feelings. The approach is rooted in the cognitive model that asserts that specific situations do not cause us to feel a certain way; rather, it is the way we *interpret* events or experiences that influences our emotions. And it is our emotions, not our thoughts, that determine our behavior, or what we *do*.

The core strategy in CBT is to first help the client link situations they experience (or have experienced) to the thoughts that arise automatically during the event. Here, it is important to understand that these *automatic thoughts* are very different from those that we develop through contemplation or active, critical examination. Rather, automatic thoughts "just happen"—popping up just under the surface, below our conscious awareness. It is the *emotion* or *feeling* tied to an automatic thought that we notice, and *that* makes us feel distressed. As an example, suppose an adolescent boy who stutters tells the clinician that walking into the cafeteria at school is stressful. The therapist then prompts him to describe the situation, and as he does, the therapist notices the boy becoming flushed and losing eye contact—clearly experiencing an emotional reaction. The clinician stops the boy and asks:

Clinician: "What is going through your mind right now?"
Teen: "I'm going to stutter when I talk at lunch."
Clinician: "What else?"
Teen: "I think that people think I'm weird when I stutter."
Clinician: "And how does that make you feel?"

This sequence of clinician questions is an example of the essential structure of CBT, one in which the therapist helps the client identify their automatic thoughts and their consequent emotions and behaviors. For example, suppose the teen answers this last question by revealing that he feels ashamed. The clinician can then probe to uncover what the boy does when he feels this way—perhaps avoiding eating lunch in the cafeteria. The focus of therapy then becomes one in which the therapist and the client problem-solve ways to break these "thinking traps" by searching for evidence to support or refute the automatic thought ("People don't like me"). In summary, the methods of CBT can be used in stuttering therapy to help a client examine connections between situations and their cognitive and emotional reactions to them—and to search for interpretations that lead to positive coping strategies.

12.7 Mindfulness

The practice of *mindfulness* has seen a significant increase over the past 20 years or so, proving to be a powerful method for improving psychological well-being.[42] More recently, practitioners and researchers have described the efficacy of incorporating mindfulness practice into stuttering treatment, finding that it improves the ability to attend to what one *is doing* at the moment (physically, cognitively, and emotionally), an essential skill in all forms of therapy.[43] Further, the act of staying in the present moment, without the continual shifting between the past and the future so common to the human experience, leads to lower levels of anxiety and time urgency (the feeling of being rushed to perform) and increased mental acuity and emotional self-regulation. For these benefits alone, mindfulness practice can be helpful for individuals who stutter and provide a stable foundation for the challenging work of therapy.

12.7.1 Acceptance and Commitment Therapy

Acceptance and commitment therapy (ACT) is an expanded version of CBT that combines (1) the process of contrasting automatic thoughts with objective observations and (2) mindfulness and personal *values* to develop a roadmap for setting treatment goals.[44] In addition to using CBT strategies, the ACT process begins with a values clarification exercise that facilitates the expression of what is important to the client. One such exercise requires them to think of a moment from the past or more recently when they felt joyful, fulfilled, or calm. They are then prompted to describe the setting: Who was there? What was happening? What were the surroundings? This activity helps the client understand the essential ingredients of situations or events that bring them feelings of contentment or ease—particular relationships, settings, activities, or topics of conversation. These are identified as the client's values and doing things to move closer to achieving them becomes the goal of therapy. For example, if relationships in general, or with specific people, are something the client values, what changes can they make to get closer to attaining more or better relationships? If some of these changes relate to stuttering, the client and clinician can discuss how doing something about stuttering may help the client initiate more social relationships. The important point is that the client may come to see that doing something about stuttering helps them to achieve something personally meaningful, not because stuttering itself needs to be changed. Just as importantly, the clinician may come to understand that their clients who stutter are able to meet their aspirational values despite, and sometimes because of, stuttering.

In addition to identifying important values and the role that stuttering plays in living them out, the ACT approach also emphasizes acceptance of stuttering as something that is an integral part of the client's past, present, and probably future life. Stuttering and the thoughts and feelings the client experiences are noticed but not evaluated, and attempts are not made to eliminate them. Instead, the client is taught how to attend to the present without judgment (*acceptance*) and make a *commitment* to flexibly *respond* (rather than react) to their thoughts, emotions, and behaviors in ways that honor their values. By doing so routinely, the client's perspective shifts from what they can do to

eliminate stuttering toward what they can do about stuttering (if anything) to *live a values-driven life*.

12.7.2 Solution-Focused Brief Therapy

The focus of this approach is on what the client wants to achieve and how to do it as opposed to closely examining the problem and its causes. The word "brief" in the title conveys the result of spending *less* time discussing the problem and *more* time talking about possible solutions; the goal of solution-focused brief therapy (SFBT) is to quickly implement a course of action and see positive results in a relatively short period of time (or relatively few therapy sessions).[45]

SFBT involves a targeted conversation in which the clinician asks questions to uncover times in the client's life when stuttering has *not* been a problem or an exception to the rule. For example, if a client who stutters is anxious about talking and potentially stuttering at parties but is not distressed about stuttering when talking in other, smaller social situations (e.g., in the break room at work), the therapist would highlight the client's interactions at work as an *exception* to the client's *usual* experience with stuttering. The clinician and client then discuss ways in which the irregularity differs from the client's typical experience with stuttering, with the therapist focusing the conversation on the strengths and abilities that the client *already* possesses and uses in those atypical situations. In this way, the therapist borrows principles from positive psychology described earlier in this chapter, bringing the client's skills to the forefront instead of trying to build new ones. In fact, it is this strategy—illuminating what is already known as opposed to what needs to be learned—that is the main reason that SFBT can be implemented over a relatively short time frame.

12.7.3 Narrative Therapy

This approach to understanding the way we think and feel about ourselves assumes that our identity is shaped by the stories that people in our lives tell about us and the ways in which we rewrite them.[46] For some people who stutter, the main theme in their story, and in turn their identity, is their stuttering and the fact that they are a person who stutters. As such, their story is described as "thin," meaning that in their minds, stuttering makes up the bulk of who they are. Narrative therapy provides a structure for expanding one's story to include multiple pieces, a "thickening" of one's identity so to speak. One of the first steps in narrative therapy for stuttering is to help the client to *externalize* stuttering by giving it a name and describing it as an entity separate from the person.[47] The client then writes about stuttering as though it were a person, describing its characteristics and their relationship with it. This is followed by another writing assignment in which the client is instructed to "Write about a time when stuttering wasn't able to boss you around" or "did not control you." Through the lens of their own stories, the client comes to see that they have experienced *typical* and *unique outcomes* related to stuttering, both resulting from a complex interaction of external and internal forces. Here, as in *SFBT*, the emphasis is on the *unique outcome* (i.e., those times when stuttering did not control you) and the internal strengths and skills the client brought to the situation that they already possess. Simply put, the goal is for the client to write a "new story" (or identity) in which stuttering occupies less space.

12.7.4 Bibliotherapy

Bibliotherapy refers to the process of reading, reflecting upon, and discussing first-person narratives. By reading and discussing the stories that people who stutter have shared about their lives, both clients and clinicians can better understand the lived experience of stuttering and increase their awareness of different ways to cope with it. For example, in a recent qualitative study, adults who stutter reported that reading and discussing the narrative *Out With It* (a memoir about stuttering written by a person who stutters) in their therapy sessions was beneficial.[48] Specifically, they reported that reading the memoir helped normalize stuttering, inspired more positive thoughts and feelings, and instilled hope for living well with stuttering in the future. Regarding change readiness, studies in behavioral health psychology have shown that bibliotherapy can move clients in Precontemplation toward Action. In our clinical experience, we have found that some clients are not ready to discuss their stuttering but are willing and open to talking about stuttering in general, at a safe distance and removed from themselves. Reading about the experiences of *others* who stutter is a way to help more guarded clients "dip their toes" in the water of openly talking about stuttering-related thoughts and feelings. Finally, it is worth mentioning that clinicians should be creative in exploring a variety of platforms for bibliotherapy. For example, clients who do not enjoy reading, or who are poor readers, can watch and discuss films such as "The Way We Talk" or "When I Stutter," TED (technology, entertainment, and design) talks or videos made by people who stutter, or listen to podcasts and audiobooks.

12.7.5 Self-Help and Support Organizations

Connecting with other people who stutter in a safe, supportive environment where stuttering is the norm, not the exception, is in and of itself therapeutic. Although not typically facilitated by speech-language pathologists, stuttering self-help or support groups can play an integral role in developing healthy coping mechanisms and social support among people who stutter of all ages. Spending time and talking with other people who stutter can help the client realize that they have options about the ways in which they think and feel about stuttering and how to live with it. A growing body of evidence indicates that participating in stuttering self-help groups increases self-acceptance and reduces feelings of shame and isolation.[49,50,51] There are many organizations that offer self-help or support events, and these events can take a variety of formats ranging from 1-hour virtual "hangouts" to multiday in-person conventions. Specific support organizations include the National Stuttering Association (NSA), FRIENDS: The National Stuttering Association for Young People who Stutter, and Stutter Social.

12.8 Selecting Therapy Approaches: Approaching Talking without Avoiding

Many people who stutter become highly adept at anticipating upcoming moments of stuttering. This can exist at the sound or word level, where speakers scan ahead when they are talking and identify a specific upcoming sound/word that they know they will stutter on. In these instances, people who stutter often employ a variety of avoidance behaviors such as changing that target sound/word with a similar word that is easier to say, using filler words to buy themselves time, or talking around the target word (i.e., circumlocuting). People who stutter also anticipate stuttering at the situation level, where they have a sense that they will stutter during a specific interaction in the future such as when introducing themselves at an upcoming party or during a forthcoming work presentation. This anticipation of impending difficulty, and the subsequent avoidance behaviors that speakers plan and carry out, contributes a great deal to their overall distress and feeling of "walking on eggshells."

One approach to helping clients approach feared sounds/words is *Stutter More Easily*, which we described previously. With this approach, clients are guided to enter moments of stuttering, and then hold and tolerate them before easing out. When practiced in a safe and supportive space, this act of staying in a moment of stuttering can be hugely desensitizing for people who stutter and can help them feel more comfortable approaching trigger sounds/words in the future. In addition to this approach, there are other ways that clients can practice approaching talking and stuttering, which we will describe in the following subsections and are outlined in ▶ Table 12.5.

12.8.1 Avoidance Reduction Therapy for Stuttering

Avoidance Reduction Therapy for Stuttering (ARTS) is a therapy approach grounded in Joseph Sheehan's pioneering theoretical and clinical work in stuttering that has been refined and modernized by Vivian Sisskin.[52,53] The *ARTS* perspective holds that attempting to *control* or *suppress stuttering* results in greater communication difficulty than the act of stuttering itself. Specifically, teens and adults who stutter have experienced many years of communication difficulty and as such, have developed idiosyncratic strategies or "tricks" to avoid and escape these disruptions. The heart of ARTS is helping clients learn to do *less* when they stutter—less control, avoidance, escape, emotional reactivity, and unhelpful thoughts that all lead to struggle behaviors. By approaching feared sounds, words, and situations, clients can communicate with greater efficiency, spontaneity, comfort, confidence, and joy.

12.8.2 Pseudostuttering

The act of stuttering, and the anticipation that leads up to it, commonly spurs a great deal of negative thoughts and feelings for teens and adults who stutter. They may be afraid of feeling "out of control," anxious of how their listener will perceive them, guilty about taking up extra time during the interaction, or shame about how they talk. These negative emotions can take hold of the speaker and deter them from approaching talking. A long-held approach for desensitizing clients to the negative emotions they have associated with the moment of stuttering is to guide them in simulating stuttering, an exercise that is commonly referred to as *pseudostuttering, voluntary stuttering*, or *purposeful stuttering* and is, in essence, a form of exposure therapy.

The primary goals of pseudostuttering are to (1) desensitize the client to the autonomic nervous system arousal (i.e., "fight or flight") and negative emotion that accompany moments of stuttering and (2) practice stuttering modification techniques such as holding, tolerating, and easing out of stuttered disruptions. Pseudostuttering in a manner that most closely simulates the client's actual stuttering has a more positive effect on affective, behavioral, and cognitive outcomes than pseudostuttering in a way that is different from how the client typically stutters.[54] As such, the client must first become physically aware of what they do when they stutter. Once the client's behavioral awareness of their stuttering pattern is adequate, they can purposefully stutter in a way that physiologically mirrors what they do during actual moments of stuttering.

It is common for a client to be confused or resistant when pseudostuttering is first introduced in therapy. Why am I being asked to stutter *more* when I have come here to learn how to stutter *less?* This is a valid concern, and as such, the clinician must present the client with a sound and clear rationale for the ways in which pseudostuttering can help them approach talking with less avoidance. As the client practices pseudostuttering in the safe space of the therapy room and gradually outside of it, the clinician must provide examples that mirror the client's unique style of stuttering. When the clinician "puts stuttering in her own mouth," he or she is not only modeling to the client what the target behavior is but also desensitizing the client to hearing and seeing stuttering, which serves to normalize their experience. In time, the emotional arousal associated with the moment of stuttering slowly dissipates and the client finds it easier to approach previously feared sounds, words, and situations.

12.8.3 Self-Disclosure

Another way to help clients learn to approach, rather than avoid, stuttering and speaking situations is to explore, role-play, and practice self-disclosure. Self-disclosure refers to instances in which people who stutter share information about their identity as a person who stutters with others, often through verbal disclosure statements. There are infinite ways to tell others about stuttering, but an example of a disclosure statement is "You might notice that I stutter; feel free to check in with me if you have any questions about it." Research has shown that disclosing stuttering is most beneficial at the beginning of a communicative interaction when presented as a neutral (rather than apologetic) statement.[55,56] Self-disclosure is also associated with social benefits for both speakers and listeners.[57,58] Specifically, individuals who stutter report that disclosing stuttering reduces fear and worry and increases feelings of authenticity, self-respect, and dignity. Further, people who stutter report that disclosing stuttering makes it easier for them to be present with their communication partners because they can "let go" of the urge to monitor whether the listener knows about their stuttering. Finally, listeners perceive speakers who disclose stuttering as more outgoing, confident, and friendly compared to those who do not disclose.[59]

Although there are several positive benefits associated with stuttering disclosure, it is important to remember that deciding whether to self-disclose (and when to do it) is a personal choice that should be made by the client. Outcomes of disclosing a stigmatized condition are not always positive, and are influenced by *how* and *why* clients choose to disclose, along with a host of other factors.[60]

12.8.4 Summary

For many teens and adults who stutter, the amount of space that negative thoughts and feelings about stuttering occupy in their minds is the primary contributor to a reduced quality of life, even more so than the behavior of stuttering itself. Even so, it is often the case that both clients and clinicians default to speech goals as the focus of therapy. The reasons for this are unclear, but likely relate to the familiarity and comfort with dealing with the observable characteristics (overt speech and stuttering patterns) rather than the unobservable (thoughts and feelings). Further, people who stutter are sometimes not consciously aware that they avoid, or that they frequently engage in negative thinking, as these ways of reacting have become habitual coping patterns. These Precontemplators are not seeking ways to change because they do not clearly see the problem, and they feel hopeless that anyone or anything can help. Working with people who stutter requires the clinician to be prepared to help the client learn ways to *intentionally* respond to stuttering, first by offering a safe place to express thoughts and feelings and second by helping them to explore strategies for changing unhelpful thoughts, feelings, and behaviors.

12.9 Putting it All Together: Two Cases

The following two cases—one a teen who stutters (Appendix 12.1) and one an adult who stutters (Appendix 12.2)—provide an opportunity for you to integrate and apply what you have learned in this chapter. After reading these case descriptions, discuss each and map out a basic therapy approach. Include major areas of focus, with a rationale based on the information provided in each case and try your hand at writing therapy goals. Consider the following questions:

1. What does the client seem *most ready* to do about stuttering? Why?
2. What additional information do you need to develop a therapy plan? How will you obtain it? For instance, are there additional assessments you would like to administer? Are there other people you would like to talk to? What questions do you want to ask the client and/or others?
3. What therapy approach(es) appear warranted and recommended for this client? Why?
4. Based on questions 1, 2, and 3, what might you and the client do in the first therapy session? Can you write two or three long- and short-term goals?

References

[1] Plexico LW, Erath S, Shores H, Burrus E. Self-acceptance, resilience, coping and satisfaction of life in people who stutter. J Fluency Disord. 2019; 59:52–63

[2] Williams D. A perspective on approaches to stuttering therapy. In: Gregory H, ed. Controversies about Stuttering Therapy. Baltimore, MD: University Park Press; 1979:241–268

[3] Wampold BE, Imel ZE, Laska KM, et al. Determining what works in the treatment of PTSD. Clin Psychol Rev. 2010; 30(8):923–933

[4] Wampold BE. How important are the common factors in psychotherapy? An update. World Psychiatry. 2015; 14(3):270–277

[5] Lambert MJ. Psychotherapy outcome research: implications for integrative and eclectic therapists. In: Norcross JC, Goldfreld MR, eds. Handbook of Psychotherapy Integration. New York, NY: BasicBooks; 1992:94–129

[6] Wampold BE, Imel ZE. The great psychotherapy debate: the evidence for what makes psychotherapy work. New York, NY: Routledge; 2015

[7] Robey RR. A meta-analysis of clinical outcomes in the treatment of aphasia. J Speech Lang Hear Res. 1998; 41(1):172–187

[8] Herder C, Howard C, Nye C, Vanryckeghem M. Effectiveness of behavioral stuttering treatment: a systematic review and meta-analysis. Contemp Issues Commun Sci Disord. 2006; 33:61–73

[9] Croft RL, Watson J. Student clinicians' and clients' perceptions of the therapeutic alliance and outcomes in stuttering treatment. J Fluency Disord. 2019; 61:105709

[10] Plexico LW, Manning WH, DiLollo A. Client perceptions of effective and ineffective therapeutic alliances during treatment for stuttering. J Fluency Disord. 2010; 35(4):333–354

[11] Prochaska JO, DiClemente CC. The transtheoretical approach: crossing traditional boundaries of therapy. Homewood, IL: Dow Jones-Irwin; 1984

[12] Prochaska JO, DiClemente CC, Norcross JC. In search of how people change. Applications to addictive behaviors. Am Psychol. 1992; 47(9):1102–1114

[13] Prochaska JO, Velicer WF, Rossi JS, et al. Stages of change and decisional balance for 12 problem behaviors. Health Psychol. 1994; 13(1):39–46

[14] Mauriello LM, Rossi JS, Fava JL, et al. Assessment of the pros and cons of stress management among adolescents: development and validation of a decisional balance measure. Am J Health Promot. 2007; 22(2):140–143

[15] Redding CA, Mundorf N, Kobayashi H, et al. Sustainable transportation stage of change, decisional balance, and self-efficacy scale development and validation in two university samples. Int J Environ Health Res. 2015; 25(3):241–253

[16] O'Hea EL, Boudreaux ED, Jeffries SK, Carmack Taylor CL, Scarinci IC, Brantley PJ. Stage of change movement across three health behaviors: the role of self-efficacy. Am J Health Promot. 2004; 19(2):94–102

[17] Shiffman S, Balabanis MH, Paty JA, et al. Dynamic effects of self-efficacy on smoking lapse and relapse. Health Psychol. 2000; 19(4):315–323

[18] Floyd J, Zebrowski PM, Flamme GA. Stages of change and stuttering: a preliminary view. J Fluency Disord. 2007; 32(2):95–120

[19] Rodgers NH, Gerlach H, Paiva AL, Robbins ML, Zebrowski PM. Applying the Transtheoretical Model to Stuttering Management Among Adolescents: Part II. Exploratory Scale Validation. Am J Speech Lang Pathol. 2021; 30(6):2510–2527

[20] Attride-Stirling J, Humphrey C, Tennison B, Cornwell J. Gathering data for health care regulation: learning from experience in England and Wales. J Health Serv Res Policy. 2006; 11(4):202–210

[21] Prochaska JO, DiClemente CC. Stages of change in the modification of problem behaviors. Prog Behav Modif. 1992; 28:183–218

[22] Miller W, Rollnick S. Motivational interviewing: helping people change. 3rd ed. New York, NY: Guilford Press; 2013

[23] Behrman A. Facilitating behavioral change in voice therapy: the relevance of motivational interviewing. Am J Speech Lang Pathol. 2006; 15(3):215–225

[24] Luterman D. Counseling Persons with Communication Disorders and their Families. 6th ed. Austin, TX: Pro-Ed; 2017

[25] Quesal R, Yaruss S. Historical perspectives on stuttering treatment: Dean Williams. Contemp Issues Commun Sci Disord. 2000; 27:178–187

[26] Zebrowski PM, Arenas RM. The "Iowa Way" revisited. J Fluency Disord. 2011; 36(3):144–157

[27] Blomgren M. Stuttering treatment for adults: an update on contemporary approaches. Semin Speech Lang. 2010; 31(4):272–282

[28] Onslow M, Costa L, Andrews C, Harrison E, Packman A. Speech outcomes of a prolonged-speech treatment for stuttering. J Speech Hear Res. 1996; 39(4):734–749

[29] O'Brian S, Onslow M, Cream A, Packman A. The Camperdown Program: outcomes of a new prolonged-speech treatment model. J Speech Lang Hear Res. 2003; 46(4):933–946

[30] Bothe AK, Davidow JH, Bramlett RE, Ingham RJ. Stuttering treatment research 1970–2005: I. Systematic review incorporating trial quality assessment of behavioral, cognitive, and related approaches. Am J Speech Lang Pathol. 2006; 15(4):321–341

[31] Guitar B. Stuttering: an integrated approach to its nature and treatment. 4th ed. Philadelphia, PA: Lippincott Williams & Wilkins; 2014

[32] Gregory HH. Controversies about stuttering therapy. Baltimore, MD: University Park Press; 1979

[33] Conture EG, Curlee RF. Stuttering and related disorders of fluency. 3rd ed. New York, NY: Thieme; 2007

[34] Constantino CD, Eichorn N, Buder EH, Beck JG, Manning WH. The speaker's experience of stuttering: measuring spontaneity. J Speech Lang Hear Res. 2020; 63(4):983–1001

[35] Van Riper C. The treatment of stuttering. Englewood Cliffs, NJ: Prentice-Hall; 1973

[36] Williams DF, Dugan PM. Administering stuttering modification therapy in school settings. Semin Speech Lang. 2002; 23(3):187–194

[37] Blomgren M, Roy N, Callister T, Merrill RM. Intensive stuttering modification therapy: a multidimensional assessment of treatment outcomes. J Speech Lang Hear Res. 2005; 48(3):509–523

[38] Williams DE. A point of view about stuttering. J Speech Hear Disord. 1957; 22(3):390–397

[39] Boyle MP. Identifying correlates of self-stigma in adults who stutter: further establishing the construct validity of the Self-Stigma of Stuttering Scale (4S). J Fluency Disord. 2015; 43:17–27

[40] Boyle MP. Assessment of stigma associated with stuttering: development and evaluation of the self-stigma of stuttering scale (4S). J Speech Lang Hear Res. 2013; 56(5):1517–1529

[41] Beck JS. Cognitive Behavior Therapy: Basics and Beyond. 2nd ed. New York, NY: Guilford Press; 2011

[42] Kabat-Zinn J. Wherever you go, there you are: mindfulness meditation in everyday life. New York, NY: Hyperion; 2005

[43] Boyle MP. Mindfulness training in stuttering therapy: a tutorial for speech-language pathologists. J Fluency Disord. 2011; 36(2):122–129

[44] Beilby JM, Byrnes ML, Yaruss JS. Acceptance and commitment therapy for adults who stutter: psychosocial adjustment and speech fluency. J Fluency Disord. 2012; 37(4):289–299

[45] Nicolas A. Solution focused brief therapy with children who stutter. Procedia Soc Behav Sci. 2015; 193:209–216

[46] DiLollo A, Neimeyer RA, Manning WH. A personal construct psychology view of relapse: indications for a narrative therapy component to stuttering treatment. J Fluency Disord. 2002; 27(1):19–40, quiz 41–42

[47] Wolter JA, Dilollo A, Apel K. A narrative therapy approach to counseling: a model for working with adolescents and adults with language-literacy deficits. Lang Speech Hear Serv Sch. 2006; 37(3):168–177

[48] Gerlach H, Subramanian A. Qualitative analysis of bibliotherapy as a tool for adults who stutter and graduate students. J Fluency Disord. 2016; 47:1–12

[49] Boyle MP. Psychological characteristics and perceptions of stuttering of adults who stutter with and without support group experience. J Fluency Disord. 2013; 38(4):368–381

[50] Gerlach H, Hollister J, Caggiano L, Zebrowski PM. The utility of stuttering support organization conventions for young people who stutter. J Fluency Disord. 2019; 62:105724

[51] Trichon M, Tetnowski J. Self-help conferences for people who stutter: a qualitative investigation. J Fluency Disord. 2011; 36(4):290–295

[52] Sheehan JG. Conflict theory and avoidance-reduction therapy. In: Stuttering: A Second Symposium. New York, NY: Harper & Row; 1975:97–198

[53] Sisskin V. Avoidance Reduction Therapy for Stuttering (ARTS®). In: Amster BJ, Klein ER, eds. More than Fluency: The Social, Emotional, and Cognitive Dimensions of Stuttering. San Diego, CA: Plural Publishing; 2018:157–186

[54] Byrd CT, Gkalitsiou Z, Donaher J, Stergiou E. The client's perspective on voluntary stuttering. Am J Speech Lang Pathol. 2016; 25(3):290–305

[55] Healey EC, Gabel RM, Daniels DE, Kawai N. The effects of self-disclosure and non self-disclosure of stuttering on listeners' perceptions of a person who stutters. J Fluency Disord. 2007; 32(1):51–69

[56] Byrd CT, Croft R, Gkalitsiou Z, Hampton E. Clinical utility of self-disclosure for adults who stutter: apologetic versus informative statements. J Fluency Disord. 2017; 54:1–13

[57] Boyle MP, Milewski KM, Beita-Ell C. Disclosure of stuttering and quality of life in people who stutter. J Fluency Disord. 2018; 58:1–10

[58] Boyle MP, Gabel R. Toward a better understanding of the process of disclosure events among people who stutter. J Fluency Disord. 2020; 63:105746

[59] Byrd CT, McGill M, Gkalitsiou Z, Cappellini C. The effects of self-disclosure on male and female perceptions of individuals who stutter. Am J Speech Lang Pathol. 2017; 26(1):69–80

[60] Chaudoir SR, Fisher JD. The disclosure processes model: understanding disclosure decision-making and postdisclosure outcomes among people living with a concealable stigmatized identity. Psychol Bull. 2010; 136(2):236–256

[61] Wampold BE, Brown GS. Estimating variability in outcomes attributable to therapists: a naturalistic study of outcomes in managed care. J Consult Clin Psychol. 2005; 73(5):914–923

[62] Wampold BE, Imel ZE, Minami T. The placebo effect: "relatively large" and "robust" enough to survive another assault. J Clin Psychol. 2007; 63(4):401–403, discussion 405–408

Appendix 12.1 Case Study: Teen

Darrius, a 13-year-old English-speaking adolescent boy, was referred to the clinic by his father, Mr. Carter. Mr. Carter reported that Darrius was experiencing increased difficulties with communication after being discharged from therapy for stuttering approximately 1 year ago. According to Mr. Carter, recently Darrius has repeatedly expressed a desire for help with stuttering.

Darrius lives at home with his mother, father, and younger sister. He enjoys reading, playing video games, science experiments, and "anything Star Wars."

During the evaluation, Darrius stated that he would like "a place to talk about my stuttering" and to "learn how to change it." Analysis of a 300-word speech sample revealed an average of 20 disfluent words per 100 words, primarily characterized by sound/syllable repetitions and sound prolongations (without airflow or voicing, i.e., blocks). These disfluencies were accompanied by several associated behaviors, including reduced eye contact and hitting his leg with his fist. Darrius appeared to be highly aware of moments of stuttering and associated behaviors, specifically describing the pounding behavior as "annoying." He added that he would "like to change it if he knew how."

The *Stuttering Severity Instrument—Fourth Edition* (SSI-4[1]) was also administered, yielding a severity rating of "severe," and placing Darrius in the 78th to 88th percentile rank compared to other children who stutter in his age range. Darrius also completed the *Overall Assessment of the Speaker's Experience with Stuttering* (OASES[2]), which assesses the adverse impact of stuttering. His overall OASES score yielded a "moderate-severe" rating, with the highest score on the "Communication in Daily Situations" subtest.

Darrius also completed the *Stage of Change* scale to assess how ready he was to do something about stuttering. His responses indicated that he is in the *Preparation* stage for overall stuttering management. For the subscale responses, he indicated that he is also in the *Preparation* stage for both (1) learning and using speech strategies or techniques for speaking more fluently and/or stuttering with less tension and struggle and (2) changing negative thoughts and feelings about stuttering, but in Precontemplation for (3) approaching talking with less avoidance.

Darrius reported that his previous therapy focused on "cancellations and slowing down," and shared that these techniques "worked for a while, but not anymore." He described his family as "helpful" and "understanding" of stuttering. When asked if he wished anything could be different about stuttering at home, Darrius shared the opinion that being told to "slow down" is not helpful but that having "more time to talk helps a lot." He described classroom presentations and small talk with same-age peers as particularly challenging speaking situations. Further, he reported that he "sometimes" gets mocked and bullied for stuttering in science class, adding that he "doesn't know what to do when that happens," so he "stays quiet." When asked if he would be interested in meeting other teens who

stutter, Darrius said it "could be embarrassing" but might also help him "feel less alone" about stuttering.

Appendix 12.2 Case Study: Adult

Sasha is a 36-year-old woman who referred herself for a stuttering evaluation. She is married, has two young children, and works as a nurse. She remembers starting to stutter around the age of 8 years after her parents separated. She had minimal speech therapy when she was growing up, and the therapy she did have was not helpful; she recalls the speech-language pathologist (SLP) pulling her out of class to practice using "easy starts" while reading aloud, despite the fact that she tended to be spontaneously fluent while reading aloud. She did not receive any therapy for stuttering during high school or college. According to Sasha, she was diagnosed with an anxiety disorder in college and has been on a daily regimen of antianxiety medication since her mid-20 s.

During the evaluation, Sasha stated that she is "exhausted" from hiding stuttering all the time. She feels like she is "walking on eggshells" during every conversation and is at a "breaking point." Analysis of a 300-word conversational speech sample revealed an average of 7 speech disfluencies per 100 words, primarily characterized by interjections including "you know" and "uh" (e.g., "It's been *you know* really hard to *you know* talk on the phone and *uh-uh-uh*-introduce myself to *you know* new people"). She occasionally produced fleeting sound/syllable repetitions during both conversational speech and oral reading. Further, Sasha consistently avoided eye contact while speaking, especially while producing sound/syllable repetitions. When probed about her pattern of stuttering and avoidance, Sasha reported that she anticipates stuttering "almost always."

The *Stuttering Severity Instrument—Fourth Edition* (SSI-4; Riley, 2009) was also administered, yielding a severity rating of "very mild," placing Sasha in the 5th to 11th percentile of other adults who stutter. She also completed the *Overall Assessment of the Speaker's Experience with Stuttering* (OASES; Yaruss), which assesses the adverse impact of stuttering. Sasha's overall OASES score yielded a "severe" rating with the highest scores on both the "Your Reactions to Stuttering" and "Quality of Life" subtests.

Sasha also completed the *Stage of Change* scale to assess how ready she is to do something about stuttering. Her responses indicated that she is in the *Contemplation* stage for stuttering management. For the subscale responses, she indicated she is in the Precontemplation stage for learning and using strategies for speaking more fluently or stuttering with less struggle, *Preparation* for changing negative thoughts and feelings about stuttering, and *Contemplation* for approaching talking with less avoidance.

During the evaluation, Sasha appeared to react negatively to the clinician's use of the word "stuttering" to describe her communication difficulty. She stated that "It's not that [stuttering]... it's some sort of panicky feeling." She does not use the words *stutter* or *stuttering* to describe herself or her pattern of speech. Sasha reported that she has never talked about her difficulty in speaking with her husband or other family members. She went on to say that "no one at work knows about my condition" and that she would like to "keep it that way."

References

[1] Riley G. Stuttering severity instrument for children and adults. 4th edition. Pro-Ed; 2009
[2] Yaruss JS, Quesal R. Overall assessment of the speaker's experience of stuttering. Stuttering Therapy Resources; 2010

Section V

Additional Treatment Considerations

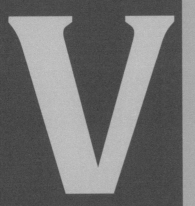

13 Language and Phonological Considerations

Nancy E. Hall, Julianne Garbarino, and Nan Bernstein Ratner

Abstract

This chapter aims to describe fundamental considerations for assessment and treatment of stuttering within the context of language and phonology, along with best practices for treating concomitant stuttering and language/phonological impairments in children. The chapter expands on what is known about treating stuttering and concomitant phonology and/or language impairment, despite a lack of research on best practices. Thus, the approach espoused in this chapter is one in which language is recognized as the structure within which speech is embedded and therefore is central to how we plan and execute therapy. Accordingly, we review principles of evidence-based practice as well as practice-based evidence while discussing potential approaches to treating the child who stutters who presents with concomitant impairments in other areas of communication. Case studies are included to illustrate possible approaches to the management of children who stutter with comorbid diagnoses.

Keywords: stuttering, fluency disorder, language delay/disorder, phonological disorder, articulation, concomitant impairment

13.1 Introduction

We know that stuttering onset typically occurs around the time that the child's language and phonological developments are undergoing substantial growth (see ▶ Chapter 1 and Bloodstein et al[1] for an overview of stuttering onset). Thus, while we do not yet know the possible role that rapid advances in language and/or phonological development plays in precipitating the onset of stuttering, it is essential that we acknowledge the interaction between what is happening in the development of linguistic processes and those involved with motor speech production. Nevertheless, we know a few things about the complexities involved in interactions among language production, phonological encoding, and both stuttering and fluency that can guide work with children who face multiple challenges in producing grammatically correct, well-articulated, and fluent utterances. See ▶ Chapter 4 for details on the connection between stuttering and speech and language.

"Language impairment is observed more frequently in children who stutter than in the general population."

The complexity involved in speech and language formulation and production requires that we be diligent in collecting as much information as we can about a youngster's linguistic and pragmatic skills as well as their fluency abilities. Some children who stutter will have co-occurring phonology and/or language deficits. Stuttering and co-occurring, clinically relevant language impairment has been documented, with language impairment observed more frequently in children who stutter than in the general population.[2,3,4,5,6] Little is known about the nature of these language concerns in children who stutter, although some

have suggested these children might represent a "subgroup" of the larger population of children who stutter.[7,8] Regardless, children who stutter who also exhibit language impairment require careful therapeutic care. A balance between addressing their linguistic deficits and facilitating their fluency must be achieved such that one is not being sacrificed for the other. In terms of co-occurring stuttering and phonological impairment, little research evidence exists to suggest that there is an established association between the two (see Sasisekaran[9] for review). That said, the clinician treating a young child who stutters would be wise to bear in mind phonological skills and phonological context in structuring treatment goals, objectives, and activities (see discussion on phonology and stuttering later).

"The clinician should consider phonological skills and phonological context when structuring treatment goals, objectives, and activities."

We also know that even children who stutter with presumably typical language skills will have difficulty maintaining fluency while attempting to construct utterances that contain newly acquired or complex language structures (see ▶ Chapter 4 and Hall et al[10] for review). Because a common hallmark of child language disorders is difficulty with encoding new materials (often measured in tangible terms by examining children's ability to store and repeat nonsense words, i.e., nonword repetition [NWR]), many children who stutter with concomitant diagnoses of language impairment may struggle to remember new linguistic information, further stressing their abilities to be fluent. Difficulties with short-term (working) memory, as well as other executive function deficits, seem to be characteristic of most children with language impairment,[11] as well as some children who stutter (see ▶ Chapter 4).[7,8] Recent work suggests, in fact, that children who stutter with better NWR skills have more favorable prognoses for spontaneous recovery.[12] Thus, the child you are treating for stuttering may have weaknesses in memory for new information which merit both evaluation and therapy planning consideration.

Most recently, efforts to understand disorders of communication, such as stuttering and impairments of language and phonology, have highlighted the integrated nature of the systems underlying speech and language production. That is, while many of us studied from textbooks that classified stuttering as a "speech disorder," it is now clear that subsystems within the language production process interact and influence one another. Although classical approaches to communication disorders demarcate some as language, and others as speech, we now know that the conventional view of discrete contrasts (e.g., speech/language or linguistic/motor) is too simplistic and overlooks dynamic relationships between these constructs. For instance, in children, utterances that are relatively longer or more complex than the child's typical productions result in destabilization of the coordinated motor actions that underlie articulatory gestures.[13,14,15,16] This may reflect weakened connectivity between brain regions in children who stutter. For example, in their study of children who stutter, Usler et al[13] showed not only reduced coordination among motor gestures for speech but also difficulty in remembering and repeating complex linguistic stimuli, evidence of cascading effects of demands on aspects of the speech/language encoding process that interact with one another. This model of interactive processes necessitates an approach to treatment that recognizes the delicate balance between reducing linguistic demands to facilitate fluency while at the same time providing appropriate language and phonology targets to allow for continued growth.

"Simply demarcating a communication disorder as either speech or language overlooks the dynamic relationship between the two."

Finally, it is worth restating that best practices for the treatment of stuttering should always occur within an ecologically valid linguistic context. Thus, the clinician must plan and execute therapy in ways that allow the child to learn "real-world" strategies for managing fluency while also supporting language and phonology at or close to the zone of proximal development—creating appropriate opportunities for the child to continue to grow linguistically while both fluency and communication are facilitated. To generalize successfully, however, all work will need to be practiced under conditions that duplicate the cognitive, linguistic, and conversational time-constraint challenges of communicating in "real-world" situations.

"All work should be practiced under conditions that duplicate the cognitive, linguistic, and conversational time-constraints of communicating in 'real-world' situations."

13.2 Intervention Principles

Taken together, research studies suggest the following important considerations in working with children who stutter who have additional difficulties with articulation/phonology, language, or both:

- We know from studies of both typically developing children and children who stutter that various levels of language demand can adversely impact children's ability to maintain fluency (see ▶ Chapter 4 for more information). Thus, when designing activities meant to work on stuttering directly, the level of language challenge that these activities may require of the child needs to be carefully considered, if the objective is to facilitate fluent speech.
- Facilitating fluency, in the context of carefully designed linguistic tasks, can be advanced by providing ample opportunity to practice the speech motor behaviors consistent with fluent speech.
- Why language demand adversely impacts the child's ability to be fluent is not well understood. However, the relationship between language or phonological demand and fluency may be modulated by the impacts that increased linguistic challenge placed on the child's speech-motor system. An increased body of experimental research supports this view, for speech-motor stability has been shown to be adversely impacted by increasing language task demand in both children and adults.[13,14,15,16]

13.3 Diagnostic Considerations

13.3.1 A Thorough Evaluation

Given the recognized potential for comorbidity of stuttering and additional communication impairments, it is wise for clinicians to conduct thorough evaluations of all children referred for fluency disorder. Our clinical impression agrees with that of Johnson et al,[17] who found that disorders impacting the "form" of children's communication (e.g., articulation, fluency) are more likely to be identified as areas of concern by adults in a child's environment than are more subtle impairments in language understanding or use. Tomblin et al agree that language disorder may be under-referred.[18] Thus, thorough assessment of children referred for concerns about stuttering is imperative for the following reasons: (1) there is a high likelihood of comorbidity among communication impairments in young children and we do not want to miss a potential disorder that merits intervention; (2) the child's language skills are relevant in planning appropriate fluency therapy activities and goals; and (3) it is possible that the child's fluency profile is actually not stuttering, but evidence of a language formulation disorder. We will discuss the challenge of differential diagnosis of stuttering and other disfluency profiles later in this chapter.

"Given the potential for concomitant clinical needs, clinicians should conduct thorough evaluations of all children referred for fluency disorder."

A final benefit of thorough language and phonological assessment of the young child who stutters is that recent research suggests differential profiles of recovery and persistence in children based on test performance at initial assessment as well as growth in language skills over time.[19,20,21,22,23] Although poorer performance on language or phonological measures cannot predict that a given child will or will not recover without intervention, presence of a frank concomitant disorder or less than average performance in areas of communication development other than fluency may be used to counsel parents on the advisability of intervention, rather than continuing to wait for the child to outgrow either the stuttering or additional lags in speech and language.

13.3.2 Differential Diagnosis

It is our clinical experience that many clinicians encounter children who they feel are excessively disfluent and may stutter; however, they are unsure. The research literature increasingly documents why making decisions in these cases may be challenging. We now know that children with histories of language delay or diagnoses of language impairment may in fact display elevated rates of disfluency, including general categories of disfluency often grouped under the rubric of "stutterlike disfluency" (SLD).[24,25,26,27,28,29,30,31] The primary behavior seen in many reports is an elevated rate of whole- or part-word disfluency.

Similarly, bilingual children may demonstrate elevated levels of SLDs. Although some of these children undoubtedly stutter (see recent review by Choo and Smith[32]), not all children do—many simply show elevated rates of behaviors that overlap between stuttering and typical disfluency.[33,34,35,36] This pattern is far from universal.[37] In fact, typically fluent children who speak a language other than English may have rates of disfluency, including SLDs, that exceed conventional thresholds typically reported by studies that have tracked English-speaking children. The reader is referred to ▶ Chapter 14 for more on stuttering and bilingual considerations.

How is the clinician to distinguish between elevated rates of disfluency and "stuttering"? In our experience, when children with language delay/disorder or bilingual children, particularly those who are older, arouse concern due to the number of disfluent episodes seen in their speech samples, two classical components of stuttering are often not observed. As noted in other places in this text, stuttering is somewhat unique among childhood communication disorders because of its tripartite constellation of affect, behavior, and cognition, the so-called ABCs of stuttering (see ▶ Chapter 1). Bilingual children show, in our experience, only one of these: behavior. The other two are rarely in evidence. The first of these is that moments of stuttering lack the tension, struggle, or awareness that characterize the speech of children who stutter, features that cross with the quality of behavior, but also intersect with the affective qualities seen in stuttering. The second is that these children do not seem to have a self-concept of speaking difficulty that we typically assign to the cognitive features of stuttering.

We do not believe that it is trivial to presume that a child stutters when in fact they merely experience fluency breakdown more often than a peer judged to be typically fluent. Disfluency in this population is likely to arise from the child's difficulty in encoding language targets. In some cases, disfluency in bilingual children can even be an indication of attrition in language proficiency (of the heritage language when in a different majority language setting).[38] Therapies for stuttering have different underlying premises and goals than what is required if disfluency is the natural by-product of a less proficient expressive language system.

13.3.3 Profiles of "Atypical" Disfluency

Some children and adults present with disfluencies that affect the medial and final parts of words (e.g., "like -ike -ike"), and these are referred to as "atypical disfluencies."[39] These disfluencies have primarily been described in case reports. In most cases, the individuals presenting with atypical disfluencies have neurodevelopmental or acquired disorders including autism spectrum disorders,[39,40] attention deficit hyperactivity disorder,[41] brain trauma,[42,43] reading disability,[41,43] and language and articulation disorders.[43] Interestingly, though, of the two school-age children with atypical disfluencies described by McAllister and Kingston,[44] one had no neurodevelopmental or acquired conditions and the other had only a history of stuttering that had resolved.

As with the elevated disfluency levels that can be associated with typical bilingual language development, consideration of the cognitive and affective features associated with atypical disfluencies seems to indicate that these disfluencies are not a type of stuttering. Children and adults presenting with these atypical disfluencies may not be aware of them,[39,43,44] which clearly contrasts with the typical presentation of stuttering, especially in older individuals. Further, these disfluencies also are not reported to be associated with increased muscle tension.[40,43,44,45] Although atypical disfluency lacks at least two hallmark features of stuttering, such behaviors have responded to traditional stuttering modification therapy that begins with work in identifying the moments in which atypical disfluencies are produced.[39]

13.4 Treatment Options

13.4.1 Principles of Evidence-Based Practice and Practice-Based Evidence

Because so few studies have been done to evaluate how best to treat the child who stutters who has a concomitant articulatory/phonological or language disorder, and because each child will inevitably present with his or her own unique mix of strengths and needs, we would like to preface this section with a few reminders about the importance, not only of principles of evidence-based practice (EBP) but also of those of practice-based evidence (PBE).

To remind, EBP combines the best available published evidence with clinical expertise and patient/client preferences or specifics.[46] PBE, in contrast, gathers data on treatments and outcomes in routine service settings.[47] Readers should be mindful that the highest ranked "evidence" in EBP is the randomized clinical trial, which typically strives to examine uncomplicated clinical cases and tends to eliminate participants with concomitant problems[48]—the topic of this chapter. Thus, in this context, PBE can be very valuable.

We acknowledge at the outset that little empirical evidence exists to guide the clinician in working with a child who stutters who has concomitant clinical needs in phonology, language, or in any other aspect of communication (e.g., a child who stutters with autism spectrum disorder, attention deficit hyperactivity disorder, or intellectual deficiency). One cannot go to Google Scholar to determine what the best approach is for a 4-year-old who stutters, has numerous phonological processes, and has poor development of phrase structure in spoken language. To the extent that a clinician finds that their caseload in a public school setting, for example, tends to have multiple parallel individualized educational plan needs across different areas of communication (e.g., fluency, phonology, language), results of intervention with this particular caseload may be more informative than numerous reports of therapy effectiveness that were conducted using less complex child client profiles. Let us take another example. One of the most widely published interventions for young children who stutter is the Lidcombe Program.[49] To date, it has been modified in many ways, including telehealth versions.[50,51] However, the program requires substantive parental training, understanding, and commitment. How might this therapy (or any other therapy) fare when the parent is not available for training, unwilling, or otherwise not able to provide the daily sessions? This is when the clinician's local success in modifying the program to suit population- or setting-specific needs is very important in monitoring progress (or lack thereof) and adjusting therapy goals and methods to suit individual children. This is the heart of PBE, which is sensitive to demographics, limitations, or advantages of specific groups of children or specific settings.

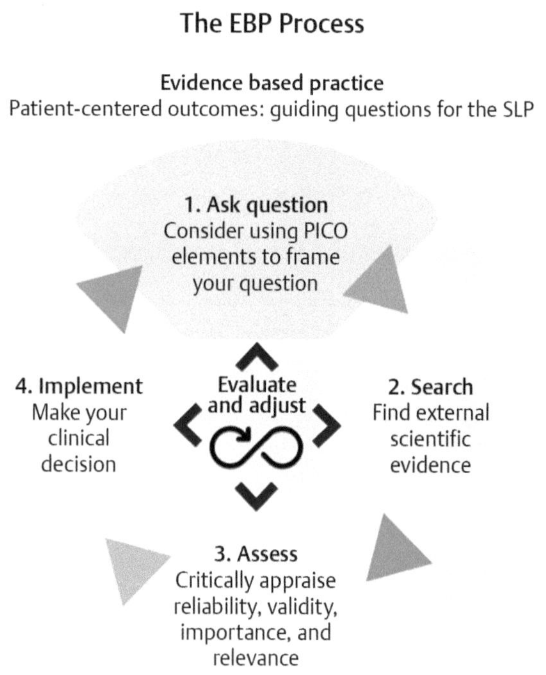

The EBP Process

Evidence based practice
Patient-centered outcomes: guiding questions for the SLP

1. Ask question
Consider using PICO elements to frame your question

Evaluate and adjust

4. Implement
Make your clinical decision

2. Search
Find external scientific evidence

3. Assess
Critically appraise reliability, validity, importance, and relevance

Fig. 13.1 The evidence-based practice cycle. (This image is provided courtesy of Chelsea G. Alexander, M.A., CCC-SLP.)

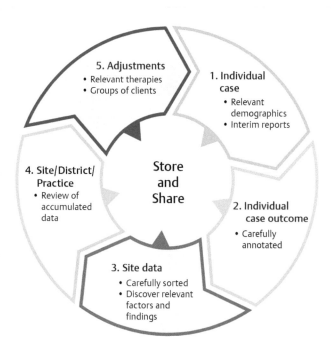

5. Adjustments
• Relevant therapies
• Groups of clients

1. Individual case
• Relevant demographics
• Interim reports

4. Site/District/ Practice
• Review of accumulated data

Store and Share

2. Individual case outcome
• Carefully annotated

3. Site data
• Carefully sorted
• Discover relevant factors and findings

13.4.2 Monitoring Outcomes

In the absence of empirical outcome or efficacy data, we can apply knowledge gleaned from basic research studies to construct and test our selection of therapy targets, their ordering, and other aspects of our approach to treatment. However, it sometimes appears that the final stage of both EBP and PBE is under-applied (see the "hub" in ▶ Fig. 13.1 and Step 5 in ▶ Fig. 13.2). This step requires us to evaluate the outcome of the treatment plan on the patient's behaviors. Even in published therapy outcome reports, close inspection of individual data can sometimes cause concern: in one report of a popular preschool treatment for stuttering, at least two children's treatment was not shifted to an alternative option after more than 90 weeks with no discernable progress.[52] That means that a single, manualized approach to treatment was employed for almost 2 years without clear evidence of a child's response to the desired criterion. The take-home message we want to convey is that even well-documented, evidence-based treatment approaches that work well for many children may not work well for an individual child. The clinician should not presume treatment effectiveness; clinicians should document progress flowing from their treatment decisions. If progress is not seen, treatment decisions need to be reconsidered. This may involve changing general approaches (e.g., whether one decides to use Lidcombe Program,[49,53] Palin Parent–Child Therapy,[54] RESTART-DCM,[55] or any other reasonably well-documented therapy), treatment goals, goal ordering, or activities. The evidence seen in the monitoring of client progress (or lack of progress) is more valuable than that reported for groups of children in a published article. How long might one wait before deciding that an

Fig. 13.2 A practice-based evidence map. (This image is provided courtesy of Chelsea G. Alexander, M.A., CCC-SLP.)

approach might not be appropriate for a particular child? As one possible strategy, we note that many reports of therapeutic change when using a program such as Lidcombe, for example, show rapid response to treatment from baseline status, often within a few weeks of therapy initiation. We suggest that a rule of thumb might be a few months (perhaps as long as 6 months), and then reevaluating why the child is not responding as anticipated.

"Even well-documented, evidence-based treatment approaches that work well for many children may not work well for an individual child."

Particularly when managing complex cases, the clinician may wish to view some therapy plans in the same way as we employ diagnostic teaching to appraise the client's response before committing to a long-term hierarchy of therapy activities. A suggested sequence of planning is as follows:

- *Use the available literature to decide how much "interference" there might be between two areas of therapy need in a single client.* Concretely, if working with a child who has an articulation disorder and also stutters, one might begin with a premise that can be drawn from the literature to date: that initial attempts at new phonological targets is unlikely to aggravate the child's fluency over and above its typical profile. Little evidence suggests a direct relationship between moments of fluency breakdown and children's misarticulations or phonological targets, although there may be an additional weight of phonetic complexity on speech production in children who stutter who also have a language disorder. In contrast, as noted in this chapter and others in this text, there is fairly strong evidence of the impacts of language targets on children's fluency and stuttering.
- *Consider possible "contradictory messages" in how therapy goals or targets are framed.* Thus, we might also think carefully about principles of articulation therapy or how we often see it applied in practice. For instance, as noted by Wolk and others,[56,57] and discussed further in the next section of this chapter, while one might overarticulate a therapy target to help the child focus on the task (e.g., full loud release of a word-final consonant, or prolongation of a sibilant in a complex cluster), such a "cue" might contrast with a potential fluency-shaping goal to use light articulatory contacts.[58,59,60]
- *Be clear (for ourselves, and for the child's benefit) about what constitutes a successful response.* We should clarify for ourselves and for the child what will be reinforced and rewarded in activities. Although it may seem straightforward, clinicians should be clear about what sorts of behaviors meet specific therapy goals. For instance, if one is working on inclusion of a grammatical marker or rectifying a sound substitution, the fluency of the response should be irrelevant. Conversely, if one is practicing speaking rate or soft contacts, we reinforce how well the child achieves those targets, rather than whether the child's utterance is grammatical, properly articulated, or even fluent. In our experience, this basic premise is sometimes difficult for families to understand, if homework will be assigned or recommended. In this sense, not every error is an opportunity to learn, much as it might seem so. For a child with multiple communication needs, it is not reasonable to expect progress across multiple aspects of communication simultaneously.

- *See what the child's responses suggest about the ways in which the child's two areas of need may interact.* In other words, be prepared to change initial assumptions. Even highly effective evidence-based interventions in our field, or in medicine or education, do not work equally well for everyone. Probably every reader of this book has experienced a so-called paradoxical reaction to something—a response that is not predicted to impact most people, but which can affect an individual. Let us go back to the premise that articulation goals will not necessarily impact fluency in an individual child. What if this turns out not to be the case? We could try a different articulation target to see if working on this goal diminishes the disfluency. Sasisekaran[9] suggests other approaches to easing the communicative load for a child whose fluency appears stressed by phonological processing load. If we continue to see that complex phonological targets disrupt fluency for a child, this is a sign that managing both sets of demands is challenging. We should then be sure that for fluency "exercises," care might be taken to load activities with targets that the child is more easily able to articulate well. Language seems to have a wider literature suggesting possible interactions between domains. We might presume at the onset that fluency targets, activities, or goals be practiced first in elicited contexts that fall comfortably within the child's expressive language skills. Only as the child masters such skills in carefully scaffolded and supported environments might we practice generalization to more difficult language targets, or unstructured spontaneous conversation.

None of this adjustment to a child's therapy planning will work well without active monitoring of possible ways in which goals interact. EBP requires adjustment around the client's responses to well-conceptualized therapy choices.

13.4.3 Therapeutic Approaches

The following section describes processes of treatment for the child who stutters with language and/or phonology concerns. Broadly speaking, structural models designed to assist in targeting priority therapy goals for fluency and language and phonology have included sequential, concurrent, and cyclic approaches (see ▶ Fig. 13.3 for illustration of considerations in deciding on a treatment approach).[59,60] We define *sequential treatment* of children with concomitant disorders as a therapy plan that targets remediation of one of the disorders ahead of the other(s). In other words, a clinician might decide to directly work on a child's articulation until better intelligibility has been achieved before direct work on fluency. In the interim, the clinician might counsel parents on indirect strategies to use when dealing with the child's fluency in the home environment. Obviously, an advantage of such an approach is that goals that might conflict or interact with one another do not; on the other hand, it might delay work on one of the child's areas of needs indefinitely. In the case of a child with language impairment, since areas of need are typically wide and almost limitless, this could defer work on fluency for quite some time.

"The session structure for targeting fluency and language and phonology goals includes sequential, concurrent, and cyclic approaches."

We define *concurrent treatment* as working with the child's multiple areas of need more or less in parallel. This might mean dividing therapy sessions into portions that each deal with an aspect of the child's fluency, language, or articulation needs. It might even involve a single activity that combines aspects of therapy goals for two areas of the child's needs, as one of the case studies below illustrates.

The third option that we describe in some detail, *cyclic treatment*, combines aspects of concurrent treatment, but defines a set period of time for work on goals before progressing to next goals on the child's long-term plan. After a predetermined period of time, the original goals are reassessed, and work continues if the child has not progressed to mastery. In the interim, the clinician relies on the impetus of initial work on the goal to aid the child to generalize outside the therapy room. We illustrate a cycles approach in detail in ► Fig. 13.4.

Sequential Approach

Treatment programs using a sequential approach start by identifying the more significant need area and treating it directly until mastery occurs before moving on to the other areas. Criticism of such an approach, particularly when used with children who stutter, includes the potential for untargeted areas to worsen or end up never being addressed.[59] This is especially true for children diagnosed with a primary language impairment, as research suggests that these children may never fully catch up to unaffected peers,[17] and one can potentially work on numerous language goals for long periods of time without reaching a point where the language "problem" appears sufficiently addressed to the point that it no longer merits therapeutic attention. Box 13.1 presents a case study involving a sequential approach to treatment.

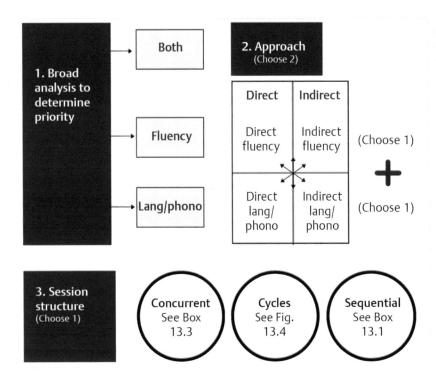

Fig. 13.3 Considerations in treatment decisions. (This image is provided courtesy of Chelsea G. Alexander, MA, CCC-SLP.)

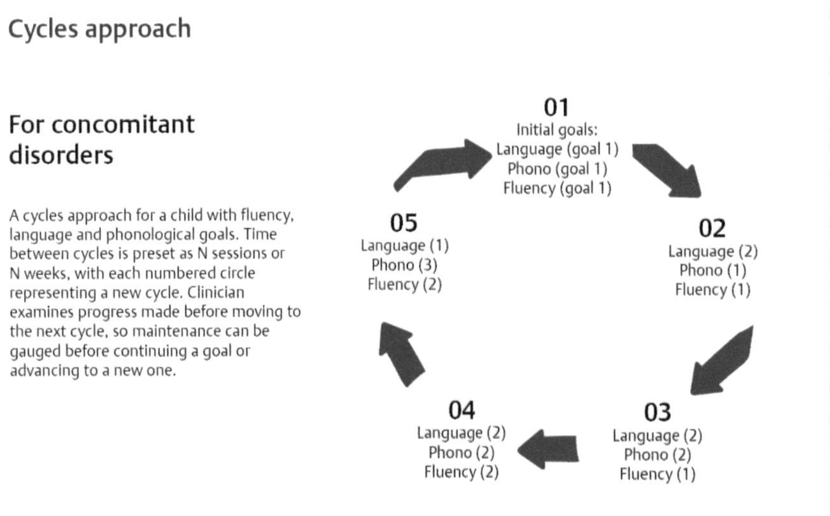

Fig. 13.4 A cycles treatment approach to fluency, language, and phonology. (This image is provided courtesy of Chelsea G. Alexander, M.A., CCC-SLP.)

Box 13.1 Case Study: Fluency, Language, and Phonology Treatment (Sequential Approach)

You are a speech-language pathologist (SLP) working at an outpatient pediatric speech department at a hospital. You have received a case history form for an upcoming evaluation, along with the child's most recent speech-language assessment (from 18 months ago), and a speech-language progress report (from 6 months ago). The client is a 12.11-year-old boy named Quinn who recently moved to your area with his family; his progress report was written to provide an update on his progress before his move. He was receiving speech therapy until he moved 6 months ago, and goals on his discharge summary indicate that he was working on (1) accurate production of /r/, (2) narrative organization, and (3) reduction in stuttering with a stuttering modification approach. Quinn's previous SLP recommended continued treatment with work in these goal areas. The case history form was completed by Quinn's mother and the goal areas indicated on his progress report matched his mother's major concerns.

Quinn's most recent speech-language evaluation is outdated, and he presents with a complex profile, so you plan to conduct a comprehensive assessment. You know that you will have to collect information about the impact of the communicative weaknesses on Quinn's life from Quinn himself, a parent, and with parent permission: (1) at least one of his current teachers at his current parochial school, who have known him for 6 months and (2) his previous SLP.

Given the complexity of Quinn's profile, you know that this assessment will be lengthy and may require more than the typically allotted 2 hours. You plan the following test battery:
- *Stuttering*:
  - Stuttering Severity Instrument, Fourth Edition (SSI-4).[61]
  - Overall Assessment of the Speaker's Experience of Stuttering-School Age (OASES-S).[62]
- *Language*:
  - Clinical Evaluation of Language Fundamentals-5 (CELF-5), Core Language Battery.[69]
  - CELF-5 Structured Writing.[63]
  - CELF-5 Reading Comprehension.[63]
  - Test of Narrative Language-2 (TNL-2).[64]
  - Expository discourse sample, using the Favorite Game or Sport Task and analyzed with the expository scoring scheme.[65]
- *Articulation/phonology*:
  - Goldman–Fristoe Test of Articulation-3 (GFTA-3).[66]
  - Speech sample with relational analysis, using TNL-2 narrative samples.
- *Related*:
  - Informal structural functional examination.
  - Hearing screening if Quinn has not passed a recent one.

After you have completed testing and interviewed Quinn, his mother, and his English/language arts teacher, a summary of your impressions is as follows. Quinn presents with overtly mild stuttering characterized primarily by fleeting part-word repetitions and prolongations, sometimes accompanied by eye blinking. Based on your structured life impact measure (the OASES-S) and client, parent, and teacher interviews, Quinn's stuttering has a moderate adverse life impact, characterized by fear of moments of stuttering, use of word substitutions to avoid stuttering, avoidance of oral class participation, and deferral to his parents to speak around new people (e.g., when ordering in a restaurant). He has made two good friends since moving and is reportedly comfortable speaking around these friends and his family members.

Results of articulation and language testing were consistent with the areas of need in his most recent speech-language evaluation. He presented with errors on /r/ in all word positions, at both the single-word level and in connected discourse, and also indicated that he wanted to learn to say /r/ so that he would sound more like his peers. All spoken and written language skills were average to above average except for narrative organization. Mild to moderate difficulty with narrative organization was apparent in the fictional expressive narratives that are part of the TNL-2 and in the expository narrative sample. These weaknesses were not identified in Quinn's writing, possibly due to the slower pace of writing compared to speaking and more opportunities for preplanning. Still, given his expressive language weaknesses, you will discuss narrative organization with his English/language arts teacher so that he or she can communicate with his team, and encourage him or her to contact you if concerns about written organization arise.

Because Quinn attends parochial school and his parents are not interested in pursuing speech-language services through his public school district, you recommend twice weekly private speech-language therapy to target (1) decreasing avoidance behaviors and cognitive reactions related to stuttering, (2) increasing his ability to use a stuttering modification approach when he desires, (3) increasing organization of expository and fictional narratives, and (4) increasing accuracy of /r/ production.

You adopt a sequential approach, meaning that you will address targets sequentially during your sessions. You believe that balancing stuttering therapy and narrative organization with this approach will be manageable, and your greater concern is addressing Quinn's residual articulation disorder while avoiding hard articulatory contacts and overarticulation. He had made some progress on /r/ production and was able to produce /r/ in the word-initial position at the word level, per his progress note, but seems to have lost all progress made on /r/ during his 6 months out of therapy. You therefore decide to (1) ask Quinn's previous SLP for tips on which strategies were effective in eliciting /r/ and (2) pay close attention to the /r/ models that Quinn will be hearing—you will be careful to use light articulatory contacts and avoid overarticulating with your models and coach Quinn and his mother, who will provide models and feedback during home practice, to do the same.

Concurrent Approach

A concurrent approach aims to address multiple areas of need within a therapy plan, although the structure of the approach may include combinations of direct and indirect treatment, or segments of individual sessions being devoted to different areas (see Box 13.3 later in the chapter for an example). When planning this type of approach, the clinician must examine the effects of directly treating one area (e.g., phonology) on the other area(s) of need (e.g., fluency). In some cases, targeting a particular phonological item, process, or linguistic structure may lead to increased tension and exacerbate stuttering behavior. Conversely, direct attention to specific fluency strategies without maintaining support for language may inadvertently reinforce the use of reduced language by the child and set the stage for limited linguistic growth.

Cyclic Approach

Finally, a cyclic approach (patterned after the successful cycles approach to phonological intervention by Hodson and Paden[67]) can be applied to the treatment of concomitant disorders in stuttering (see Box 13.4 later in the chapter for an example). In this approach, a schedule is set up whereby each area of need receives direct intervention in its own cycle, which is alternated with other cycles targeting the other areas of need individually. What makes the cycles approach unique is that the clinician works on a skill or a series of skills for a predetermined period of time, rather than to a predetermined level of accuracy. For example, the clinician may decide that a set of goals will be worked on during a cycle consisting of eight sessions, after which some goals will be dropped and others added, regardless of the child's progress toward mastery of selected targets. A primary principle of this approach is that recently learned concepts will generalize outside of direct instruction and practice sessions, even during cycles addressing different targets. A graphic illustration of a potential cycles approach with a child having fluency, articulation, and language goals is shown in ▶ Fig. 13.4. As shown, the program includes returning to prior targets to assess possible generalization toward desired treatment outcomes, or to reestablish behaviors and bolster learning, should that be necessary. If the child has consolidated some learning toward mastery of a particular therapy goal in the interim, then the clinician can select new goals from the child's areas of need.

13.4.4 Linguistic Context

Addressing stuttering in young children requires careful analysis of the linguistic context in which fluency and communication strategies are embedded. In addition to consideration of the phonologic, syntactic, semantic, and pragmatic characteristics of therapeutic activities and techniques, the clinician must continually examine and reexamine language production skills, the potential for tradeoffs between various developmental domains that may be competing for resources, and whether or not targeted strategies are serving to advance fluency development. It is recommended that the clinician use a philosophy of "communicative effectiveness" while determining priority goals for a child who stutters with language and/or phonology deficits. Importantly, intelligibility in speech and language production includes managing speech rate, phonological accuracy, lexical retrieval, language formulation, and pragmatic demands, as well as incorporating strategies to reduce tension. Following

the determination of an overall approach (i.e., addressing individual components sequentially or concurrently), the clinician must structure the linguistic context. Standard practice is to implement hierarchies for teaching new skills and reinforcing mastery of old skills. Hence, the introduction of fluency-facilitating strategies is done within the context of established linguistic constructions. Once new fluency behaviors, such as reduced speaking rate and easy starts, have been introduced, they can be practiced in many different linguistic contexts, which can be modified to help a youngster learn language concepts without having to formulate or draw on linguistic skills not yet acquired. For example, the use of carrier phrases with words from different categories can help with practicing fluent speech while learning basic concepts (Box 13.2). As the child gains success with the fluency strategies, additional language targets can be introduced and practiced.

"Addressing stuttering in young children requires careful analysis of the linguistic context in which fluency and communication strategies are embedded."

Box 13.2 Example Linguistic Context for Practicing Fluency Strategies

Fluency skills to practice	Carrier phrases	Language concept
Easy starts Reduced rate	*This boy is _____.* *I put the block _____.*	Emotion: "happy," "angry" Position: "on top," "next to"

13.4.5 Treating Concomitant Stuttering and Phonology

Evidence-based protocols for treating concomitant stuttering and phonology are yet to be developed. At present, debate continues as to whether children who stutter are at greater risk of phonological impairment,[9] and yet, it is clear that such children do show up on clinician's caseloads.[2,3,4,5,6] Consequently, best practice principles are based primarily on the recommendations of experienced professionals. The most comprehensive model for addressing phonology in children who stutter is based on the work of Wolk and colleagues.[56,57] According to this model, phonology is best addressed indirectly in children who stutter to minimize the potential for exacerbating stuttering because of heightened pressure and tension in speech production, which occurs as children attempt to achieve correct sound production. The resulting approach involves directly targeting fluency using techniques such as speech rate reduction, prolonged speech techniques, and light articulatory contacts; teaching children about and modeling contrasts (e.g., differences between stops and fricatives, or between tense and loose); incorporating parent involvement; and using group therapy settings. Box 13.3 presents a case example of the treatment of concomitant stuttering and phonological impairment in the context of a concurrent approach.

"Children who stutter with phonological impairment do show up on clinician's caseloads."

Box 13.3 Case Study: Stuttering and Phonological Impairment (Concurrent Approach)

You are the SLP at a special education preschool and have been contacted about a 3.6-year-old boy named Kaden. His parents bring him in for an assessment because they are concerned that he is stuttering. When you approach the family to walk them to the assessment room, you hear Kaden talking to his dad, and notice that you understand very little of his speech.

When you enter the assessment room, you ask Kaden to play with his mom while you speak with his dad to collect case history information. You intermittently stop and listen to Kaden's speech. You hear part-word repetitions with one to two extra iterations and brief prolongations. You estimate that his speech is about 25% intelligible. Given this presentation, you plan to complete a comprehensive battery in the 2 hours you have for the assessment. Because you know that your time with the family is limited, you make sure to record a speech and language sample. You know that spending about 20 minutes collecting a speech and language sample for later analysis is efficient, as you can use the sample to obtain information about three key areas: articulation, language, and fluency.

- *Stuttering*:
  - SSI-4.[61]
  - Communication Attitude Test for Preschool and Kindergarten Children Who Stutter (KiddyCAT).[68]
- *Language*:
  - CELF-Preschool 2nd Edition (CELF-P2), Core Language Test.[69]
  - Language sample, with planned analyses including mean length of utterance (MLU), Brown's morpheme/stages analysis.[70,71,72]
- *Articulation/phonology*:
  - GFTA-3.[65]
  - Speech sample, with independent and relational analyses.
- *Oral-motor*:
  - Informal structural functional examination.

In the parent interview, you collect information about Kaden's speech-language and developmental history, risk factors related to persistent stuttering, and his parents' concerns about his communication and view of his communicative strengths. You also find out that Kaden recently passed a hearing screening at his pediatrician's office.

Highlights from your assessment:
- Structural functional examination results were within normal limits.
- Articulation skills were at the 1st percentile for his age, per the GFTA-3. He demonstrated fronting, stopping, cluster reduction, prevocalic voicing, liquid gliding, and final consonant deletion.
- KiddyCAT results indicated generally positive communicative attitudes, but some perception of talking being difficult.
- SSI-4 results indicated that Kaden stuttered on 4% of syllables, with mean duration of his longest three moments measured at about 0.5 seconds, with no concomitant behaviors. This corresponds to the mild stuttering range.
- CELF-P2 receptive language and expressive language indices were both within the average range.
- Computation of MLU, Index of Productive Syntax (IPSyn), Developmental Sentence Scoring (DSS), and other language sampling measures was not possible because Kaden only produced 43 fully intelligible utterances in the 20-minute sample (out of 155 total utterances). Further, you were concerned that MLU computed based on fully intelligible utterances would be deflated and inaccurately represent his abilities, as it was Kaden's longer utterances that were more likely to be unintelligible. Using the entire 155-utterance sample, you heard production of present progressive -*ing*, *on*, *in*, irregular past tense (e.g., *went*), uncontractible copula, articles *a* and *the*, third person irregular (e.g., *has*), and the uncontractible auxiliary. You did not hear possessive -*s*, regular past tense -*ed*, third person singular -*s*, contractible copula, or contractible auxiliary—all morphemes that may be impacted by his articulation skills.
- *Parent interview:* You found that Kaden lives with his mother, father, older brother (5.5 years old), and younger sister (1.1 years old). His stuttering began when he was 3.4 years old, which means that he has been stuttering for 2 months. He and his brother compete for talking time. Review of his case revealed both risk factors for persistent stuttering (male sex, speech sound disorder) and positive prognostic indicators (negative family history of persistent stuttering, onset before turning 4, <6 months since onset, and average language skills).

A summary of your impressions is that Kaden presents with a severe phonological disorder, mild stuttering, and age-appropriate language skills, though his expressive skills were difficult to assess given the severity of his phonological disorder. Although stuttering was the concern that brought him to you, his poor phonological skills are having a far greater impact on his communicative success than his mild stuttering, which is accompanied by generally positive communicative attitudes. Given this presentation, you recommend direct therapy focusing on suppression of phonological processes, accompanied by parent counseling to address stuttering.

Based on this assessment, you recommend a concurrent approach. Phonological skills will be addressed with direct therapy, with initial goals targeting final consonant deletion and prevocalic voicing, as these syllable-level processes were judged to have the most substantial impact on intelligibility. Additionally, final consonant deletion made it difficult for Kaden to produce age-appropriate morphemes. For instance, one initial phonological goal may be the following:

Kaden will produce final singleton consonants in one- and two-syllable words, at the single-word level, in 80% of opportunities across three consecutive sessions.

You will be careful to use light articulatory contacts in your models and avoid over-articulation and full release of stop consonants; you will coach Kaden's parents to do the same.

(Continued)

Indirect parent therapy will begin with counseling and education and may address the advice below. Your goals will be adjusted as you get to know the family and their routines and specific needs better over time.

- Allow turn-taking, and permit Kaden (and all siblings) to have sufficient "floor" time to express what they would like to.
- Establish 10 minutes of one-on-one protected talking time every day, for Kaden and one of his parents (this can be done with his siblings as well).
- Continue to support the development of positive attitudes toward communication.
- Adult models of slower, easier speech.
- Ensure that the parents understand that it is okay to acknowledge Kaden's stuttering.
- Monitor Kaden's stuttering and attitudes toward speaking over time.

Kaden's phonological repertoire is currently so limited that the relationship between stuttering and phonology is difficult to assess. As his phonological skills improve, this relationship should be monitored.

13.4.6 Treating Concomitant Stuttering and Language

As indicated in our discussion of assessment considerations, determining a profile of linguistic skills and how stuttering behavior is related to those skills will help in identifying therapeutic priorities for children with concomitant stuttering and language. A hierarchy of language targets should be developed in concert with fluency targets. According to Hall, fluency treatment may be introduced in the context of reduced linguistic demand to establish new speaking behaviors, such as reduced speaking rate and easy starts.[73] That said, once established, it is best to introduce new language behaviors while supporting fluency through the use of routine speaking tasks and practiced structures (e.g., carrier phrases). To expand a youngster's morphosyntactic repertoire while simultaneously managing fluency, the clinician will need to take advantage of times when speech is reasonably fluent. Likely, with certain fluency-facilitating behaviors having been established, there will be periods in which the child is relatively fluent, and linguistic targets can be addressed directly. See Box 13.4 for a case example of stuttering and language impairment in the context of a hybrid approach involving cycles principles in conjunction with occasional concurrent targets.

"A hierarchy of language targets should be developed in concert with fluency targets."

Box 13.4 Case Study: Stuttering and Language Impairment (Concurrent and Cycles Approach)

You are a private practice SLP and have been working twice a week with Ethan, a 3.11-year-old boy with a receptive–expressive language disorder. You have been treating him since he was 3.4 years old, at which time his language skills were approximately at the 2.5-year-old level. Receptive language goals have included increasing comprehension of wh-questions and directions containing multiple steps, as well as sentences with increasingly advanced concepts and syntax. Expressive goals have targeted production of sentences containing basic concepts such as spatial terms, use of the copula and auxiliary, production of the irregular past tense, and production of more complex wh-question types such as *why*, *how*, and *when*.

Over a period of several weeks, it has become apparent to you and Ethan's mother, who brings her son to his sessions, that he has begun to stutter. He primarily produces repetitions but also produces sound prolongations and blocks. You already have information about his language profile and will update this information with formal testing when he is 4.4 years old, after 1 year of therapy. To gather information about Ethan's stuttering, you complete the SSI-4,[61] which indicates moderate stuttering. You judge his language skills to be insufficient for completion of a formal attitudes measure, so you informally interview Ethan instead and continue to discuss his reactions to stuttering with his mother. He stomps his feet during moments of stuttering. His mom reports additional signs of frustration occurring at home, including crying, shouting, and "shutting down" during periods of increased stuttering. He has several risk factors for persistent stuttering, including male sex, and below-average language skills.

You know that addressing Ethan's language skills is still important because (1) he is still about 6 months behind age expectations and (2) greater language growth is related to greater likelihood of recovery from stuttering.[19] However, you also feel that immediately addressing Ethan's stuttering is important because of his frustration and that it should take precedence over his language skills for the first few weeks. You adopt a hybrid concurrent and cycles approach. You begin with modeling easy speech in person and include a substantial parent counseling component focused on environmental modifications. Your first aim is to decrease Ethan's frustration with his speech, as you feel that expressive language therapy will be less effective until this is achieved. Thus, you plan to spend several weeks on fluency exclusively. After you have decreased Ethan's frustration level, you will return to language therapy and adopt a concurrent approach. During all phases of treatment, you use language targets that are already in Ethan's repertoire when modeling fluency behaviors. You will use periods when Ethan is more fluent and less frustrated to implement direct language therapy. You will also increase your parent counseling component for language and teach Ethan's mother to increase modeling and recasting with language targets.

13.5 Conclusions

Treatment outcome studies, whether in stuttering or other conditions, tend to focus on the responses of groups to specific treatment approaches. Not infrequently, children with concomitant disorders are not included in either basic research studies or treatment outcome reports. When included, it is often difficult to ascertain what impact other communication difficulties might have had on the child's therapeutic progress.

In the real world, particularly if children who stutter are thoroughly evaluated, we can expect a proportion of children who stutter on any caseload to require additional goals that involve language, articulation/phonology, or both. Although specific published guidance in working with these children is still scant, we believe that clinicians who have an understanding of commonly observed interactions between fluency and certain task demands, who carefully monitor the child's response to therapy planning decisions, and who are willing to adjust therapy goals or approaches in response can assist these children in making progress toward multiple communicative goals.

13.6 Definitions

Concurrent approach: A therapeutic approach that addresses multiple areas of need at the same time.

Cycles approach: A therapeutic approach that uses a cyclic structure for targeting goals such that each goal is worked on by itself within a larger structure in which other goals may be addressed.

Ecologically valid: That which is or can be applied in real-life settings.

Evidence-based practice: An approach to clinical services that combines the best available research evidence with practitioner expertise and family/client values in making clinical decisions.

Practice-based evidence: An approach to clinical services that uses data and outcomes from routine clinical practice to make therapeutic decisions.

Sequential approach: A therapeutic approach that addresses one target area for remediation prior to another.

Zone of proximal development: Those skills that are close to being mastered, those that are between what a child can do without help and that which can be done with guidance.

References

[1] Bloodstein O, Bernstein Ratner N, Brundage SB. A handbook on stuttering. San Diego, CA: Singular; 2021

[2] Blood GW, Seider R. The concomitant problems of young stutterers. J Speech Hear Disord. 1981; 46(1):31–33

[3] Homzie MJ, Lindsay JS, Simpson J, Hasenstab S. Concomitant speech, language, and learning problem in adult who stutterers and in members of their families. J Fluency Disord. 1988; 13:261–277

[4] St. Louis KO, Murray CD, Ashworth MS. Coexisting communication disorders in a random sample of school-aged stutterers. J Fluency Disord. 1991; 16:13–23

[5] Arndt J, Healey EC. Concomitant disorders in school-age children who stutter. Lang Speech Hear Serv Sch. 2001; 32(2):68–78

[6] Blood GW, Ridenour VJ, Qualls CD, Hammer CS. Co-occurring disorders in children who stutter. J Commun Disord. 2003; 36(6):427–448

[7] Anderson JD, Ofoe LC. The role of executive function in developmental stuttering. Semin Speech Lang. 2019; 40(4):305–319

[8] Ofoe LC, Anderson JD, Ntourou K. Short-term memory, inhibition, and attention in developmental stuttering: a meta-analysis. J Speech Lang Hear Res. 2018; 61(7):1626–1648

[9] Sasisekaran J. Exploring the link between stuttering and phonology: a review and implications for treatment. Semin Speech Lang. 2014; 35(2):95–113

[10] Hall NE, Wagovich S, Bernstein Ratner N. Language considerations in developmental stuttering. In: Conture EG, Curlee RF, eds. Stuttering and Related Disorders of Fluency. 3rd ed. New York, NY: Thieme; 2007:153–167

[11] Henry LA, Botting N. Working memory and developmental language impairments. Child Lang Teach Ther. 2017; 33:19–32

[12] Spencer C, Weber-Fox C. Preschool speech articulation and nonword repetition abilities may help predict eventual recovery or persistence of stuttering. J Fluency Disord. 2014; 41:32–46

[13] Usler E, Smith A, Weber C. A lag in speech motor coordination during sentence production is associated with stuttering persistence in young children. J Speech Lang Hear Res. 2017; 60(1):51–61

[14] Usler ER, Walsh B. The effects of syntactic complexity and sentence length on the speech motor control of school-age children who stutter. J Speech Lang Hear Res. 2018; 61(9):2157–2167

[15] Sasisekaran J, Basu S, Weathers EJ. Movement kinematics and speech accuracy in a nonword repetition task in school-age children who stutter. J Commun Disord. 2019; 81:105916

[16] Smith A, Goffman L, Sasisekaran J, Weber-Fox C. Language and motor abilities of preschool children who stutter: evidence from behavioral and kinematic indices of nonword repetition performance. J Fluency Disord. 2012; 37(4): 344–358

[17] Johnson CJ, Beitchman JH, Young A, et al. Fourteen-year follow-up of children with and without speech/language impairments: speech/language stability and outcomes. J Speech Lang Hear Res. 1999; 42(3):744–760

[18] Tomblin JB, Records NL, Buckwalter P, Zhang X, Smith E, O'Brien M. Prevalence of specific language impairment in kindergarten children. J Speech Lang Hear Res. 1997; 40(6):1245–1260

[19] Leech KA, Bernstein Ratner N, Brown B, Weber CM. Preliminary evidence that growth in productive language differentiates childhood stuttering persistence and recovery. J Speech Lang Hear Res. 2017; 60(11):3097–3109

[20] Leech KA, Bernstein Ratner N, Brown B, Weber CM. Language growth predicts stuttering persistence over and above family history and treatment experience: response to Marcotte. J Speech Lang Hear Res. 2019; 62(5): 1371–1372

[21] Hollister J, Van Horne AO, Zebrowski P. The relationship between grammatical development and disfluencies in preschool children who stutter and those who recover. Am J Speech Lang Pathol. 2017; 26(1):44–56

[22] Lee SB, Lee DY, Sim HS, Yim DS. The potential usage of language skills for predicting recovery from persistent group in Korean speaking children who stutter. Commun Sci Disord. 2019; 24:141–153

[23] Kefalianos E, Onslow M, Packman A, et al. The history of stuttering by 7 years of age: follow-up of a prospective community cohort. J Speech Lang Hear Res. 2017; 60(10):2828–2839

[24] Hall NE, Yamashita TS, Aram DM. Relationship between language and fluency in children with developmental language disorders. J Speech Hear Res. 1993; 36(3):568–579

[25] Hall NE. Language and fluency in child language disorders: changes over time. J Fluency Disord. 1996; 21:1–32

[26] Hall NE. Speech disruptions in pre-school children with specific language impairment and phonological impairment. Clin Linguist Phon. 1999; 13: 295–307

[27] Boscolo B, Bernstein Ratner N, Rescorla L. Fluency of school-aged children with a history of specific expressive language impairment. Am J Speech Lang Pathol. 2002; 11(1):41–49

[28] Guo LY, Tomblin JB, Samelson V. Speech disruptions in the narratives of English-speaking children with specific language impairment. J Speech Lang Hear Res. 2008; 51(3):722–738

[29] Finneran DA, Leonard LB, Miller CA. Speech disruptions in the sentence formulation of school-age children with specific language impairment. Int J Lang Commun Disord. 2009; 44(3):271–286

[30] Steinberg ME, Ratner NB, Gaillard W, Berl M. Fluency patterns in narratives from children with localization related epilepsy. J Fluency Disord. 2013; 38 (2):193–205

[31] Befi-Lopes DM, Cáceres-Assenço AM, Marques SF, Vieira M. School-age children with specific language impairment produce more speech disfluencies than their peers. CoDAS. 2014; 26(6):439–443

[32] Choo AL, Smith SA. Bilingual children who stutter: convergence, gaps and directions for research. J Fluency Disord. 2020; 63:105741

[33] Byrd CT, Bedore LM, Ramos D. The disfluent speech of bilingual Spanish-English children: considerations for differential diagnosis of stuttering. Lang Speech Hear Serv Sch. 2015; 46(1):30–43

[34] Byrd CT. Assessing bilingual children: are their disfluencies indicative of stuttering or the by-product of navigating two languages? Semin Speech Lang. 2018; 39(4):324–332

[35] Eggers K, Van Eerdenbrugh S, Byrd CT. Speech disfluencies in bilingual Yiddish-Dutch speaking children. Clin Linguist Phon. 2020; 34(6):576–592

[36] Leclercq AL, Suaire P, Moyse A. Beyond stuttering: speech disfluencies in normally fluent French-speaking children at age 4. Clin Linguist Phon. 2018; 32(2):166–179

[37] Brundage SB, Rowe H. Rates of typical disfluency in the conversational speech of 30-month-old Spanish-English simultaneous bilinguals. Am J Speech Lang Pathol. 2018; 27 3S:1287–1298

[38] Hansen L, Gardner J, Pollard J. The measurement of fluency in a second language: evidence from the acquisition and attrition of Japanese. In: Visgatis E, ed. On JALT'97: Trends & Transitions Tokyo: Japan Association for Language Teaching; 1998:37–45

[39] Sisskin V, Wasilus S. Lost in the literature, but not the caseload: working with atypical disfluency from theory to practice. Semin Speech Lang. 2014; 35(2):144–152

[40] Scaler Scott K, Tetnowski JA, Flaitz JR, Yaruss JS. Preliminary study of disfluency in school-aged children with autism. Int J Lang Commun Disord. 2014; 49(1):75–89

[41] Evans DL, Owens KL. Word-final repetition in an adult with attention-deficit/hyperactivity disorder: a case report. Perspect ASHA Spec Interest Groups. 2019; 4:615–623

[42] Van Borsel J, Geirnaert E, Van Coster R. Another case of word-final disfluencies. Folia Phoniatr Logop. 2005; 57(3):148–162

[43] van Borsel J, van Coster R, van Lierde K. Repetitions in final position in a nine-year-old boy with focal brain damage. J Fluency Disord. 1996; 21:137–146

[44] McAllister J, Kingston M. Final part-word repetitions in school-age children: two case studies. J Fluency Disord. 2005; 30(3):255–267

[45] Brejon Teitler N, Ferré S, Dailly C. Specific subtype of fluency disorder affecting French speaking children: a phonological analysis. J Fluency Disord. 2016; 50:33–43

[46] Bernstein Ratner N. Selecting treatments and monitoring outcomes: the circle of evidence-based practice and client-centered care in treating a preschool child who stutters. Lang Speech Hear Serv Sch. 2018; 49(1):13–22

[47] Barkham M, Mellor-Clark J. Bridging evidence-based practice and practice-based evidence: developing a rigorous and relevant knowledge for the psychological therapies. Clin Psychol Psychother. 2003; 10:319–327

[48] Ruscio AM, Holohan DR. Applying empirically supported treatments to complex cases: ethical, empirical, and practical considerations. Clin Psychol. 2006; 13:146–162

[49] Jones M, Onslow M, Packman A, et al. Randomised controlled trial of the Lidcombe programme of early stuttering intervention. BMJ. 2005; 331(7518):659–663

[50] Wilson L, Onslow M, Lincoln M. Telehealth adaptation of the Lidcombe Program of Early Stuttering Intervention: five case studies. Am J Speech Lang Pathol. 2004; 13(1):81–93

[51] Lewis C, Packman A, Onslow M, Simpson JM, Jones M. A phase II trial of telehealth delivery of the Lidcombe program of early stuttering intervention. Am J Speech Lang Pathol. 2008; 17(2):139–149

[52] Guitar B, Kazenski D, Howard A, Cousins SF, Fader E, Haskell P. Predicting treatment time and long-term outcome of the Lidcombe Program: a replication and reanalysis. Am J Speech Lang Pathol. 2015; 24(3):533–544

[53] Trajkovski N, O'Brian S, Onslow M, et al. A three-arm randomized controlled trial of Lidcombe Program and Westmead Program early stuttering interventions. J Fluency Disord. 2019; 61:105708

[54] Millard S, Edwards S, Cook FM. Parent–child interaction therapy: adding to the evidence. Int J Speech Lang Pathol. 2009; 11:61–67

[55] de Sonneville-Koedoot C, Stolk E, Rietveld T, Franken M-C. Direct versus indirect treatment for preschool children who stutter: the RESTART randomized trial. PLoS One. 2015; 10(7):e0133758

[56] Wolk L. Intervention strategies for children who exhibit coexisting phonological and fluency disorders: a clinical note. Child Lang Teach Ther. 1998; 14:69–82

[57] Byrd C, Wolk L, Davis B. Role of phonology in childhood stuttering and its treatment. Stuttering and Related Disorders of Fluency. New York, NY: Thieme Medical Publishing; 2007

[58] Ramig PR, Bennett EM. Working with 7- to 12-year-old children who stutter: ideas for intervention in the public schools. Lang Speech Hear Serv Sch. 1995; 26:138–150

[59] Bernstein Ratner N. Treating the child who stutters with concomitant language or phonological impairment. Lang Speech Hear Serv Sch. 1995; 26: 180–186

[60] Logan KJ, LaSalle LR. Developing intervention programs for children with stuttering and concomitant impairments. Semin Speech Lang. 2003; 24(1): 13–20

[61] Riley GD. Stuttering severity instrument. 4th ed. San Diego, CA: Pro-ed; 2009

[62] Yaruss JS, Coleman C, Quesal RW. Overall Assessment of the Speaker's Experience of Stuttering-School Age. McKinney, TX: Stuttering Therapy Resources, Inc.; 2016

[63] Wiig EH, Semel E, Secord WA. Clinical evaluation of language fundamentals. 5th ed. Bloomington, MN: Pearson Assessments; 2013

[64] Gillam RB, Pearson NA. Test of narrative language. 2nd ed. San Diego, CA: Pro-ed; 2017

[65] Heilmann J, Malone TO. The rules of the game: properties of a database of expository language samples. Lang Speech Hear Serv Sch. 2014; 45(4):277–290

[66] Goldman R, Fristoe M. Goldman-Fristoe Test of Articulation. 3rd ed. Bloomington, MN: Pearson Assessments; 2015

[67] Hodson BW, Paden EP. A Phonological approach to remediation: targeting unintelligible speech. Pro-Ed Austin, TX; 1991

[68] Vanryckegehem M, Brutten G. KiddyCAT: Communication Attitude Test for Preschool and Kindergarten Children Who Stutter. San Diego, CA: Plural Publishing; 2007

[69] Semel E, Wiig EH, Secord WA. Clinical evaluation of language fundamentals preschool. 2nd ed. Bloomington, MN: Pearson Assessments; 2004

[70] Brown R. A first language: the early stages. Cambridge, MA: Harvard University Press; 1973

[71] Lee LL, Canter SM. Developmental sentence scoring: a clinical procedure for estimating syntactic development in children's spontaneous speech. J Speech Hear Disord. 1971; 36(3):315–340

[72] Altenberg EP, Roberts JA, Scarborough HS. Young children's structure production: a revision of the index of productive syntax. Lang Speech Hear Serv Sch. 2018; 49(4):995–1008

[73] Hall NE. Lexical development and retrieval in treating children who stutter. Lang Speech Hear Serv Sch. 2004; 35(1):57–69

Further Readings

Bernstein Ratner N. Selecting treatments and monitoring outcomes: the circle of evidence-based practice and client-centered care in treating a preschool child who stutters. Lang Speech Hear Serv Sch. 2018; 49(1):13–22

Byrd CT. Assessing bilingual children: are their disfluencies indicative of stuttering or the by-product of navigating two languages? Semin Speech Lang. 2018; 39(4): 324–332

Sasisekaran J. Exploring the link between stuttering and phonology: a review and implications for treatment. Semin Speech Lang. 2014; 35(2):95–113

Sisskin V, Wasilus S. Lost in the literature, but not the caseload: working with atypical disfluency from theory to practice. Semin Speech Lang. 2014; 35(2): 144–152

14 Bilingual and Multicultural Considerations

Courtney Byrd, Kia Noelle Johnson, and Julie Fortier-Blanc

Abstract

In this chapter, we explore the relationship between typically fluent speech and stuttering in both mono- and multilingual individuals. General information and characteristics regarding bilingualism will be presented along with the inherent difficulties encountered when using English monolingual guidelines for assessing stuttering in bilingual speakers. Suggestions are made to help clinicians accurately diagnose those who do stutter. Treatment issues with bilingual populations will be discussed including ways to better adapt our intervention with these speakers. We take into account multicultural considerations and how best to incorporate them when assessing and treating culturally diverse children and adults. Together, these learning outcomes will ensure that you are equipped to provide quality care to persons who stutter from culturally and linguistically diverse (CLD) backgrounds.

Keywords: stuttering, bilingualism, bilingual, multilingualism, multilingual, multicultural, assessment, treatment

14.1 Introduction

Stuttering is a multifactorial speech disorder that is present in speakers of all languages and cultures. Although we may perceive that a person stutters when they speak Spanish, French, or another language, there are some unique challenges that the speech-language pathologist faces when working with bilingual individuals. In particular, speech disfluencies are more frequent when facing linguistic uncertainty, for example, when trying to retrieve the right word or sentence structure to express a thought or idea, and bilinguals are more likely to face this uncertainty given that they are navigating between languages. This may result in an increase in the production of both typical speech disfluencies and those considered to be stuttering-like, thus compromising the accurate diagnosis of stuttering in bilingual speakers.[1]

The purpose of this chapter is to explore the dimensions of stuttering that are unique to the ever-growing population of bilingual and multicultural speakers. In the follow sections, we examine the difficulties encountered when distinguishing stuttering from the disfluent speech often produced by speakers of more than one language. Before launching into the focus of the chapter, we will first describe basic concepts and key terms to provide a framework, and give some general knowledge regarding bilingualism.

14.1.1 Basic Concepts

For the purpose of this chapter, we will consider *bilingualism* as the regular use of two or more languages in daily life.[2] We need to keep in mind that bilingualism is on a continuum and that bilingual speakers are not simply two monolingual speakers in one person. Why? Because to differing degrees, their knowledge, exposure, and use of a language are actually spread across their two languages.

When bilingual speakers are described as being *dominant* in one language, it means that they have more advanced skills in that language than they do in the other. As such, they can read, write, and speak more proficiently in their dominant as opposed to their nondominant language. Bilinguals can also be described as *balanced bilinguals*, meaning they have relatively equal skills in each of the languages they speak.

Another term that is inherent to bilingualism is *linguistic uncertainty*. A speaker whose linguistic knowledge is comprised of more than one language will have higher linguistic uncertainty. On the one hand, they may have less knowledge in the language they are using to express themselves while also having more options for what they want to say and how they could say it, given that their overall language abilities are broader and more complex.

Over the last 40 years, the rate of bilingualism has doubled, with at least 23% of the U.S. population speaking two languages; a rate that is projected to double in the next four decades. Thus, in the years ahead, the United States (U.S.) bilingual population will be more comparable to that of traditionally bilingual populations, where at least 40% of the population speaks a second language. Immigration is one factor that has contributed to this rise, in addition to the relearning of other languages, and the increase in dual language immersion programs. That said, the United States' consideration of mandating English as the national language in addition to some states adopting English as the official language may have kept the country's bilingual population lower than that of other countries. In fact, until the last two decades, families that immigrated to the United States focused on learning English and adapting to American culture resulting in the loss of their native languages and culture.

Countries such as Canada have two official languages and some, such as Belgium and Switzerland, have three. Canada, as with other countries, has legislation that governs the use of languages in schools, commerce, and places of work. Thus, the importance of bilingualism is likely to be very different and more complex in other countries than it is in the United States.

The laws of a country are sometimes written to protect a language and a culture. For example, in the Canadian province of Quebec there is legislation stating that French is the official language. This has helped preserve the French language and culture from slowly disappearing among the largely English-speaking population of North America. There is also federal legislation being written to preserve the rights of French-speaking residents outside of Quebec. These laws will guarantee access to judicial services in French, and encourage bilingualism in both French and English throughout the country. The Canadian census survey that is taken every 4 years includes a large number of questions relating to the status of languages and bilingualism in the country. This information helps the government assess how the issues surrounding languages and bilingualism are evolving over time, and plays a role in adjusting linguistic policies. The issues surrounding bi- and multilingualism are complex and often associated with highly emotional points of view that are at times difficult to resolve.

It is interesting to note that a bilingual speaker is able to use only one (*codes*) language when talking with a monolingual speaker, but will easily alternate between two languages during a conversation with another bilingual person who speaks the same two languages. This is referred to as *code-switching*, wherein speakers will use the word or sentence structure or expression in the language that comes to mind first, as it is less cognitively demanding and thus easier and faster to communicate. Therefore, when you listen to bilingual speakers talking together, you might often hear them saying part of a sentence or word in one language and the rest of the sentence in another language, alternating between languages as they speak.

Culture includes race, religion, and ethnicity, amongst other factors and is reflected in one's values and the way one thinks, communicates, and interacts. Whereas bilingualism is defined as a speaker of two languages, *multiculturalism* is defined as a person belonging to more than one culture coexisting together. Although monolingual speakers can be influenced by more than one culture, it is likely that multiple cultures influence the daily communication of bilingual speakers. The distinctions in these influences should be taken into account when completing our assessment and when developing individual treatment plans. It is important to understand that for children to connect with their families, they need to be able to speak the languages of their household. This means that any recommendation to speak one language exclusively—for example, English—may be detrimental to the child's connection with their community. For every individual we assess, we must consider the parts that contribute to the person as a whole.

Finally, in many countries worldwide, including the United States, there are speakers who speak more than two languages and, thus, are considered to be *multilingual*. However, the information in this chapter will largely focus on bilinguals, as the vast majority of the limited research completed to date has focused on this area. Nevertheless, readers should assume that the factors discussed in the present chapter will likely apply to multilinguals as well.

14.2 Speech, Language, and Fluency in Bilingual Speakers

Although it is beyond the scope of this chapter to discuss speech and language development in bi- and multilingual populations, there are interesting findings that highlight the uniqueness of these speakers. Clinicians commonly report difficulties determining whether children who speak more than one language present with a communication *disorder* or a *difference*.[3,4] Bilingual children sometimes speak less and are not as grammatically accurate as monolingual speakers. This is a direct result of the complexity of navigating more than one language, and this difference in the acquisition and use of a language is often misinterpreted as a disorder.[5] In fact, researchers have since learned that this "silent period" is not representative of a deficit, but instead reflects children internalizing the languages they are learning to speak. The following quote draws attention to this probability[6]: "There are great individual differences within and between the two languages of bilingual children and current assessment instruments are not designed to differentiate differences from true disabilities in these children."

In terms of speech fluency, while additional research is needed, it seems that bilingual speakers are naturally more disfluent. This is most likely related to the linguistic uncertainty they experience when deciding which words to say and in what language they will say it. This increase in the frequency of disfluency may make these children more vulnerable to be identified as stuttering.

Presently, researchers report that the positive benefits of being bilingual far outweigh any misperceived disadvantages. For example, learning a second language can increase multitasking skills and improve memory and the ability to focus. Bilingualism has also been shown to contribute to a cognitive advantage in aging, with studies showing that bilingual speakers may be less likely to develop neurological diseases such as dementia and Alzheimer's disease. Finally, being bilingual allows one a view of other cultures in ways that can expand our horizons and provide a new and different window into the world.

14.3 Challenges in Identifying Stuttering in Bilingual Speakers

Recent research suggests that typically developing bilingual children are not only more likely to be misidentified as exhibiting a language deficit but also more likely to be mislabeled as being a child who stutters. This increased likelihood of false-positive identification, or rather inaccurately identifying the presence of a disorder in a typically developing child, may be explained by the following factors: (1) use of monolingual guidelines for stuttering assessment; (2) a misperception of bilingualism as a risk factor for onset and persistence of stuttering; (3) inconsistency in the description of bilingualism; and (4) an assumption that stuttering and typical speech disfluency are related to language dominance. We consider each of these in the following sections.

14.3.1 Use of Monolingual Guidelines for Stuttering Assessment

Multiple studies confirm that speech-language pathologists can use monolingual English guidelines to accurately assess stuttering in non-English monolingual speakers of other languages such as Dutch, French, and German.[7,8,9] Yet, some have indicated that they may not be applicable to all languages, for example, Spanish.[10] Nevertheless, we cannot assume that these monolingual English guidelines, effectively used with monolingual Dutch speakers, for example, will also apply to bilingual Dutch-English speakers. This is because the use of these guidelines with bilingual speakers does not consider the possibility that bilinguals may have either limited or exceptional proficiency in both languages. In essence, they have many more choices to make when speaking, and the result of selecting among those choices is elevated levels of disfluency.[11,12]

While reading this chapter, you may be thinking: *hasn't it been proven that clinicians can listen to speakers whose language they do not speak and still be able to accurately identify stuttering?* The short answer is yes, but the long answer is no.

For example, it has been shown that speech-language pathologists can identify stuttering in adults whose language they do not understand.[13,14] It has also been shown that they can identify stuttering severity in bilingual speakers with high levels of accuracy, even when they are unfamiliar with the language.[15,16,17,18] That said, discriminating whether disfluencies are typical or atypical in bilingual speakers may prove to be more challenging.

When clinicians are asked to listen to samples of bilingual children who do and do not stutter, they accurately identify those children who actually stutter. However, they also inaccurately identify the typically fluent bilingual child to be stuttering. In essence, there is likelihood that clinicians will not be able to differentiate stuttering children from typically fluent children who are producing disfluencies that are the natural by-product of speaking two languages. *Why is this so?* To find out, researchers asked the clinicians to share what influenced their decisions about whether a bilingual child was stuttering or normally disfluent.[19] As shown in ▶ Table 14.1, practitioners stated that although they heard no tension in the disfluencies, they did hear monosyllable word, sound, and syllable repetitions or what is commonly categorized as stuttering-like disfluencies. In addition to reporting these types of disfluency, they judged that they were produced at a frequency that would be indicative of stuttering in monolinguals.

Unfortunately, by using these monolingual English guidelines with bilingual children, clinicians falsely identified typically fluent Spanish-English speaking children as stuttering. Thus, it seems that the conventionally used metric for monolingual English-speaking children of 3 stuttering-like disfluencies per 100 syllables as indicative of stuttering may be too stringent a criterion for the bilingual population.[20]

14.3.2 Speech Disfluencies Produced by Bilingual Children Who Do Not Stutter

In order to better understand the factors that increase the likelihood of misperceiving a typically fluent bilingual child as stuttering, researchers have explored the speech of nonstuttering

bilingual children. Their aim was to clarify or help determine what is typical versus atypical in bilingual speakers when compared to monolingual English speakers. An analysis of the speech disfluencies produced by 18 typically fluent bilingual Spanish-English children between 5 and 6 years of age demonstrated that they produced stuttering-like disfluencies that exceeded 3 per 100 syllables. In fact, if the monolingual English-speaking guidelines had been applied, most would have been classified as children who stutter despite the fact that no child, parent, teacher, or clinician expressed concern regarding their fluency.[11]

Similar results were found for 59 typically developing Yiddish-Dutch speaking children ranging from 6 to 10 years of age. The number of stuttering-like disfluencies produced by these children was higher in both languages than the standard guidelines would allow.[21] This shows that the use of our current monolingual English guidelines for assessment of stuttering in bilingual speakers should be adapted so as to avoid false-positive identification of stuttering in these children.

In summary, clinicians are able to identify stuttering in individuals even when they do not speak their language. However, given the high rates of disfluencies produced by speakers of more than one language, typically fluent bilinguals, particularly children, may be more likely to be inaccurately identified as stuttering. Thus, our guidelines for determining stuttering in bilinguals need to be stricter, especially when it comes to frequency of disfluencies and the presence of sound, syllable, and word repetitions in their speech. This broader view will help us better differentiate stuttered speech from typical speech disfluency in these speakers and advance our understanding of how stuttering manifests in bilinguals.

14.3.3 Misperception of Bilingualism as a Risk Factor for Stuttering

When clinicians are asked to identify factors that might contribute to the onset and development of stuttering, it is surprising to see

Table 14.1 Identification, description, and examples in English and Spanish of the types of speech disfluencies considered to be stuttering-like disfluency (SLD) versus nonstuttering-like disfluency (non-SLD) or typical in nature

SLD	Description	Examples
Monosyllabic word repetition	Repetition of a monosyllabic word	And (they) they were looking El búho (lo) lo persiguió
Sound repetition	Repetition of a sound within a word. Typically occurs at the beginning of a word	The (dª) dog started playing (Sª) se metió en la canasta
Syllable repetition	Repetition of a syllable within a word. Typically occurs at the beginning of a word	Out of the (buª) bucket Se enojó (muª) mucho
Non-SLD	Description	Examples
Revision	Word usage or grammatical error correction	His (frog) dog also came along (La rana mayor) la rana bebé
Unfinished word	Abandoned or not completed word	His (frª) dog came along Fueron (a busª) a ver que era el sonido
Phrase repetition	Repetition of a phrase within an utterance	(A squeaky) a squeaky sound (Con las) con las avispas
Interjection	Filler words or nonlinguistic sounds used within an utterance	(Um) what is this? La rana trató de (ah) tomar la leche
Polysyllabic word repetition	Repetition of a polysyllabic (more than one syllable) word	He was (playing) playing around (Para) para evitar la rana

ª Adapted from Byrd et al,[11] and Ambrose and Yairi.[20]

how many are concerned that speaking more than one language puts a child at risk of developing stuttering. This phenomenon was observed using a web-based survey completed by 207 speech-language pathologists who were members of the American Speech-Language-Hearing Association (ASHA).[22] Preliminary results indicate that more than a quarter of the speech-language pathologists polled view bilingualism as a risk factor. However, there are no data to support this risk.

One of the most commonly cited historical studies suggesting that bilingualism may increase the risk was completed in 1937 by Travis et al.[23] This study, along with a more recent one in 2009 by Howell et al,[24] has methodological concerns that resulted in their findings being disproven and in the case of Howell et al. even recanted.[1,11,25]

Think about this: If speaking more than one language increased the likelihood that you would develop stuttering, then there would be higher rates of stuttering in countries where there are higher rates of bilinguals, but there are not. Additionally, if you reflect back to the beginning of this chapter, there are numerous advantages to being bilingual and, for many children, speaking more than one language is the only means of communicating with members of their family and connecting to their culture.

14.3.4 Inconsistency in the Description of Bilingualism

The vast majority of investigations in stuttering and bilingualism have considered bilingualism as a categorical label with the idea that a person is or is not bilingual.[26,27] This is misleading because bilingualism is on a continuum, and performance on speech and language tasks will fluctuate depending on language dominance and proficiency.[2,28,29] In addition, the frequency of disfluency will most likely be affected by these factors.

Thus, in both clinical practice and research, it is not enough to simply describe an individual who stutters as bilingual because we need to consider the *language history, function,* and *proficiency* across the languages they speak. This will paint a truer picture of bilingualism and enable us to compare bilinguals who stutter with greater accuracy.

As shown in ► Table 14.2, *language history* is defined as the age and conditions in which the speaker was exposed to their second/non-native language (L2). The first/native language is labeled L1. *Language function* is defined as the amount or frequency that each language is currently used across specific settings such as at home, school, or work, in various contexts (e.g., monologue or narrative, dialogue or conversation) or with different conversational partners. *Language proficiency* is defined as the speaker's overall ability to speak and understand each language in verbal and written form.

Two systematic reviews of the stuttering literature revealed that the vast majority of studies simply referred to the participant as bilingual, without providing more insight into the language history, function, and proficiency.[26,27] This means that despite the increase in the *quantity* of research examining the nature of stuttering in bilinguals, the *quality* of the descriptors used to characterize their bilingualism remains insufficient and inconsistent. Thus, one should interpret the findings of any research in stuttering among bilingual speakers with caution

Table 14.2 Characterizations of language history, language function, and language proficiency

Factor	Characterization
Language history	Age or years since first exposure
	Order of acquisition
	Languages exposed to at home
	Languages taught at school
	Years of formal language instruction
Language function	Amount of use per language
	Languages currently spoken in different environments
	Languages spoken with different people (family, friends, etc.)
Language proficiency	Subjective or objective ability to speak, comprehend, read, and/or write in a language

Note: List items and definitions are identical to Coalson et al[25] and Werle et al.[26]

given the manner in which bilingualism has been defined in the literature.[26,27]

14.3.5 Assumption That Stuttering is Related to Language Dominance

To date, there have been conflicting results from studies examining the relationship between stuttering and the language dominance of bilingual speakers. Certain studies have found similar amounts of stuttering in both languages, while others have reported that some bilingual speakers produce more stuttering in one language when compared to the other.

Why is this so? Some have argued that the differences are related to the grammatical structure of the language being spoken. Others have argued the difference may be related to linguistic uncertainty. It seems intuitive that linguistic uncertainty only occurs when one's knowledge and use of the language spoken is reduced when compared to one's second language. However, research has not proven this to be true. In fact, there is uncertainty when there are more options, and also when there are fewer options. This means that bilinguals may be more disfluent because they are selecting among many choices, or they may be more disfluent because they are struggling with too few choices.

Importantly, many clinicians have noticed from experience that the relationship between language dominance and stuttering can be different from one speaker to the other and is difficult to predict. This is also true for typically fluent bilinguals. For this reason, regardless of whether the differences in speech disfluencies and/or stuttering are related to the grammatical structure of the language or linguistic uncertainty, it is critical to collect samples in each of the languages a child or adult speaks when conducting a stuttering evaluation.

14.4 Culturally and Linguistically Sensitive Assessment of Stuttering

Whether a child or adult speaks one, two, or more languages, clinicians must seek to identify and understand the similarities and differences between their own cultural influences and the client's, because these factors contribute to clinical decisions and the client's response to those decisions. For example, a *clinician* might identify with a culture in which verbal interactions occur regardless of the perceived status or gender of a conversational partner. The *client*, however, may be from a culture that restricts verbal interactions with conversational partners that are of a perceived higher status or a different gender. This discrepancy between conversational styles could create a perception that either the clinician or the client is being rude or inappropriate during the clinical exchange.

It is important that clinicians continue to educate themselves on the culture(s) with which their clients identify, particularly as it relates to stuttering. At the same time, one should never assume that individuals who identify with the same culture(s) will present with the same cultural expression. As our personal experience grows, so should our knowledge regarding the distinctions across different cultures as well as the individual differences among people within the same culture. This will enable clinicians to conduct a culturally responsive assessment as well as consider the influence of culture on intervention. The following section provides strategies for the assessment and treatment of stuttering when working with culturally and linguistically diverse (CLD) individuals.

14.4.1 Formal Assessment of Stuttering

There are a number of commonly used assessment tools to determine the presence and/or severity of stuttering in both children and adults. When we use these instruments in our clinical practice, we need to consider their appropriateness from both a linguistic and cultural viewpoint.

For example, was the assessment tool normed on a sample that represents the cultural background of the client? Was the tool designed for use with individuals who speak more than one language? The fact that many stuttering assessment instruments do not consider cultural or language diversity does not generally devalue their effectiveness, nor diminish their reliability or validity. Nevertheless, clinicians should consider the impact of culture and be cautious when interpreting the assessment results.

For example, one of the most commonly used stuttering assessments is the Stuttering Severity Instrument, Fourth Edition (SSI-4).[28] The SSI-4 was normed on children and adults recruited from California public schools, private practice, and university and community clinics. Although the manual does not provide guidance for speakers of languages other than English, this measure can be used if considering only those speech disfluencies produced with atypical timing and tension that are clearly indicative of stuttering. Since typically fluent bilinguals produce more stuttering-like disfluencies than their monolingual peers, it is critical that only those produced in a tense, arrhythmic manner be computed in the SSI-4. Otherwise, typically disfluent bilinguals may be erroneously identified as presenting moderate to severe stuttering.

The Communication Attitude Test for Preschool and Kindergarten Children who Stutter (KiddyCAT)[29] is another commonly used assessment tool that examines the perceptions and attitudes of kindergarteners and preschool-age children about stuttering in general and their own stuttering in particular. There is no specific guidance provided for the use of this tool with a CLD child. For example, in some cultures, children are not encouraged to openly share their feelings and attitudes with others and instead may have a tendency to agree with an elder so as to not show disrespect. When this tendency carries over into the test setting, the child may be looking for opportunities to guess which answer the examiner expects rather than providing a valid response. *So what do you do about this?* You can complete this assessment in each language the child speaks. And as you learn more about the child's cultures, you will become more apt at determining how their responses may be influenced by culture, independently of stuttering.

The Test of Childhood Stuttering (TOCS)[30] is a standardized assessment tool that measures stuttering in children through a variety of speaking contexts. The authors of the TOCS have intentionally included information regarding the ethnicity of the sample used to norm the test, which includes children of the following race and ethnic groups: White, African-American, Asian/Pacific Islander, American Indian/Eskimo/Aleut, and Hispanic. The authors also clearly state that this tool is not appropriate for use with children who have limited English proficiency.[30]

Since its development, the validity and reliability of the TOCS have been examined for use in other languages, specifically Persian and Arabic,[31,32] but the cross-linguistic reliability and validity require further investigation. As with the SSI-4, clinicians should attend only to disfluencies associated with tension or atypical timing.

The Overall Assessment of the Speakers Experience of Stuttering (OASES) is used to determine the adverse impact of stuttering on an individual's life.[33,34] Originally published in English, the OASES in its initial form did not lend itself to being used with CLD individuals. However, since that time, the authors have made considerable strides in broadening the application of their test. The OASES has been translated and validated for use with Spanish, German, Dutch, Hebrew, and Portuguese speakers.[35,36,37] Because the impact of stuttering on quality of life can vary depending on language and culture, it is again important to evaluate this in each of the languages that the person speaks.

14.4.2 Informal Assessment of Stuttering

With any CLD person suspected of stuttering, combining the results of both formal and informal assessment of stuttering is necessary to minimize cultural biases. Instead of relying heavily on the frequency of speech disfluencies to render a diagnosis of stuttering, a good starting point is simply to reflect on the question, "Does the speaker sound like a person who stutters?" The clinician's perception and judgment are important components to a stuttering evaluation and are very helpful when assessing these individuals.

A high frequency of disfluencies is a common characteristic of stuttering; however, there are reasons other than stuttering that can explain a high frequency of speech disfluencies. One is that there is a greater cognitive demand placed on bilingual speakers as they navigate more than one language. Another, from a strictly cultural perspective, may be the purposeful use of a significantly high number of interjections or word repetitions solely for purposes of expression. This is commonly seen in

African-American speakers and sometimes in French speakers. It is clear that a diagnosis of stuttering in either case would be inappropriate.[1,38]

Although it is not always easy to differentiate these behaviors from stuttering, obtaining narrative and conversational samples in each of the languages the person speaks during the assessment process is an important step. Subsequently, by focusing less on the overall frequency and more on the types of disfluencies and especially the manner in which they are produced, the clinician can make a more accurate diagnosis. An in-depth discussion about centering the stuttering assessment on *how* a person stutters and their *response* to stuttering, as opposed to *how much* they stutter, is presented in ▶ Chapter 9 of this text. By attending to those disfluencies that sound like stuttering and are associated with tension, it will be simpler to distinguish stuttering from repetitions the speaker is using to emphasize a point, or those related to the speaker's effort to determine the word and the language they will use to communicate.

In addition to the speech disfluencies produced across speaking samples, the assessment of nonverbal behaviors is common practice in evaluations of all persons who stutter. With CLD individuals, there may be large differences in the way that nonverbal behaviors are used and interpreted, especially in terms of what is considered acceptable or unacceptable within that culture. The nonverbal behavior most critical to consider during a stuttering assessment is eye contact.

For example, persons from western cultures (i.e., North America and Europe) generally establish some eye contact with a conversational partner regardless of age or gender. However, in Middle Eastern, Asian, African, Latin American, and American Indian cultures, any direct eye contact is considered inappropriate, rude, or threatening depending on the gender or age of their conversational partner.[39,40] This behavior can greatly influence an assessment of stuttering because that lack of eye contact could be misinterpreted as a secondary behavior, perhaps signaling habitual avoidance. So it is essential that the clinician familiarizes themselves with what is considered appropriate in that person's culture in order to determine whether the individual's eye contact is related to stuttering or to cultural influences.

14.5 Additional Cultural Considerations

14.5.1 Age and Gender

Age and gender are two additional factors that can indirectly influence the presentation of speech disfluencies. For example, in middle-class, mainstream cultures, it is assumed that children are appropriate conversation partners for adults, especially when these adults are their parents. Thus, it is common during the assessment to observe the conversation between a child and his or her parent(s) in order to obtain a sample of typical language use.

However, in some cultures such as in traditional Asian families, it can be considered inappropriate to expect conversational interactions between parents and their children.[41] These children have often learned that they are expected to speak when spoken to and rarely initiate a new conversation topic with persons they perceive to be of higher status. Thus, if they are placed in a conversational setting with their parents or a clinician during a fluency evaluation, their verbal output may be limited. One likely explanation is that the child is limiting their speech to shorter, less complex utterances to mask the occurrence of stuttering. However, it is also possible that the clinician uses their own culturally based expectations to assume the child to be reserved about speaking due to their stuttering *rather than* their culture. A clinician who is culturally aware of these possibilities would prepare the evaluation in a way that minimizes these potential biases. Ideally, one way is to include a clinician who is of the same cultural background and possibly the same gender as the client to assist with the assessment.

14.5.2 Conversational Style

Conversational style is another aspect of communication that has the potential to impact service delivery to CLD individuals. Specifically, in some cultures (e.g., African-Americans, Hispanics, French and French-Canadians), speakers interrupt each other frequently during conversation. These interruptions are not intended to be negative to the flow of conversation, but instead indicate active participation and emotional involvement on the part of the speaker during communication. Sometimes they are also used as a strategy to gain the conversational floor. These interruptions may also be associated with disfluencies such as word or sound repetitions at the beginning of utterances. Again, they do not indicate the presence of stuttering. These disfluencies may be interpreted as a way of showing spontaneity or interest in the conversation and be considered by certain cultures as a fashionable way of talking. Although some speakers are naturally more disfluent than others, it is also possible that certain cultures have a higher tolerance for disfluencies.

Speakers of some cultures talk with what could be called a culturally appropriate rate of speech. Their speech is rapid when compared to the typical rate expected for mainstream speakers. Both a rapid rate of speech and a high proportion of interruptions in a person who stutters are common findings, but this way of speaking is also appropriate and perceived positively in some cultures. Unfortunately, it may also exacerbate stuttering in those who actually do stutter, particularly children. When speaking rapidly, there is less time available to make changes, so modifying stuttering becomes more difficult and challenging.

In this situation, the clinician should educate the client and their conversational partners, such as the family, on the negative impact these features may have on stuttering. In the case of a child, it may be necessary to reassure the parent that making small changes to lower the number of interruptions or decrease speech rate used in conversation will not take away from their child's cultural identity, but is necessary in order to progress in stuttering treatment.

14.5.3 Views on the Cause of Stuttering

Finally, there is considerable variability in how cultures view the etiology and treatment of stuttering. For example, a historical etiological belief within African-American culture is that stuttering is the result of an evil spirit or the will of a higher power.[38] Others may think that the problem is psychological in nature and firmly believe it is rooted in difficult family relationships or personality traits such as shyness. When clinicians are faced with such strong and resilient beliefs, they should be respectful of them while also providing clinical education to the family or client. It is best for clinicians to send the message that the information given is another viewpoint on stuttering that is more research based. This attitude is more helpful than giving the impression that there is a correct versus incorrect way of viewing stuttering.

Now that we have reviewed the data regarding the nature of disfluent speech production in speakers of more than one language, and the relevant formal and informal assessment considerations, it is time for you to review the case study (Box 14.1 and Box 14.2) and apply what you have learned by answering the reflection questions.

Box 14.1 Case Study

Matthew is a 5-year-old English-Spanish bilingual child. His parents are seeking a professional opinion after Matthew's kindergarten teacher raised concern about his speech fluency. Matthew began learning English first, which is the language spoken at home. But, at the age of 4 years, he began attending a dual-language preschool where he was first introduced to Spanish. According to Matthew's parents, he only speaks Spanish in school.

He reportedly began exhibiting speech disfluencies at 3.5 years of age, but his parents report them to have been less frequent and less noticeable at that time. However, over the 6 months, his mother and the teacher have noticed an increase in frequency of speech disfluencies, which has coincided with an increase in his exposure and use of Spanish. His parents report noticing it most often when he is excited or when others "speak over him." His parent noted further that his teacher hears the "stuttering" in English when Matthew responds to questions in class or is explaining something, but considers it less noticeable when Matthew is speaking Spanish.

Conversational and narrative samples collected in Spanish and English demonstrated that across both sample types and languages, Matthew produced an average of 30 speech disfluencies per 100 spoken words. Of these disfluencies, more than 3% were stuttering-like in nature and specifically included repetitions of sounds, syllables, and words. The remaining disfluencies produced were non-stuttering-like in nature and consisted of interjections, revisions, and phrase repetitions. None of the speech disfluencies were produced with atypical tension.

Box 14.2 Case Study Reflection Questions

- Based on the details provided, what is your assessment recommendation for Matthew?
- What support would you directly provide to the parents?
- What role—if any—is bilingualism playing in Matthew's case?
- Are there any additions that you would make to the assessment protocol? If so, what and why?
- What recommendations would you provide to Matthew's teacher?
- Matthew's parents ask if they should transition to just communicating with Matthew in his native language only. What is your response and rationale for your response?

14.6 Considerations for Intervention

Similar to assessment tools, most therapeutic strategies and programs for stuttering have been developed for, and often by, monolingual speakers of English. Many speech-language pathologists working with bilingual children and adults who stutter have modified therapy on a trial-and-error basis in order to effect change in their client's stuttering. The first question that arises is whether or not we should treat stuttering in all languages spoken by the individual. The answer is yes, as much as possible.

As we have seen earlier, stuttering is not distributed equally across the languages a person speaks. An individual may stutter more in one language and much less in the other. However, treating stuttering in all of the languages the person speaks is not always easy. Sometimes the clinician is unable to speak the language of the client, or the client does not speak the clinician's language very well and an interpreter will be needed. Although having an interpreter, preferably within the family, is ideal, it may not be possible. In such cases, keeping explanations to a minimum and modeling behavioral therapy strategies (e.g., reduced rate) are most helpful. Since clinicians are able to correctly perceive disfluencies in different languages, especially when a diagnosis of stuttering is established, it is also possible for them to give feedback to clients when they are practicing in a language different from the clinician's.

When teaching specific behaviors in therapy, some clients and/or their parents may express resistance due to different culturally-based interpretations. For example, slowing the rate of speech, especially in adolescents and adults, may meet resistance. This is true even for monolingual speakers of English, but cultural interpretations regarding the perception of the slower speaker may differ. For example, some seem to value speaking rapidly and often perceive these speakers favorably as quick thinkers, active, and interesting people. Conversely, they may view a person who speaks more slowly as less intelligent and uninteresting. To encourage use of any sort of rate reduction strategy, the clinician must establish rapport with the client and, if applicable, their parents. The therapeutic alliance is critical regardless of culture, and perhaps more essential when the treatment requires behaviors that do not culturally align. Speech-language pathologists should take the time to discuss the rationale for using any therapy technique with the client, and work together to determine ways to help the client feel more comfortable.

The nature of parental participation may be another issue that has to be confronted when treating young children who stutter from a different cultural background and their parents. Current intervention practices tend to rely heavily on parents both in and out of therapy, to help carry out both therapy procedures and practice sessions. For example, the Lidcombe Program[42] teaches parents to distinguish between stuttered speech and typical speech disfluency. They are then coached to provide feedback to a set proportion of fluent and stuttered utterances during daily parent–child interactions and, ultimately, to request the child reproduce their stuttered utterances more "smoothly."

In contrast, the Dutch RESTART-DCM program (see https://restartdcm.nl/wp-content/uploads/2019/01/RESTART-DCM.Method.-English-met-app.pdf) and Palin Parent–Child Interaction Therapy[43] indirectly target the reduction of specific fluency disrupters in the child's environment. The parent and child engage in daily interactions, but without the child directly asked to modify their speech. A randomized clinical trial of Lidcombe compared to RESTART-DCM therapies showed negligible outcome differences for speakers of more than one language.[45] More detailed discussion of both Lidcombe and RESTART-DCM can be found in ▶ Chapter 10 of this text.

Recently, research has shown similar results from these two distinct programs. This is likely because there are common factors driving the outcomes. It has been speculated that the component common to both approaches, which contributes most to outcomes, is the daily interaction between parent and child, where the parent takes the time to listen to the child prior to responding. Nevertheless, regardless of the approach used, parental involvement is essential in the treatment of childhood stuttering. Although this is the case, some parents across some cultures may have a more formal relationship with their children, some do not feel comfortable engaging in play with their child in a professional setting, and still others may think that it is inappropriate for them to carry out therapy activities with their child. Fortunately, it is often possible through sensitive guidance to facilitate the parents openness to their involvement and to help them acquire the necessary skills to work effectively with their child.

In some cases, because cultural resistance is so strong, speech-language pathologists may need to modify intervention, so it relies more on the clinician than on the parent. When this happens, the clinician should inform the parents that due to these cultural restraints the course of treatment may be longer, and the outcomes may differ from what has been documented in the cases where parents played a more significant role.

Ideally, therapy should be completed in all of the languages that the child speaks. However, there is evidence that generalization of results across languages can occur in fluency therapy.[46] It should be noted, however, that these generalizations are restricted to the behavioral aspects of stuttering and do not extend to the cognitive (i.e., thoughts) and affective (feelings) aspects. In other words, learning to produce an easy onset at the beginning of a word is a behavioral strategy that has been shown to transfer to another language without practice in that other language. This makes sense intuitively, as learning to open your mouth slightly and making lighter articulatory touches and a breathier start to their utterances are strategies that can be used across many spoken languages. That said, these behavioral gains are often not maintained in the long term for either language, especially in adults.

More recently, there are data focusing on overall communication such as eye contact, using gestures, and smiling slightly while speaking to express a positive affect, rather than focusing on fluency and/or reduction of stuttering, with results replicated in CLD populations. This work showed a significant decrease in the negative impact of stuttering on the person who stutter's overall quality of life. In addition, there was a significant increase in communication competencies, social skills, self-advocacy, and positive communication attitudes for children aged 4 years through adults older than 90 years. As is demonstrated in this video clip, of the final treatment session of a Spanish-speaking adult who stutters (along with his interpreter), improvements in functional outcomes such as reducing speech avoidance, talking openly about stuttering, and using more competent communication skills are significant.

In summary, although there are inherent challenges in serving the multicultural and multilingual population, communication is critical across all cultures, and all languages. Thus, the focus should be on helping them to communicate freely and competently. Treatment may take longer, be more demanding for the clinician who must adapt and be creative, and often may not be as perfect as was hoped. However, for the speech-language pathologist, the CLD client will provide many satisfying moments as well as opportunities to learn and grow as a clinician, and as a person.

14.7 Conclusion

This chapter has provided an overview of the progression of research centered on the role of bilingualism and multilingualism as they relate to the assessment of stuttering, the impact on treatment, and cultural considerations to be made throughout service delivery. The findings to date have highlighted a major challenge for clinicians to accurately identify behaviors that differentiate typical disfluency, language learning, language impairment, and stuttering in monolingual and bilingual speakers. The data have also shown that typically fluent bilinguals and those who stutter are often much more disfluent than their monolingual counterparts because they are navigating between languages. This raises the question of how best to adapt our monolingual English guidelines to this population in order to enhance our differential diagnosis of these speakers.

From a theoretical perspective, additional research exploring the overlapping and distinguishing behaviors could serve to demonstrate the relative contribution of linguistic planning and speech motor control to the different manifestations of disfluent speech. As cultural and linguistic awareness and bilingual and multilingual populations increase, it is expected that this area of knowledge and research will expand. Thus, clinicians should be prepared to continue educating themselves in this area as findings emerge and evolve. Nevertheless, the information given in this chapter has provided readers with an evidence-based starting point with regard to the key differentiating characteristics, areas of overlap, and other critical assessment and treatment considerations.

References

[1] Byrd CT. Assessing bilingual children: Are their disfluencies indicative of stuttering or the by-product of navigating two languages? Semin Speech Lang. 2018; 39(4):324–332

[2] Grosjean F. Studying bilinguals: Methodological and conceptual issues. In: Bhatia TK, Ritchie WC, eds. The Handbook of Bilingualism. Cambridge: Cambridge University Press; 2004:32–63

[3] Blom E, Boerma Tessel. Effects of language impairment and bilingualism across domains: vocabulary, morphology and verbal memory. Linguist Approaches Biling. 2017; 7(3–4):277–300

[4] Grimm A, Schulz P. Specific language impairment and early second language acquisition: the risk of over- and underdiagnosis. Child Indic Res. 2014; 7(4): 821–841

[5] Paradis J, Genesee F, Crago MB. Dual language development and disorders: a handbook on bilingualism and second language learning. Baltimore, MD: Brookes Publishing Company; 2011

[6] Gutiérrez-Clellen VF, Simon-Cereijido G. Using language sampling in clinical assessments with bilingual children: challenges and future directions. Semin Speech Lang. 2009; 30(4):234–245

[7] Boey RA, Wuyts FL, Van de Heyning PH, De Bodt MS, Heylen L. Characteristics of stuttering-like disfluencies in Dutch-speaking children. J Fluency Disord. 2007; 32(4):310–329

[8] Leclercq A-L, Suaire P, Moyse A. Beyond stuttering: speech disfluencies in normally fluent French-speaking children at age 4. Clin Linguist Phon. 2018; 32(2):166–179

[9] Natke U, Sandrieser P, Pietrowsky R, Kalveram KT. Disfluency data of German preschool children who stutter and comparison children. J Fluency Disord. 2006; 31(3):165–176

[10] Watson JB, Byrd CT, Carlo EJ. Effects of length, complexity, and grammatical correctness on stuttering in Spanish-speaking preschool children. Am J Speech Lang Pathol. 2011; 20(3):209–220

[11] Byrd CT, Bedore LM, Ramos D. The disfluent speech of bilingual Spanish-English children: considerations for differential diagnosis of stuttering. Lang Speech Hear Serv Sch. 2015; 46(1):30–43

[12] Rincon C, Johnson KN, Byrd C. An introductory examination of speech disfluencies in Spanish–English bilingual children who do and do not stutter during narratives. Perspect ASHA Spec Interest Groups. 2020; 5(1):131–141

[13] Einarsdóttir J, Ingham RJ. Have disfluency-type measures contributed to the understanding and treatment of developmental stuttering? Am J Speech Lang Pathol. 2005; 14(4):260–273

[14] Van Borsel J, Medeiros de Britto Pereira M. Assessment of stuttering in a familiar versus an unfamiliar language. J Fluency Disord. 2005; 30(2):109–124

[15] Bosshardt H-G, Packman A, Blomgren M, Kretschmann J. Measuring stuttering in preschool-aged children across different languages. Folia Phoniatr Logop. 2015; 67(5):221–230

[16] Cosyns M, Einarsdóttir JT, Van Borsel J. Factors involved in the identification of stuttering severity in a foreign language. Clin Linguist Phon. 2015; 29(12):909–921

[17] Hoffman L, Wilson L, Copley A, Hewat S, Lim V. The reliability of a severity rating scale to measure stuttering in an unfamiliar language. Int J Speech Lang Pathol. 2014; 16(3):317–326

[18] Lee AS, Robb MP, Ormond T, Blomgren M. The role of language familiarity in bilingual stuttering assessment. Clin Linguist Phon. 2014; 28(10):723–740

[19] Byrd CT, Watson J, Bedore LM, Mullis A. Identification of Stuttering in Bilingual Spanish-English-Speaking Children. Contemp Issues Commun Sci Disord. 2015; 42:72–87

[20] Ambrose NG, Yairi E. Normative disfluency data for early childhood stuttering. J Speech Lang Hear Res. 1999; 42(4):895–909

[21] Eggers K, Van Eerdenbrugh S, Byrd CT. Speech disfluencies in bilingual Yiddish-Dutch speaking children. Clin Linguist Phon. 2020; 34(6):576–592

[22] Byrd CT, Haque AN, Johnson K. Speech-language pathologists perception of bilingualism as a risk factor for stuttering. J Commun Disor Deaf Studies Hear Aids. 2006; 4(2):1000158

[23] Travis LE, Johnson W, Shover J. The relation of bilingualism to stuttering: a survey of the East Chicago, Indiana, schools. J Speech Disord. 1937; 2(3):185–189

[24] Howell P, Davis S, Williams R. The effects of bilingualism on stuttering during late childhood. Arch Dis Child. 2009; 94(1):42–46

[25] Coalson GA, Peña ED, Byrd CT. Description of multilingual participants who stutter. J Fluency Disord. 2013; 38(2):141–156

[26] Werle DR, Byrd C, Coalson G. Description of multilingual participants who stutter: an update 2011–2018. Comm Disord Q. 2019; 42(1):50–57

[27] Riley G, Bakker K. SSI-4: Stuttering Severity Instrument. Austin, TX: PRO-ED; 2009

[28] Vanryckeghem M, Brutten EJ. KiddyCat: Communication Attitude Test for Preschool and Kindergarten Children Who Stutter. San Diego, CA: Plural Publishing Incorporated; 2007

[29] Gillam RB, Logan KJ, Pearson NA. TOCS: Test of Childhood Stuttering. Austin, TX: Pro-Ed, 2009

[30] Naderi S, Shahbodaghi MR, Khatonabadi A, Dadgar H, Jalaei SH. Translation of the test of childhood stuttering into Persian and investigation of validity and reliability of the test. Journal of Modern Rehabilitation. 2011; 5(2):29–34

[31] Abdou R. Assessment of Egyptian children who stutter using the standardized Arabic form of the Test of Childhood Stuttering. Egypt J Otolaryngol. 2015; 31(3):180–187

[32] Yaruss JS, Quesal RW. Overall Assessment of the Speaker's Experience of Stuttering (OASES): documenting multiple outcomes in stuttering treatment. J Fluency Disord. 2006; 31(2):90–115

[33] Yaruss JS, Quesal RW. Overall Assessment of the Speaker's Experience of Stuttering (OASES). McKinney, TX: Stuttering Therapy Resources; 2016

[34] Stuttering Therapy Resources. Frequently Asked Questions. 2018. Available at: https://www.stutteringtherapyresources.com/menu-oases#frequently-asked-questions

[35] Bleek B, Reuter M, Yaruss JS, Cook S, Faber J, Montag C. Relationships between personality characteristics of people who stutter and the impact of stuttering on everyday life. J Fluency Disord. 2012; 37(4):325–333

[36] Koedoot C, Versteegh M, Yaruss JS. Psychometric evaluation of the Dutch translation of the Overall Assessment of the Speaker's Experience of Stuttering for adults (OASES-A-D). J Fluency Disord. 2011; 36(3):222–230

[37] Robinson TL, Jr, Crowe TA. Culture-based considerations in programming for stuttering intervention with African American clients and their families. Lang Speech Hear Serv Sch. 1998; 29(3):172–179

[38] Roseberry-McKibbin Celeste. Multicultural students with special language needs. Oceanside, CA: Academic Communication Associates; 2014

[39] Nishishiba M. Culturally mindful communication: essential skills for public and nonprofit professionals. New York, NY: Routledge; 2018

[40] Klein MD, Chen D. Working with children from culturally diverse backgrounds. Albany, NY: Delmar; 2001

[41] Harrison E, Onslow M. (2010). The Lidcombe program for preschool children who stutter. Treatment of stuttering: Established and emerging interventions; 2010:118–140

[42] Kelman E, Nicholas A. Palin Parent-Child Interaction Therapy for Early Childhood Stammering. Abingdon, UK: Routledge; 2020

[43] de Sonneville-Koedoot C, Stolk E, Rietveld T, Franken MC. Direct versus indirect treatment for preschool children who stutter: the RESTART randomized trial. PLoS One. 2015; 10(7):e0133758

15 Pharmacological Considerations for the Treatment of Stuttering

Lisa LaSalle, Angharad Ames, and Gerald Maguire

Abstract

Pharmacological considerations for adults who stutter are important for an interprofessional team to address. This chapter provides information that speech-language pathologists need to know about pharmacotherapy for adults who stutter. We begin with a dopamine hypothesis about stuttering—how persistent developmental stuttering is likely a hyperdopaminergic condition similar to Tourette's syndrome. Background is provided as to how neurotransmitter reuptake, the placebo effect, and safety play a role in medication development. A historical perspective is then added, spanning the earlier use of haloperidol to the present use of newer, second-generation dopamine antagonists. New investigatory medications such as ecopipam are included. Second-generation dopamine antagonists currently used to treat stuttering with the lowest adverse drug reaction profiles include six medications (e.g., asenapine), presented in a table format. Adverse drug reactions are also considered, as they occur with all medications, but can be minimized with careful dosage decisions. Stuttering, for the purpose of this chapter, will include (1) persistent developmental stuttering, whether comorbid/co-occurring or not; (2) exacerbated stuttering (i.e., paradoxical effects); and (3) acquired stuttering (i.e., iatrogenic effects) versus serendipitous stuttering amelioration that may occur when individuals who stutter are medicated for a co-occurring condition. We then discuss the effect of medications prescribed for other conditions on both persistent developmental stuttering and acquired stuttering. Future directions include new medications, and combining support/self-help group, behavioral treatment, and/or pharmacotherapy is recommended. Treatment options arise from the informed client's wishes in both an evidence-based practice and a cost–benefit type framework. Finally, we believe that pharmacological considerations for adults who stutter are where our ethics, counseling, scope of practice, and interprofessional practice intersect to provide the best possible treatment options.

Keywords: persistent developmental stuttering, medication, dopamine, hyperdopaminergic condition, dopamine antagonists, pharmacotherapy, interprofessional practice, speech-language pathologists and psychiatrists, comorbidity, necessity–concerns framework

15.1 Introduction

The purpose of this chapter is to provide pharmacological considerations for individuals who stutter. We define pharmacotherapy as treatment of a client/patient with medications, thus requiring medical professionals (e.g., physicians or psychiatrists). We have focused especially on adults who stutter, but we included several pediatric case reports. We have excluded pharmacological considerations for individuals younger than 18 years, as pharmacotherapy for stuttering in children and adolescents may not be effective or advisable.[1] Compared to children and teens, adults who stutter (AWS) are the most likely age of individuals seeking pharmacotherapy. In general, AWS are likely to seek pharmacotherapy if their stuttering severity is moderate to severe, and/or if they have experienced relatively negative impacts of stuttering on their quality of life, despite behavioral treatments.

Based on criteria such as stuttering severity and being a nonresponder to speech therapy, medication is an option for AWS. Providing access to self-help/support groups and to behavioral speech fluency/stuttering modification treatment for individuals who stutter are other important options. Providing all evidence-based options when requested is an obligation that falls upon the speech-language pathologist (SLP). Ideally, individuals who stutter would consult with an interprofessional practice team to determine treatment options.

The third author of this chapter, Dr. Gerald Maguire, is a person who stutters, a researcher of stuttering, and a psychiatrist. He served as chair of the National Stuttering Association, and he believes that acceptance of stuttering by the person who stutters is the first step in the treatment of stuttering in AWS. Based on his experience over the years, Dr. Maguire views medication as an important adjunct to available fluency shaping, stuttering modification, and support/self-help group services for AWS. When considering treatment for stuttering, he believes that SLPs are the primary helpers and that treatment options including medication should be at the client's discretion and involve appropriate education for the AWS.[2] The authors of this chapter believe that combining evidence-based treatments in a comprehensive, synergistic way is best for individuals who are seeking help for their stuttering.

Thus, by way of introduction, a brief coverage or reminder of evidence-based practice (EBP) is in order. For the present chapter, EBP involves applying the body of peer-reviewed literature to the pharmacological (as well as other) options for those who stutter. However, EBP also considers the clinician(s)' expertise and the informed wishes of the client/patient who stutters. The first author recalls attending a panel discussion of stuttering specialists who stutter. One speaker recounted his experience in taking an antianxiety medication in attempts to speak more fluently in his presentation, only to have the medication wear off before getting his turn at the microphone! This anecdote highlights the informed wishes of this individual to take a medication that would assist him in stuttering symptom alleviation, at least for the presentation. It also addresses the phenomena of both pharmacodynamics (i.e., what a medication does to the body, in this case presumptively decrease anxiety) and pharmacokinetics (i.e., what the body does to the medication, including metabolism and the wearing-off of its effects). Dr. Ehud Yairi, another person who stutters, an SLP and a researcher of stuttering, has expressed that "the search of the person who stutters for a relief, if not a complete cure, is understandable."[3] This chapter is written in that spirit.

We also believe that a type of cost–benefit model, specifically the necessity–concerns framework, is one helpful way to understand how people perceive medications.[4] People tend to focus on either or both the *necessity* (i.e., benefits) of maintaining one's health or quality of life with medications and the *concerns* (i.e., costs) toward the adverse effects or "side effects" of those medications. The necessity–concerns framework helps explain how people exhibit individual differences in their cognitive and affective perception of medication or pharmacotherapy. The model assumes that people perceive that when costs outweigh benefits, negative beliefs toward medication occur. Conversely, people may decide that benefits of a medication outweigh its costs, thus viewing medications relatively positively. Such individual differences regarding people's attitudes about medications could cluster together into at least four subgroups. For example, one subgroup could be *accepting* (high necessity, low concerns), another *ambivalent* (high necessity, high concerns), *indifferent* (low necessity, low concerns), and still another *skeptical* (low necessity, high concerns). This necessity–concern framework could be applied to a vast range of medications administered to treat a range of human conditions.[4,5] Persistent developmental stuttering is one of those human conditions.

Findings from 18- to 65-year-old individuals who stutter (*n* = 226), using an international Beliefs about Medication Questionnaire indicated that pharmacotherapy was as equally sought out as was speech therapy. In these survey results, 16% responded as being *accepting* in their beliefs about medication, whereas 27% were *indifferent*, 24% *ambivalent*, and 33% *skeptical*.

Those who were *accepting* in their medication beliefs, as might be expected, were most likely to seek pharmacotherapy for their stuttering. Furthermore, the *ambivalent* and *indifferent* participants who stutter were significantly more likely to seek pharmacotherapy than were the *skeptical* participants who stutter.[6] It would seem helpful for the clinician to know that almost one out of five (16%) AWS might be accepting, that is, they have low concerns about the cost aspect of pharmaceuticals and feel a high necessity for alleviating/ameliorating to stutter symptoms. In this way, clinicians can be better prepared to frame discussion with their clients regarding pharmacological considerations. We can further appreciate that the one out of three AWS who are skeptical about medications might be so for various reasons (e.g., acceptance of one's stuttering; knowing that medications cross the blood–brain barrier; encountering problems with access to quality health care and thus access to medication, out-of-pocket costs of medication, etc.).

15.2 Stuttering and the Dopamine Hypothesis

In order to explain why medication might alleviate stuttering symptoms, we will present basic information about a neurological timing/programming deficit, likely to be present in AWS. This presumed deficit is what the medication is designed to act upon. After all, medicine at its simplest level is the use of a compound reasoned to alleviate symptoms. It is important to understand what is referred to as a mechanism of action (MOA), that is, biochemically, how the medication produces its pharmacological effect. A medication's MOA describes how the chemical structure of the medication/compound binds to molecular targets, such as the enzyme or receptor. It is not the purpose of this chapter to provide comprehensive coverage of such processes. Indeed, basic overviews of pharmacodynamics and pharmacokinetics specific to stuttering have been previously presented, for example, by Ludlow[7] and Saxon and Ludlow.[8]

Recent available evidence suggests that the basal ganglia and white matter tract development is abnormal in those who stutter.[9,10,11,12,13] The over-activation of the basal ganglia circuits (i.e., the red nucleus, pedunculopontine nucleus, subthalamic nucleus, and substantia nigra) in AWS during speech tasks supports the likelihood that stuttering is associated with a hyperactive dopaminergic system.[14] Dopamine is one of six major types of neurotransmitters. Each neurotransmitter is presented with its type and function in ▶ Table 15.1.

Skilled motor movements, such as speaking, are highly interconnected with the basal ganglia, cerebellum, and other subcortical and cortical regions, so much so that the neurological/neuropharmacological "juries are still out." That is, we do not yet know where in the basal ganglia/white matter tract specific deficits of developmental stuttering would be found,

Table 15.1 The six major neurotransmitters relevant to this chapter. These six transmitters are listed, in alphabetical order, within three main categories of monoamines, amino acids, and others, such as acetylcholine (Ach). Peptides are considered as neurotransmitters, but excluded here

Neurotransmitter	Function
Monoamines	
Dopamine	Regulates various behaviors (e.g., goal-directed behaviors, especially pleasurable goals, food, sex, and social interaction); used by neurons for both voluntary and involuntary movements; role in integration of focus and memory
Norepinephrine	Regulates modulation/regulation of vigilance, arousal, attention, learning, memory, motivation, and mood; increases oxygen to the brain; increases heart rate; shuts down metabolic processes; "stress/fight or flight hormone"
Serotonin (5-hydroxytryptamine)	Regulates various behaviors (e.g., sleep, wakefulness, eating); role in regulating many bodily functions (e.g. digestion, blood clotting)
Amino acids	
Gamma-aminobutyric acid (GABA)	Inhibition of *postsynaptic* neuron; present in ~40% of all synapses; has a role in allowing us to calm ourselves as well as inhibits feelings of being overwhelmed; perhaps related to emotional regulation
Glutamate	Excitation of *postsynaptic* neuron; present in ~90% of all synapses; promotes the firing of an action potential
Other	
Acetylcholine (ACh)	Sends and receives signals among motor neurons and muscle cells; motor neurons release ACh in order to activate muscles; it has a role in attention, arousal, and memory

"...especially against the backdrop of a developing linguistic and nervous system in children."[15]

Brain imaging studies of AWS have been enlightening, but findings from these studies are likely to show compensatory effects of stuttering, not pure etiology of stuttering. And yet, for 33- to 34-month-old children who are at the typical age to have just begun to stutter,[16] it does not yet seem feasible to use brain imaging techniques on them, given their difficulties cooperating with procedures that restrict their activities/movements. With that background, we present three findings that pertain to (1) dopamine metabolism, (2) excessive release of dopamine, and (3) dopaminergic genes.

First, *dopamine metabolism* is implicated in persistent developmental stuttering.[10,17] Dopamine is a monoamine catecholamine neurotransmitter. To unpack that definition, like other neurotransmitters (e.g., serotonin, norepinephrine), dopamine is a compound with a *single* amine group in its molecule (i.e., a monoamine). Dopamine is also a hormone produced in the adrenal gland, sent to our bloodstream when we are physically or emotionally stressed (i.e., a catecholamine). Dopamine functions in our learning, attention, movements, emotions and reward/motivation systems, and possibly even fear.[18]

Understanding the actions of agonists and antagonists is prerequisite knowledge to the metabolism of dopamine. Agonists are chemicals that *bind* to a receptor, which produces a biological response. Antagonists, however, *block* the action of the agonist. *Thus, dopamine receptor blockers are synonymous with dopamine antagonists.* There are five types of dopamine receptors, D1, D2, D3, D4, and D5. When a neurotransmitter binds to a receptor, an extracellular signal converts to an intracellular signal, which then changes target neurons. ▶ Table 15.2 shows the specific genes and chromosomes that encode each of these dopamine receptors, their distinct functions, the rank ordering of how abundant each dopamine receptor type is, and where each receptor tends to be found.

Second, AWS, when compared to adults who do not stutter (AWNS), *exhibit excessive release of dopamine* into the striatum (i.e., the caudate nucleus and putamen). As a group, AWS exhibit a disproportionately increased amount of activity in the substantia nigra, and excessive release of dopamine in the striatum.[14,17,19] In an early (1997) example of these types of findings, positron emission tomography (PET) imaging of the brains of AWS showed an increase in fluorodopamine (FDOPA, specifically 6-FDOPA) activity in the caudate tail. The caudate, as well as the putamen (which are both components of the basal ganglia), contains cells on which D1 and D2 receptors are located. The location of these two dopamine receptors on components of the basal ganglia suggests that dopamine plays a role in the pathophysiology of stuttering.[20]

Third, empirical findings indicate that *dopaminergic genes* (i.e., possibly SLC6A3 and DRD2 and GNPTAB) are associated with stuttering, further supporting the dopamine hypothesis of stuttering.[21,22,23] Genetic findings and interpretations are presented in a cautionary manner, as further research is needed to support or refute these claims. It also helps one's understanding of the pharmacodynamics of stuttering to know about common conditions with *over-sufficient* dopamine levels (e.g., schizophrenia) as well as *insufficient* dopamine levels (e.g., Parkinson's disease [PD]). For instance, stuttering could be a comorbid or concomitant disorder for those with schizophrenia and PD, or stuttering could result from a dopamine agonist medication (i.e., iatrogenic), either when stuttering is acquired for the first time or when a worsening of developmental stuttering occurs.

The MOA of the medication prescribed for schizophrenia targets the *over-sufficiency* of dopamine (i.e., the medication *decreases* dopamine availability as a mechanism for alleviating schizophrenic symptoms, such as disorganized speech, or flat affect). An example of pharmacotherapy for schizophrenia would be to prescribe D2 antagonists, those that block the D2 receptor, or affect other receptors, such as the serotonin and histamine receptors. For example, the medication aripiprazole, often prescribed for schizophrenia, is both a serotonin and a D2 partial agonist. Partial agonists bind to or activate a receptor in an incomplete manner, in an analogous way to a door open

Table 15.2 Dopamine receptor types. Each of the *five dopamine receptors* (i.e., D1–D5) are listed in numerical order, followed by the genes/chromosomes encoding each, and the presumed function of each dopamine receptor. The rightmost columns are the "abundancy rating," i.e., the rank ordering of how abundant each dopamine receptor type is in the cerebral cortex, and "cortical location of high density," i.e., the place in the brain where each type of dopamine receptor is found neuroanatomically

Dopamine receptor	Gene encoding	Function	Abundancy rating	Cortical location of high density
D1	Gene 5q31–q34	attention, impulse control, learning, locomotion, memory, motor activity, regulation of renal function, regulation of the reward system	1st	striatum, nucleus accumbens, olfactory bulb, and substantia nigra
D2	On chromosome 11	attention, learning, locomotion, memory, neuronal development, sleep, fear	2nd	striatum, external globus pallidus, core of nucleus accumbens, hippocampus, amygdala, and cerebral cortex
D3	On chromosome 3	attention, cognition, impulse control, sleep, fear	3rd	striatum, external globus pallidus, core of nucleus accumbens, hippocampus, amygdala, and cerebral cortex
D4	On chromosome 11	attention, cognition, impulse control, sleep, fear	5th	striatum, external globus pallidus, core of nucleus accumbens, hippocampus, amygdala, and cerebral cortex
D5	On chromosome 4	attention, cognition, decision-making, learning, motor activity, regulation of renal function, regulation of the reward system	4th	striatum, nucleus accumbens, olfactory bulb, and substantia nigra

halfway as opposed to a full entrance to a receptor, which would be the case with a full agonist.

In contrast to schizophrenia, for PD, the substantia nigra produces an *under-sufficiency* of dopamine. This results in the person with PD exhibiting such symptoms as bradykinesia, festination, micrographia, resting tremor, shuffling gait, and postural instability.

Dopamine agonist medications for PD *increase* dopamine availability as a mechanism for alleviating PD symptoms. To treat PD pharmacologically, physicians prescribe medications such as carbidopa and levodopa together (i.e., carbidopa–levodopa). In this case, levodopa is converted into dopamine, while carbidopa's MOA decreases to some extent the peripheral side effects of dopamine.[24,25] Carbidopa–levodopa has been reported to both exacerbate developmental stuttering and cause acquired stuttering,[26,27] thus providing further support for the dopamine hypothesis of persistent developmental stuttering.

Another condition that can be misdiagnosed as stuttering, and occasionally co-occurs with stuttering, is Tourette's syndrome (TS). Like persistent developmental stuttering and schizophrenia, TS likely has a hyperdopaminergic etiology. Like stuttering, TS has a vocal fluency disruption component (i.e., vocal tics), a likely genetic predisposition (i.e., in the case of TS, the ASH1 L gene), childhood onset, and a prevalence of less than or about 1%. There is one other commonality between persistent developmental stuttering and TS that, to our knowledge, has not yet been pointed out in the literature. This is the commonality that individuals who stutter and those with TS both tend to show poor time estimation, which is likely a hyperdopaminergic function. Such poor time estimation involves the perception that time is moving faster than real time, which has been observed in both those who stutter[28,29,30] and in those with TS.[31] We will return to medications designed for TS and stuttering-related findings.

However, the next section follows from the hyperdopaminergic condition aspect of stuttering and TS, and it addresses a "two-loop" hypothesis about how speech output fluency might be facilitated via neurotransmitters such as dopamine and GABA.

15.3 Stuttering and the "Two-loop" Hypothesis of Speech Output

There is a large body of evidence that the basal ganglia are implicated in stuttering. Yet, the basal ganglia are basically motor nuclei, and they comprise almost all of the gray matter of the cerebrum, with the exception of the thalamus, which is primarily sensory (i.e., only motoric in a secondary feedback manner). The function of the basal ganglia is to plan and execute movements, and the basal ganglia serve as the main relay station for the extrapyramidal motor system. ▶ Table 15.3 shows, first, the breakdown of the three largest motor nuclei in the basal ganglia (i.e., caudate nucleus, putamen, and globus pallidus) and their related structures (i.e., subthalamic nucleus, substantia nigra, and centromedian [thalamic] nucleus). Many indirect (i.e., inhibitory) and direct (i.e., excitatory) pathways exist among the thalamus, basal ganglia/related structures, parietal lobe, premotor, primary, and supplementary cortices, to one another. When dopaminergic neurons in the substantia nigra no longer function, the indirect pathway is suppressed, halting the direct pathway as well. The result of this dysfunction is inhibition of the thalamocortical neurons, causing hypokinetic movement disorders such as PD. Regarding stuttering, Chang and colleagues provide support for Alm's early speculations that the excessive dopaminergic dysfunction is either (1) in the indirect pathway, thus increasing motor activation due to decreased inhibition, or (2) in the direct pathway, thus decreasing motor activation due to decreased excitation.[9]

The "two-loop timing theory of speech output" suggests an outer linguistic loop and an inner motoric loop. Borrowing from this inner and outer loop theory allows us to understand how dopamine blockers might facilitate speech fluency in AWS. The second part of ▶ Table 15.4 breaks down the function and implicated brain regions for this hypothesis.

We have adapted this original "two-loop speech theory" considered by Foundas and colleagues to fit with a hyperdopaminergic view of stuttering.[32] The inner motoric loop is speculated to be abnormal in adults with persistent developmental stuttering. To overcome this deficit, individuals who stutter need to access an outer loop through fluency-enhancing activities like choral speech during reading, where the linguistic load is low (see ▶ Chapter 1). Because dopamine *decreases* the activity of the putamen and caudate nucleus (i.e., the striatum), a dopamine receptor blocker type of medication would increase the activation of the striatum, thereby increasing speech fluency. Another treatment possibility is to administer a medication that affects the inhibitory neurotransmitter gamma-aminobutyric acid (GABA), in attempts at facilitating speech fluency. Enhancing

Table 15.3 Basal ganglia background. The nuclei and related structures of the basal ganglia and the two-loop timing theory of speech output, based on Foundas et al,[32] where the inner linguistic loop is in the corpus striatum and cortex

Basal ganglia: three largest motor nuclei			Basal ganglia: three related structures
Lentiform nucleus	Caudate nucleus	Corpus striatum	Subthalamic nucleus (STN)
	Putamen		Substantia nigra (SN)
	Globus pallidus (GP)		Centromedian nucleus (CMS; thalamic)

Table 15.4 Two-loop timing theory of speech output. The nuclei and related structures of the basal ganglia and the two-loop timing theory of speech output, based on Foundas et al,[32] where the inner linguistic loop is in the corpus striatum and cortex

	Function	Brain regions implicated
Inner linguistic loop	Motor programming and activation of vocal and speech mechanism (phonatory/articulatory movements)	Corpus striatum and cortex
Outer linguistic loop	Phonological, lexical/semantic, syntactic functions; selecting/self-monitoring speech sounds (auditory verbal info)	Perisylvian regions: Broca's and Wernicke's areas

GABA and reducing dopamine would facilitate fluency even during spontaneous speech through the inner loop, even though the linguistic and resulting motoric load is high, and especially so under time pressure.[17]

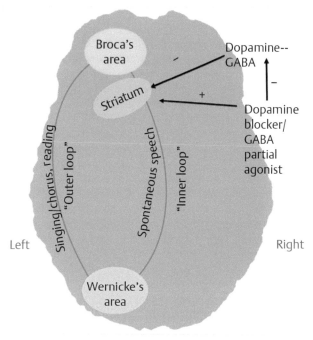

Fig. 15.1 Dopamine pathways. The authors speculate that fluency-enhancing behaviors like singing, choral speaking, and reading allow for accessing a compensatory "outer loop" when the "inner loop" is deficient in people who stutter. As can be seen here, when prescribing (+) a dopamine blocker or a GABA partial agonist, dopamine and GABA are reduced (–) as input to the striatum, and fluency facilitation can occur even during spontaneous speech/"inner loop" production.

▸ Fig. 15.1 is a graphic overview of the neurotransmitter pathway possibilities between Broca's and Wernicke's areas in the frontal and temporal lobes of the left hemisphere.

Additional data will help us to better understand whether (1) (in)direct pathways are related to these inner and outer loops, (2) synchrony of the loops matter for fluency facilitation, and (3) perception and production operate autonomously in spontaneous speech, and how that informs these neurotransmitter pathway possibilities.

15.4 Background Pertaining to Pharmacotherapy for Stuttering

Three background areas need explanation before the history of pharmacology and stuttering: (1) a neuropharmacological impact on neurotransmitters known as reuptake, (2) limiting or controlling the placebo effect, and (3) four phases of clinical trials (e.g., pagoclone).

15.4.1 Neuropharmacological Impact on Neurotransmitters: Reuptake

Neurotransmitters (e.g., dopamine, GABA) travel from the cell body down the axon and reenter the axon by endocytosis (i.e., transporting molecules into the cell by taking them inside the cell membrane). Alternatively, the neurotransmitter can reenter the presynaptic neuron by being taken back up by the same neurons that released them at the synaptic junction, a process known as "reuptake." ▸ Fig. 15.2 shows this reuptake process and reuptake ports, as might occur with serotonin, dopamine, or other neurotransmitters. If the needed transport molecules are not available, then neurotransmitter reuptake does not occur, causing the neurotransmitter to accumulate in the

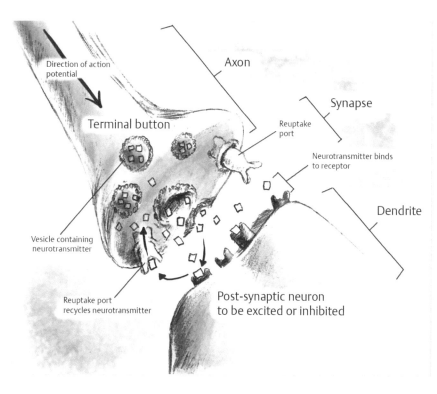

Fig. 15.2 Neurotransmitter reuptake process. Some neurotransmitters will bind to the receptors on the postsynaptic neuron, but others will be recycled through reuptake ports. (This image is provided courtesy of Isaac Rodriguez, University of Redlands Biochemistry student.)

synaptic junction. This would then increase the excitability of the neuron. Pharmacological agents that are reuptake inhibitors would then bring about this presumed effect.

15.4.2 Limiting or Controlling the Placebo Effect

To understand the historical context of pharmacological options for those who stutter, we next introduce the placebo effect. Researchers want to minimize the placebo effect, as it is one type of threat to internal validity. When a study has good internal validity, the independent variable (e.g., a medication) appears to be the only variable affecting the dependent variable or outcome (e.g., stuttering frequency). An individual who stutters perceiving that "this medication will be beneficial for me" could be a nuisance variable affecting the outcome.[33]

The placebo effect in pharmacology means that patients could perceive and self-report symptom improvement without ever being administered the actual medication. Research design for controlling the placebo effect includes randomly administering either a fake/sham pill or the real one (e.g., "2.5 mg/d of olanzapine *or* identical placebo for the first 4 weeks"[34]).

Appropriate statistical methods help us to ascertain if it is the medication and not the placebo that causes the change in outcome. Placebo administration in medication designs are important. The importance of placebos in COVID-19 vaccine development became one of many familiar news stories in 2020. Here are two examples of placebo use pertaining to stuttering. First, barbiturates have shown no beneficial effects over placebo in stuttering frequency outcomes.[35] Olanzapine, however, showed a statistical difference from placebo in improving patients' self-ratings of stuttering (22% change from baseline with olanzapine versus 1% change from baseline with placebo).

15.4.3 Four Phases of Clinical Trials and the Example of Pagoclone

An overview of the four phases (i.e., I–IV) of clinical trials allows for the appreciation of the role of "safety" in the development of any medication.

Phase I studies evaluate the safety of medications, typically take several months to complete, and most experimental medications/drugs pass this phase of testing.

Phase II studies, following phase I, attempt to determine whether or not the drug has the desired effect. Phase II studies often last up to 2 years, require statistical power, and thus often include more than 100 participants. Most phase II studies involve randomized, placebo trials, and are double-blinded. Double-blind or blinded means that neither the patients nor the researchers know who has received the experimental drug. At the end of the double-blind phase, participants are invited to enroll in open-label extension studies. This type of study involves giving all participants the "experimental drug." As part of the open-label extension study, both participants and investigators are made aware that the experimental drug is being used.

Phase III involves a large-scale test lasting several years. It elucidates the medication's benefits and all side effects or adverse drug reactions (ADRs) for the U.S. Food and Drug Administration (FDA) as well as for the pharmaceutical corporation producing the drug. Placebos may or may not be used in phase III trials, and the actual medication might be offered to a patient receiving placebo after a certain time span. Successful phase III completion allows a pharmaceutical corporation to request FDA approval for marketing a medication.

Finally, *phase IV* or "post marketing surveillance trials" are run in order to compare the medication with alternative medications, to estimate long-term effectiveness, impact on quality of life, and to determine cost-effectiveness. The authors of this chapter have been considering medications that are without specific FDA indications for treating stuttering. The absence of FDA approval is not equal to the absence of medication/drug safety and efficacy. FDA approval is a branding of sorts.

One example of a medication tested on individuals who stutter that illustrates the application of the four phases of a clinical trial is that of pagoclone. Pagoclone is an anxiolytic (antianxiety) agent belonging to the class of nonbenzodiazepines that binds with high affinity to the GABA-A receptor, acting as a partial agonist. Pagoclone was under development by two pharmaceutical companies as an investigational therapy for panic disorder in 1996 to 2000. Indevus later acquired the rights to test the medication for the pharmacological treatment of stuttering.

Pagoclone showed early efficacy for stuttering amelioration in the largest pharmacological trial of stuttering conducted to date. Researchers in 2010 assessed the safety, tolerability, and effectiveness of pagoclone during 8 weeks of double-blind treatment followed by a 1-year open-label extension in patients who stutter. It was an 8-week, 16-center, randomized clinical trial, double-blind study, followed by a 1-year open-label extension. Participants had persistent developmental stuttering. Pagoclone was administered twice daily to 88 patients, with matching placebo given to 44 patients. Participants reduced percent syllables stuttered (%SS) by 19% from baseline in contrast to only a 5% SS reduction with placebo. Then 40% SS reduction from baseline was observed during open-label treatment, after 1 year of treatment with pagoclone. Headache (12.5% pagoclone patients, 6.8% placebo patients) was the most reported ADR.[36,37]

Next, a phase II trial of pagoclone for treating stuttering enrolled over 330 participants who stutter in just 2 weeks with no formalized advertising for the trial. Although this provided convincing evidence for the interest and need in this population for advanced treatment options, the phase II results yielded a high placebo response, which, as a result, did not pass the stringent criteria stated earlier for Indevus to proceed with investing financially and further developing pagoclone for stuttering. The primary endpoint in the study was the percentage of syllables stuttered, which revealed great variability from visit to visit and a high placebo response with all subjects overall, showing improvement compared to baseline on this metric. However, the social anxiety levels of individuals on active therapy showed a marked improvement over placebo. The experience with pagoclone serves as a prime example of the need for more valid instruments for measuring stuttering response over time. With pagoclone, there was a strong interest from the community, and stuttering amelioration benefits were at least initially observed.[36,37]

15.5 Medications for Stuttering: A Historical Perspective

Presently, there are no medications approved by the FDA for the treatment of stuttering. Investigation is ongoing into the utility of already-developed medications in the treatment of stuttering. Several classes of medications have been studied in this way, and multiple medications have demonstrated positive results in the treatment of stuttering. Medications, however, are not always prescribed for symptoms that they were labeled or designed to treat. Specifically, physicians have and will prescribe a medication to treat a symptom, complaint, or condition in a manner *not* specified in the FDA's insert (i.e., approved packaging label required for each prescription drug marketed in the United States, i.e., "off-label"). Indeed, this is a prescription procedure that also occurs for stuttering.

Historically, pharmacotherapy for the treatment of stuttering as a symptom or as a condition has been conducted without specific FDA indications. Many helpful overviews exist on this topic of medications for stuttering.[3,5,35,38,39,40,41] For example, Brady reviewed 102 papers (1940s to 1990) and concluded that the pharmacological agents administered to AWS span a wide spectrum, including, for example, carbon dioxide, beta blockers (e.g., propranolol), calcium channel blockers (e.g., verapamil), stimulants (e.g., methylphenidate), sedatives (e.g., benzodiazepines), tranquilizers (e.g., meprobamate), and neuroleptics/antipsychotics (e.g., haloperidol).[35] For example, in one case study, propranolol was reported to decrease stuttering by 50% from baseline.[42] In another case study, propranolol nearly completely eliminated stuttering in a male adolescent patient who reported a late onset of stuttering at age 10 years.[43] In his 1991 narrative review of pharmacological treatments for stuttering in adults, Brady predicted that calcium channel blocking agents and cholinergic medications (i.e., those inhibiting, facilitating, enhancing or mirroring the action of acetylcholine) would show promise,[34] but no recent investigations have yet supported or refuted this possibility. Calcium channel blockers, such as verapamil, have been shown in at least a couple studies to demonstrate only limited efficacy in treating stuttering.[44,45]

The remainder of the chapter will refer to many different medications and drug classes. To help readers locate, in one place, the various brand names of these medications as well as the intended and unintended effects of each, we have included ▶ Table 15.5, which provides an alphabetized list and an explanation of each medication included in this chapter.

Beyond the challenge of the heterogeneity of stuttering, there are specific challenges involved in analyzing and synthesizing the stuttering pharmacotherapy literature to date. The first challenge is that when case studies naming a medication or recreational drug (e.g., "severe stuttering and motor tics responsive to cocaine")[46] are reported to show serendipitous fluency-exacerbating or fluency-enhancing effects,[47] researchers would not ethically/legally try them out with AWS. As another example, the antidepressant fluoxetine (Prozac) was reported to enhance fluency in at least one case of an AWS.[48] Such findings may encourage physicians to prescribe fluoxetine to a patient with stuttering to see if the drug has a similar effect on their stuttering, but presumably would do so if the patient also presented with depression.

We might learn that a certain medication improves, worsens, or even brings on an incident of stuttering based on its incidental effects. For example, anticholinergic medications (i.e., medications that block the actions of the neurotransmitter acetylcholine), such as tricyclic antidepressants, have been found to cause some people to begin stuttering.[35] Observing these findings, a clinician might reason that the opposite, cholinergic medications (i.e., those that enhance the actions of acetylcholine) would alleviate stuttering, but such reasoning could be fallacious. Another specific challenge is that there is no standard outcome measure for stuttering frequency across medication studies. Some employ outcomes such as %SS (i.e., stuttering frequency), whereas other studies report only such measures as time speaking fluently, which aims at the same construct as stutter frequency, but also includes stutter duration in the same measure. The present authors suggest that the best way to tackle these challenges is to engage in safe, scientific, scope of practice viewpoints. Historical perspectives provide us with a variety of "lessons learned" regarding pharmacological considerations for AWS.

Since about the mid-1990s, as alluded to earlier, there is increasing evidence for an association between basal ganglia activity and stuttering. Speculations on the association between basal ganglia and stuttering are based on findings from studies of brain lesions, neurodevelopment, and fluency-enhancing conditions (e.g., Delayed Auditory Feedback, appropriate for those with severe stuttering during reading tasks[49]).[10,50,51,52] By the onset of the 21st century, some were surmising a hyperdopaminergic condition in individuals who stutter. At present, the only effective way to reduce dopamine activity is through blocking the dopamine receptors via the MOA of a given medication. Such blocking of dopamine receptors is accomplished by employing a medication with low to no side effects or adverse reactions. The hypothesis taking shape by around the year 2004 was that D2 antagonist medications enhance or facilitate fluency because they compensate for excessive dopamine in individuals who stutter.[17,19,20,34,40]

Prior to 1990, before researchers investigated the dopamine hypothesis, most research studies reported on first-generation medications, such as dopamine antagonists (i.e., neuroleptics; typical antipsychotics, e.g., haloperidol) as the primary fluency-enhancing medications. Unfortunately, these first-generation, dopamine antagonistic medications that block dopamine are potentially associated with a variety of adverse effects, such as sexual dysfunction, dysphoria, extrapyramidal symptoms, and tardive dyskinesia. These adverse side effects obviously act to decrease patient/client tolerability and long-term adherence.[53,54,55,56]

In 1995, Gordon et al published results about the use of clomipramine, a medication that works, in part, by blocking the reuptake of serotonin in the neuronal synapse. They found that clomipramine had a fluency-enhancing effect in adults who stuttered.[57] Gordon et al's findings suggest that, in addition to dopamine antagonists, there might have been a therapeutic role for serotonin-related or serotonergic medications.[57,58] During this same time period, sertraline (Zoloft), which is classified as a selective serotonin reuptake inhibitor (SSRI), was found to both alleviate[59] and induce[60] stuttering symptoms.

A decade later in 2005, Stager and her colleagues examined two medications: (1) pimozide, a first-generation dopamine

Table 15.5 A listing of substances/medications referred to at least once in the present chapter. For each of these listed substances/medications, we provide corresponding brand names, medication category, and if prescribed (i.e., not recreational), we give the primary indications, presumed mechanisms of action, and adverse drug reactions

Medication/substance	Brand name	Medication category	Primary indications	Off-label uses	Mechanisms of action (MOA)	Other effects, side effects, and ADRs
Alcohol (ethanol)	Many names: beer, wine, distilled spirits (liquor)	Depressant/psychoactive	ND; the oldest and most common recreational substance	N/A, but alcohol use is a risk factor for other pharmacological considerations	GABA is increased; glutamate, glycine, acetylcholine, and serotonin affected	Mood lift; euphoria; decreased anxiety; increased sociability; sedation; cog/memory/motor/sensory impairment; generalized depression of CNS
Apomorphine	Uprima	Antiparkinsonism; emetic	Parkinson's disease	DSx: minimal data; Alcoholism; Heroin addiction	D2 partial agonist; serotonin antagonist	Movement disorders; nausea; depression; risk-taking behaviors; psychosis
Aripiprazole[a]	Abilify	2nd-generation atypical antipsychotic	Schizophrenia, bipolar disorder	DSx; Depression; Irritability in children; Tourette's syndrome	Engages at the dopamine receptor (D2); partial agonist of the serotonin 5-HT1A receptor	>ASx; ESx; >Dizziness, insomnia, akathisia, activation, nausea, vomiting, weight gain, sedation
Asenapine[a]	Saphris	2nd-generation atypical antipsychotic	Schizophrenia, mania in bipolar disorder	>DSx: 60–75% improvement on CGI; Depression	Partial agonist at serotonin (5-HT1A) receptors; all other targets, an antagonist	Less weight gain than other atypical antipsychotics; sedation, dizziness, extrapyramidal symptoms, akathisia, dizziness
Baclofen	Lioresal	Muscle relaxant	Muscle spasticity (e.g., spinal cord injury)	>IDS; Alcohol dependence	GABA-B receptor agonist	Drowsiness, dizziness, weakness, fatigue, headache, nausea/vomiting, urinary retention or constipation
Cannabis	Marijuana THC/CBD	Recreational and medicinal	Nausea from chemotherapy seizure disorders	Tourette's syndrome	THC indirectly increases dopamine release by activating cannabinoid receptor	Short- vs. long-term/chronic use effects; perceptual/memory effects (e.g., time perception); relaxation; increased appetite
Carbidopa-levodopa	Sinemet	Antiparkinsonism	Parkinson's disease	ND	Converts to dopamine due to decarboxylase	>ESx; ASx; Movement disorders; nausea; depression; risk-taking behaviors; psychosis
Chlorpromazine	Thorazine	1st-generation typical antipsychotic	Schizophrenia, bipolar disorder, ADHD behavioral problems	Chronic hiccups	Antiserotonergic; antihistaminic	>ASx, movement problems, sleepiness, dry mouth, low blood pressure upon standing, weight gain, tardive dyskinesia
Clomipramine	Anafranil	Tricyclic antidepressant	OCD, panic disorder, major depressive disorder, and chronic pain	>DSx: minimal data	Reuptake inhibitor of serotonin and norepinephrine	dry mouth, constipation, loss of appetite, sleepiness, weight gain, sexual dysfunction, and trouble urinating
Clonidine	Catapres	Hypotensive agent	High blood pressure, ADHD, addiction/drug withdrawal	>DSx: minimal data	Alpha-2A adrenergic receptor agonist; inhibitory via preventing secretion of norepinephrine	dry mouth, dizziness, headaches, and sleepiness
Clozapine	Clozaril	2nd-generation atypical antipsychotic	Schizophrenia symptoms w/o improvement	ND	Binds to serotonin and dopamine receptors; serotonin antagonist	>ASx; >many side effects that span from lowered white blood cell count to cardiac toxicity
Cocaine	Coke; "pinch of coca leaves" in original 1886 Coca-Cola recipe	Recreational stimulant	ND	>IDSs; Occasional medical needs for numbing	Inhibits reuptake of serotonin, norepinephrine, and dopamine; high concentrations of all three neurotransmitters	Perceptual changes; agitation or intense emotions; fast heart rate, sweating, and large pupils; high blood pressure or body temperature

Table 15.5 (Continued) A listing of substances/medications referred to at least once in the present chapter. For each of these listed substances/medications, we provide corresponding brand names, medication category, and if prescribed (i.e., not recreational), we give the primary indications, presumed mechanisms of action, and adverse drug reactions

Medication/substance	Brand name	Medication category	Primary indications	Off-label uses	Mechanisms of action (MOA)	Other effects, side effects, and ADRs
Dextroamphetamine sulfate, dextroamphetamine saccharate, etc.	Adderall	Stimulant	ADHD, narcolepsy	ND	Increases activity of dopamine and norepinephrine	>ESx Physical and psychological effects
Deutetrabenazine	Austedo	Vesicular mono-amine transporter 2 (VMAT2) inhibitor	Chorea associated with Huntington's disease and tardive dyskinesia	ND	An isotopic isomer of tetrabenazine in which six hydrogen atoms have been replaced by deuterium atoms; slows metabolism for less frequent dosing	ND
Ecopipam	SCH-39166	Benzazepine derivative	Schizophrenia	>DSx Tourette's syndrome, pathological gambling	Selective dopamine D1/D5 receptor antagonist	Mild sedation; restlessness; anxiety
Fluoxetine	Prozac	Antidepressant (SSRI)	Depression, OCD, bulimia	ND	Inhibits serotonin reuptake in the synapse; metabolites of fluoxetine also act as serotonin reuptake inhibitors	>AS indigestion, trouble sleeping, sexual dysfunction, loss of appetite, dry mouth, rash, and abnormal dreams
Haloperidol	Haldol	1st-generation typical antipsychotic	Schizophrenia, tics in Tourette's syndrome, bipolar disorder	>DSx; >agitation; acute psychosis; hallucinations (alcohol withdrawal)	High-affinity dopamine D2 receptor antagonism	Significant extrapyramidal symptoms
Lithium (salts)	Many names; in lemon-lime soda that would later become 7-Up (1929)	1st-generation typical antipsychotic	Bipolar; major depressive disorder that does not respond to antidepressants	Alzheimer's disease (to slow progression)	Unknown MOA; interacts with many receptors, decreasing norepinephrine release; increasing serotonin synthesis	>EDSx; ASx Increased urination, shakiness of the hands, and increased thirst
Lurasidone[a]	Latuda	2nd-generation atypical antipsychotic	Schizophrenia, bipolar disorder, depression	>DSx Behavioral disturbances in children and adolescents	Antagonist of D2 and D3 receptors and many of the serotonin receptors (not 5-HT2C receptor)	Sedation, weight gain, akathisia
Meprobamate	Equanil	Anxiolytics; antianxiety	Short-term relief of anxiety; similar to valium "Mother's little helper" (Rolling Stones, 1966)	ND	Binds to GABA-A receptors, unknown of MOA	>ASx Drowsiness, headache, sluggishness, unresponsiveness, or coma
Methylphenidate	Ritalin	Stimulant	ADHD, narcolepsy	ND	Blocking dopamine and norepinephrine reuptake	Sleep problems; decreased appetite; anxiety; weight loss
Olanzapine[a]	Zyprexa	2nd-generation atypical antipsychotic. Antidepressant	Schizophrenia, bipolar disorder, treatment-resistant depression, acute agitation associated with schizophrenia	ND	Higher affinity for 5-HT2A serotonin receptors than D2 dopamine receptors	>ASx Weight gain, movement disorders, dizziness, feeling tired, constipation, and dry mouth. Paradoxical and metabolic effects
Pagoclone	Pagoclone	Novel anxiolytic	Panic and anxiety	>DSx: 19% reduction from baseline of %SS in placebo and 40%↓ open label	GABA-A selective receptor modulator; partial agonist	Headache; sedation
Paroxetine	Paxil	Antidepressant (SSRI)	Depression, OCD, PTSD, panic disorders; anxiety disorders	>DSx Premature ejaculation; hot flashes	Selective serotonin (5-HTP) reuptake inhibit; binds to serotonin transporter; inhibits norepinephrine reuptake	Drowsiness, dry mouth, loss of appetite, sweating, trouble sleeping, and sexual dysfunction
Phenothiazine	Agrazine	See derivative chlorpromazine				

Table 15.5 (Continued) A listing of substances/medications referred to at least once in the present chapter. For each of these listed substances/medications, we provide corresponding brand names, medication category, and if prescribed (i.e., not recreational), we give the primary indications, presumed mechanisms of action, and adverse drug reactions

Medication/substance	Brand name	Medication category	Primary indications	Off-label uses	Mechanisms of action (MOA)	Other effects, side effects, and ADRs
Pimozide	Orap	1st-generation/typical antipsychotic	Tourette's syndrome and resistant tics	>IDSx	Antagonist of the D2, D3, and D4 receptors and the 5-HT7 receptor. High affinity for the D2 receptor	Akathisia, tardive dyskinesia, and, more rarely, neuroleptic malignant syndrome
Propranolol	Abilify	2nd-generation/atypical antipsychotic	Schizophrenia, bipolar disorder	>DSx; >autism-related irritability; >depression; >tic disorders	D2 partial agonist; serotonin antagonist	>ASx Movement disorders; tardive dyskinesia; restlessness; nausea
Quetiapine[a]	Seroquel	2nd-generation/atypical antipsychotic	Schizophrenia; bipolar disorder	>DSx	Norepinephrine activity	Weight gain; sedation; dizziness
Risperidone	Risperdal	2nd-generation/atypical antipsychotic	Schizophrenia, bipolar disorder, autism-related irritability in children	>DSx Behavioral disturbances in children, adolescents, and dementias	More pronounced serotonin than dopamine antagonism; antagonist of D1 and D5; antagonist of D2 family (D2, D3, and D4) receptors	Weight gain (common), sedation (common), prolactinemia, dose-dependent EPS, dizziness, insomnia, and anxiety. May increase risk of diabetes and hyperlipidemia
Sertraline	Zoloft	Antidepressant (SSRI)	Depression; OCD; PTSD; premenstrual dysphoria; social anxiety disorder	ND	SSRI with a high affinity for the dopamine transporter	>ASx Digestion; sexual dysfunction; troubles with sleep; risk of suicide; antidepressant discontinuation syndrome
Theophylline (1, 3-dimethylxanthine)	Many names	Bronchodilator; methylxanthin; found in tea and cocoa; like caffeine	Respiratory diseases: chronic obstructive pulmonary disease (COPD) and asthma	ND	Nonselective adenosine receptor antagonist; A1, A2, and A3 receptors equally	>ASx Nausea, diarrhea, increase in heart rate, abnormal heart rhythms, and CNS excitation
Valbenazine	Ingrezza	Vesicular monoamine transporter 2 (VMAT2) inhibitor	Tardive dyskinesia	>DSx Tourette's syndrome	Causes reversible reduction of dopamine release by selectively inhibiting presynaptic VMAT2	Sleepiness; tachycardia
Venlafaxine	Effexor	Antidepressant-SNRI	Depression; anxiety; panic disorder; social phobia	ND	Blocking transporter "reuptake" proteins for serotonin and norepinephrine	>ASx Loss of appetite, constipation, dry mouth, dizziness, sweating, and sexual problems
Verapamil	Calan	Calcium channel blocker	High blood pressure, angina	>DSx: minimal data Migraines	Blocks voltage-dependent calcium channels	Low blood pressure, nausea; constipation
Ziprasidone	Geodon	2nd-generation/atypical antipsychotic	Schizophrenia, bipolar disorder	>DSx; 38% decrease in SSI score from baseline	Affects D2 receptors, serotonin, and epinephrine/norepinephrine to a high degree, unsure of MOA	Dizziness, drowsiness, dry mouth, twitches

Abbreviations: ADHD, attention deficit hyperactivity disorder; ADRs, adverse drug reactions; ADS, adverse drug reactions; ASx, acquired stuttering; CBD, cannabidiol; CGI, clinical global impressions; CNS, central nervous system; DSx, decrease in stuttering; ESx, exacerbated stuttering; GABA, gamma-aminobutyric acid; IDSx, incidental decrease in stuttering (i.e., was not predicted, but found); ND, no data; OCD, obsessive compulsive disorder; PTSD, posttraumatic stress disorder; SNRI, serotonin–norepinephrine reuptake inhibitor; SSRI, selective serotonin reuptake inhibitor; Sx, stuttering; THC, tetrahydrocannabinol.

Note: ASx, DSx, ESx, and IDSx are marked with a >. Only one or several example brand names are given. Recreational substances are italicized.

Primary indications: Disorders for which the Food and Drug Administration (FDA) has approved the medication to treat, a designation that is based on the availability of specific empirical data that demonstrate the medication's ability to reduce symptoms measurably and significantly when compared to placebo (sugar pill) or another substance.

Off-label: The use of a medication in treating a disease for which it does not hold FDA approval, but for which there may be evidence of efficacy that does not meet the particular requirements of the FDA (>designates uses for DSx vs. other off-label uses).

Mechanisms of action (MOA): The ways a substance works on a molecular level to cause a specific outcome.

[a] Also included in ▶ Table 15.6.

blocker, similar to haloperidol (originally studied in 1997), and (2) paroxetine, an SSRI commonly used to treat depression and anxiety. Both pimozide and paroxetine had been shown to improve mood and anxiety, which Stager et al reasoned could be fluency enhancing.[61,62] These researchers investigated the effects of medications on the speech-related anxiety of 11 AWS as well as the associations between anxiety and fluency changes. Several important findings and interpretations emerged from this study. First, pimozide was associated with significantly more time speaking fluently on the telephone and significantly shorter average stutter duration compared to baseline. However, generalized and speech-related anxiety did not differ from baseline. Half (3/6) of the participants experienced depression and one-third (2/6) experienced "mood alteration." As many as 16 other types of side effects were reported by the participants taking pimozide (e.g., prolactin elevation or "prolactinemia" and cardiac conduction abnormalities). For the five AWS who were administered paroxetine throughout the study, there was no significant fluency improvement observed, and withdrawal from paroxetine was associated with severe side effects (e.g., increased anxiety, nausea, blurred vision).[62]

Given the fact that paroxetine is like clomipramine in that both inhibit the reuptake of serotonin, it was remarkable that fluency effects differed: clomipramine was fluency-enhancing in previous studies,[57,58] but paroxetine was not, in the Stager et al study. Stager and colleagues reasoned that this difference was because clomipramine is less selective of a serotonin reuptake inhibitor than is paroxetine, and clomipramine affects dopamine metabolism more so than it blocks serotonin reuptake. Based on their findings, Stager et al concluded that dopaminergic mechanisms are more important than serotonergic mechanisms to explain changes in dysfluency in adults with persistent developmental stuttering.[62]

ADRs, known to most laypersons as "side effects," are a key concern when initiating pharmacotherapy in AWS, or for any human condition, for that matter, and for good reason. For example, in 1997, Bloch et al found that four out of seven (57%) men who stuttered and who adhered to prescribed pimozide began to develop what the authors termed "marked depressive symptoms." Although these researchers reported no association between these ADRs and the specific dose of pimozide, ADRs resolved when pimozide was discontinued.[61]

Prior to the 1990s, so-called first-generation medications were mainly used to treat hallucinations and delusions in schizophrenia (i.e., antipsychotics, e.g., haloperidol). In the 1990s to early 2000s, newer medications emerged, labeled as second-generation medications. These second-generation medications showed promise by having fewer extrapyramidal ADRs (e.g., tremor, parkinsonism) in the individuals for whom they are prescribed. In addition to blocking dopamine receptors, these second-generation antipsychotics also blocked serotonin receptors. Risperidone and olanzapine were the two main second-generation medications, both of which appeared to be fluency-enhancing in AWS[20,40,63,64] as well as in children who stutter.[65] In order to understand this set of studies of second-generation medications, we underscore the importance of dosage amounts, in what exact milligram (mg) dosage. Participants who stutter in some studies exhibited what could be considered paradoxical effects (i.e., risperidone-induced stuttering when risperidone is intended to treat stuttering), and dosages exceeding 4 mg could be responsible.[66,67]

Maguire and associates in 1999 to 2000 were the first to publish data about risperidone's effect on stuttering. They conducted a randomized, double-blind, placebo-controlled study on the efficacy of risperidone in 16 AWS. Eight participants received placebo, and eight received risperidone (0.5 mg once daily at night, gradually increased to 2 mg/d). Findings indicated significant reductions in stuttering frequency from baseline (i.e., 50% decrease) for the risperidone group (n = 8) compared to the placebo group (n = 8). Given what we know about the importance of the dosage administered, it is noteworthy that five participants responded best to only 0.5 mg of risperidone per day. Notably, stuttering recurred when doses were increased to 2 mg for these five participants. The remaining three participants spoke most fluently at 2-mg doses.[63,64]

Although the focus in this chapter is on adults, a child case study illustrates the beneficial effects of proper dosage of risperidone. The case was a 4-year-old boy with a familial history of bipolar disorder. He presented with severe aggressive behaviors (i.e., temper tantrums, biting, kicking) that did not resolve with behavioral treatment. The boy also stuttered severely, so his doctor administered 0.25 mg of risperidone. One week later, the boy reportedly returned with improved behavior and complete remission of the stuttering. His physician further reported that discontinuing by tapering off the risperidone led to a return of the boy's stuttering, although not to the severity documented prior to treatment.[68] Although it is possible that changing nonspeech behaviors (e.g., aggressive behaviors, in this case study) led to improvement in the child's speech fluency, finding that it was a rapid change suggests that the dopamine blocker medication was responsible. In summary, several studies have shown the fluency facilitation effects of risperidone in individuals who stutter.[68,69,70]

Olanzapine, also a second-generation dopamine blocker, has been effective in reducing symptoms of stuttering. Support for olanzapine's efficacy are based on findings from both individual/case and group studies. We provide one example of each here. In an older case study of a 37-year-old veteran with psychosis and stuttering associated with postconcussive syndrome, this man's stuttering showed noticeable improvement after initiation of olanzapine.[71] An example of a group study took place in 2004 when Maguire and associates studied 23 AWS who completed a 12-week, randomized, double-blind, placebo-controlled trial conducted at two separate sites. Participants received either placebo or olanzapine (2.5 mg titrated to 5 mg) and they were closely monitored for ADRs. Stuttering severity and associated socio-emotional and cognitive symptoms were significantly improved as compared to placebo on doses between 2.5 and 5 mg, but an average of 5 kg in weight gain was observed. It should be noted that olanzapine has both a different tolerability profile and a different ADR profile than risperidone. More recently in 2013, a team of researchers in Tehran, Shaygannejad and associates, published a randomized control trial (single-blind) comparing the effects of olanzapine to haloperidol in 93 individuals who stutter, between 10 and 50 years of age. They found that olanzapine, when compared to haloperidol (i.e., a first-generation medication), was associated with a significantly greater reduction in stuttering score from baseline. These researchers expressed caution that olanzapine could worsen stuttering in patients who are on antidepressants or who have preexisting brain pathology. Regarding ADRs, they also noted that olanzapine is associated with weight gain, but that sedation effects are lower than with haloperidol.[72]

Ziprasidone, asenapine, aripiprazole, and lurasidone are examples of alternative second-generation dopamine *antagonist* medications with seemingly more tolerable ADR profiles than olanzapine.[73,74,75,76] A recent case report demonstrated that ziprasidone may be an effective, well-tolerated medication for treating stuttering.[73] Asenapine, a newer dopamine antagonist medication, has been reported to be less associated with significant weight gain and metabolic side effects. Furthermore, in a limited open-label trial study, three participants who were administered asenapine demonstrated improved fluency when on a well-tolerated dose.[74] Aripiprazole is another unique medication that acts as a partial D2 agonist, acts on certain serotonin receptors, and is FDA approved for TS in children and adults. There are published case reports of aripiprazole demonstrating its safety and efficacy in treating stuttering[75,77,78] including, again, in efficacious dosages.[79] However, the potential side effect of akathisia (i.e., a state of restlessness and agitation) limits its tolerability.[78] Lurasidone is another newer dopamine antagonist that, in a small open-label study in individuals with stuttering, showed improvement in reported stuttering symptoms.[76,80]

In general, the tolerability of second-generation dopamine blockers varies among individuals. A reasonable approach would be for a physician to prescribe lurasidone or aripiprazole as first-line medications in order to minimize the risks of weight gain and metabolic abnormalities. Based on findings of peer-reviewed studies as well as the authors' experience, ▶ Table 15.6 presents the top six choices for a psychiatrist or physician to consider when deciding about second-generation dopamine antagonist medications for a patient who stutters. In our determination of such choices, we have given careful consideration to each medication's primary indications and ranked each ADR from minimal to significant. Other considerations in ▶ Table 15.6 involve the relative strength of efficacy, also ranked from minimal to clinically significant.

Another line of research regarding dopamine-blocking medications for stuttering involves ecopipam. Ecopipam blocks dopamine D1 receptors and thus has a lowered risk of extrapyramidal symptoms than do medications that block D2 receptors. Furthermore, ecopipam is not associated with weight gain, a common consequence of olanzapine and other second-generation dopamine antagonists. Maguire and associates in 2019 published preliminary findings of a phase I, open-label experimental study of ecopipam, suggesting the need for a future double-blind and randomized control clinical trials (i.e., phase II–type studies).[82] In this phase I study, five men with moderate to very severe stuttering participated. They were administered an initial dose of 50 mg of ecopipam daily at bedtime. If this dose was well tolerated and there was no reported improvement in their symptoms of stuttering, it was increased to 100 mg. If there was reported difficulty tolerating

Table 15.6 A listing of *second-generation* dopamine antagonist medications with evidence in treating stuttering. For each medication are listed the relative strength of efficacy of drugs (RSED), primary indications, potential advantages, and potential adverse drug reactions (ADRs) or side effects

Name	RSED	Primary indications	Potential advantages	Potential ADRs/side effects
Aripiprazole (Abilify)	+ +	Schizophrenia, bipolar disorder, depression, autism-related irritability in children, Tourette's syndrome in children	Lower risk of weight gain and sedation compared to other meds, comparatively safer in diabetes and *dyslipidemia*. Serotonergic activity may help co-occurring anxiety and depression symptoms	Weight gain + sedation + akathisia + + + dizziness, insomnia, nausea, vomiting
Asenapine (Saphris)	+ +	Schizophrenia, mania in bipolar disorder	Mild to moderate risk of weight gain compared to other meds. May have some antidepressant actions	Weight gain + sedation + + akathisia + Extrapyramidal symptoms (EPS), dizziness
Lurasidone (Latuda)	+ +	Schizophrenia, bipolar depression, behavioral disturbances in children and adolescents (off-label)	Less weight gain compared to other meds, lower risk of prolactinemia compared to risperidone. May enhance serotonin levels, which may help co-occurring depressive symptoms	Weight gain + sedation + + akathisia +
Olanzapine (Zyprexa)	+ + +	Schizophrenia, bipolar disorder, treatment-resistant depression, acute agitation associated with schizophrenia	Although metabolic side effects may be significant, it is otherwise well tolerated. May enhance treatment of co-occurring depressive symptoms	Weight gain + + + sedation + + dizziness Dry mouth
Quetiapine (Seroquel)	+ +	Schizophrenia, bipolar disorder, depression, behavioral disturbances in children/adolescents (off-label), behavioral disturbances in Parkinson's disease (off-label)	No motor side effects or prolactinemia. Active metabolite has norepinephrine activity, which may help improve depressive symptoms Some evidence of improving anxiety and insomnia associated with mood disturbances	Weight gain + + sedation + + + dizziness
Risperidone (Risperdal)	+ + +	Schizophrenia, bipolar disorder, autism-related irritability in children, behavioral disturbances in children, adolescents, and dementias (off-label)	Less sedation and weight gain than some other medications (olanzapine)	Weight gain + + sedation + + hyper-prolactinemia Dose-dependent EPS, dizziness, insomnia, anxiety. May increase risk of diabetes and hyperlipidemia

Note: +, + +, and + + + indicate minimal, moderate, and significant strength of efficacy, respectively.

100 mg of ecopipam, the dosage was reduced to 50 mg per day. At 4 weeks and at 8 weeks post-baseline, stuttering and ecopipam tolerability was assessed, and no ADRs were of concern.

Most germane to the present discussion, ecopipam was associated with a significant reduction in stuttering frequency in %SS. Participants with moderate stuttering made significant fluency gains in reading and spontaneous speech; however, those with very severe stuttering at baseline exhibited smaller reductions, that is, a more modest 4- to 8-point reductions in the Stuttering Severity Instrument, Fourth Edition scores. Findings indicated that ecopipam, compared to baseline, was associated with the following changes: (1) reduced %SS in both reading and spontaneous speaking; (2) faster completion of oral reading; (3) reduced duration of instances of stuttering; (4) improved attitudes as per the use of the Overall Assessment of the Speaker's Experience of Stuttering.[81] Findings were taken to support the need for a larger sample, double-blind, randomized, controlled clinical trial to examine the efficacy of ecopipam in treating stuttering.[82,83,84]

15.6 The Effect of Medications Prescribed for Other Conditions on Stuttering

Given that many medical conditions are treated with pharmacotherapy, it is no surprise that individuals who stutter may be prescribed medications for conditions other than stuttering. In some cases, the condition for which an individual is medicated is a condition unrelated to stuttering. In other cases, medications may be prescribed for conditions that more commonly co-occur with stuttering and are more related to overall communication and educational progress, such as attention deficit hyperactivity disorder (ADHD). When we assess clients/patients known to stutter or suspected to be stuttering, we ask them to report medication(s) that they take and the dosages per day. This helps determine whether medications known to be associated with the onset or exacerbation of stuttering symptoms (i.e., iatrogenic) are part of the individual's diagnostic profile. Conversely, as we have reviewed earlier, medications could also be associated with amelioration of stuttering symptoms. Stuttering symptom amelioration could either be planned by the client's/patient's health caregiver/provider or could occur in a serendipitous manner.

The conditions discussed in this section that appear to have some medication relationship to stuttering are as follows: (1) schizophrenia, bipolar, anxiety, and major depressive disorder; (2) TS; (3) ADHD; and (4) infections (e.g., strep). In 2015, Lustig and Ruiz published guidelines for SLPs on drug-induced movement disorders (DIMDs) including cautions about medications prescribed for various conditions.[85] Parkinsonism or extrapyramidal symptoms are a potential iatrogenic result of certain neuroleptic or antipsychotic medications, an important topic that we turn to next.

15.6.1 Parkinsonism versus Parkinson's Disease and "Stuttering"

Earlier in the chapter, we explained how dopamine antagonists are often the medications of choice to help treat stuttering.

However, movement abnormalities (e.g., tremor, changes in tone, rate) are potential ADRs associated with the use of dopamine antagonists. DIMDs are characterized by a variety of symptoms (e.g., tremors, spasms, extrapyramidal symptoms). DIMDs are involuntary movements that may occur shortly after the medication is administered; may be delayed by weeks, months, or even years; and vary in severity (i.e., mild to severe). DIMDs are iatrogenic and take many forms, but can be categorized into two types:

- Extrapyramidal symptoms, which include akathisia (i.e., agitation, restlessness), dystonia (i.e., involuntary muscle contractions), and dyskinesia (i.e., difficulties with muscle movement). Likely, the ADR leading to acquired stuttering or even exacerbated developmental stuttering is an iatrogenic concern related to dyskinesia.
- Parkinsonianlike symptoms, which occur when there is no formal, previous diagnosis of PD but there is observation of delayed motor initiation, slow completion, gait shuffling/stooped posture, micrographia (i.e., tiny handwriting), muscle rigidity, and/or tremor. The drug-induced tremor is often less severe than that which occurs in PD. Also, the *intentional* tremor type (e.g., when the patient tries to point to something or lift a spoonful of food) is more often found in parkinsonism. In contrast, *resting* tremor type (e.g., when the patient's hand shakes when it is lying in their lap) is more often found in PD.[85]

Other DIMDs and/or related ADRs associated with parkinsonism include excessive fatigue, difficulty multitasking, altered breathing patterns, bradykinesia (i.e., slowed facial movements), and tardive dyskinesia (i.e., involuntary body or facial movements such as rapid blinking or facial contortions). DIMDs occur more frequently in women than in men and have more of a sudden onset in parkinsonism, as opposed to gradual, progressive onset associated with actual PD. DIMDs can include any number of distinct types of speech disfluencies or prosodic disturbances.[86,87,88,89] If a patient presenting with drug-induced parkinsonism were to be put on levodopa for a presumed PD diagnosis, the parkinsonism/extrapyramidal symptoms are not likely to resolve. This result helps the medical professional infer that the parkinsonism is likely drug induced/DIMD.[85] Just as dopamine antagonists often alleviate stuttering symptoms, administering a dopamine agonist such as carbidopa–levodopa can worsen stuttering or increase speech disfluencies.[26,27]

15.6.2 Schizophrenia, Bipolar Disorder, Major Depressive Disorder, and Stuttering

Since 1954, neuroleptics (e.g., chlorpromazine) prescribed for symptoms of schizophrenia have been reported to induce extrapyramidal symptoms (e.g., tremor) as well as stuttering-like behaviors (e.g., physically tense sound repetitions).[90,91] For example, one report indicated that phenothiazine was prescribed for two schizophrenic patients (35- and 40-year-old men). An ADR reportedly followed from this administration of phenothiazine whereby both patients began to "stutter."[92] The brevity of many of the case studies makes it difficult to determine what the acquired stuttering symptoms would have sounded like when they first began. Findings from these types of case studies are relevant for SLPs because it helps them be aware that parkinsonism and extrapyramidal symptoms are the primary ADR of dopamine antagonists.[85,93,94]

Consistent with previously mentioned ADRs regarding drug-induced stuttering, there are at least two case study reports on the worsening of stuttering being associated with lithium.

Lithium is a substance used primarily to treat bipolar depression. Lithium is also used to treat a variety of other psychiatric illnesses, without specific FDA indications to do so. At present, lithium's MOA is not entirely known. It is presumed to function by displacing sodium and calcium ions. Such displacement affects neurotransmitters, and thus it may impact the dopaminergic as well as serotonergic, cholinergic, noradrenergic systems. Common side effects of lithium are lightheadedness and tremor.

One related case study reports on an adult male patient with developmental stuttering. This patient had previously been treated with fluoxetine (Prozac) for suspected depression, and he was later put on lithium for diagnosed bipolar disorder. When administered lithium, his stuttering became worse. When lithium was discontinued, his stuttering returned to his prior baseline level.[95]

Another case was reported of a 10-year-old boy with a history of developmental stuttering, bipolar disorder not otherwise specified (NOS), ADHD, and conduct disorder with recurrent suicidal ideations and increased physical aggression. He had been administered lithium 150 mg/d at bedtime for bipolar disorder, which was later increased to 900 mg twice daily. During the time of the 150 to 1,800 mg/d dose adjustment, the boy's stuttering worsened severely, but when the dose was reduced to a divided dose of 600 mg in the morning and 900 mg in the evening, his stuttering returned to baseline. The authors surmised that the worsening of his fluency was an ADR of lithium at higher doses. This 10-year-old patient was on stable doses of other medications (i.e., risperidone, clonidine), a peptic ulcer medication (famotidine) and the supplement melatonin, so it was unlikely that one of these contributed to his stuttering exacerbation.[96,97] Again, it is important with these case studies of co-occurring stuttering plus multiple medications for psychiatric conditions for the clinician to know details about the other medications prescribed and adhered to and, of course, to know about the client's exacerbation of stuttering. Such knowledge helps medical professionals attempt to reverse such concerns (e.g., exacerbation of stuttering). For cases like this 10-year-old boy, SLPs are an integral part of the team to help describe the stuttering onset, its progression, and severity.

15.6.3 Anxiety Disorders and Stuttering

Individuals who stutter could be treated for a co-occurring social anxiety disorder, or a generalized anxiety disorder. Joseph LeDoux, a well-respected researcher on the topic of emotion, claims that fear is a state of awareness of being in harm's way, whereas anxiety is an emotion or worry involving the possibility that threat(s) will cause harm. LeDoux contributed to the decision made by the Diagnostic Statistical Manual, Fifth edition (DSM-5) committee to retract and reorganize certain categories related to anxiety disorders. Now there is a "fear and anxiety disorder" category in the DSM-5 including Generalized Anxiety Disorders (i.e., maladaptive feelings about future threats), Panic Disorders (i.e., including panic attacks; somatic), and Posttraumatic Stress Disorder (PTSD). LeDoux considers fear and anxiety disorders to be the most prevalent psychiatric disorder in the United States, affecting as many as one-fifth of Americans, and with a diagnosis 20 times more frequently occurring than schizophrenia. Complicating this picture of fear and anxiety disorders is that it can co-occur (i.e., be comorbid) with other disorders in the DSM-5 such as major depressive disorder.[98]

Social anxiety has been investigated as it relates to persistent developmental stuttering. For example, Blumgart et al introduced a study by explaining that social anxiety may be considered primary (i.e., existing without particular social impetus) or secondary (i.e., developing because of stuttering experiences). AWS, when compared to AWNS, have been reported to exhibit significantly higher prevalence of social phobia (i.e., 50/200 or 25% of AWS in their study identified with social phobia). Although one cannot rule out the possibility that stuttering contributes to social phobia, these researchers cautioned that health care professionals need to treat social phobia in AWS, whether it is primary or secondary.[99]

Prevailing pharmacotherapy for anxiety and depression include the use of SSRIs (e.g., fluoxetine) and serotonin-norepinephrine reuptake inhibitors (SNRIs, e.g., venlafaxine). These SSRI and SNRI drugs work by blocking the proteins that are responsible for gathering leftover serotonin and norepinephrine, respectively.

Medications, of course, are just one element of the treatment for anxiety. Counseling or talk therapy is another critical element in the treatment of anxiety.[98] Meditation is another.[100] For about one out of five individuals who stutter who seek out medications,[6] medications can be effective in reducing anxiety/social phobia symptoms coinciding with or coming from chronic stuttering. Of course, following scope of practice guidelines, only a physician can prescribe and change dosage of medications. The professionals whose scope of practice it is to treat primary social anxiety, such as psychiatrists, psychologists, and clinical social workers, would perhaps recommend talk therapy and medication. We concur with authors who assert that we achieve the best outcomes of speech treatment when a co-occurring primary disorder of social anxiety is also treated.[99]

Iverach and colleagues investigated the relationship between mental disorders and stuttering treatment outcomes. These researchers reported that the only subgroup of adult participants who maintained stuttering treatment benefits for 6 months was comprised of the participants *without* a mental disorder. Most importantly, Iverach et al reported that the presence of anxiety disorders was associated with situational avoidance following treatment.[101]

These findings suggest that the high rate of relapse often found for AWS may be, in part, due to the presence of anxiety or other disorders. Specifically, such disorders may be associated with avoidance of speech practice and social encounters that may, in turn, contribute to reduced maintenance of the gains made initially in speech treatment.[101] Iverach et al's findings exemplify how stuttering and co-occurring disorders interact across time. These interactions require the development of a treatment plan and the services of an interprofessional practice team that fits this trajectory. Such a team and an associated dynamic treatment plan might involve stuttering modification/fluency-shaping approach counseling and/or medication management to achieve the best outcome for the client/patient.

What might help treat social anxiety disorder may not lead to a decrease in stuttering. Antianxiety GABA receptor agents or anxiolytics, such as benzodiazepines and barbiturates, have been investigated with the idea that by reducing co-occurring anxiety, they might alleviate stuttering. Although these anxiolytics have been shown to reduce anxiety in the short term, they have not demonstrated an ability to improve speech fluency, nor do GABA receptor medications show any benefits over and above that of placebo.[35,102,103] Furthermore, there is evidence that anxiolytic agents may be associated, at least with certain dosages, with acquired, drug-induced stuttering. Researchers of veterans from the Iraq and Afghanistan wars performed careful work separating out the effects of PTSD and traumatic brain injury (TBI) from the effects of medications that they were prescribed. These researchers reported that anxiolytics were the most likely, and dopamine receptor blockers the least likely, to trigger acquired stuttering.[104]

15.6.4 Tourette's Syndrome and Stuttering

For reducing signs and symptoms of TS, clonidine is a medication that has some demonstrated efficacy. It has been hypothesized that clonidine may show similar efficacy in treating stuttering. However, findings from school-aged children who stutter in a study by Althaus and colleagues did not support this hypothesis. Specifically, these researchers reported a nonsignificant difference between clonidine and placebo in terms of their effects on objective measures of stuttering as well as subjective symptom ratings by parents and teachers.[105] These findings suggest that although TS and stuttering are similar conditions, it is not a simple matter of prescribing the same medication at the same dosage for both disorders and expecting significantly improved outcomes of, say, vocal tics and stuttering respectively. Also, further research of medications like clonidine in AWS rather than in children who stutter may be warranted.[105] Findings such as these suggests that although TS and stuttering are similar conditions, it is not a simple matter of prescribing the same medication at the same dosage for both disorders.

15.6.5 Attention Deficit Hyperactivity Disorder and Stuttering

Medications for ADHD fall into two categories, stimulants (e.g., mixed amphetamine salts–see dextroamphetamine sulfate or Adderall in ▶ Table 15.5) and nonstimulants (e.g., atomoxetine or Strattera). Only a scant literature on (non)stimulants and stuttering is available. One report suggested that stimulant medication may worsen stuttering symptoms. This was a case of a 10-year-old boy with stuttering, ADHD, and TS, wherein the boy demonstrated increased stuttering, tic behaviors, social anxiety, and communication-related frustration shortly after starting dextroamphetamine sulfate. This medication was then discontinued, and he was started on atomoxetine. Subsequently, he demonstrated a 63% reduction in disfluency rate and a 51% reduction in the proportion of speech behaviors typical of stuttering. Unfortunately, the change in medications was also associated with an increase in impulsivity and a decrease in attention and focusing in the academic setting. This case highlights the dilemma that often arises in treating co-occurring disorders.[106]

Beginning as early as 1996 when methylphenidate (Ritalin) was a common medication for ADHD, no significant differences were reported between an on- and off-methylphenidate conditions in the speech rate and overall speech fluency for individuals with ADHD who had no co-occurring developmental stuttering.[107] Finally, there is one anecdotal report of a preschooler who was treated for stuttering and speech sound disorder with behavioral concerns. The report indicated that the child "ceased to stutter after the right prescriptive match was found to treat his ADHD" (p.11)."[108] More research is sorely needed in regard to the comorbidity of ADHD and stuttering. Recent findings from Choi et al suggest that language skills are an important variable to consider with stuttering and ADHD genetic predisposition, as they found significantly lower language scores and positive family histories of ADHD in a normally fluent (control group) of children when a positive family history of stuttering was reported.[109]

15.6.6 Autoimmune Conditions and Stuttering

The onset of stuttering can result as an autoimmune condition triggered by an infection, as first reported in a 2010 case study. A 6-year-old boy with no family history of stuttering experienced a sudden onset of stuttering approximately 1 month after a documented streptococcal infection (i.e., "strep throat"). The medical team thought that stuttering symptoms could be a manifestation of *pediatric autoimmune neuropsychiatric disorder associated with streptococcal infections* (*PANDAS*), which is an uncommon, but important, sequelae of streptococcal infections in some children.

PANDAS is characterized by a waxing–waning course, with proposed involvement of the basal ganglia, and neuropsychiatric symptoms that often involve ticlike motions. At the time of diagnosis of PANDAS, the boy's parents declined antibiotics. Reportedly, the acute onset of sound and syllable repetitions and blocking was followed by facial grimaces and head twitches/ticlike behaviors 3 months later. According to the report, the boy continued to have a positive rapid *streptococcus* antigen test 5.5 months after initial diagnosis. Next, he was administered amoxicillin/clavulanic acid (800 mg/d for 10 days), and stuttering symptoms resolved within 2 weeks. At that time, streptococcal throat culture was negative, and the course of antibiotics was complete. The authors stated the possibility that in the process of combating the infection, a cross-reaction could occur between antibodies and antigens. The speculation the authors offered was that this cross-reaction interferes with the developing basal ganglia.[110,111] The postulation that PANDAS may be a cause for at least some forms of stuttering has now essentially been confirmed by recent research (Alm et al[112]), bringing forth the model to screen children at onset of stuttering for such a possible cause.

To conclude, from the above coverage of co-occurrence of conditions with stuttering, it appears that a key part of assessment of an individual known or suspected to stutter is to gather information on medications, dosage, and adherence. This information should help the SLP rule in or rule out ADRs including DIMDs and other medication effects. Equally important is the need to report to a medical provider stuttering onsets that occur suddenly with the onset/diagnosis of another condition and/or when medication is administered. Thus, knowing when to refer to (or consult with) a medical provider is an important skill for an SLP. Thus far, this section has been centered on *prescriptions* including antipsychotics (i.e., some causing DIMDs), antidepressants, antianxiety medications, as well as those for TS, ADHD, and even antibiotics. *Nonprescribed*, recreational drugs and self-medicating behaviors are also worthy of mention.

15.7 Recreational Drugs and Self-medicating Behaviors and Stuttering

Results of two large sample studies of AWS indicate that neither AWS from the community nor AWS on a waitlist to receive speech therapy exhibit greater substance-use disorders (e.g., alcohol use and abuse) than matched controls.[113,114] However, a paucity of literature exists on the potential effects of recreational substances (e.g., marijuana) on stuttering.[114] This is because so-called Schedule I drugs, such as cocaine and marijuana,[46,115] are difficult to study scientifically due to state/federal regulations. Thus, most reports of effects of recreational drugs on stuttering have so far come from case reports.

One example of such a case study involved a 16-year-old adolescent boy who presented with persistent developmental stuttering with a family history of stuttering, cannabis dependence, and a conduct disorder. Speech therapy was sought to help improve his overall communication skills, so that he could achieve healthier relationships. Abstinence from marijuana became the focus of the speech therapy approach. The authors reported that after the teen decreased his use of marijuana, but did not stop use completely, his normal and stuttered disfluencies were fewer. The authors noted that the client became more critical about and responsive to his own treatment, which appeared to motivate him to try longer periods of abstinence from marijuana usage.[115]

15.8 Future Directions in Pharmacological Options for Adults Who Stutter

By now, the reader might have correctly inferred the following. Although we know quite a lot about pharmacological options for AWS and related studies, there is far more we do not know. Many studies, including those cited here, have various interpretative as well as methodological flaws that we can improve upon, going forward.[39,116] Systematic reviews and letters to the editor exchanges often include controversies over the tolerability of medications and how much quality-of-life improvement could be expected from pharmacotherapy.[39,116,117,118] Furthermore, correlation between a medication and either increases or decreases in stuttering should not be assumed to infer a causal relation between the medication and stuttering. Certainly, the onset of a medication and the onset of stuttering or relative

fluency can be remarkable. However, an individual patient/client may be adhering to multiple medications and/or self-medicating, circumstances that may contribute to or indeed cause changes in speech fluency. In short, there are always other factors to be considered besides the more obvious ones. For example, therapy including antibiotic and anti-inflammatory treatments could be warranted for some patients who stutter. Discussions about medications and treatments require rapport and trust-building between clinicians and their clients or patients who stutter. Certainly, ASHA's (American Speech-Language-Hearing Association) guidelines for ethics, counseling, interprofessional practice, and scope of practice all apply to this important topic. The more we involve ourselves with understanding new classes of medications, the more these considerations (e.g., ethics, counseling) continue to be critically important.

We see several future directions as promising. The first is a class of relatively new medications, known as vesicular monoamine transporter 2 (VMAT2) inhibitors, such as valbenazine and deutetrabenazine. These medications work by decreasing the synthesis of dopamine through the inhibition of VMAT2. VMAT2 is a transport protein responsible for packaging dopamine into vesicles, from which dopamine is then released by neurons into the central nervous system. VMAT inhibitors have shown efficacy in treating TS, tardive dyskinesia, and abnormal movements associated with Huntington's disease.[82,83]

Research is now underway to determine whether these medications are safe and may assist in the treatment of stuttering. Of course, study of these medications would require the applications of all the ethical and legal guidelines stipulated by the Institutional Review Board for Human subjects as well as phases I to IV of randomized controlled trials previously mentioned. Second, perhaps there is value in further study of a protein known as homovanillic acid (HVA), which is necessary for dopamine metabolism to occur. Results of an early study hold promise for further understanding of the presence of HVA in preschool and school-age children who stutter.[119]

In terms of interprofessional practice, we as SLPs can offer valuable information to our colleagues and our clients who stutter about how, for example, TS is and is not similar to stuttering. We can offer AWS the information included in this chapter and help them better appreciate and understand the available information on medications and stuttering. Following the guidelines for SLP scope of practice established by the ASHA, the SLP needs to be careful, cautious, and circumspect when a client who stutters asks us about dosage or efficacy of a medication that he or she is already prescribed, or when we are asked about the appropriateness of particular medications for stuttering. Instead of directly responding to such client inquiries, the SLP must refer the client who stutters to colleagues in psychiatry, neurology, or other appropriate branches of the medical profession.

The authors of this chapter are an interprofessional team of an SLP, psychiatrist/person who stutters, and a psychiatry resident, and we have enjoyed sharing our knowledge bases. We believe that the ideal future direction for AWS might follow these steps:

1. Complete the research phases necessary to get a safe, tolerable, low/no ADR medication designed for AWS.

2. Complete the randomized control trials needed to improve the efficacy and efficiency of behavioral treatment, for example, of stuttering modification and fluency-shaping treatment approaches.

3. Where possible, appropriately blend (1) +(2) with any additional treatments needed if there are conditions co-occurring with stuttering (e.g., talk therapy/Cognitive Behavior Treatment/Acceptance Commitment Therapy for anxiety). Others concur with us that the best option for AWS is to combine behavioral treatments with pharmacotherapy, when warranted, in interprofessional practice.[7,38,41,104]

15.9 Conclusions

In closing, we would like to underscore the importance of the informed wishes of the client when considering pharmacological options: Has the client had self-help or support group experiences? How severe is the stuttering? What is the apparent impact of stuttering on the person's quality of life? Medications are one therapeutic path that we could recommend be accompanied by behavioral treatment and/or talk therapy, as our fields of study progress. We have presented here guiding principles so that clinicians can best help individuals who stutter when we consider pharmacological options and pharmacological effects.

15.10 Definitions

Adherence: Refers to taking medications correctly; whether a patient who is prescribed a medication gets the prescription filled, remembers to take the correct dosage of medication on time, while understanding and following any specific directions about the medication (e.g., take with food).

Adverse drug reactions (ADR): Also called side effects or adverse drug events (ADE); such effects are unwanted, unexpected, or dangerous responses to a drug. ADRs can be of a gradual or sudden onset.

Affinity: The extent to which, or strength with which, a **ligand** (**defined below**) binds to a receptor at any given concentration of that ligand.

Agonist: A substance that binds to a receptor to induce a chemical physiologic response.

Akathisia: A state of agitation, distress, and restlessness that is an occasional side effect of antipsychotic and antidepressant medications.

Antagonist: A substance that blocks a receptor, thereby preventing agonists from acting at the receptor; blocker medications.

Anticholinergic: That which blocks the action of acetylcholine in the central and peripheral nervous systems.

Antiemetic: A medication that prevents vomiting.

Anxiolytics: Substances that produce a reduction in anxiety.

Apomorphine: A medication that is a dopamine receptor agonist; can be used to treat advanced Parkinson's disease.

Barbiturates: Sedative and sleep-inducing medications; derivative of barbituric acid.

Basal ganglia: Basal nuclei, consisting of the corpus striatum (i.e., caudate nucleus and putamen) and global pallidus (▶ Table 15.3).

Benzodiazepines: Anxiolytic medications with addictive properties that work by acting as an agonist at the GABA-A receptor; Food and Drug Administration (FDA) indicated for treatment of panic attacks and alcohol withdrawal syndrome; nonbenzodiazepines are similar without the addictive properties, and are prescribed for anxiety and for sleep.

Blood–brain barrier (BBB): The means by which the central nervous system (CNS) is isolated from surrounding tissues. The inner layer of BBB involves a tightly sealed, continuous capillary endothelial cell layer, the middle layer, a basal lamina surrounding the endothelial cell layer, and on the outermost layer, astrocytic processes that envelope the capillary. Molecules that are too large and/or those smaller molecules that are not easily transported by the endothelial cells are blocked from entering the CNS due to the protection of the BBB. Lipid-soluble (i.e., fat-soluble, not water-soluble, like aspirin or amoxicillin) molecules are endothelial cell transported and thus cross the BBB. Most medications discussed here are lipid soluble and thus cross the BBB.

Bradykinesia: Slowness of movement; a cardinal manifestation of Parkinson's disease.

Blinded study: An experimental study in which subjects do not know if they are receiving a treatment or placebo (and are thus "blinded"), to reduce the bias that such knowledge might have on the subjects' responses.

Catecholamine: An amine class including several neurotransmitters—dopamine, norepinephrine and serotonin—produced in the adrenal glands and elsewhere in the sympathetic nervous system.

Cholinergic: That which precipitates or enhances the action of acetylcholine in the central and peripheral nervous systems.

Dopamine: A neurotransmitter of the catecholamine class with many functions, for example, learning, attention, reward, and motivation-related pathways in the brain. See ▶ Table 15.1 and ▶ Table 15.2 for more explanation of dopamine compared to other neurotransmitters and types of dopamine, respectively.

Downregulation: The process by which consistent overstimulation of a receptor on a cell leads the cell to produce fewer of the receptors, thereby leading to a marked reduction in the number of receptors that are available.

Drug-induced parkinsonism: A type of DIMD (see drug-induced movement disorders, DIMDs), this is motor system dysfunction caused by medications that deplete dopaminergic activity in the nigrostriatal pathway of the brain (such as D2 receptor blockers). Symptoms associated with DMID mimic those of Parkinson's disease, but differ in important ways (e.g., onset).

Dyskinesia: Abnormality or impairment of voluntary movement, typically due to neurological disease or a side effect of a medication.

Dyslipidemia: Abnormal amount, usually elevated, of lipids, such as cholesterol or triglycerides, in the blood.

Dysphoria: A general unease or dissatisfaction with one's life.

Dystonia: abnormal muscle tone resulting in muscular spasm and/or abnormal posture, typically due to neurological disease or a side effect of a medication.

Extrapyramidal system: Composed of fibers or tracts that do not directly course through the pyramidal tract of the medulla, but are responsible for motoric control; includes the indirect pathways from the cortex, feedback loops, and the descending pathways that are auditory-visual-vestibular.

Extrapyramidal symptoms: Symptoms such as tremors, involuntary movements, and muscle contractions belonging to Parkinson's disease and parkinsonism (see drug-induced parkinsonism), these can be associated with dopamine blockers.

Festination: A characteristic of Parkinson's disease; the tendency, when performing repetitive movements, to speed up the movement and perform it with decreased amplitude.

First-generation antipsychotic medications: Primarily used to treat hallucinations and delusions in disorders such as schizophrenia, these are also called "typical" antipsychotics, as they are an older class of antipsychotics than second-generation or "atypical" antipsychotics.

Fluorodopamine (F-DOPA): A fluorinated form of levodopa (L-DOPA). When parkinsonism is suspected, F-DOPA is used as a radiotracer for positron emission tomography (PET) to image the dopaminergic nerve terminals in the striatum.

GABA-A receptor: A receptor at which the primary endogenous inhibitory neurotransmitter gamma-aminobutyric acid (GABA) is an agonist; it is also the site of agonist actions of alcohol, barbiturates, and benzodiazepines.

Heterogeneity of stuttering: The high degree of behavioral, symptomatic, etc., variability within and across people who stutter. Such variability may be caused or manifested by differences in the onset, development, and maintenance of stuttering. For example, such variation may be observed when a person who stutters exhibits differences in stuttering duration, frequency, severity, and types of disfluency (i.e., sound prolongations, sound/syllable repetition, etc.) from one speaking or reading task to the next, or from one day or week to the next, without any apparent or known reason for doing so.

Homovanillic acid (HVA): An organic *compound* (specifically a catecholamine and a metabolite) included when considering neurotransmitters such as epinephrine and dopamine. HVA is the product of the action of first monoamine oxidase and then catechol-O-methyltransferase on dopamine. HVA is associated with dopamine levels in the brain.

Iatrogenic: Greek for the concept of "bringing forth by a healer." This concept or word refers to effects that result from health care professionals' use of products or services with the intent of gaining health benefits, but which negatively affects some behavior/condition of the patient (e.g., a worsening of developmental stuttering or acquired stuttering).

Internal validity: The degree to which the independent variable is responsible for affecting the dependent variable in research design; related to limiting nuisance variables like *placebo effect*.

Ligand: A substance that binds to a receptor.

Mechanism of Action (MOA): Also known as mode of action (MOA); this refers to how a substance acts upon or binds to specific molecular targets (e.g., receptor, enzyme). An MOA is a logical or reasoned attempt to explain how a medication/agent yields a reported or observed pharmacological effect.

Micrographia: The condition of having progressively smaller handwriting or abnormally small, cramped handwriting; commonly associated with neurodegenerative disorders of the basal ganglia, such as Parkinson's disease.

Necessity-concerns: Somewhat similar to the notion of cost-to-benefits ratio, this notion suggests that adherence to a treatment is influenced by one's implicit beliefs regarding personal *need* for the treatment and implicit *concerns* about the potential adverse effects of the treatment.

Neuroleptics: Antipsychotics; effects can be both intended (e.g., reduction in confusion and agitation) or unintended ADRs (e.g., a state of apathy, lack of initiative, and limited range of emotion).

Nucleus accumbens: A region in the brain that is a component of the basal ganglia. it has a significant role in the cognitive processing of motivation, aversion, reward, and reinforcement.

"Off-label": The use of a medication to treat a disorder or symptom, for which it does not have an FDA indication.

"Open-label" extension study: An investigation planned to occur after a double-blind, randomized controlled drug trial has occurred and before requesting FDA approval. These types of studies append to, or extend, a randomized controlled clinical trial. No blinding is used in these types of studies and all parties (i.e., patient and physician) are aware of the treatment groups (i.e., "open label"). Such open-label studies are sometimes referred to as "unblinded." Unblinding means that the participant and/or study team is told which treatment the participant received during the trial, and the medicine is under an investigational new drug license.

Paradoxical drug effects: Alterations in observing an opposite clinical effect (e.g., exacerbating stuttering symptoms) than the desired clinical effect (e.g., ameliorating stuttering symptoms).

Parkinson's disease: A progressive disease of the nervous system caused by the destruction of cells that are responsible for producing dopamine in the substantial nigra of the midbrain, leading to characteristic motor system dysfunction, hallmarked by tremor, difficulty initiating movement, slowness of movement, and difficult walking.

Pediatric autoimmune neuropsychiatric disorder associated with streptococcal infections (PANDAS): A clinical diagnosis in children, roughly from about 3-year-olds to puberty, in which health care providers use diagnostic criteria to determine the presence of such concerns as obsessive compulsive disorder (OCD) or a tic disorder (i.e., Tourette's syndrome), or both. PANDAS can be associated with group A beta-hemolytic strep infection, such as a positive throat culture for strep or history of scarlet fever, and with neurological abnormalities, such as physical hyperactivity or unusual, jerky movements that are not in the child's control. PANDAS can have a very abrupt onset or be associated with worsening of symptoms (i.e., no lab tests can diagnose PANDAS, but blood tests may be ordered to determine if there was a prior strep infection).

Pedunculopontine nucleus: Part of the reticular activating system, this nucleus is located in the brainstem, in the upper pons. this nucleus has two divisions of subnuclei, the *pars compacta* of cholinergic neurons and the *pars dissipata* of mostly glutamatergic neurons.

Persistent developmental stuttering: Developmental stuttering (that typically onsets in childhood) that has not resolved spontaneously, or which persists despite speech therapy.

Pharmacodynamics: Described as what a drug does to the body versus what the body does to the drug (i.e., pharmacokinetics), this is the study of the physiologic/molecular and biochemical effects of substances. Subtopics relating to pharmacodynamics include receptor sensitivity, receptor binding, post-receptor effects, and chemical interactions. Pharmacodynamics can be affected by physiologic changes due to aging, drug interactions, and a given disorder or disease.

Pharmacokinetics: Described as what the body does to the drug versus what a drug does to the body (i.e., pharmacodynamics), this is the study of the process of the uptake of the substance, when effects of a medication wears off, what biotransformations the medications undergo, and how their metabolites are distributed in tissues and eliminated.

Pharmacotherapy: Medical treatment with pharmacologic agents (medications), sometimes referred to as drug therapy.

Placebo: A sham or an inert substance or treatment intended to have no benefits therapeutically (e.g., sugar pills, saline injections); such substances are important with regard to research design considerations. Placebos are typically provided to volunteer participants in phase III portion of a randomized controlled trial for a medication to determine whether the medication is more effective therapeutically than the substance having no known benefit; see *internal validity*/controlling placebo effect.

Prolactinemia: A state of elevated levels of the hormone prolactin, which is produced by the pituitary gland and is responsible for breast development during pregnancy.

Red nucleus: Part of the extrapyramidal motor system in the basal ganglia along with the substantia nigra, this nucleus is in the tegmentum of the midbrain; it is termed "red" because in cadaver views it is pale pink, due to ferritin and hemoglobin (i.e., iron); functions in motor coordination and in the gait of primates.

Schedule-I drugs: A classification of drugs used by the U.S. drug enforcement agency (DEA) for drugs that have no currently accepted medical use and a high potential for abuse (e.g., heroin, cannabis).

Schizophrenia: A psychotic illness hallmarked by delusional beliefs, hallucinations, blunted affect, and a variety of other symptoms.

Second-generation antipsychotic medications: Primarily used to treat hallucinations and delusions in disorders such as schizophrenia, these are also called "atypical" antipsychotics. Compared to first-generation "typical" antipsychotics, second-generation antipsychotics are newer in the origins and usage.

Social anxiety disorder: Also called social phobia, a psychiatric diagnosis characterized by fear and anxiety of being evaluated negatively by other people, marked impairment in everyday functioning and significant distress.

Substantia nigra: Latin for "black substance," named as such because it appears darker than adjacent regions due in part to elevated dopaminergic neuron levels. it is part of the extrapyramidal motor system, together with the red nucleus, produces and sends dopamine to the striatum.

Subthalamic nucleus: Thought to be part of the extrapyramidal motor system in the subthalamus of the basal ganglia, this nucleus is a small and lens-shaped nucleus, and its function is unknown.

Tardive dyskinesia: A rare but serious side effect of neuroleptic medications that is characterized by involuntary and uncontrollable movements of the face or body (e.g., sticking one's tongue out); risk of occurrence increases with length of time of neuroleptic use.

Tricyclic antidepressants: An early class of antidepressant medications, which often have broad indications beyond depression (e.g., pain, insomnia) and which are associated with many side effects, especially anticholinergic effects.

References

[1] Boyd A, Dworzynski K, Howell P. Pharmacological agents for developmental stuttering in children and adolescents: a systematic review. J Clin Psychopharmacol. 2011; 31(6):740–744

[2] Maguire GA, Wither LG. Without hesitation: speaking to the silence and the science of stuttering. New York, NY: National Stuttering Association; 2010

[3] Yairi E, Seery CH. Stuttering: Foundations and clinical applications. Upper Saddle River, NJ: Pearson; 2015

[4] Horne R, Weinman J. Patients' beliefs about prescribed medicines and their role in adherence to treatment in chronic physical illness. J Psychosom Res. 1999; 47(6):555–567

[5] Tibaldi G, Clatworthy J, Torchio E, Argentero P, Munizza C, Horne R. The utility of the necessity–concerns framework in explaining treatment non-adherence in four chronic illness groups in Italy. Chronic Illn. 2009; 5(2):129–133

[6] McGroarty A, McCartan R. Beliefs and behavioural intentions towards pharmacotherapy for stuttering: a survey of adults who stutter. J Commun Disord. 2018; 73:15–24

[7] Ludlow CL. Neuropharmacology of stuttering: concepts and current findings. In Bernstein Ratner N, Tetnowski J, eds. Current issues in Stuttering Research and practice. London: Lawrence Erlbaum Associates; 2006:239–254

[8] Saxon KG, Ludlow CL. A critical review of the effect of drugs on stuttering. in: Conture EG, Curlee RF, eds. Stuttering and Related Disorders of fluency. New York, NY: Thieme; 2007:277–293

[9] Chang SE, Guenther FH. Involvement of the cortico-basal ganglia-thalamocortical loop in developmental stuttering. Front Psychol. 2020; 10:3088:

[10] Alm PA. Stuttering and the basal ganglia circuits: a critical review of possible relations. J Commun Disord. 2004; 37(4):325–369

[11] Giraud AL, Neumann K, Bachoud-Levi AC, et al. Severity of dysfluency correlates with basal ganglia activity in persistent developmental stuttering. Brain Lang. 2008; 104(2):190–199

[12] Lu C, Ning N, Peng D, et al. The role of large-scale neural interactions for developmental stuttering. Neuroscience. 2009; 161(4):1008–1026

[13] Lu C, Peng D, Chen C, et al. Altered effective connectivity and anomalous anatomy in the basal ganglia-thalamocortical circuit of stuttering speakers. Cortex. 2010; 46(1):49–67

[14] Watkins KE, Smith SM, Davis S, Howell P. Structural and functional abnormalities of the motor system in developmental stuttering. Brain. 2008; 131(Pt 1):50–59

[15] LaPointe LL. Atlas of neuroanatomy for communication science and disorders. New York, NY: Thieme; 2011

[16] Ambrose NG, Yairi E. Normative disfluency data for early childhood stuttering. J Speech Lang Hear Res. 1999; 42(4):895–909

[17] Maguire GA, Riley GD, Yu BP. A neurological basis of stuttering? Lancet Neurol. 2002; 1(7):407

[18] Fadok JP, Dickerson TM, Palmiter RD. Dopamine is necessary for cue-dependent fear conditioning. J Neurosci. 2009; 29(36):11089–11097

[19] Metzger FL, Auer T, Helms G, et al. Shifted dynamic interactions between subcortical nuclei and inferior frontal gyri during response preparation in persistent developmental stuttering. Brain Struct Funct. 2018; 223(1):165–182

[20] Wu JC, Maguire G, Riley G, et al. Increased dopamine activity associated with stuttering. Neuroreport. 1997; 8(3):767–770

[21] Chen H, Wang G, Xia J, et al. Stuttering candidate genes DRD2 but not SLC6A3 is associated with developmental dyslexia in Chinese population. Behav Brain Funct. 2014; 10(1):29

[22] Lan J, Song M, Pan C, et al. Association between dopaminergic genes (SLC6A3 and DRD2) and stuttering among Han Chinese. J Hum Genet. 2009; 54(8):457–460

[23] Han TU, Root J, Reyes LD, et al. Human GNPTAB stuttering mutations engineered into mice cause vocalization deficits and astrocyte pathology in the corpus callosum. Proc Natl Acad Sci U S A. 2019; 116 (35):17515–17524

[24] Li BD, Cui JJ, Song J, et al. Comparison of the efficacy of different drugs on non-motor symptoms of Parkinson's disease: a network meta-analysis. Cell Physiol Biochem. 2018; 45(1):119–130

[25] Armstrong MJ, Okun MS. Diagnosis and treatment of Parkinson disease: a review. JAMA. 2020; 323(6):548–560

[26] Anderson JM, Hughes JD, Rothi LJ, Crucian GP, Heilman KM. Developmental stuttering and Parkinson's disease: the effects of levodopa treatment. J Neurol Neurosurg Psychiatry. 1999; 66(6):776–778

[27] Louis ED, Winfield L, Fahn S, Ford B. Speech dysfluency exacerbated by levodopa in Parkinson's disease. Mov Disord. 2001; 16(3):562–565

[28] Jezer M. Stuttering: A life bound up in words. New York, NY: Basic Books; 1997

[29] Ezrati-Vinacour R, Levin I. Time estimation by adults who stutter. J Speech Lang Hear Res. 2001; 44(1):144–155

[30] Barasch CT, Guitar B, McCauley RJ, Absher RG. Disfluency and time perception. J Speech Lang Hear Res. 2000; 43(6):1429–1439

[31] Inagawa T, Ueda N, Nakagome K, Sumiyoshi T. Time estimation in a case of Tourette's syndrome: effect of antipsychotic medications. Neuropsychopharmacol Rep. 2020; 40(2):198–200

[32] Foundas AL, Bollich AM, Feldman J, et al. Aberrant auditory processing and atypical planum temporale in developmental stuttering. Neurology. 2004; 63(9):1640–1646

[33] Haynes WO, Johnson CE. Understanding Research and Evidence-Based Practice in Communication Disorders: A Primer for Students and Practitioners. Boston, MA: Pearson; 2009

[34] Maguire GA, Riley GD, Franklin DL, Maguire ME, Nguyen CT, Brojeni PH. Olanzapine in the treatment of developmental stuttering: a double-blind, placebo-controlled trial. Ann Clin Psychiatry. 2004; 16(2):63–67

[35] Brady JP. The pharmacology of stuttering: a critical review. Am J Psychiatry. 1991; 148(10):1309–1316

[36] Maguire G, Franklin D, Vatakis NG, et al. Exploratory randomized clinical study of pagoclone in persistent developmental stuttering: the EXamining Pagoclone for peRsistent dEvelopmental Stuttering Study. J Clin Psychopharmacol. 2010; 30(1):48–56

[37] Ingham RJ. Comments on article by Maguire et al: pagoclone trial: questionable findings for stuttering treatment. J Clin Psychopharmacol. 2010; 30(5):649–650, author reply 650–651

[38] Ratner NB, Tetnowski JA. Current issues in Stuttering Research and Practice. New York, NY: Psychology Press; 2014

[39] Bothe AK, Davidow JH, Bramlett RE, Franic DM, Ingham RJ. Stuttering treatment research 1970–2005: II. Systematic review incorporating trial quality assessment of pharmacological approaches. Am J Speech Lang Pathol. 2006; 15(4):342–352

[40] Maguire GA, Yu BP, Franklin DL, Riley GD. Alleviating stuttering with pharmacological interventions. Expert Opin Pharmacother. 2004; 5(7): 1565–1571

[41] Guitar B, McCauley RJ. Treatment of stuttering: established and emerging interventions. Baltimore, MD: Lippincott Williams & Wilkins; 2010

[42] Cocores JA, Dackis CA, Davies RK, Gold MS. Propranolol and stuttering. Am J Psychiatry. 1986; 143(8):1071–1072

[43] Kymissis P, Martin E. Antistuttering medication? J Am Acad Child Adolesc Psychiatry. 1990; 29(5):840

[44] Brady JP, Price TR, McAllister TW, Dietrich K. A trial of verapamil in the treatment of stuttering in adults. Biol Psychiatry. 1989; 25(5):630–633

[45] Brumfitt SM, Peake MD. A double-blind study of verapamil in the treatment of stuttering. Br J Disord Commun. 1988; 23(1):35–40

[46] Linazasoro G, Van Blercom N. Severe stuttering and motor tics responsive to cocaine. Parkinsonism Relat Disord. 2007; 13(1):57–58

[47] Brady JP. Drug-induced stuttering: a review of the literature. J Clin Psychopharmacol. 1998; 18(1):50–54

[48] Kumar A, Balan S. Fluoxetine for persistent developmental stuttering. Clin Neuropharmacol. 2007; 30(1):58–59

[49] Foundas AL, Mock JR, Corey DM, Golob EJ, Conture EG. The SpeechEasy device in stuttering and nonstuttering adults: fluency effects while speaking and reading. Brain Lang. 2013; 126(2):141–150

[50] Braun AR, Varga M, Stager S, et al. Altered patterns of cerebral activity during speech and language production in developmental stuttering. An H2(15)O positron emission tomography study. Brain. 1997; 120(Pt 5): 761–784

[51] De Nil LF, Kroll RM, Kapur S, Houle S. A positron emission tomography study of silent and oral single word reading in stuttering and nonstuttering adults. J Speech Lang Hear Res. 2000; 43(4):1038–1053

[52] Fox PT, Ingham RJ, Ingham JC, et al. A PET study of the neural systems of stuttering. Nature. 1996; 382(6587):158–161

[53] Burns D, Brady JP, Kuruvilla K. The acute effect of haloperidol and apomorphine on the severity of stuttering. Biol Psychiatry. 1978; 13(2): 255–264

[54] Prins D, Mandelkorn T, Cerf FA. Principal and differential effects of haoperidol and placebo treatments upon speech disfuluencies in stutterers. J Speech Hear Res. 1980; 23(3):614–629

[55] Spehr W, Andresen B, Pascher W. The impact of long-time, low-dosage haloperidol therapy on anxiety proneness. Agressologie. 1981; 22(D):33–36

[56] Wells PG, Malcolm MT. Controlled trial of the treatment of 36 stutterers. Br J Psychiatry. 1971; 119(553):603–604

[57] Gordon CT, Cotelingam GM, Stager S, Ludlow CL, Hamburger SD, Rapoport JL. A double-blind comparison of clomipramine and desipramine in the treatment of developmental stuttering. J Clin Psychiatry. 1995; 56(6): 238–242

[58] Stager SV, Ludlow CL, Gordon CT, Cotelingam M, Rapoport JL. Fluency changes in persons who stutter following a double blind trial of clomipramine and desipramine. J Speech Hear Res. 1995; 38(3):516–525

[59] Costa D, Kroll R. Stuttering: an update for physicians. CMAJ. 2000; 162(13): 1849–1855

[60] Christensen RC, Byerly MJ, McElroy RA. A case of sertraline-induced stuttering. J Clin Psychopharmacol. 1996; 16(1):92–93

[61] Bloch M, Stager S, Braun A, et al. Pimozide-induced depression in men who stutter. J Clin Psychiatry. 1997; 58(10):433–436

[62] Stager SV, Calis K, Grothe D, et al. Treatment with medications affecting dopaminergic and serotonergic mechanisms: effects on fluency and anxiety in persons who stutter. J Fluency Disord. 2005; 30(4):319–335

[63] Maguire GA, Gottschalk LA, Riley GD, Franklin DL, Bechtel RJ, Ashurst J. Stuttering: neuropsychiatric features measured by content analysis of speech and the effect of risperidone on stuttering severity. Compr Psychiatry. 1999; 40(4):308–314

[64] Maguire GA, Riley GD, Franklin DL, Gottschalk LA. Risperidone for the treatment of stuttering. J Clin Psychopharmacol. 2000; 20(4):479–482

[65] Lavid N, Franklin DL, Maguire GA. Management of child and adolescent stuttering with olanzapine: three case reports. Ann Clin Psychiatry. 1999; 11 (4):233–236

[66] Yadav DS. Risperidone induced stuttering. Gen Hosp Psychiatry. 2010; 32 (5):559.e9–559.e10

[67] Lee HJ, Lee HS, Kim L, Lee MS, Suh KY, Kwak DI. A case of risperidone-induced stuttering. J Clin Psychopharmacol. 2001; 21(1):115–116

[68] van Wattum PJ. Stuttering improved with risperidone. J Am Acad Child Adolesc Psychiatry. 2006; 45(2):133

[69] Generali JA, Cada DJ. Risperidone: stuttering. Hosp Pharm. 2014; 49(3): 242–243

[70] Tavano A, Busan P, Borelli M, Pelamatti G. Risperidone reduces tic-like motor behaviors and linguistic dysfluencies in severe persistent developmental stuttering. J Clin Psychopharmacol. 2011; 31(1):131–134

[71] Catalano G, Robben DL, Catalano MC, Kahn DA. Olanzapine for the treatment of acquired neurogenic stuttering. J Psychiatr Pract. 2009; 15(6):484–488

[72] Shaygannejad V, Khatoonabadi SA, Shafiei B, et al. Olanzapine versus haloperidol: which can control stuttering better? Int J Prev Med. 2013; 4 Suppl 2:S270–S273

[73] Munjal S, Schultheis G, Ferrando S. Ziprasidone for the treatment of stuttering. J Clin Psychopharmacol. 2018; 38(4):404–405

[74] Maguire GA, Franklin DL, Kirsten J. Asenapine for the treatment of stuttering: an analysis of three cases. Am J Psychiatry. 2011; 168(6):651–652

[75] Tran NL, Maguire GA, Franklin DL, Riley GD. Case report of aripiprazole for persistent developmental stuttering. J Clin Psychopharmacol. 2008; 28(4): 470–472

[76] Charoensook J, Maguire GA. A case series on the effectiveness of lurasidone in patients with stuttering. Ann Clin Psychiatry. 2017; 29(3):191–194

[77] Bharadwaj A, Andrade C. Efficacy of aripiprazole in severe, persistent, socially- and occupationally-impairing developmental stuttering. Asian J Psychiatr. 2020; 48:101861

[78] Hoang JL, Patel S, Maguire GA. Case report of aripiprazole in the treatment of adolescent stuttering. Ann Clin Psychiatry. 2016; 28(1):64–65

[79] Naguy A, Moodliar S, Elsori DH, Alamiri B. Dose-dependent aripiprazole-induced stuttering in a child with mild intellectual disability. Am J Ther. 2020

[80] Maguire GA, Nguyen DL, Simonson KC, Kurz TL. The pharmacologic treatment of stuttering and its neuropharmacologic basis. Front Neurosci. 2020; 14:158

[81] Yaruss JS, Quesal RW. Overall Assessment of the Speaker's Experience of Stuttering (OASES): documenting multiple outcomes in stuttering treatment. J Fluency Disord. 2006; 31(2):90–115

[82] Maguire GA, LaSalle L, Hoffmeyer D, et al. Ecopipam as a pharmacologic treatment of stuttering. Ann Clin Psychiatry. 2019; 31(3):164–168

[83] Sreeram V, Shagufta S, Kagadkar F. Role of vesicular monoamine transporter 2 inhibitors in tardive dyskinesia management. Cureus. 2019; 11(8):e5471

[84] Niemann N, Jankovic J. Real-world experience with VMAT2 inhibitors. Clin Neuropharmacol. 2019; 42(2):37–41

[85] Lustig A, Ruiz C. Drug-induced movement disorders. Perspect Neurophysiol Neurogenic Speech Lang Disord. 2015; 25(2):70–77

[86] Alvarez MV, Evidente VG, Driver-Dunckley ED. Differentiating Parkinson's disease from other parkinsonian disorders. Semin Neurol. 2007; 27(4):356–362

[87] Perez Lloret S, Amaya M, Merello M. Pregabalin-induced parkinsonism: a case report. Clin Neuropharmacol. 2009; 32(6):353–354

[88] Thanvi B, Treadwell S. Drug induced parkinsonism: a common cause of parkinsonism in older people. Postgrad Med J. 2009; 85(1004):322–326

[89] Rachamallu V, Haq A, Song MM, Aligeti M. Clozapine-induced microseizures, orofacial dyskinesia, and speech dysfluency in an adolescent with treatment resistant early onset schizophrenia on concurrent lithium therapy. Case Rep Psychiatry. 2017; 2017:7359095

[90] Steck H. Extrapyramidal and diencephalic syndrome in the course of largactil and serpasil treatments. Ann Med Psychol (Paris). 1954; 112(2 5):737–744

[91] Steck H. Extrapyramidal syndrome in chlorpromazine and serpasil therapy; clinical symptomatology and therapeutic role. Encephale. 1956; 45(4):1083–1089

[92] Nurnberg HG, Greenwald B. Stuttering: an unusual side effect of phenothiazines. Am J Psychiatry. 1981; 138(3):386–387

[93] Claxton KL, Chen JJ, Swope DM. Drug-induced movement disorders. J Pharm Pract. 2007; 20(6):415–429

[94] Shin HW, Chung SJ. Drug-induced parkinsonism. J Clin Neurol. 2012; 8(1):15–21

[95] Netski AL, Piasecki M. Lithium-induced exacerbation of stutter. Ann Pharmacother. 2001; 35(7–8):961

[96] Sabillo S, Samala RV, Ciocon JO. A stuttering discovery of lithium toxicity. J Am Med Dir Assoc. 2012; 13(7):660–661

[97] Gulack BC, Puri NV, Kim WJ. Stutter exacerbated by lithium in a pediatric patient with bipolar disorder. Ann Pharmacother. 2011; 45(10):e57

[98] LeDoux JE. Anxious: using the brain to understand and treat fear and anxiety. New York, NY: Viking; 2015

[99] Blumgart E, Tran Y, Craig A. Social anxiety disorder in adults who stutter. Depress Anxiety. 2010; 27(7):687–692

[100] Harris D. Meditation for Fidgety Skeptics: A 10% Happier How-to Book. 1st ed. New York, NY: Spiegel & Grau; 2017

[101] Iverach L, Jones M, O'Brian S, et al. The relationship between mental health disorders and treatment outcomes among adults who stutter. J Fluency Disord. 2009; 34(1):29–43

[102] Novák A. Results of the treatment of severe forms of stuttering in adults. Folia Phoniatr (Basel). 1975; 27(4):278–282

[103] Sedláčková E. A contribution to pharmacotherapy of stuttering and cluttering. Folia Phoniatr (Basel). 1970; 22(4):354–375

[104] Norman RS, Jaramillo CA, Eapen BC, Amuan ME, Pugh MJ. Acquired stuttering in veterans of the wars in Iraq and Afghanistan: the role of traumatic brain injury, post-traumatic stress disorder, and medications. Mil Med. 2018; 183(11–12):e526–e534

[105] Althaus M, Vink HJ, Minderaa RB, Goorhuis-Brouwer SM, Oosterhoff MD. Lack of effect of clonidine on stuttering in children. Am J Psychiatry. 1995; 152(7):1087–1089

[106] Donaher J, Healey EC, Zobell A. The effects of ADHD medication changes on a child who stutters. Perspect Fluen Fluen Disord. 2009; 19(3):95–98

[107] Radant HJ. The Effect of Ritalin on the Speech Rate and Fluency of Individuals with Attention Deficit Hyperactivity Disorder. Eau Claire, WI: University of Wisconsin–Eau Claire; 1996

[108] Graham CG. The effect of ADHD on the treatment of stuttering. Perspect Fluen Fluen Disord. 2006; 16(2):10–12

[109] Choi D, Conture EG, Tumanova V, Clark CE, Walden TA, Jones RM. Young children's family history of stuttering and their articulation, language and attentional abilities: an exploratory study. J Commun Disord. 2018; 71:22–36

[110] Maguire GA, Viele SN, Agarwal S, Handler E, Franklin D. Stuttering onset associated with streptococcal infection: a case suggesting stuttering as PANDAS. Ann Clin Psychiatry. 2010; 22(4):283–284

[111] Maguire GA, Yeh CY, Ito BS. Overview of the diagnosis and treatment of stuttering. J Exp Clin Med. 2012; 4(2):92–97

[112] Alm PA. Streptococcal infection as a major historical cause of stuttering: data, mechanisms, and current importance. Front Hum Neurosci. 2020; 14 (389):569519

[113] Iverach L, Jones M, O'Brian S, et al. Mood and substance use disorders among adults seeking speech treatment for stuttering. J Speech Lang Hear Res. 2010; 53(5):1178–1190

[114] Heelan M, McAllister J, Skinner J. Stuttering, alcohol consumption and smoking. J Fluency Disord. 2016; 48:27–34

[115] Oliveira CCCd, Scivoletto S. Relationship between abstinence from marijuana and speech fluency in an adolescent with stuttering: implications for speech therapy and psychiatric treatment. Rev CEFAC. 2014; 16(2):660–662

[116] Bothe AK, Davidow JH, Bramlett RE, Ingham RJ. Stuttering treatment research 1970–2005: I. Systematic review incorporating trial quality assessment of behavioral, cognitive, and related approaches. Am J Speech Lang Pathol. 2006; 15(4):321–341

[117] Meline T, Harn WE. Comments on Bothe, Davidow, Bramlett, Franic, and Ingham (2006). Am J Speech Lang Pathol. 2008; 17(1):93–97, author reply 98–101

[118] Bothe AK, Franic DM, Ingham RJ, Davidow JH. Pharmacological approaches to stuttering treatment: reply to Meline and Harn (2008). Am J Speech Lang Pathol. 2008; 17(1):98–101

[119] Mohammadi H, Joghataei MT, Rahimi Z, Faghihi F, Farhangdoost H. Relationship between serum homovanillic acid, DRD2 C957 T (rs6277), and hDAT A559V (rs28364997) polymorphisms and developmental stuttering. J Commun Disord. 2018; 76:37–46

Section VI

Related Fluency Disorders

VI

16 Cluttering: Etiology, Symptomatology, Identification, and Treatment

Kathleen Scaler Scott, Hilda Sønsterud, and Isabella Reichel

Abstract

The purpose of this chapter is to provide updated information on cluttering, a fluency disorder that is often misunderstood and misdiagnosed. Updated definitions and research findings will be presented to provide latest information about the best clinical practices. The chapter begins with a case study of a teenager who is referred for an evaluation due to decreased speech intelligibility. The case is woven throughout the chapter to illustrate all aspects of client management: initial referral, evaluation and differential diagnosis, treatment, and education of the client, family members, and other professionals. The case reflects the challenges a clinician often encounters with a client's resistance to treatment. As the chapter illustrates, part of this resistance may be due to the nature of cluttering symptoms, and partly due to prior missed diagnoses and failed treatments. The chapter provides background on how our knowledge of cluttering has evolved, and the need for it to continue in the future. Additionally, methods for evaluation, differential diagnosis, and treatment of cluttering are presented. Background on the past and present state of cluttering research provides the context for what we do and do not know about cluttering, and for making the best decisions in treatment. The overall focus is to help the clinician better understand how to (1) identify cluttered speech and (2) treat the client with cluttering in a holistic manner, based upon symptom presentation.

Keywords: cluttering, fast speech, fluency, intelligibility, disfluencies, over-coarticulation, pausing, speech rate

16.1 Introduction

The Referral: Peter

Peter was a high school junior who was concerned about his grade on a recent classroom presentation. His history teacher stated that he spoke too fast and wanted him to correct this issue for his next presentation. Peter, an honors student, was frustrated at what he felt was his inability to control his rate. He also did not agree that he spoke quickly. His parents noted that he did speak fast at times, which made him difficult to understand. When Peter's parents would tell him to slow down, he would respond that they should, "Listen faster." He said that no one else was telling him that they could not understand his speech.

Peter's mother was frustrated and wanted to help her son. She did an online search for "fast speech." The term "cluttering" came up. She read the description and wondered if this could be her son's problem. She called a speech-language clinician who specialized in cluttering to inquire about a possible evaluation. Before we delve into the evaluation, the reader will need some background information on how cluttering came to be defined as it is today.

16.1.1 Common Characteristics of Cluttering: Past and Present

History

Experts have discussed the topic of cluttering for much longer than most people are aware. A description of this history will demonstrate how in different time periods, and in different parts of the world, characteristics associated with cluttering were similar. We begin by sharing information about the well-known Demosthenes, the Greek orator, who lived more than 300 years before the common era (384–322 BC). People working in the field of fluency disorders might know that Demosthenes stuttered, but fewer people know about his cluttering, which was characterized at the time by reduced intelligibility, weak voice, short breaths, and an inability to focus on the main point of discourse.[1] The famous actor and voice teacher, Satyros, reportedly "cured" Demosthenes of his cluttering. It is worth questioning what "cured" meant in this context since even in the present day we have no documentation of people being "cured" of cluttering.

The first complete book devoted to cluttering was titled "Das Poltern" (German word for cluttering[2]). In this book, Richard Luchsinger explained cluttering as a "mismatch" between a speaker's intention (i.e., what they want to say) and their ability to produce it (i.e., control of speech production). Another pioneering book by Deso Weiss, "Cluttering," was published in 1964.[1] Weiss explained cluttering as a central language imbalance. Weiss' holistic perspective on the treatment of cluttering influenced the work of many researchers and clinicians around the world.

Current Definition of Cluttering

Original definitions of cluttering described the speaker as someone with a "syndrome" who was messy and disorganized, or constantly interrupting conversation.[1] Because this description was so broad, however, it became difficult to distinguish cluttering from other communication disorders.

In a quest to uncover the distinctive features of cluttering, core symptoms upon which fluency experts could agree were identified.[3,4,5,6] These were the symptoms that stood out when an expert said, "I know cluttering when I hear it." These symptoms were always present (albeit not always in the same speaking situations) in cluttering. Based on the data of 15 participants who cluttered (ranging in age from 11 to 37 years), the most commonly occurring symptoms of cluttering were identified, resulting in the lowest common denominator (LCD) definition of cluttering (note that the parenthetical numbers in the definition refer to the notes that appear directly underneath it)[6]:

Definition

Cluttering is a fluency disorder wherein segments of conversation (1) in the speaker's native language (2) typically are perceived

*as too fast overall (3), too irregular (4), or both. The segments of rapid and/or irregular speech rate **must** further be accompanied by one or more of the following: (a) excessive "normal" disfluencies (5); (b) excessive collapsing (6) or deletion of syllables; and/or (c) abnormal pauses, syllable stress, or speech rhythm* (pp. 241–242).

    Notes
1. *Cluttering must occur in naturalistic conversation, but it need not occur even a majority of the time. Clear but isolated examples that exceed those observed in normal speakers are sufficient for a diagnosis.*
2. *This may also apply to the speaker's mastered and habitual non-native language, especially in multilingual living environments.*
3. *This may be true even though syllable rates may not exceed those of normal speakers.*
4. *Synonyms for irregular rate include "jerky," or "spurty."*
5. *These disfluencies are often observed in smaller numbers in normal speakers and are typically not observed in stuttering.*
6. *Collapsing includes, but is not limited to, excessive shortening, "telescoping," or "over-coarticulating" various syllables, especially in multisyllabic words.*

Under this definition, speech that is *rapid sounding* or "*perceived as too fast overall*" is a mandatory criterion for a diagnosis of cluttering. Note that although this criterion is mandatory, the speaker does not have to present with a rapid or irregular rate in all or even most speaking situations (see note 1 above).[6] People who clutter may be perceived as having a rate that is more rapid than average, yet objective measures of speech rate do not often exceed the average. Thus, there is something else about cluttering that makes the listener perceive the rate as "fast."[7] One widely held hypothesis is that speakers with cluttering are speaking at a rate that is too fast for their speech production system to handle.[8] Such a challenge results in a communication breakdown that sounds "too fast" to the listener.[8] The resulting symptoms that come with a "too fast" rate may be what makes the listener say, "That person speaks quickly!"

It is important to note that cluttering may occur in people with additional diagnoses. One of the most commonly reported co-occurring disorders in cluttering is stuttering. Some of the other co-occurring diagnoses may include but are not limited to expressive and/or receptive language disorder, attention deficit hyperactivity disorder, and autism spectrum disorder. Not all individuals with cluttering have these diagnoses, and not everyone with these diagnoses exhibits cluttering. To avoid confusing symptoms of cluttered speech with symptoms of other disorders, the clinician is advised to focus on the criteria in the LCD definition above. Symptoms related to other disorders, such as a receptive and/or expressive language disorder or stuttering, should be further evaluated as potential concomitant diagnoses.

Prevalence

The exact prevalence of cluttering is uncertain. However, because there is such a lack of understanding about cluttering among many professionals, both combined stuttering/cluttering and pure cluttering (i.e., cluttering without any additional disorders; see the section "Co-Occurring Symptoms/Disorders" below) are likely underdiagnosed. Experts estimate that fewer than 5% of cases referred for stuttering exhibit "pure cluttering,"[9]

although a more recent study found the prevalence to be approximately 1.2% among Dutch and German adolescents.[10] Research has further revealed that approximately 40% of individuals with Down syndrome exhibit excessive disfluencies and 12 to 19% of these individuals were subsequently diagnosed with cluttering or mixed cluttering/stuttering.[11]

16.2 Diagnostic Considerations

The LCD definition allows the practicing clinician to differentiate cluttered speech from characteristics that might be related to other disorders. However, careful attention to differential diagnosis is still required when diagnosing cluttering.

Talking with Peter's Parents

Peter's mother was convinced that her son was cluttering, but Peter's dad was skeptical. Peter had been evaluated by his school clinician and did not meet the school's criteria for any services. The parents asked for a conference call with the speech-language clinician who specialized in cluttering. During that call, the clinician asked for Peter's speech history. Peter was a "late talker" who received services as a preschooler for articulation difficulties. Peter's parents could not recall the sounds Peter had worked on. Peter's dad reported that when Peter was younger, his speech sounded like someone who had a hearing impairment. His mother did not have this perception. Peter's parents believed that when Peter slowed down, his speech was clear. Both agreed that his speech could sound "mumbled" at times. Peter's parents reported that Peter argued that their inability to understand him was due to their inadequate hearing.

Peter's mother wanted to schedule an evaluation as soon as possible. She felt that even though Peter was not expressing any perceived problems, his frustration when others asked him to repeat or commented on his speech was becoming very apparent. She felt this frustration was carrying over into other activities, causing Peter to "shut down" and communicate less. His father was more hesitant. He knew that Peter was resistant to pursuing help with his speech, and he wanted to make sure that Peter was going to get an accurate diagnosis without more wasted time. Peter's dad was concerned that too many attempts in the "wrong direction" would close his son off to the idea of treatment.

16.2.1 Important Background Information

When determining whether cluttering is the issue, the clinician should be cautious, as there are many factors that can contribute to decreased speech intelligibility. Given the statement about potential issues with prosody (i.e., client's possible history of sounding like he had a hearing impairment) and previous work on speech sounds, the clinician considered a possible diagnosis of mild childhood apraxia of speech. Peter's parents said this diagnosis had never been brought up to them. There were no current articulation errors. Due to the mention of prosody, the clinician also wanted to rule out any resonance issues that might be contributing to decreased intelligibility. Peter's dad's concern about too many efforts in the wrong direction was not unfounded; many adults who clutter report frustration with wasted time and efforts with inaccurate diagnoses.[12,13]

16.2.2 Continuous or Intermittent Rapid or Irregular Speech Rate

In making a diagnosis of cluttering, the clinician wanted to ensure that Peter had the mandatory speech characteristic for people with cluttering: his speech sounds fast at least some of the time. If Peter never sounded fast, there would be no support for a diagnosis of cluttering. It is important to note that just as in stuttering, cluttering does *not* have to occur each time the speaker talks to warrant a diagnosis. In fact, under the LCD definition, the cluttered moments do *not* even have to occur most of the time.[6] Just as you will read elsewhere in this book that stuttering is situational, so too is cluttering. The clinician also wanted to ensure that Peter had at least one of the following difficulties: excessive "normal" disfluencies, excessive moments of over-coarticulation, and/or atypical pauses.

16.2.3 Excessive "Normal" Disfluencies

Normal disfluencies (NDs; i.e., nonstuttering disfluencies) are defined as interjections (e.g., "uh," "um," etc.), multisyllabic word repetitions without tension, phrase repetitions, and revisions. These should be contrasted with stuttering-like disfluencies, which consist of within-word repetitions, prolongations, and blocks (see ▶ Chapter 1).

NDs can come from many different sources, such as helping a speaker gather their thoughts or retrieve a word. However, if NDs are used "excessively," speakers are likely to transmit their messages inefficiently. In this case, difficulties with retrieval/ language organization, which may require language treatment, must be ruled out. Language testing can help ascertain this question objectively. The clinician's informal assessment of the speaker's performance during reading, conversation, retelling a story, and monologue samples is also crucial for a comprehensive evaluation of cluttering. Does the speaker use NDs when less language formulation is required, such as when reading? Does the speaker use vague terms or need additional time to formulate the remaining part of the sentence? Is the speaker's message disorganized and difficult to follow?

People who stutter may use excessive numbers of NDs to escape or avoid moments of stuttering. This does not, by default, make them people with cluttering. However, if a speaker has a propensity to stutter and clutter, then establishing the root cause of the excessive NDs is necessary for the accurate diagnosis and effective management of cluttering. If someone has a combination of stuttering and cluttering, and engages in stuttering avoidance behaviors, the stuttering avoidance must be addressed first. Objective testing and an interview will help identify whether the speaker has symptoms of cluttering and/or stuttering, including use of NDs as stuttering avoidance.

16.2.4 Excessive Moments of Over-Coarticulation

A hallmark cluttering symptom is that the client's speech often sounds "mumbled." This is the listener's perception of over-coarticulation, whereby the speaker runs one word into the next one, blending sounds or syllables so that some sounds and/or syllables are deleted (this is also referred to as telescoping). This is likely a consequence of the speaker speaking at a rate that is too fast for their system to handle.[8] However, additional speech disorders might cause this lack of clarity. To differentiate a severe articulation or phonological disorder from cluttering, the clinician must consider, for example, whether the client is dropping syllables due to a phonological disorder (e.g., weak syllable deletion and/or final consonant deletion) or over-coarticulation. The clinician must also consider whether speech errors or distortions are due to apraxia of speech, dysarthria, or perhaps a severe vocalic /r/ distortion, as all these disorders can impact intelligibility.

An important distinction the clinician must consider during an assessment is that if a client's over-coarticulation is due to cluttering, then decreasing the rate by inserting natural pauses will eliminate or significantly reduce symptoms. Although reducing rate should also decrease some of the symptoms of dysarthria and/or apraxia of speech, the motor patterns exhibited by these disorders will remain. Additionally, even with a reduced rate, phonological disorders and/or articulation errors will continue to be present on a fairly consistent basis. Unlike other speech sound disorders, with cluttering decreased intelligibility will often be correlated with an increased rate rather than with the ability to correctly produce specific sounds or words. This is not to say that those who clutter may not have words that they find difficult to produce (often multisyllabic words), but rather that this correlation links more to rate than to the ability to correctly produce specific words or sounds.

The clinician should also rule out any type of resonance issue, such as cul-de-sac resonance. Resonance issues are *not* characteristic of cluttering and should be differentiated from cluttering as a cause of decreased intelligibility. Such issues are related to differences in the structure and/or function of the velopharyngeal mechanism. In those instances, evaluation by a craniofacial team is warranted.

16.2.5 Atypical Pauses

Atypical pauses are those which occur in places not expected syntactically. It has been suggested that people who clutter do not pause as much as typical speakers.[14] Therefore, if they speak past the point of natural pauses, when they finally do pause, the pauses are likely to occur in linguistically atypical places. The clinician should ensure that such pauses are not caused by avoidance or anticipation of stuttering or word finding and/or language formulation problems. ▶ Fig. 16.1 summarizes the key differential diagnosis procedures that need to be considered when assessing cluttering.

16.2.6 Co-occurring Symptoms/ Disorders

As previously indicated, cluttering commonly co-occurs with other diagnoses, such as attention deficit hyperactivity disorder, receptive/expressive language disorder, speech sound disorder, autism spectrum disorder, stuttering, and/or learning disorders.[15] Thus, it is important to evaluate and consider these diagnoses in addition to cluttered speech. Clinicians should conduct a comprehensive assessment of other speech and language skills (e.g., language, articulation, pragmatics, etc.)

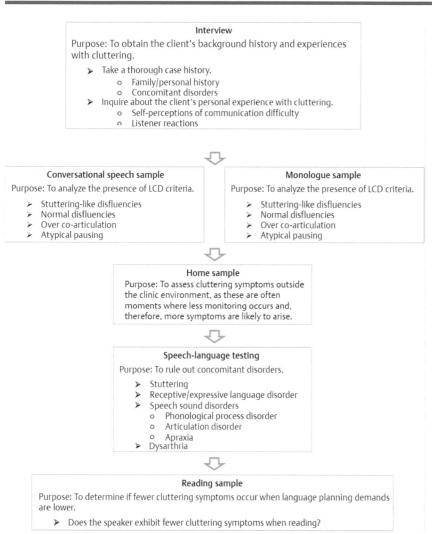

Fig. 16.1 Evaluation procedures. (This image is provided courtesy of Paula Thomson.)

using norm-referenced standardized tests or informal measures to identify coexisting symptoms/disorders that may also require treatment.

It is important to understand the potential interaction between cluttering and other coexisting disorders. For example, when a person who clutters speaks at a rate that is faster than their system can handle, cluttering is triggered. If someone who stutters and clutters speeds up to avoid stuttering, they often end up speaking at a rate that is faster than their system can handle, thereby triggering cluttering. Therefore, the root "trigger" for the increased speed in this case is avoidance of stuttering. On the other hand, some individuals who both stutter and clutter state that if they begin to clutter, they may feel increased pressure to speak fluently and clearly, resulting in increased stuttering.[16] When there is overlap of symptoms in these ways, this should be taken into consideration in intervention. A summary of differential diagnostic considerations is outlined in ▶ Table 16.1.

Peter's Evaluation and Results

After the clinician explained the procedures for differentiating cluttering from other disorders, Peter and his parents were ready to pursue the evaluation. To guide the process of differential diagnosis, it was necessary to obtain a detailed case history and to collect speech samples in various contexts.

The clinician began the evaluation by asking Peter how he felt about his speech. Peter said that he was frustrated that others could not understand him. Even though he had told his parents the opposite, he told the clinician that others asked him to repeat frequently, and he really did not understand why. He felt misunderstood by his teacher, who told him he needed to slow down. Peter felt annoyed and discouraged by this feedback and said that sometimes it was easier to avoid speaking in certain situations.

A conversational sample was taken to analyze for the presence of stuttering-like disfluencies, NDs, over-coarticulation, and/or atypical pausing. Peter was asked to speak about baseball, since he was passionate about this topic and research has shown that monologues tend to elicit more moments of over-coarticulation in school-age children who clutter.[17] Peter did not exhibit stuttering, and both he and his parents denied any family history of stuttering. Peter recalled that his articulation treatment in elementary school focused on the production of /r/. At that time, the clinician had concluded that Peter had symptoms that made her initially consider a language disorder, such as multiple revisions, but he never qualified for services based on the results of standardized testing.

Peter currently scored within the average range on an articulation test, as well as on tests examining word finding and language organization. Peter's parents provided a sample of Peter's

Table 16.1 Key differential diagnosis procedures to consider when assessing for possible cluttering

Potential cluttering symptom	Other things to rule out	What to ask in history and/or interview with client/family	What to test in evaluation
Nonstuttering disfluencies (revisions, interjections, restarts)	• Language disorder • Avoiding stuttering • Trying to find a word due to bi-/multilingualism	• Any history of language disorder? • Any history of stuttering? • Does the client speak other languages? How proficient is the client in the other language(s)?	• Tests focusing on word finding and language organization • Monologue speech sample to subjectively evaluate efficiency of message and stuttering versus nonstuttering disfluencies
Over-coarticulation	• Articulation disorder • Apraxia of speech/ dysarthria	• Does the client have difficulty articulating sounds? • Is there a history of apraxia of speech? Any history of neurological disorder? • When client slows rate, is the speech clear, or not completely clear?	• Articulation tests and tests of apraxia or dysarthria if suspected • Have client speak with and without pauses to evaluate impact of adjusting rate on overall clarity
Atypical pauses	• Stopping to avoid stuttering on a word • Stopping to think of a word or way to say something	• Any history of stuttering? • Any difficulty finding words or organizing thoughts?	• Checklists/surveys/interviews about speech, possible avoidance of stuttering • Objective testing of word finding and language organization • Subjective evaluation of efficiency of message in language samples

conversational speech, prerecorded before the evaluation. The clinician explained that this sample was important, since in-clinic samples may not always show the symptoms of cluttering. The clinician also asked Peter's parents if there was a family history of rapid rate and/or unclear speech. Peter's mother recalled that her brother had a speech pattern where others were constantly asking him to repeat what he said or asking him to stop mumbling. She now wondered whether Peter's uncle had cluttering as well.

Peter was asked to read a passage at a rapid rate, during which over-coarticulation was evidenced. The clinician then presented Peter with the same reading passage marked with vertical slashes at commas and periods to indicate where he should pause. With the natural pauses inserted, over-coarticulation was no longer a symptom, and Peter's speech became clear. When asked to discuss baseball, Peter exhibited multiple phrase and word repetitions without tension. The clinician concluded that these NDs sounded "excessive" because it took Peter much longer to get his point across than if he did not exhibit so many NDs. When shown how to include natural pauses in a second monologue, Peter exhibited only a few NDs. Peter exhibited several instances of atypical pauses during conversation and a monologue, but these also abated when Peter used natural pausing.

At this point, Peter's speech fit the required criteria of rapid-sounding rate and all three breakdowns in intelligibility (either of speech or of message): excessive over-coarticulation, an excessive number of NDs, and atypical pausing. None of these symptoms were present all the time in Peter's speech; rather, they presented themselves at different times in various speaking contexts. At times, a combination of symptoms (i.e., "clusters"), such as an excessive number of NDs and over-coarticulation, was noted, as has been documented in speakers who clutter.[18]

Upon gathering the diagnostic information just described, the clinician compared Peter's history and his speech samples to the LCD definition. This is the most basic way to diagnose cluttering. In addition to the basics presented above, a variety of additional tools can help with identifying cluttering symptoms.

Once the clinician feels comfortable diagnosing cluttering according to the LCD symptoms, he or she may want to consider using these additional tools (see ▶ Table 16.2). These tools, however, should not be used as the sole means of diagnosing cluttering, especially considering that most, if not all, of the characteristics identified in these tools may not be present in all people who clutter. Rather, when combined with a thorough examination of the core features of cluttering under the LCD definition, these tools should be used to help the clinician identify concomitant characteristics. Additionally, having a better understanding of these other characteristics, if present, may inform treatment planning, as will be discussed later in this chapter.

16.2.7 Patterns of LCD Symptoms

To design better treatment, it is important to identify patterns among those who clutter. The clinician should consider which cluttering symptoms are most predominant and, therefore, need to be prioritized in treatment. In addition to rapid-sounding speech, many people who clutter present with (1) overarticulation, (2) excessive NDs, or (3) a combination of both, with one pattern predominant. Understanding the patterns will drive treatment decisions. For more information on differentiating between "motor" and "sensory" cluttering subtypes, see Ward,[9] and for "syntactic" and "phonological" cluttering subtypes, see van Zaalen et al.[19,20] For testimony by people who clutter about their experiences with syntactic and phonological subtypes of cluttering, see Exum et al.[16]

Discussion of Peter's Evaluation Results

After the evaluation, Peter and his parents met with the clinician to discuss the findings. Although Peter's mother was relieved to have a definitive diagnosis for her son, Peter's father was still skeptical about the diagnosis. "How much do we really understand about this disorder of cluttering anyway? What research is there to back it up? And what are the options for treatment?"

Table 16.2 Additional assessment measures for cluttering

Cluttering Assessment Program (CLASP)[61]	• Determines a speaker's talking time versus duration of cluttering • Assesses duration of cluttering episodes as well as cluttering severity by calculating the percentage of cluttering within overall speaking time • Free downloadable software program created by Bakker[61]
Fluency Assessment Battery (FAB)[19]	• Comprehensive instrument designed to evaluate speech fluency, rate, and intelligibility • Assesses structure during reading, spontaneous speech, and story retelling • Phonological and diadochokinetic tasks measure the ability of speakers to produce multisyllabic phrases accurately, smoothly, and at an appropriate rate
Predictive Cluttering Inventory (PCI)[62]	• Assesses characteristics associated with speech (i.e., "speech motor") and concomitant symptoms (i.e., "pragmatics," "language and cognition," "motor coordination and writing problems," etc.)
Checklist of Cluttering and Associated Features (COCAF-4)[9]	• Assesses through a checklist, which, in addition to lowest common denominator (LCD) features (e.g., speech rate and speech fluency), includes some nonspeech features in the areas of attention, language, motor control, and writing
Overall Assessment of the Speaker's Evaluation of Stuttering (OASES)[63]	• Assesses life impact for individuals who stutter (for e.g., anxiety). This test is currently being modified for those who clutter; in the meantime, OASES can be used to gather life impact of cluttering
Brief Cluttering and Stuttering Questionnaire (BSQ)[19]	• Assesses clients who present with a combination of stuttering and cluttering, focusing on the impact of each disorder to determine priorities for intervention planning • Ten-question semi-structured interview designed to assist the clinician in better understanding clients

Source: Table design by Paula Thomson.

Table 16.3 Web-based resources for cluttering

International Cluttering Association	• https://sites.google.com/view/icacluttering/home
Too Fast for Words	• https://toofastforwords.com/
The Stuttering Homepage	• https://web.mnsu.edu/comdis/kuster/stutter.html
Facebook Cluttering Speech Group	• https://www.facebook.com/groups/56339307698
Stuttering Foundation	• https://www.stutteringhelp.org/
International Fluency Association	• https://www.theifa.org/
American Speech-Language-Hearing Association	• https://www.asha.org/
International Stuttering Association	• https://www.isastutter.org/
Mindfulness Assessment: Five Facet Mindfulness Questionnaire (FFMQ), Mindful Attention Awareness Scale (MAAS), Child and Adolescent Mindfulness Measure (CAMM), etc.	• https://www.ruthbaer.com/academics/index.html

Source: Table design by Paula Thomson.

16.3 Cluttering Research: Past and Present

Much of the early cluttering research has suffered from various methodological shortcomings. A special edition of the *Journal of Fluency Disorders*, published in 1996, featured articles relating solely to the cluttering disorder, and included discussions on its characteristics, diagnosis, assessment, and treatment. Upon reviewing this edition, Richard Curlee[21] called for "more systematic, better controlled research." Specific flaws were identified in many of the studies, including a lack of consensus in defining cluttering, the inclusion of participants who had both cluttering and other disorders, and small sample sizes. Although progress had been made in cluttering research,[22] more progress was clearly needed.

The call for progress was taken seriously. Over the last 25 years, cluttering has, indeed, gained more attention, as more studies focusing solely on cluttering have been published. Publications about fluency disorders have more commonly been including information about cluttering. In 2007, the First World Conference on Cluttering was held in Bulgaria in honor of Deso Weiss. This conference brought together, for the first time, researchers, clinicians, and people who clutter, and resulted in the creation of the International Cluttering Association. The association has been instrumental in spreading awareness about the symptoms, prevalence, diagnosis, and treatment of cluttering around the world, taking significant steps to end the long-standing era when cluttering was considered an "orphan"[1] in the field of speech-language pathology.[23] They also continue to address challenges in the field of cluttering, such as further refining the cluttering definition.[24] See ▸ Table 16.3 for web-based resources focused on cluttering awareness (see also Further Readings).

With a more streamlined definition of cluttering, research methodology has improved. And objective data continue to be collected and analyzed, improving our understanding of differential diagnosis (e.g., cluttering vs. stuttering), cluttering characteristics (e.g., speech rate and rate variability),[7,20,25] the topography of cluttering moments,[18] and the neural correlates of cluttering.[26] These studies represent a start to improved cluttering research, yet more replication is needed to draw firm conclusions.

There are still challenges in conducting cluttering research. For example, it is difficult to examine "pure" cluttering because few participants exhibit cluttering with no other diagnoses.

This leads to a catch-22: we need larger sample sizes to have enough power to find statistically significant effects (if present), but the larger the sample, the more likely it is that the participants will have one or more concomitant diagnoses.[27] We must also be cautious in defining cluttering too broadly so that we do not overdiagnose, but at the same time, it should be broad enough so as to not overlook clients who have cluttering. Cluttering research and theory must continue to overcome these challenges.

16.4 Treatment Options for Cluttering

Just as we used the LCD definition to identify the mandatory symptoms of cluttering, so too can we use it to develop a plan to treat cluttering symptoms. As a perceived rapid and/or irregular speech rate is the primary criterion for a cluttering diagnosis,[6] rate is a primary area to address.[8] Treatment of speech rate means first increasing awareness and then implementing strategies to regulate rate. At the same time, direct work on over-coarticulation may be needed. For long-term success, working on self-regulation in increasingly complex environments is needed. One option to consider in treatment is the "synergistic approach,"[28] which means that working on one area of cluttering will decrease symptoms in another area. For example, pausing may help reduce both the symptoms of over-coarticulation and an excessive number of NDs. In the same manner, by emphasizing sounds and syllables, a client may reduce their speech rate, which could, in turn, reduce other cluttering symptoms. Finally, working on symptoms of co-occurring disorders that might have an impact on the efficiency of communication should be considered. We will elaborate on these treatment options in the following sections.

16.4.1 Treatment of LCD Symptoms

Speech Rate Awareness and Regulation

Treatment for cluttering has generally focused on helping clients regulate their speech rate.[28,29,30,31,32] There are many ways in which this can be accomplished. For example, clients can insert natural pauses into their speech[33] or use pacing devices and/or analogies (e.g., slowing down when driving on a curvy road).[9,30] In a case study examining the use of pausing and overemphasis in articulation in a teenager, both strategies were found to reduce symptoms of over-coarticulation, although pausing was used more often in carryover than overemphasis.[34] Placing pauses in natural places may eliminate the symptom of atypical pausing. However, some people with cluttering who have atypical pauses may be unaware of the grammatical rules for where pauses should naturally occur in sentences. These individuals may benefit from a review of the grammatical rules for more natural pause placement during conversational speech.

To work on speech rate and other LCD symptoms, a client must have awareness of these symptoms. Active self-monitoring is often difficult for many people who clutter, resulting in a failure to notice specific symptoms of cluttering as they occur. Although in some cases, such as Peter's, there is a general lack of awareness, in others there is *general awareness* but a lack of awareness

of *specific* moments of cluttering.[35] Being aware of one's speech rate and/or lack of clarity can improve communication effectiveness, as the speaker can quickly repair breakdowns when they occur.[33]

In clinical settings, we can observe improved speech clarity when clients increase levels of effortful attention to their speech. Awareness of fast articulatory rate or inadequate speech clarity can be taught by integrating "contrasting exercises," in which the client is first asked to contrast an extremely fast and an extremely slow speech rate, and then identify speech rates that fall in between extremely fast and extremely slow. As the person who clutters becomes more aware of how fast or how unclear their speech feels, they become more aware of these symptoms during conversations, allowing them to repair cluttering moments. It is also important to teach clients to become knowledgeable about the symptoms that tend to trigger their cluttering, so that they can proactively monitor their speech rate and clarity, as discussed below.

The clinician can have people who clutter record themselves speaking using a mobile phone, iPad, or other electronic devices to increase awareness both within and beyond the clinical setting. These recordings can document progress and management over time. Audio recordings can also be used in awareness training. This method can be aversive for some clients at first, so it should be introduced gradually when needed. For example, with audio-visual feedback training using Praat software, clients learn how to monitor their speech, visually represented as a waveform, for rate, fluency, pitch, and prosody, as well as pause placement and duration. The effectiveness of this training was evaluated in a recent study.[36] Findings indicated that participants not only improved their speech, language, and monitoring skills but also became more confident and satisfied with their interactional skills.[36]

People who clutter may have difficulty with the perception of their speech rate.[8,37] Helping people with cluttering gain insight that they may perceive their speech rate differently than the listener may help them see the importance of improving their monitoring skills during practice. For example, even though the person who clutters may perceive their rate to be "extremely slow," this impression may not mirror the listener's perception. It may be helpful for clients to consider speech rate as falling on a 10-point scale, with 1 being too slow, 5 "just right," and 10 too fast.[15] Clients can practice speaking at a slightly slower than average rate (e.g., a 3 or 4 on the 10-point scale) in the clinic, and then work toward regulating rate, with the ultimate goal being for them to use an average rate in everyday speaking situations. Keeping the overall concept the same, the range along the 10-point scale can be adjusted to the clinician's preference, such as from 1 to 6.[38,39]

Some experts believe that difficulties with speech monitoring may be related to inconsistent eye contact.[15] Although some adult clients do not like to be interrupted and asked to repeat words, other clients have said, "I really wish they would just tell me that my speech is unclear." Thus, the speaker may not always receive the feedback they need to repair breakdowns in conversation. In these situations, tuning in to subtle (and often unconscious) signals from the listener about a communication breakdown necessitates steady eye contact. Yet even when their pragmatic skills are within normal limits, we have found that many people who clutter may not maintain consistent eye

Table 16.4 Treatment technique: options for approaching a speaking situation

Proactive	Reactive
Definition: using strategies in specific, challenging situations where an individual may clutter	Definition: using strategies predominantly when a moment of cluttering occurs
Example(s): presentations, formal speaking situations, large gatherings	Example(s): applying the strategy to a moment of cluttering within conversation
Being *proactive* in using strategies, having an established communication plan	Being *reactive* in using strategies, having a plan on the "backburner"

Source: Table design by Paula Thomson.

contact. Difficulty maintaining eye contact may be manifested for a variety of reasons: (1) not feeling confident as a communicator due to prior negative experiences, (2) being uncomfortable with making and/or maintaining eye contact, and (3) having difficulty organizing thoughts while also maintaining eye contact. Learning to proactively initiate eye contact while speaking will help the speaker "catch" confusion on the listener's face sooner rather than later, which allows them to make the appropriate repair before the speaker gets too far into the conversation.[33] On the other hand, some people who clutter are acutely aware of listener feedback, noticing things such as the listener moving closer to them and/or looking intently at their mouth when speaking. Nevertheless, if they are unaware that the listener is having difficulty following them, increasing eye contact may help them to become more proactive in repairing communication breakdowns. A summary of the proactive and reactive approaches to managing speech is outlined in ▶ Table 16.4.

NDs and Over-Coarticulation

Although excessive NDs and over-coarticulation may abate with rate regulation and/or pausing alone, some clients need more direct work. If excessive NDs do not decrease with rate regulation alone, the clinician should consider targeting language organization. Although pausing to regulate speech rate may reduce or eliminate over-coarticulation for some speakers, others may continue to have difficulty with over-coarticulation if they rush the words in between the pauses. To increase clarity of speech when over-coarticulation difficulties remain, clients can be taught to emphasize sounds, syllables, and/or words by focusing on clear and accurate productions of the (1) overall phrase or sentence, (2) first few words of a sentence, and/or (3) last few sounds of a word (e.g., emphasizing consonant blends at the ends of words, such as "st" in "first" or "last" and "nt" in "can't" or "don't").

16.4.2 Improving Self-Regulation

Once the person who clutters becomes more aware of their fast speech rate and accompanying symptoms of excessive NDs, over-coarticulation, and/or atypical pauses, they must work toward regulating their speech in everyday speaking situations. Just as stuttering treatment may involve the simulation of moments of stuttering, cluttering treatment may include simulating moments of cluttering.[15] Part of the goal of simulation in stuttering treatment is to desensitize the individual who stutters to the moment of stuttering. The goal of simulating moments of cluttering, on the other hand, is to help the person

who clutters to concentrate on how it *feels* to increase speaking rate, over-coarticulate, and/or produce excessive NDs. The objective in simulating and identifying cluttering, along with practicing repair strategies, is to help the client learn how to: (1) identify when these moments occur earlier during real-life speaking situations and (2) react to these moments by adjusting their speech (e.g., adding pauses, overemphasizing sounds) in a way that does not interfere with ongoing communication.

In more recent years, mindfulness-based approaches have been shown to be helpful in the therapeutic setting, including stuttering therapy.[40,41,42,43,44,45,46] Due to the connection between mindfulness, self-awareness, and self-regulation, the assessment of self-awareness in individuals who clutter may be beneficial for treatment planning and maintenance. Based on the Western conceptualization of mindfulness and the work of Baer,[40] mindfulness involves intentionally focusing on one's internal and external experiences in the present moment. We have chosen to use the concept broadly, with the intention of cultivating awareness or focusing attention to thoughts, feelings, and sensations as they arise. Several questionnaires designed to measure mindfulness or related variables have been developed and may be downloaded at no cost (▶ Table 16.3). We have found that introducing and implementing awareness-based exercises to increase awareness and communication skills can be helpful for people who clutter.[38,39] In a recent study,[47] it was found that mindfulness indirectly targeted the self-regulation skills of a person with cluttering. Future research of awareness-based approaches with larger samples of individuals who clutter is needed.

16.4.3 Treatment of Concomitant Symptoms/Disorders

If language organization difficulties are identified by standardized testing and/or by observing symptoms subjectively, then work on those symptoms is warranted. Further, since cluttering and stuttering frequently co-occur, it is important for the clinician to understand how to treat both disorders. For example, if a client with stuttering and cluttering is speeding up to hide stuttering and this triggers their cluttering, as previously discussed, it would be important to prioritize work on avoidance and address negative thoughts and feelings about stuttering. Considering that stuttering moments often occur after pauses, and pauses are frequently used to regulate rate in cluttering, people with both disorders may need to be taught how to manage moments of stuttering after pauses using stuttering modification strategies (see ▶ Chapters 11 and 12).

Although they may not have the same pragmatic deficits as others with communication disorders, such as in autism spectrum disorder, people who clutter may not provide all the relevant information needed for listeners to understand them during communication exchanges.[48] These clients may, therefore, benefit from working on how to better communicate from a linguistic and/or social point of view. In a dyad, both partners must be able to notice and interpret nonverbal signals, body language, and vocal information that signal when messages are unclear.

16.4.4 Treatment of Affective and Cognitive Components of Cluttering

Communication with people who clutter brings to the fore their emotional reactions to the challenges they experience when interacting with the people around them. The first empirical studies.[49,58] examining affective and cognitive aspects of cluttering were conducted using qualitative research (a semi-structured interview). People who clutter reported feelings of frustration, shame, sadness, fear, and avoidance of certain social situations in response to their cluttering. They also described having difficulty accepting their disorder and had to learn how to deal with the consequences.

Many famous neural scientists have demonstrated that the mind consists of thoughts and emotions, which work together to influence reasoning and decision-making processes. An understanding of the link between thinking and feeling is needed to succeed in stuttering and cluttering intervention.[50] Bar-On's[51] emotional intelligence model can provide clinicians with the tools to address any feelings of sadness, frustration, and incompetence, and self-defeating thoughts that an individual who clutters may experience. Reichel[50] adapted five of Bar-On's emotional intelligence competencies to benefit individuals who clutter: (1) emotional self-awareness, (2) impulse control, (3) reality testing, (4) empathy, and (5) interpersonal relationships. These competencies can help people with cluttering to enhance their awareness of emotions and communication behaviors, become self-controlled, assess situations realistically, resolve conflicts in interpersonal relationships, and consider the feelings and reactions of listeners to their speech.

16.4.5 Cluttering and the Working Alliance

The concept of the working alliance has its roots in psychodynamic theory. Bordin[52] described the "working alliance" as the degree to which the client and clinician are engaged in collaborative, purposeful work. Bordin's model of the working alliance includes the dimensions of therapy goals, therapy tasks, and the bond between client and clinician. We believe that clinicians who are effective in forming alliances with persons who clutter may have better therapy outcomes. The establishment of a strong *working alliance*, in which the client and clinician develop an emotional bond and work together to develop treatment goals and tasks, can go a long way toward facilitating change.[52] This may be particularly important to cluttering treatment. That is, therapy should focus on providing a clear rationale for the joint selection of treatment tasks, and these tasks should be assessed and integrated into what really matters for each person.[53,54] As with any communication disorder, the clinician

needs to be sensitive to each individual client's profile, needs, values, motivation, and responses.

Keep in mind, however, that the preferences and goals of individuals who clutter may become clearer with improvements in self-awareness and self-regulation throughout therapy.[54] The treatment may also be influenced by unique intrapersonal and contextual factors. Therefore, the clinician should be open to a continued dialogue about the need for goal revision throughout treatment.

16.5 Future Directions in Cluttering

As mentioned earlier, progress has been made in better understanding the nature and treatment of cluttering. Today speech-language pathology students are receiving more information about cluttering in their fluency courses than they did even 10 years ago. This is remarkable considering that at one time experts would not even acknowledge the existence of cluttering as a valid diagnostic category.

Despite this progress, more work needs to be done. This can begin by educating the public to recognize the signs and symptoms of cluttering, and where to go for diagnostic evaluation and treatment. While getting the consumer to professionals who can evaluate and differentially diagnose cluttering from other communication disorders is one challenge, making clinicians more knowledgeable about cluttering is another. Many myths surround cluttering, and as long as these myths persist, clinicians will face uncertainty about how to diagnose and treat cluttering.

Based on survey studies, most schools of higher education provide weak academic preparation and limited clinical training in cluttering. Most university faculty report that cluttering is addressed in less than 2 hours in fluency disorders courses, which is considerably less than what most other communication disorders receive.[55] Clearly there is a need for more time spent on cluttering.[56]

In fact, some university programs in various countries (e.g., Germany, Hungary, Israel, the Netherlands, Norway, Russia, United States, etc.) have dedicated courses in cluttering. As awareness of cluttering and its pernicious consequences on communication, social interactions, and quality of life has increased, establishing independent courses in cluttering—or at least teaching more than what is currently being taught in most universities—becomes imperative.[56,57]

Peter's Treatment: Addressing all Aspects of Cluttering
Peter and his parents felt that the clinician answered all their questions about cluttering, and they were ready to commit to treatment. Because Peter reported that he did not think there was anything wrong, the clinician began by talking about communication breakdowns in general, rather than his own communication.[33] This "normalizing" approach helped Peter break his defensiveness toward examining his speech. Eventually, Peter noticed more and more when communication breakdowns occurred in his own speech. Peter learned that to avoid misunderstanding, it is necessary to repair communication breakdowns, and that this is done by speakers every day. Peter learned to use strategies that involve natural communication, rather than feeling different. In this way, the treatment changed from "fixing"

the problem to building confidence in his ability to communicate efficiently and effectively with others.[33]

As Peter began treatment, his clinician asked him about previous strategies he tried and how they worked. Peter indicated that he had been uncomfortable with the exercises he did with his previous clinician because he did not understand how they could help. He said that he had practiced "tongue twisters," but he could not explain why they did this. Peter and his new clinician proceeded to work on natural strategies such as pausing to regulate rate, emphasizing all sounds and syllables, and tuning in to listener feedback. Peter learned to proactively look for communication breakdowns and repair these breakdowns in natural ways, such as by inserting more typical pauses when he found himself speaking too quickly. As the clinician developed a rapport with Peter, Peter revealed more about his feelings. He said that in the course of their work together, he had become increasingly aware of his speech difficulties. Peter's mother had told him that she now thought his uncle was a person with cluttering and encouraged Peter to speak with him. Peter and his uncle had a talk about their speech. Peter's uncle spoke of times in his life when others asked him if he was "stupid" or "drunk" and/or told him to "stop mumbling." Peter's uncle felt he had not been considered for a promotion at work, despite his qualifications, due to his poor communication skills. He never had a diagnosis, and never understood why others judged him so negatively. As a result of this discussion, Peter's uncle began to seriously consider seeking an evaluation himself. Peter said that this talk made him realize the extent to which he had been hiding the frustration and anxiety he had been feeling about his speech for years.

Talking with Peter's Previous School Clinician

The clinician asked Peter for permission to contact the school clinician who had worked with Peter in the past. When the current clinician told the former school clinician about the cluttering diagnosis, the former clinician said, "Oh that makes sense. You know I often wondered if Peter cluttered. However, I really didn't learn much about fluency disorders in graduate school, let alone cluttering. And, working in a school, I see about two cases of stuttering a year. So, I don't feel confident about my work with fluency disorders." The current clinician said she understood and suggested that the school clinician consider continuing education in fluency disorders. The school clinician responded, "I think about this all the time. However, it has often been difficult for me to justify using my continuing education on fluency disorders when I have so many clients in language and articulation. I will consider it, though." The school clinician went on to say that she had considered cluttering as a potential diagnosis for Peter, but discounted it after her colleague had said,

"Well, he doesn't sound fast all of the time, does he?" The school clinician was unaware that many who clutter do so only situationally. She also said that she considered a cluttering diagnosis for a different student, but she again discounted it when the student's mother came to school one Monday morning saying, "He didn't do it all weekend." Peter's clinician asked, "Well, if you had a client with an articulation disorder that only occurred in certain contexts, and the parent didn't see any of those contexts over the weekend, would you declassify the child of the articulation disorder?" "Ooooh," the school clinician responded. "I never thought of it that way."

Peter's clinician went through the LCD definition of cluttering with the school clinician, showing her how the mandatory criterion is perceived rapid rate rather than measured rapid rate, and how cluttering does not have to occur in all situations to be diagnosed. The school clinician also admitted that she would have a hard time working with Peter because he did not acknowledge that he had a communication disorder, and therefore, even if he did have a disorder, there was no functional impact on his communication or quality of life. The clinician acknowledged that Peter often said he was not impacted by his speech. However, when examining his frustration about others asking him to repeat and/or to slow down, it seemed that Peter was, in fact, negatively impacted by his fast and unintelligible speech. The clinician indicated that formal checklists measuring the impact of cluttering on a speaker are under development. Additionally, Peter's clinician told the school clinician about a study in which adults who clutter were interviewed about their experience living with cluttering.[58] One theme that emerged from this study was that when the adults were teens, they did not want to acknowledge that cluttering was an issue. It eventually took someone outside of their family, such as a supervisor at work or school, to tell them that their communication needed to be improved. This was the trigger that finally inspired them to look for treatment. Thus, Peter's behavior is typical for someone who clutters, especially teens.[16,59,61]

16.6 Conclusions

Has there been a great deal of progress regarding the field of cluttering? Yes. Is there much further to go? Yes. Educating the public and clinicians to identify the disorder and conducting well-controlled research to examine the characteristics of cluttering are still needed. As a future or current clinician or researcher interested in cluttering, we thank you for learning more. As this chapter illustrates (see ▶ Table 16.5 for a summary of the key points), people like Peter and his family are

Table 16.5 Summary of key points

- To be classified as a person who clutters, the individual must meet the criteria listed in the lowest common denominator (LCD) definition
- An individual who clutters may not necessarily exhibit symptoms of cluttering in all speaking situations
- Formal assessment measures should not be the only tools used to diagnose cluttering
- Self-regulation of speech rate and intelligibility are successful treatment strategies for individuals who clutter when combined with other strategies
- Treatment strategies fall into two categories: proactive and reactive. Proactive strategies are used when a speaker wants to monitor full-time to avoid a communication breakdown, while reactive strategies are used to respond to and manage moments of cluttering without constant monitoring
- As in all areas of fluency treatment, a working alliance allows for more productive teamwork to help the client manage cluttering
- Cluttering research continues to advance as awareness of cluttering increases and the definition tightens

Source: Table design by Paula Thomson.

eagerly awaiting your knowledge to help them to overcome challenges related to cluttering, and to clear the path for marching triumphantly along an ever-widening road to successful communication.

16.7 Definitions

Atypical pause: A pause in speaking that is not within grammatical boundaries.

Cluttering: A fluency disorder characterized by a rapid- and/or irregular-sounding rate of speech and breakdown in intelligibility in at least one of the following three areas: excessive normal disfluencies, excessive over co-articulation, and/or excessive atypical pauses.

Emotional intelligence: There are two contrasting models of emotional intelligence. First, the *ability model* focuses on the emotional and cognitive relationship and is comprised of four categories: the ability to perceive emotions, the ability to use emotions to facilitate thought, the ability to understand emotions, and the ability to manage emotions. Second, the *mixed model* combines mental abilities with other characteristics of a person, such as motivational and interpersonal qualities, similar to personality traits.

Mindfulness: Mindfulness involves intentionally bringing one's attention to the internal and external experiences occurring in the present moment.

Over-coarticulation: When sounds or syllables are blended in excess so that to the listener, syllables or sounds are perceived as deleted and/or collapsed. Also known as telescoping.

Self-regulation: The ability to monitor and control one's speech rate and/or clarity.

Speech awareness: Knowledge of how one's speech is coming across in terms of clarity of message and words.

Working alliance: The working alliance represents a proactive collaboration of a client and a clinician and includes three processes: the emotional bond, the agreement on the goal of treatment, and the extent to which the client and clinician consider the treatment tasks as relevant.

References

[1] Weiss D. Cluttering. Englewood Cliffs, NJ: Prentice-Hall; 1964

[2] Luchsinger R. Poltern. Charlottenburg, DE: Manhold Verlag; 1963

[3] St. Louis KO, Myers F, Bakker K, Raphael L. Understanding and treating cluttering. In: Conture E, Curlee R, eds. Stuttering and Related Disorders of Fluency. 3rd ed. New York, NY: Thieme; 2007

[4] St. Louis KO. On defining cluttering. In: Myers FL, St. Louis KS, eds. Cluttering: A Clinical Perspective. Kibworth, UK: Far Communications; 1992:37–53

[5] St. Louis KO. A tabular summary of cluttering subjects in the special edition. J Fluency Disord. 1996; 2:337–343

[6] St. Louis KO, Schulte K. Defining cluttering: the lowest common denominator. In: Ward D, Scaler Scott K, eds. Cluttering: Research, Intervention and Education. East Sussex, UK: Psychology Press; 2011

[7] Kisenwether J, Scaler Scott K, Williams S, Moon R, Postiglione S. An alternative rate of speech measure for individuals who clutter. Poster presented at the Joint World Congress of the International Cluttering Association (ICA), International Fluency Association (IFA), and International Stuttering Association (ISA), Hiroshima, Japan, July 13, 2018

[8] Bakker K, Myers FL, Raphael LJ, St. Louis KO. A preliminary comparison of speech rate, self-evaluation, and disfluency of people who speak exceptionally fast, clutter, or speak normally. In: Ward D, Scaler Scott K, eds. Cluttering: Research, Intervention and Education. East Sussex, UK: Psychology Press; 2011

[9] Ward D. Stuttering and cluttering: frameworks for understanding and treatment. 2nd ed. New York: NY. Psychology Press; 2017

[10] Van Zaalen Y, Reichel I. Prevalence of cluttering in two European countries: a pilot study. Perspect ASHA Spec Interest Groups. 2017; 2:42–49

[11] Van Borsel J, Vandermeulen A. Cluttering in Down syndrome. Folia Phoniatr Logop. 2008; 60(6):312–317

[12] Kissagizlis P. An interview with Peter Kissagizlis: cluttering and me. Paper presented at the International Stuttering Online Conference, Mankato, MN, April 14–May 5, 2010. Available at: https://www.mnsu.edu/comdis/ica1/papers/kissagizlisc.html. Accessed May 2, 2020

[13] Wilhelm R. Too Fast for Words: How Discovering that I Don't Stutter but Clutter Changed My Life. Nijmegen, NL: Big Time Publishers; 2020

[14] Scaler Scott K, Harris A, St. Louis KO. Spectrographic features and SLP diagnoses of one sample of cluttering. Poster presented at the Annual Convention of the American Speech-Language Hearing Association, Chicago, IL, November 17, 2018

[15] Scaler Scott K. Fluency Plus: Managing Fluency Disorders in Individuals with Multiple Diagnoses. Thorofare, NJ: SLACK, Inc.; 2018

[16] Exum T, Absalon C, Smith B, Reichel IK. People with cluttering and stuttering have room for success. Paper presented at the International Stuttering Online Conference, Mankato, MN, April 14–May 5, 2010. Available at: https://www.mnsu.edu/comdis/ica1/papers/exumc.html. Accessed May 2, 2020

[17] Scaler Scott K. Cluttering symptoms in school-age children by communicative context: a preliminary investigation. Int J Speech Lang Pathol. 2020; 22(2):174–183

[18] Myers FL, Bakker K, St Louis KO, Raphael LJ. Disfluencies in cluttered speech. J Fluency Disord. 2012; 37(1):9–19

[19] Van Zaalen Y, Reichel IK. Cluttering: current views on its nature, assessment and treatment. Bloomington, IN: iUniverse; 2015

[20] Van Zaalen-Op 't Hof Y, Wijnen F, De Jonckere PH. Differential diagnostic characteristics between cluttering and stuttering: part one. J Fluency Disord. 2009; 34(3):137–154

[21] Curlee R. Cluttering: data in search of understanding. J Fluency Disord. 1996; 21:367–372

[22] Myers F. Annotations of research and clinical perspectives on cluttering since 1964. J Fluency Disord. 1996; 21:187–200

[23] Reichel I. Introduction to the forum on cluttering: rays of hope shine around the world. Perspect ASHA Spec Interest Groups. 2019; 4:1566–1577

[24] Myers F, Bakker K, Cook S, Reichel I, St. Louis K, van Zaalen Y. A clinical conceptualization of cluttering. Committee report: International Cluttering Association Ad-hoc Committee on Defining Cluttering, Columbia, SC, July 30, 2018. Available at: https://sites.google.com/view/icacluttering/home?authuser=0. Accessed May 26, 2021

[25] Van Zaalen Y, Wijnen F, Dejonckere P. Differential diagnostic characteristics between cluttering and stuttering, part two. J Fluency Disord. 2009; 34:146–154

[26] Ward D, Connally EL, Pliatsikas C, Bretherton-Furness J, Watkins KE. The neurological underpinnings of cluttering: some initial findings. J Fluency Disord. 2015; 43:1–16

[27] Scaler Scott K. Quandaries in cluttering: current issues and potential solutions. Paper presented at the Joint World Congress of the International Cluttering Association (ICA), International Fluency Association (IFA), and International Stuttering Association (ISA), Hiroshima, Japan, July 15, 2018

[28] Myers FL, Bradley CL. Clinical management of cluttering from a synergistic framework. In: Myers FL, St. Louis KS, eds. Cluttering: A Clinical Perspective. Kibworth, UK: Far Communications; 1992

[29] St. Louis KO, Raphael LJ, Myers FL, Bakker K. Cluttering updated. ASHA Lead. 2003; 8(21):4–22

[30] Ward D, Scaler Scott K. Cluttering: Research, Intervention and Education. East Sussex, UK: Psychology Press; 2011

[31] Bennett Lanouette E. Intervention strategies for cluttering disorders. In: Ward D, Scaler Scott K, eds. Cluttering: Research, Intervention and Education. East Sussex, UK: Psychology Press; 2011

[32] Myers FL. Treatment of cluttering: a cognitive-behavioral approach centered on rate control. In: Ward D, Scaler Scott K, eds. Cluttering: Research, Intervention and Education. East Sussex, UK: Psychology Press; 2011

[33] Scaler Scott K, Ward D. Managing cluttering: a comprehensive guidebook of activities. Austin, TX: Pro-Ed., Inc.; 2013

[34] Healey K, Nelson S, Scaler Scott K. A case study of cluttering treatment outcomes in a teen. Procedia Soc Behav Sci. 2015; 193:141–146

[35] Van Zaalen Y, Wijnen F, Dejonckere P. The assessment of cluttering: Rationale, tasks, and interpretation. In: Ward D, Scaler Scott K, eds. Cluttering: Research, Intervention and Education. East Sussex, UK: Psychology Press; 2011

[36] Van Zaalen Y, Reichel I. Clinical success using the audio-visual feedback training for cluttering. Perspect Glob Issues Commun Sci Relat Dis. 2019; 4 (6):1589–1594

[37] Garnett EO, St. Louis KO. Verbal time estimation in cluttering. Contemp Issues Commun Sci Disord. 2014; 41:196–209

[38] Hoff K, Sønsterud H. Er det løpsk tale – og hva kan gjøres? Del I [Is it cluttering: and what can we do about it? Part I]. Nor Tidsskr Logop. 2012; 2: 26–33

[39] Hoff K, Sønsterud H. Er det løpsk tale – og hva kan gjøres? Del II [Is it cluttering: and what can we do about it? Part II]. Nor Tidsskr Logop. 2012; 3: 24–29

[40] Baer RA. Mindfulness training as a clinical intervention: a conceptual and empirical review. Clin Psychol. 2003; 10(2):125–143

[41] Boyle MP. Mindfulness training in stuttering therapy: a tutorial for speech-language pathologists. J Fluency Disord. 2011; 36(2):122–129

[42] Plexico LW, Sandage MJ. A mindful approach to stuttering intervention. Perspect Fluen Fluen Disord. 2011; 21(2):43–49

[43] Cheasman C, Simpson S, Everard R. Stammering Therapy from the Inside: New Perspectives on Working with Young People and Adults. Guildford, UK: J&R Press; 2013

[44] Emge G, Pellowski MW. Incorporating a mindfulness meditation exercise into a stuttering treatment program. Comm Disord Q. 2019; 40(2):125–128

[45] Sønsterud H, Halvorsen MS, Feragen KB, Kirmess M, Ward D. What works for whom? Multidimensional individualized stuttering therapy (MIST). J Commun Disord. 2020; 88:106052

[46] Palasik S, Jaime H. The clinical application of acceptance and commitment therapy with clients who stutter. Perspect Fluen Fluen Disord. 2013; 23: 54–69

[47] Littlewood F, Ward D. A mindfulness approach to cluttering therapy: a single case study. Paper presented at the Oxford Dysfluency Conference, Oxford, UK; September 20, 2017

[48] Teigland A. A study of pragmatic skills of clutterers and normal speakers. J Fluency Disord. 1996; 21(3–4):201–214

[49] Van Zaalen Y. Reichel I. A qualitative study on the cognitive and affective aspects of cluttering. Presented at the Joint World Congress of the International Cluttering Association (ICA), International Fluency Association (IFA), and International Stuttering Association (ISA), Hiroshima, Japan, July 16, 2018

[50] Reichel IK. Treating the person who stutters and clutters. Proceedings of the First World Conference on Cluttering, Katarino, Bulgaria, May 12–14, 2010:99–107

[51] Bar-On R. Emotional and social intelligence: insights from the emotional quotient inventory. In: Bar-On R, Parker JDA, eds. The Handbook of Emotional Intelligence: Theory, Development, Assessment, and Application at Home, School, and in the Workplace. San Francisco, CA: Jossey-Bass; 2000

[52] Bordin ES. The generalizability of the psychoanalytic concept of the working alliance. Psychother.. 1979; 16(3):252–260

[53] Sønsterud H, Kirmess M, Howells K, Ward D, Feragen KB, Halvorsen MS. The working alliance in stuttering treatment: a neglected variable? Int J Lang Commun Disord. 2019; 54(4):606–619

[54] Sønsterud H. The importance of the working alliance in the treatment of cluttering. Perspect ASHA Spec Interest Groups. 2019; 4:1568–1572

[55] Scott KS, Grossman HL, Tetnowski JA. A survey of cluttering instruction in fluency courses. Proceedings of the First World Conference on Cluttering, Katarino, Bulgaria, May 12–14, 2010:171–179

[56] Reichel I. Multinational highlights on cluttering curricula. Paper presented at: the International Conference Fluency Disorders: Theory and Practice, Katowice, PL, August 30, 2016

[57] Reichel I, Bakker K. Global landscape on cluttering. Perspect Fluen Fluen Disord. 2009; 19(2):62–66

[58] Scaler Scott K, St. Louis KO. Consumer issues: self-help for people with cluttering. In: Ward D, Scaler Scott K, eds. Cluttering: Research, Intervention and Education. East Sussex, UK: Psychology Press; 2011

[59] Dewey J. My experiences with cluttering. Paper presented at the International Stuttering Online Conference, Mankato, MN, October 22, 2005. Available at: https://www.mnsu.edu/comdis/isad8/papers/dewey8.html. Accessed May 2, 2020

[60] Kvenseth H. Cluttering: Helene's personal experiences. Proceedings of the First World Conference on Cluttering, Katarino, Bulgaria, May 12–14, 2010:50–53

[61] Bakker K, St. Louis KO, Myers F, Raphael L. A freeware software tool for determining aspects of cluttering severity. Poster presented at Annual Convention of the American Speech-Language Hearing Association. San Diego, CA, November 18, 2005

[62] Van Zaalen Y, Wijnen F, Dejonckere PH. The predictive cluttering inventory—Dutch revised, part two. J Fluency Disord. 2009; 34(3):147–154

[63] Yaruss JS, Quesal RW. Overall Assessment of the Speaker's Experience of Stuttering (OASES). McKinney, TX: Stuttering Therapy Resources, Inc.;2016

Further Readings

Scaler Scott K. Fluency plus: managing fluency disorders in individuals with multiple diagnoses. Thorofare, NJ: SLACK, Inc.; 2018

Scaler Scott K, Ward D. Managing Cluttering: A Comprehensive Guidebook of Activities. Austin, TX: Pro-Ed., Inc.; 2013

Van Zaalen Y, Reichel IK. Cluttering: Current Views on Its Nature, Assessment and Treatment. Bloomington, IN: iUniverse; 2015

Ward D. Stuttering and Cluttering: Frameworks for Understanding and Treatment. 2nd ed. New York, NY: Psychology Press; 2017

Ward D, Scaler Scott K. Cluttering: A Handbook of Research, Intervention and Education. New York, NY: Psychology Press; 2011

Wilhelm R. Too Fast for Words: How Discovering that I Don't Stutter but Clutter Changed My Life. Nijmegen, NL: Big Time Publishers; 2020

17 Acquired Stuttering: Etiology, Symptomatology, Identification, and Treatment

Catherine Theys and Luc F. De Nil

Abstract

Although stuttering typically has its onset in early childhood, stuttering speech disfluencies can also develop later in life, most often in adulthood. In this case, they are referred to as acquired stuttering. The most common subtypes of acquired stuttering are acquired neurogenic and functional (psychogenic) stuttering. The onset of acquired neurogenic stuttering is associated with a known or suspected neurological condition. Understanding the nature of this condition, as well as how it may affect speech fluency and other aspects of communication is an important aspect of diagnosis and treatment. In contrast, acquired functional stuttering is associated with traumatic emotional or psychological events, usually in the absence of an underlying neurological disorder. Because of the complex nature of acquired stuttering, clinical intervention needs to start with a comprehensive assessment in order to differentially diagnose the type of stuttering, and to differentiate stuttering from other speech and language disorders that may affect speech fluency, such as apraxia of speech and aphasia. A comprehensive assessment will allow the clinician to plan for the most effective, evidence-based and individualized intervention approach for their clients. After reading this chapter, the clinician will be able to identify the characteristics of acquired stuttering, what important elements to include in an assessment, and the clinical intervention options available to speech-language pathologists.

Keywords: stuttering, acquired stuttering, acquired neurogenic stuttering, acquired functional stuttering, psychogenic stuttering, feigned stuttering, factitious stuttering, malingered stuttering

17.1 Introduction

17.1.1 Definition

Acquired stuttering is a speech fluency disorder that is characterized by an acquired onset of stuttered disfluencies. This short and straightforward definition highlights the most important aspects of this fluency disorder. First, the onset of stuttering is acquired, as opposed to developmental. It most often starts in adulthood, typically in people with no previous history of developmental stuttering. Second, the key speech characteristic is the presence of stuttered disfluencies. These disfluencies include repetitions of sounds, syllables, and monosyllabic words, prolongations, and blocks, and are discussed in more detail in ▶ Chapter 1. Third, it is a speech fluency disorder. The disfluencies are not thought to be due to acquired language formulation problems (i.e., aphasia) and are uncharacteristic of the type of disfluencies that may be associated with other acquired speech disorders such as apraxia of speech or dysarthria, although some people with acquired stuttering will present with co-occurring speech and language problems.

17.1.2 Subtypes

Acquired stuttering is used here as an umbrella term, covering neurogenic, functional (psychogenic), and factitious subtypes of stuttering. In this chapter, we will primarily use the term acquired neurogenic stuttering to refer to stuttering onset following a neurological lesion or disorder. This terminology avoids potential confusion with developmental stuttering, which is increasingly also seen as resulting from atypical brain functioning.[1] In line with current trends in neurological classifications,[2] and as discussed in more detail in the section "Acquired Functional Stuttering," we will use the term acquired functional stuttering for the subtype traditionally referred to as psychogenic stuttering. Finally, we will use the terms factitious stuttering and malingering to refer to cases where an individual deliberately feigns stuttering symptoms. The two latter conditions are defined in ▶ Table 17.1 and are only addressed briefly in this chapter due to the feigned nature of the stuttering disfluencies.[3]

Most of the literature on acquired stuttering consists of case reports, although several studies with larger samples have been published. For this chapter, information on 188 case studies, 362 people from group studies, and 175 people from questionnaire studies was reviewed. Most of the published case studies had a neurogenic onset of stuttering (n = 156, 83%). Functional (psychogenic) stuttering was reported less often (n = 21, 11%). Reports on feigned stuttering were relatively sparse (n = 11, 6%), possibly due to the uncertainties associated with this diagnosis.[4] Therefore, the information presented in this chapter reflects the proportionally larger knowledge base that is available for acquired neurogenic stuttering compared to other subtypes of acquired stuttering.

17.2 Etiology

17.2.1 Acquired Neurogenic Stuttering

Acquired neurogenic stuttering is characterized by the onset of stuttered disfluencies following a neurological event or disease. Stroke is the most common cause of acquired neurogenic stuttering, accounting for half of the reported cases.[5,6] This is followed by traumatic brain injury (TBI) and neurodegenerative diseases.[5,7] Parkinson's disease is the most frequently reported neurodegenerative disease associated with acquired neurogenic stuttering,[8,9] but other neurodegenerative diseases such as Alzheimer's dementia,[10] motor neuron disease,[11] and multiple sclerosis[12] can also result in acquired stuttering. In addition, an acquired onset of stuttering can occur following other neurological conditions such as encephalitis,[13] brain tumours,[14] and epileptic seizures.[15] The onset of acquired neurogenic stuttering has also been reported following surgery for deep brain stimulation, although the reported effects are variable. In most people, the presence or severity of acquired stuttering remains unchanged during deep brain stimulation on and off periods.[16]

Table 17.1 Key definitions

Term	Definition	Synonym
Acquired stuttering	A speech fluency disorder characterized by an acquired onset of stuttering disfluencies	Adult-onset stuttering. This term ignores the fact that acquired stuttering can also occur in younger persons
Acquired neurogenic stuttering	A subtype of acquired stuttering that occurs when the onset of stuttering is related to a neurological event or disease	Neurogenic stuttering. This term does not specifically refer to the acquired onset of dysfluencies
Acquired functional stuttering	A subtype of acquired stuttering that is the result of underlying psychopathological factors, often in response to an emotional trauma.	Psychogenic stuttering. In line with current trends in neurological classifications, the term acquired functional stuttering is now preferred
Factitious stuttering	A subtype of acquired stuttering that occurs when a person intentionally feigns stuttering symptoms in the absence of any obvious external secondary gain. It is considered symptomatic of an underlying psychopathology	Feigned stuttering. This term does not differentiate between factitious and malingered stuttering
Malingered stuttering	A type of stuttering that occurs when a person intentionally feigns stuttering symptoms to obtain an external tangible benefit such as financial compensation, avoiding work, or another responsibility. Malingering is considered a nonmedical condition and is therefore usually not considered an acquired disorder	Feigned stuttering. This term does not differentiate between factitious and malingered stuttering

However, for some patients, especially those with preexisting stuttering, turning on the stimulation can result in increased stuttering, while turning it off can lead to a decrease in stuttering.[17] Still others may show improvements in stuttering when the deep brain stimulation is activated.[18] Finally, acquired neurogenic stuttering can begin subsequent to the use of recreational and therapeutic medical drugs.[19] Some have argued that "drug-induced stuttering" should be considered separate from other forms of acquired neurogenic stuttering, primarily because stuttering typically ceases when the drug is no longer administered or the dosage has been adjusted.[20] We continue to include drug-induced stuttering under the general umbrella of acquired neurogenic stuttering. This is because therapeutic drugs, often administered as treatment for other health conditions, may result in changes in brain functioning, which in turn can lead to the onset of stuttering. As such, this etiology is not fundamentally different from other neurological conditions that affect brain functions, especially given that even in those other neurological disorders, stuttering is not necessarily a chronic condition.[21]

Acquired neurogenic stuttering often has a sudden onset following neurological events such as strokes and TBI. Gradual onsets are more commonly reported in people with neurodegenerative diseases,[5] and sometimes an onset of acquired stuttering can be the first presenting symptom of an underlying neurodegenerative disease.[11] Although intervals of more than 1 month have been reported between the occurrence of brain damage and stuttering onset, such longer periods make it harder to establish a causal relationship between the stuttering and underlying neurological disorder.[22] Most individuals with acquired neurogenic stuttering have no history of preexisting developmental stuttering, but in some cases, complete or partial recovery from childhood stuttering was reported prior to the lesion or disease onset. In those cases, preexisting developmental stuttering may worsen or return in the presence of acquired neurological conditions.[23] For example, recurrence of childhood stuttering was the first symptom of Alzheimer's-like dementia in one reported case.[24] While one may argue that such cases should not be considered acquired neurogenic stuttering, we

do include them because of the direct link between the onset of the lesion or the disease and the reoccurrence or worsening of stuttering.

The age of onset of acquired neurogenic stuttering varies and is typically consistent with the age ranges associated with the underlying neurological disorder. In a prospective group study of 17 patients with neurogenic stuttering following stroke, the median age was 72 years (range: 51–87 years).[21] A similar mean age of 72 years (range: 56–85 years) was reported for people who developed acquired neurogenic stuttering following various neurodegenerative diseases,[5] while individuals with extrapyramidal diseases were somewhat younger—around 61 years—at the time of stuttering onset.[8] Consistent with the typical occurrence of TBI in younger individuals,[25] the age of acquired stuttering onset following TBI is lower, with averages of 35 and 47 years reported across studies.[26,27]

Although most people develop acquired neurogenic stuttering as adults, it can also occur in children. We found 12 reports of acquired neurogenic stuttering in children between 2 and 16 years of age. Their stuttering occurred following stroke, TBI, tumor resection, encephalitis, or drug ingestion. For some children, the onset of the stuttering occurred immediately following the neurological event,[28] while for others, the relationship between the onset of stuttering and the underlying event was less obvious. In these latter cases, the stuttering had a gradual onset over a number of years,[29] occurred months after the stroke,[30] or was linked to the lesion retrospectively.[31] Although the nature of acquired neurogenic stuttering in itself does not preclude it from affecting younger people, the differential diagnosis from developmental stuttering can be difficult in children, especially considering that the neurological event could act as a trigger for the onset of developmental stuttering.[6]

Lesion Localization

Investigating the localization of the brain lesion(s) underlying acquired neurogenic stuttering can provide information about the neural networks that support fluent speech production.[26,32] A review of the literature published prior to 2003 suggested

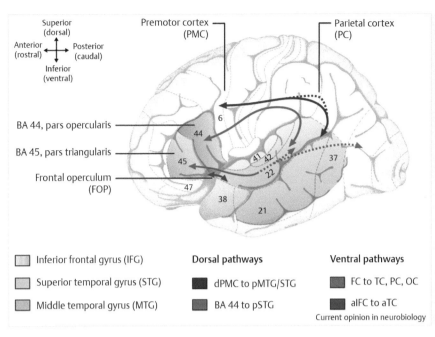

Fig. 17.1 Overview of cortical areas and white matter pathways involved in language production in the left hemisphere. In additional to cortical areas, dorsal and ventral white matter pathways are displayed (a, anterior; BA, Brodmann area; d, dorsa; FC, frontal cortex; OC, occipital cortex; p, posterior; TC, temporal cortex). (Reproduced with permission from Friederici et al.)[87]

that neurogenic stuttering can be associated with lesions in almost every part of the brain, with the possible exception of the occipital lobe.[33] However, with recent advancements in brain imaging techniques, and the availability of more group-level data, a more localized pattern of lesions has started to emerge. This pattern is remarkably consistent across the different etiological subgroups of neurogenic stuttering.

One group study investigated lesion data of 10 people who developed stuttering following TBI,[26] and another study focused on 20 people who started stuttering following stroke.[34] Both report lesions in the inferior frontal white matter (▶ Fig. 17.1), internal capsule, and basal ganglia (e.g., putamen and caudate nuclei; ▶ Fig. 17.2) to be significantly associated with acquired neurogenic stuttering. However, there was more left-sided lesion involvement for the stroke group (▶ Fig. 17.3), while more bilateral involvement was present in the TBI group. These findings overlap with those on the neural changes that occur in Parkinson's disease, as Parkinson's disease is characterized by loss of dopamine-synthesizing cells in the substantia nigra, which results in dysfunction in the motor loop mediated by the putamen.[35] Finally, reports on drug-induced stuttering have pointed to an onset of acquired stuttering following drugs that influence the dopaminergic neurotransmitter system.[19]

In summary, many case reports and group studies point to an important role of the basal ganglia systems and their interactions with the frontal cortex in the onset of acquired neurogenic stuttering.[28] However, the neural changes leading to an acquired onset of stuttering are certainly not restricted to these areas, and future research will need to clarify how these changes lead to disruptions in the neural networks that support speech fluency.

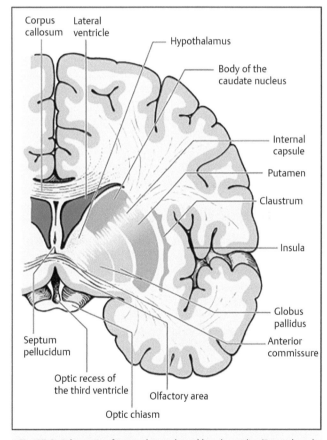

Fig. 17.2 Schematic of internal capsule and basal ganglia. (Reproduced from Bähr M, Frotscher M. Topical Diagnosis in Neurology: Anatomy, Physiology, Signs, Symptoms. 6th Edition. Stuttgart: Thieme; 2019.)

Prevalence

Although acquired stuttering, both neurogenic and functional, occurs more frequently than previously thought, comprehensive prevalence and incidence data are not yet available. To date, only one study with stroke patients has directly collected prospective prevalence data for acquired neurogenic stuttering in that patient population.[21] In this study, 319 patients were

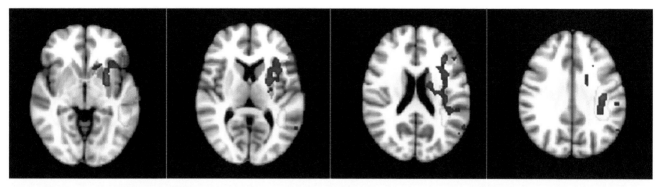

Fig. 17.3 Brain areas associated with stroke-induced neurogenic stuttering. Areas in *red* show the corticobasal ganglia-cortical network that is significantly associated with lesions in people with neurogenic stuttering compared to nonstuttering stroke controls. For reference purposes, the inferior frontal gyrus, superior temporal gyrus, striatum, and superior longitudinal fasciculus are overlaid in *blue*, *green*, *pink*, and *yellow*, respectively. (Reproduced with permission from Theys et al.[34])

screened for speech disfluencies over a 1-year period following their stroke. In the acute phase, 17 (5%) of the 319 stroke patients presented with more than 3% stuttering disfluencies. For 8 (47%) of these 17 patients, the stuttering persisted more than 6 months following the stroke.

Preliminary data on the occurrence of acquired neurogenic stuttering following Parkinson's disease suggest that the prevalence ranges from 4 to 57%. In a study of 280 people with Parkinson's disease, 15 participants (5%) reported stuttering. Four of these 15 participants had preexisting developmental stuttering, suggesting that the stuttering was first observed following the onset of Parkinson's disease in 11 of the 280 participants (4%).[36] In another study, 12 of 21 participants (57%) with Parkinson's disease exhibited more than 3% stuttering disfluencies during a reading task.[37] Future studies linking prevalence of stuttering with the different stages of Parkinson's disease are necessary to further clarify this relationship.

17.2.2 Acquired Functional Stuttering

Although acquired stuttering is typically associated with a known neurological lesion or disease, this is not always the case. Individuals, usually adults, may develop stuttering symptoms in the absence of an obvious physical medical condition. Traditionally, this condition has been known as psychogenic stuttering, reflecting the belief that the onset is found in an underlying psychological condition such as stress or emotional trauma. According to some, psychogenic stuttering can best be understood as a form of conversion reaction, a psychiatric term originally coined by Freud to indicate a condition by which unresolved unconscious conflict is converted into overt neurological symptoms.[38] However, there are a number of problems with the label "psychogenic stuttering." For one, it is based on a dualistic mind–body approach that may not reflect our current understanding of human behavior. It also suggests that the absence of a direct physical medical explanation implies a psychological origin of the disorder. Finally, it does not capture the fact that patients with a diagnosed physical disease may also develop stuttering in response to the stress and emotional trauma associated with their disease.[38] In fact, in a study of 69 people with diagnosed psychogenic stuttering, 20 also showed evidence of neurological disease.[39] As a result, the more

agnostic term "functional disorder" has become more commonly used in the neurological literature[40] and adopted in the Diagnostic and Statistical Manual of Mental Disorders, Fifth Edition (DSM-5).[41] The use of "functional" rather than "psychogenic" focuses more on the behavioral manifestation than the presumed etiology of the disorder. Importantly, this term has also been shown to be more acceptable to clients, an important predictor for tolerance of the diagnosis as well as treatment outcome.[42] Therefore, we will use the term *acquired functional stuttering* in this chapter.

Primarily based on clinical reports and retrospective studies, acquired functional stuttering is equally common among males and females.[39,43] Although it may be the sole or main complaint for some individuals, it is often associated with other motor, sensory, or cognitive complaints such as headaches, fatigue, or unilateral weakness. A history of previous psychiatric symptoms is reported in approximately one-third of the cases with functional stuttering, and in only 5% of patients who demonstrate functional stuttering with co-occurring neurological disease.[39] The age at onset of acquired functional stuttering is variable, but averaged around 45 years, both for people with and without co-occurring neurologial conditions.[39]

Precise epidemiological data for acquired functional stuttering are not yet available. Some indirect information can be gleaned from the fact that functional motor symptoms are relatively common among movement disorder patients, with prevalence ranging from 15 to 62%.[44] In one study, 16.5% of individuals who were seen for functional neurological disorders at a general movement disorders clinic also demonstrated functional speech and voice disorders, with half (8.25%) of them experiencing stuttering.[45] This suggests that functional speech disorders, particularly stuttering, may be more common than previously thought.

17.3 Symptomatology

17.3.1 Acquired Neurogenic Stuttering

Historically, when describing the symptomatology of acquired neurogenic stuttering, the focus has been on identifying characteristics that differ from those seen in developmental stuttering.[23] However, recent evidence has shown considerable overlap between characteristics of neurogenic stuttering and those typically seen in people with developmental stuttering. As a result, even experienced speech-language pathologists cannot always reliably differentiate the etiologies based on observable speech characteristics alone.[46] Nevertheless, the typical onset in adulthood and the presence of an associated neurological condition are often clear indicators to support a diagnosis of acquired neurogenic stuttering.

Speech Characteristics

The key speech characteristics of acquired neurogenic stuttering are the following: repetitions of sounds, syllables, and monosyllabic words; prolongations; and blocks. Repetitions were the most common disfluency type in the literature on stroke-induced stuttering. Most cases had more than one disfluency type, with one-third reporting a combination of repetitions, prolongations, and blocks.[6] In people with stuttering following TBI, stuttering disfluencies frequently occur in a cluster with more typical disfluencies such as interjections.[47] Although it has previously been suggested that stuttering disfluencies in acquired neurogenic stuttering are not restricted to word-initial syllables,[23,48] a recent review has shown that they almost always occur at the beginning of words.[6] In addition, a direct comparison of reading samples of 5 people with stroke-induced stuttering and 35 people with developmental stuttering found no difference in the location of within-utterance disfluencies.[49]

The frequency of stuttering disfluencies varies widely across cases and speech tasks. As one extreme, a person stuttered on 95% of words following a history of seizures.[50] However, for most people with acquired neurogenic stuttering, the frequency of stuttering disfluencies is considerably lower, ranging from 2 to 52% stuttered syllables (SS) during conversation in two studies focusing on stroke.[27,34] Interestingly, frequencies of stuttering disfluencies during conversation and monologue have been shown to be highly correlated, while such a relationship was not present with reading.[21] Sentence repetition also consistently led to a lower frequency of stuttering disfluencies compared to conversation and reading tasks.[28] Following TBI, similar variability in the occurrence of stuttering disfluencies has been shown, both between patients and between speech tasks, with disfluencies ranging from 18 to 29% during monologue and 11 to 58% during conversation.[27] People with co-occurring aphasia and apraxia of speech following stroke have also been shown to present with higher frequencies of stuttering compared to those who do not present with these disorders. No such relationship has been found with co-occurring dysarthria or cognitive problems.[21]

Changes in stuttering disfluencies during fluency-inducing conditions also highlight the heterogeneity in this population. Reading adaptation occurs in approximately half of the people with neurogenic stuttering following stroke and TBI,[6,27] and in at least two-thirds of people with stuttering following Parkinson's disease.[37] Choral reading can lead to significant reductions in stuttering disfluencies in people with Parkinson's disease,[51] but mixed results are reported for other etiologies.[52] Most reports indicate a marked reduction in stuttering during singing.[52]

Nonspeech Characteristics

It has previously been suggested that nonspeech, or concomitant, behaviors are not typically associated with moments of disfluency in acquired neurogenic stuttering.[23] Recent studies, however, have shown that the presence of such behaviors in acquired neurogenic stuttering is not unusual. Information on nonspeech behaviors was reported in only 86 of the 156 cases with acquired neurogenic stuttering that were reviewed for this chapter. Approximately half of those cases (n = 41, 48%) reported the presence of nonspeech behaviors such as facial grimacing, neck tension, and aversion of eye gaze. While it could be assumed that the occurrence of nonspeech behaviors is associated with the frequency of disfluencies, a one-on-one relationship between disfluencies and nonspeech behaviors is not always present. In some individuals, the concomitant behaviors can increase over time while the stuttering disfluencies remain unchanged,[10] whereas for others, nonspeech behaviors may persist even after speech fluency has been regained.[53]

Absence of negative speech-related emotions has also long been regarded as a characteristic of acquired neurogenic stuttering.[23] Unfortunately, this characteristic is not always addressed explicitly in published reports. Of the 156 cases we reviewed, only 50 commented on the presence or absence of speech-associated emotions and of these close to 70% showed evidence of such reactions varying from slight annoyance[8] to being anxious about their speech,[54] and feeling miserable and afraid of speaking.[50] This is consistent with speech-language pathologist reports of emotional responses such as frustration, irritation, fear, crying, and anger in reaction to the stuttering in 62% of stroke patients, 82% of TBI patients, but only in 33% of people with a neurodegenerative onset of stuttering.[5] Especially following stroke or TBI, speech attitudes can be similar to those typically seen in adults with developmental stuttering, and can be significantly more negative than those reported for people with typical fluency.[27]

17.3.2 Acquired Functional Stuttering

Acquired functional stuttering may be characterized by features that resemble those of developmental or acquired neurogenic stuttering,[55] although characteristics can also be atypical.[56] Video examples of people with acquired functional stuttering can be found in Chung et al (case 3)[55] and in Baizabal-Carvallo and Jankovic.[45]

Speech Characteristics

The largest retrospective study of acquired functional stuttering to date was conducted by Baumgartner and Duffy.[39] Their observations were based on 49 individuals diagnosed with acquired functional stuttering without accompanying neurological disease and 20 who received an additional diagnosis of neurological disease. Speech disfluencies were primarily characterized by sound or syllable repetitions (80% of all cases). Prolongations (27% of cases) and blocks (18% of cases) were also observed but much less frequently. Of the nine patients for whom reading adaptation was assessed, eight showed an absence of this effect. The most relevant feature supporting a functional diagnosis was a rapid improvement of stuttering symptoms in 70% of these cases following one to two sessions of speech therapy.

Most reported cases were diagnosed with functional stuttering because of a lack of a known neurological etiology.[55,57,58] One person developed frequent sound-syllable repetitions in addition to posttraumatic stress disorder, insomnia, and cognitive impairments, after being injured in an active war zone.[57] Another adult male developed stuttering characterized by frequent repetitions and blocks, with no periods of fluent speech. Known fluency-enhancing conditions, such as choral or whispered speech and reduced auditory feedback, did not result in increased fluency. Neuropsychological and medical tests did not point to any abnormal findings or potential organic cause.[58]

One of the authors of this chapter (CT) worked with a woman who had a sudden onset of stuttering while in hospital for acute stroke. Her speech was characterized by bizarre stress patterns, final-word repetitions, and multisyllabic repetitions. It was concluded that her stuttering most likely was a psychological reaction to distressing information that she received about her home situation while she was admitted to hospital. Her disfluencies subsided immediately when the home situation was addressed. Another individual seen by the second author (LDN) demonstrated very severe stuttering, primarily characterized by sound-syllable repetitions and blocks, on almost every word during speaking and reading, accompanied by significant struggle behavior. His stuttering had started following a minor car accident. Although medical examination immediately following the accident did not show any evidence of whiplash or any other neurological lesions, there were obvious psychological stressors in his personal life coinciding with the development of stuttering, and the stuttering was considered to be functional in nature.

Together, these cases show that many speech characteristics are similar to those reported for acquired neurogenic stuttering earlier, or developmental stuttering in previous chapters. However, atypical features such as final-word multisyllabic repetitions and absence of islands of fluency can also occur.

Nonspeech Characteristics

Concomitant behaviors, such as facial grimacing and obvious muscle tension in the orofacial area and extremities, were observed in a majority of individuals reported in the study by Baumgartner and Duffy.[39] These behaviors can occur infrequently in some clients[57] but can also present as severe struggle behavior[58]—as was the case for the man who started stuttering following a minor accident described earlier. The woman with an onset of functional acquired stuttering following stroke described earlier did not seem bothered by or aware of her stuttering, which is consistent with the suggestion that some people with acquired functional stuttering may present with "la belle indifference."[56] Overall, the presence of atypical struggle behaviors and emotional reactions, in addition to atypical speech behaviors, can be considered an important observation leading to the identification of acquired functional stuttering.[39]

17.4 Diagnostic Considerations

17.4.1 General Considerations

When assessing an individual with possible acquired stuttering, the speech-language pathologist will need to consider a number of different aspects as part of their evaluation (see

▶ Table 17.2). In addition, two general issues need to be considered. First, it is important to determine whether the observed stuttering disfluencies are newly developed or the continuation or reemergence of previously present developmental stuttering. Knowledge of any preexisting fluency disorder needs to be explored as it may result in a better understanding of the nature of the disorder and could influence the nature and direction of any recommended intervention. Second, it needs to be assessed whether the observed acquired stuttering is neurogenic, functional, or feigned in nature. This may be a somewhat more difficult question to answer as the relationship between the presence or absence of a neurological lesion or illness and subsequent acquired stuttering is not always straightforward. Differential diagnosis becomes increasingly more difficult the longer the interval between the diagnosis of the neurological lesion or disease and the onset of stuttering. Furthermore, individuals with a medically diagnosed neurological lesion or disease may still develop acquired functional stuttering as a result of their psychological reactions to the disease, or to other distressing life events occurring around the same time as the disease. Cases of acquired stuttering also have been reported where the absence of any clear neurological symptoms initially led to a diagnosis of functional stuttering, which later had to be revisited when it became apparent that there was an underlying neurological condition for which the onset of stuttering was one of the first observable symptoms.[11]

Table 17.2 Components for acquired stuttering

1. Detailed case history

a) Medical and other assessment reports
b) Onset and development of speech and language disorders
c) Onset and development of speech fluency problems
d) History of developmental stuttering
e) Impact of stuttering
f) Treatment history

2. Cognitive assessment

a) MMSE or MOCA

3. Speech and language assessment

a) Aphasia (e.g., BDAE, CAT, BNT)
b) Dysarthria (e.g., FDA-2)
c) Apraxia of speech (e.g., ABA)

4. Speech fluency assessment

a) Spontaneous speech (e.g., picture description, monologue, dialogue)
b) Reading (e.g., single words, sentences, continuous text)
c) Semiautomatic speech (e.g., counting, days of the week)
d) Stuttering severity (e.g., SSI-4)
e) Concomitant behaviors (e.g., struggle, avoidance)
f) Speech-related attitudes (e.g., S-24, SSC)
g) Quality of life (e.g., OASES, CPIB)

5. Trial intervention

6. Summary of findings and diagnosis

7. Treatment recommendations

Abbreviations: ABA, Apraxia Battery for Adults; BDAE, Boston Diagnostic Aphasia Examination; BNT, Boston Naming Test; CAT, Comprehensive Aphasia Test; CPIB, Communicative Participation Item Bank; FDA, Frenchay Dysarthria Assessment, Second Edition; MMSE, Mini-Mental State Examination; MOCA, Montreal Cognitive Assessment; OASES, Overall Assessment of Speakers' Experiences of Stuttering; SSC, Speech Situation Checklist; SSI-4, Stuttering Severity Instrument, Fourth Edition.

The differential diagnosis of acquired neurogenic versus functional stuttering can be complex and is an ongoing dynamic process that needs to be continuously reassessed as more information becomes available to the clinician.

17.4.2 Assessment Protocol

Case History

A full assessment of acquired stuttering needs to start with a comprehensive case history. A good place to start would be the medical file, if available, which normally includes information on the medical diagnosis and disease history. Special attention should be given to the time of disease onset and any fluctuations in the symptomatology, such as changes in severity, since onset. Typically, the medical file will also include details on past and current medication, so their potential impact on speech and language can be investigated. Details on brain imaging, other medical tests, and personal history could provide a deeper insight into potential causal factors for the acquired stuttering. For instance, the absence of neurological deficits may be indicative of acquired functional stuttering, especially if associated with stressful emotional variables in the client's personal life.

In addition to the medical information, the speech-language pathologist should probe the history of speech and language development, with special emphasis on the presence of developmental stuttering and whether recovery occurred. Particular attention should be given to previous stuttering treatment the client may have received, including the use of self-management strategies (e.g., avoidance, speech rate changes). If the client has a history of developmental stuttering, the speech pathologist would need to clarify whether the onset of a neurological lesion or disease resulted in a reemergence, an increase, or a decrease of previous stuttering disfluencies. Another component of the case history to explore is the impact of the speech disfluencies on the client's quality of life and their self-perceptions of the stuttering and general communication competence. Much of this information can be obtained during the interview with the client and/or significant others.

Cognitive Assessment

The speech-language pathologist should also assess the client's cognitive abilities, especially since some stuttering intervention techniques require a level of self-monitoring of or insight into stuttering that may be difficult for clients with cognitive deficits. In clients with acquired neurogenic stuttering, it is likely that results from either the Mini-Mental State Examination (MMSE)[59] or the Montreal Cognitive Assessment (MOCA)[60] are included in their medical file as these are the most common assessment tools used by medical professionals, but they can also be administered by a speech-language pathologist. The MMSE is a short test, probing different areas of cognitive function: orientation, registration, attention and calculation, recall, and language. The MOCA aims to test cognitive abilities in clients with mild cognitive impairments regardless of etiology and may be more sensitive to the clients typically seen by the speech-language pathologist for acquired stuttering.

Speech and Language Assessment

Clients with acquired neurogenic stuttering often have other speech and/or language disorders such as aphasia (including word-finding difficulties), dysarthria, apraxia of speech, and palilalia. Many of these disorders may lead to fluency disruptions in speech, which can resemble features of acquired stuttering. Therefore, a thorough speech and language assessment is necessary for differential diagnosis and intervention planning. Clinical manuals and textbooks of acquired language and speech disorders provide extensive information on available test instruments, both norm based and informal, that can be used with this population. Some of the most commonly used instruments are the Boston Diagnostic Aphasia Examination (BDAE)[61] and the Comprehensive Aphasia Test (CAT).[62] The CAT also includes a cognitive section and a disability questionnaire to address the impact of the disorder. To assess word finding, tests such as the Boston Naming Test (BNT)[63] could be used. The Frenchay Dysarthria Assessment (FDA)[64] and the Apraxia Battery for Adults (ABA)[65] can be used to guide the assessment of dysarthria or apraxia of speech, respectively. However, the results of these tests should be interpreted with caution, given that the diagnostic profiles for these speech disorders are a topic of debate.[66,67] Of course, not all clients will need to complete each of these tests and the speech-language pathologist should tailor the assessment protocol to the client's needs and the underlying disorder(s) that is believed to have led to the stuttering.

Speech Fluency Assessment

A detailed analysis of the typical and stuttering speech disfluencies observed in the client's speech during various speech tasks such as reading of single words, sentences and text, picture description, monologue, conversation, and semiautomatic serial speech (e.g., days of the week, months of the year, counting) is an essential component of an assessment for acquired stuttering. Ideally, speech samples should be collected at multiple time points and in different speech situations (e.g., in the clinic and at home).

The most common test for stuttering severity is the Stuttering Severity Instrument, Fourth Edition (SSI-4),[79] which measures stuttering frequency, duration of longest stutters, and physical concomitants. These scores combine to yield an overall severity score ranging from very mild to very severe. However, the clinician should be aware that stuttering frequency may change, sometimes dramatically, over time and across different speech situations and tasks. Furthermore, the scores on the SSI-4 may not reflect the effects of coping strategies, such as word avoidances, or techniques learned in intervention (e.g., gentle onset, slowed speech, or voluntary stuttering), on stuttering frequency. Therefore, the SSI-4 should only be used as an approximate estimate of observable stuttering severity at the time of testing, not as a general some indication of some invariant core stuttering severity.

Nonspeech Behaviors

In addition to a detailed analysis of the speech fluency behavior, the speech-language pathologist should also note the presence of concomitant behaviors, such as avoidance, escape, and struggle behaviors. Although the absence of these behaviors has traditionally been viewed as characteristic of acquired neurogenic stuttering, more recent studies and reviews discussed earlier in this chapter have shown that nonspeech behaviors are often present in this population.

Speech-Related Attitudes and Quality of Life

The psychological and emotional reactions of individuals with acquired stuttering should also be assessed. Again, contrary to initial assertions, research has since shown that many people with acquired neurogenic stuttering develop negative speech attitudes similar to those with developmental stuttering. Indeed, acquired stuttering can have a significant impact on the individual's quality of life. Instruments, originally developed for the assessment of developmental stuttering, can be used or adapted for use with clients with acquired stuttering. These can include questionnaires such as the Overall Assessment of Speaker's Experience of Stuttering (OASES),[68] the Modified Erickson Scale of Communication Attitudes (S-24),[69] and the Speech Situation Checklist (SSC).[70] Other instruments, such as the Communicative Participation Item Bank (CPIB),[71] aim at assessing the impact of communication disorders on a person's self-perceived communicative participation and can also provide useful assessment information.

Trial Intervention

Clinicians are encouraged to implement one or more trial interventions during the assessment session. Such interventions can consist of producing words or short sentences with slowed or stretched speech, using modeled gentle onset during picture naming or single word reading, chorus reading, and speaking under delayed auditory feedback. The main purpose of trial interventions is to provide insight into the variability of the speech fluency disorder, which may guide intervention planning. It also serves as a motivator for the client who may become aware, sometimes for the first time, that stuttering is not invariant and that clinical intervention can modify severity. Finally, as we have discussed in the section on acquired functional stuttering, the implementation of successful intervention strategies during the initial assessment may help differentiate between neurogenic and functional forms of acquired stuttering.

Summary of Findings and Diagnosis

At the end of the assessment, the clinician should attempt to determine a diagnosis. Formulating a diagnosis, even if we acknowledge that it may be modified as additional information becomes available, is important. It will give the clinician and other clinical service providers a better understanding of the observed disorder and will guide the formulation of an intervention plan. However, not every assessment necessarily will result in a diagnosis of acquired stuttering. Although the assessment is often motivated by the perception, either by the client, the clinician, or someone else, that the speech disfluencies are suggestive of stuttering, the clinician must leave open the possibility that the disfluencies may not represent acquired stuttering but rather are symptomatic of other speech or language disorders. Even if the disfluencies are indicative of stuttering, they may coexist with other speech and language disorders.[6] Considering the possibility that acquired stuttering may very well co-occur with other communication disorders is necessary to avoid underdiagnosis and thus a lack of focused treatment for the fluency problems. Even if the clinician is confident about a diagnosis of acquired stuttering, it may not always be possible to determine the precise nature of the acquired disfluencies. For instance, the clinician may have insufficient information to determine with certainty whether the problem is neurogenic or functional in nature. In this case, a full descriptive summary of the findings would be the best approach to provide a complete picture of the characteristics of the disorder to guide future intervention or to communicate to other clinical service providers.

Additional Assessment Considerations for Acquired Functional Stuttering

The assessment and diagnosis of acquired functional stuttering can be complex and requires input from other clinical medical and neuropsychological experts. Furthermore, because the diagnosis of a functional disorder is often primarily based on the absence of an organic cause, the speech-language pathologist should always consider the possibility that an organic neurological cause for the stuttering may become apparent later.

Differential diagnosis requires that the clinician look beyond the obvious speech characteristics and include additional information, where available, especially from the case history, medical and psychiatric examination, and neuropsychological tests.[72] For example, Baumgartner and Duffy[39] reported that 35% of their patients with acquired functional stuttering (without co-occurring neurological disease) had a prior diagnosis of a related or unrelated functional disorder.

Typical characteristics of a functional disorder include excessive manifestation of the behavioral symptoms, inconsistencies with the typical behavior expected in the organic disorder, relative lack of variability in how the behavior manifests itself, severe struggle behavior, and a previous diagnosis of functional disorders.[44] Additional signs include suggestibility and distractibility of the patient in the manifestation of their symptoms and the potential for rapid reversibility and improvement of the symptoms.[55] Normal or near-normal speech fluency within one or two therapy sessions occurred for 77% of clients with functional stuttering without an accompanying neurological condition, and for 63% of clients with such a condition.[39] One of the often referred to characteristics of functional acquired stuttering is "la belle indifference" whereby the client has no obvious concern about the stuttering or its impact. However, this may also be present in neurological disorders and can sometimes be influenced by personal or cultural expectations, such as stoic attitudes toward disease.[44] ▶ Table 17.3 summarizes questions that a clinician may consider when differentiating acquired neurogenic and functional disorders.[44,73] The answers to these questions may not always be sufficient to arrive at a differential diagnosis. However, the more questions answered affirmatively, the more confident a clinician can be of a functional origin to the observed disfluencies.

Table 17.3 Questions to guide the differential diagnosis of acquired neurogenic versus functional stuttering

Question	Rationale
1. Is there a history of other functional disorder diagnoses?	Many individuals with a functional disorder have had similar diagnoses in the past
2. Are there psychologically significant events that may help explain the onset and presence of stuttering?	These may provide an indication of psychological factors underlying the stuttering. In addition, remission and reoccurrence of stuttering can coincide with fluctuations in those events
3. Is there no clear neurological event that precedes the onset of stuttering?	A functional disorder is more likely if there is no known event or if the lag time is very long
4. Is there evidence of secondary gain associated with the presence of stuttering?	This may point to a functional disorder, but malingered stuttering may also need to be considered in this case
5. Are the findings from the oral-motor examination inconsistent with expected outcomes for motor speech disorders or stuttering?	If they are, a functional explanation should be considered
6. Is the speech pattern incongruent with what we know about stuttering?	Atypical speech symptoms should raise suspicions of a functional disorder
7. Do the speech disfluencies and concomitant behaviors look exaggerated or excessive?	This should also raise suspicions of a functional disorder
8. Does the speech deficit show extreme fluctuations across speech tasks or emotional content?	Fluctuations in disfluencies, especially during fluency-inducing conditions, can be expected in acquired neurogenic stuttering. However, if such fluctuations are extreme—from normal speech to severely disordered speech—they may be indicative of functional stuttering
9. Can the presence or severity of the speech deficit be influenced by suggestion?	In some individuals with functional stuttering, the suggestion by the clinician that a task will be difficult or easy may affect the observed severity
10. Is the severity of the speech deficit susceptible to distraction?	The presence or severity of functional stuttering may change significantly, for example, if the conversation changes from a formal to a more casual interaction with the clinician
11. Is the speech deficit reversible?	The fact that stuttering can often be dramatically reversed successfully during one or a few sessions has been considered the strongest evidence for functional stuttering

Source: Adapted from Duffy[73] and Carson et al.[44]

Additional Assessment Considerations for Feigned Stuttering

The diagnosis and management of people with factitious and malingered stuttering is challenging due to the lack of definitive objective assessments of deception. It also needs to be considered carefully, as it can have significant medicolegal implications and, if misdiagnosed, can prevent someone from accessing necessary treatment.[74] Therefore, the diagnosis should be made in collaboration with a person experienced with mental health disorders, and a speech-language pathologist who is familiar with the typical presentation of the feigned disease. This will help identify several red flags for malingering, such as inconsistent presentation style (e.g., changes in openness when asked about specifics of symptoms), atypical symptoms (e.g., extreme presentation), internal inconsistencies (e.g., when asked to elaborate on case history), and external inconsistencies (e.g., differences between self-report and directly observed behaviors). Nonresponse to treatment can also raise suspicions.[74] This last factor is especially interesting, as it contrasts with the rapid response to treatment often seen in acquired functional stuttering.

Even when all the steps above have been followed, it may not be possible to differentially diagnose neurogenic, functional, and feigned stuttering with certainty.[32,53,75] Notwithstanding the underlying etiology, people who are negatively affected by acquired speech disfluencies should be offered personalized treatment for their fluency problems.

17.5 Treatment Options

17.5.1 General Considerations

To date, no intervention programs or strategies have been developed specifically for treating acquired neurogenic or functional stuttering. Our knowledge of the range of treatment approaches and their effectiveness, or lack thereof, has come primarily from published case studies, sometimes reflecting the clinician's repeated attempts at finding an intervention that works. In addition, a number of published larger-scale clinical survey studies shed some light on common clinical approaches and their possible outcomes.[5,76,77] Although the absence of evidence-based guidelines for treatment certainly reflects the lack of clinical research in this population, it also may reflect the complex nature of acquired stuttering and its unique presentation in persons who often experience co-occurring motor speech or language disorders resulting from neurological injury or disease. Despite the lack of firm guidelines, there are several principles that can guide the clinician in deciding what intervention strategy to use.

First, not all individuals who develop acquired neurogenic stuttering require treatment. The presence of stuttering may be temporary and natural recovery may occur, especially in the early stages following a neurological injury. For example, of 14 people identified with neurogenic stuttering in the acute phase following stroke, 6 recovered from their stuttering symptoms within 6 months.[21] Also, the clinician should evaluate the presence and severity of stuttering within the context of other speech, language, and cognitive difficulties the person may be experiencing. Sometimes treating other disorders is a priority and focusing on the stuttering may not be appropriate or necessary at that stage in the individual's care. In addition, some individuals may not experience the presence of stuttering as unduly disruptive in their daily communication. Stuttering treatment often requires a high degree of motivation on the part of the client, as well as the necessary cognitive, metalinguistic, and motor skills to monitor and modify speech. If the client is not able or ready to bring these skills to the treatment or is not overly concerned about the stuttering, it may be better to focus on other aspects of communication or delay starting stuttering therapy until the client is ready.

Second, the clinician should not only focus their treatment on the speech disfluencies but also address the individual's experiences with stuttering and communication. In the case of chronic acquired stuttering following brain lesions, the goal of treatment should be to limit the severity of stuttering, optimize communication and quality of life, and help the individual with acceptance of residual speech fluency disruption. This is especially the case when working with clients with neurodegenerative disorders, where the speech problems can be expected to worsen over time.

Third, the goal setting, evaluation, and subsequent decision-making regarding the direction of treatment should be done collaboratively between the clinician and the client. To the extent possible, it should also involve important people in the client's environment, such as partners and other individuals who provide support during recovery. As part of the intervention, the clinician should always provide clients and their support networks with the necessary self-management skills to continue working on maintaining and improving the progress made once treatment is scaled back or terminated.

Fourth, individuals with acquired neurogenic stuttering may experience cognitive difficulties, mobility issues, as well as other physical and mental limitations. Therefore, it is important for the speech-language pathologist to be an integral part of the care team for the client, and coordinate their intervention in consultation with the other health professionals involved in the client's care. Referrals to other services will need to be considered where necessary (e.g., for clients who could benefit from mental health counseling or need advice regarding occupational support).

17.5.2 Treatment Approaches

With these general considerations in mind, there are a number of different treatment approaches that can be used for people with acquired stuttering.

Speech Intervention

Most clinical interventions for acquired neurogenic stuttering consist of treatment techniques typically used for developmental stuttering. Survey results from 81 clinicians showed that most chose a fluency-shaping approach, consisting primarily of teaching a slow speech rate and easy onset, or a combination of both. Far fewer listed a stuttering modification approach or a

focus on acceptance and relaxation, as their preferred intervention.[76] Other surveys found that clinicians preferred to use an eclectic approach, consisting of a combination of slowed speech rate and counselling,[77] or fluency-shaping and stuttering modification approaches.[77] Treatment outcomes are mostly reported as being positive, although these results may be influenced by spontaneous recovery, and are based on subjective clinical impressions rather than documented measures.[5,76,77]

Although stuttering intervention techniques for developmental stuttering are often used with individuals with acquired neurogenic stuttering, and can result in positive outcomes, the clinician needs to be aware of the influence of other processing difficulties that the client may experience. For instance, to achieve speech rate control, clients must be able to monitor their speech and manage their rate consistently, which may be challenging for individuals with motor speech disorders and cognitive deficits. In those cases, the use of self-pacing techniques, such as a pacing board, a toggle switch, or finger tapping may be useful.[23] Other common management approaches for dysarthria, such as rhythmic cueing and increasing loudness, which often result in a slower speech rate, could also be used.[73]

Altered Auditory Feedback

Some clinicians have commented on the effectiveness of delayed auditory feedback in treating clients with acquired neurogenic stuttering. However, the results are variable. Decreases in stuttering frequency have been reported in some cases with stuttering following TBI,[78] but no change or an increase in disfluencies has been reported in clients with stroke-induced stuttering.[79] When present, positive effects did not transfer to speech outside the clinic setting.[78] Further clinical research, especially focusing on long-term effects, is needed before any conclusions can be drawn about the usefulness of altered auditory feedback. Whether altered auditory feedback can be used effectively as a treatment will also depend on the client's tolerance for the technology. Clinically, we have noticed that some clients, especially those with concomitant cognitive problems or those suffering from headaches, may find the auditory distortion caused by the altered feedback to be fatiguing and, as a result, have a very low tolerance for this approach.

Drug Treatment

Although medication is typically not prescribed for the treatment of acquired neurogenic stuttering, there have been several reports describing the effects of various therapeutic drugs. In some cases, the stuttering may have resulted from the use of medications,[75] such that once changed, a significant reduction in stuttering occured.[80] In individuals with Parkinson's disease, a direct relationship exists between the length and dosage of L-Dopa treatment and the occurrence and severity of stuttering.[81] Clearly, a careful case history, including a detailed history of drug treatment, is a critical part of the assessment of acquired stuttering. If the clinician has reason to believe that drug treatment may be one of the factors affecting the presence or severity of stuttering, they should consult with the appropriate medical professionals to consider whether adjustments to the drug treatment, such as stopping its use, adjusting the dosage, or switching to another drug, would be appropriate.

Surgical Intervention

Surgical treatment for acquired stuttering is currently not recommended. However, knowledge of the potential impact of surgical intervention on stuttering is important as part of mapping out clinical speech intervention. Most studies that have investigated the link between neurosurgical treatment and acquired stuttering have been done in Parkinson's disease, in particular regarding the effects of deep brain stimulation (DBS). Reports range from onset of stuttering following DBS to worsening of preexisting stuttering to reemergence of developmental stuttering.[16,82] When the onset or severity of stuttering may be related to a medical intervention, speech therapy should be postponed until it is clear that modifying the medical intervention (e.g., changing the medication or making adjustments to the DBS, if deemed appropriate by the treating physician) does not result in any significant improvements in speech fluency.[73]

Additional Treatment Considerations for Acquired Functional Stuttering

As stated earlier, symptomatic treatment of the functional stuttering behavior, as early as the initial assessment session, may result in dramatic changes in the severity of stuttering. However, the speech-language pathologist should keep in mind that there is not a one-size-fits-all approach to treatment.

One of the important elements of treatment for acquired functional stuttering is the acknowledgment of the disorder and how the clinician communicates the nature of the disorder to the client. The clinician needs to make it clear that they take the problem seriously and explain that the diagnosis is based on the behavioral features that the client is showing and experiencing, rather than the absence of certain features (i.e., no known organic cause at the time of diagnosis).[2] The use of the term "functional stuttering," rather than "psychogenic stuttering," often makes it easier for clients to accept the diagnosis and the proposed treatment. It is also important to help the client find appropriate ways to explain the diagnosis and potentially rapid improvement to others in their social circle.

With regard to specific approaches to dealing with acquired functional stuttering, a symptomatic approach focusing on substituting a new speech pattern for the stuttering behavior appears to be the most successful approach in many cases,[72] especially when accompanied by a strong belief by the client, and supported by the clinician, that they can and will recover from stuttering. Nevertheless, the clinician needs to acknowledge and accept that treatment may not always be successful.[58] For instance, cognitive behavioral therapies have been proven to be successful for treating functional disorders,[83] but may not be an acceptable intervention to all clients.[2] The clinician should also be aware that functional stuttering may co-occur with other speech disorders or cognitive communication concerns, which may need to be addressed as well in treatment. The speech-language pathologist should acknowledge the limits of their intervention skills, refer if appropriate, collaborate regularly, and effectively coordinate treatment with other professionals, such as neurologists or mental health providers, involved in the client's care.

Additional Treatment Considerations for Feigned Stuttering

A multidisciplinary team approach is always necessary for people who are feigning acquired stuttering, whether this is factitious stuttering or malingering. Tactfully and nonjudgmentally presenting with inconsistencies in the presentation of the symptoms to the client and offering them a face-saving way out could be a successful approach.[74] Reviews of different intervention approaches with individuals with factitious disorders or malingering showed that both supportive confrontational (e.g., discussing inconsistencies in symptoms) and nonconfrontational (e.g., medication) approaches may be useful, although not always successful, and that long-term follow-up and support are usually required.[84,85] As with acquired functional stuttering, it is important to help the client explain the presence of the behavior as well as the potentially rapid change in the behavior to others in their environment.

17.6 Case Study

17.6.1 Background

B. was a 79-year-old woman without a history of developmental stuttering. An example of her speech prestroke can be seen in ▶ Video 17.1. One month after this video was recorded, B. had a left occipital infarct, followed by a left total anterior circulation stroke a month later. Following the strokes, she was diagnosed with expressive and receptive aphasia, apraxia of speech, and cognitive impairments. Her expressive language was characterized by perseverations, semantic and phonemic paraphasias, word-finding difficulties, impaired writing, and mild disfluencies. Her receptive language was mildly impaired, characterized by greater difficulty understanding complex topics.

B. received 4 months of speech-language therapy, focusing on word finding, easy onset speech, naturalness techniques, and slowing down her speech rate. She was able to follow the speech-language pathologist's models for easy onset speech, naturalness techniques, and slowed speech; however, she could not use these techniques independently and therefore did not show notable improvements in her speech. Six months later, B. experienced epileptic seizures, followed by an increase in part-word repetitions, monosyllabic word repetitions, phrase repetitions, and blocks. During therapy, easy onset techniques were trialed as well as naturalness techniques, with little success. Five months after the seizures, B. was referred to an aphasia group. Although she chose not to attend this group because she was embarrassed by her disfluencies, she did agree to individual sessions.

17.6.2 Assessment

Assessments were carried out over two sessions, 1.5 months apart, to allow monitoring of her disfluencies over a longer period of time before starting intervention. The assessment sessions aimed to collect information on (1) speech fluency during different speech tasks; (2) co-occurring speech, language, and cognitive problems; (3) impact of the communication problems; and (4) possible treatment techniques.

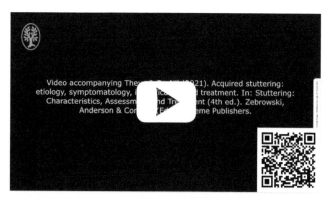

Video 17.1 This video provides supporting information for the case study in the chapter. The selected video clip shows B. while having a spontaneous conversation with a reporter for a TV interview. This interview was recorded 1 month before B.'s first stroke and provides evidence of her fluent speech prestroke.

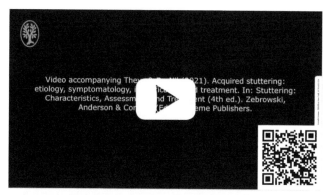

Video 17.2 This video provides supporting information for the case study in the chapter. The selected video clip shows B. while having a spontaneous conversation with the speech-language pathologist during the first assessment session. It shows the occurrence of stuttering disfluencies poststroke.

For the fluency assessment, speech samples were collected during conversation and monologue. During conversation, stuttering disfluencies occurred on 42% of syllables (▶ Video 17.2). The participant's concomitant behaviors consisted of facial movements (e.g., jaw clenching) and movements of the extremities (e.g., fist clenching and arm moving). These nonspeech behaviors were mild and not distracting. Stuttering severity, as measured with the SSI-4[86] was moderate. B. displayed negative emotions and attitudes in reaction to her speech. When talking about how she felt, she said, "I told them to just forget about me."

Assessment for co-occurring disorders started with the CAT.[62] The CAT results showed difficulties in all modalities of language and cognition. To assess the impact of her communication difficulties on daily life, the Disability and Impact subtests from the CAT were attempted, as was the CPIB,[71] but the answers were considered unreliable due to the comprehension difficulties.

Next, different treatment techniques were trialed. B.'s fluency improved dramatically during singing, unison speech, and sentence repetition. During spontaneous conversation, her speech was very fast paced and rushed. She could not slow down her speech rate on request. When asked to tap along while speaking to slow down her speech rate, she became distracted by her finger movements. However, when visual support for the tapping was provided in the form of a makeshift pacing board, she was able to slow down her speech rate and speak in a rhythm, which led to a marked improvement in her fluency.

17.6.3 Treatment

Treatment sessions took place once a week for 1 hour. The treatment was split into two blocks, with a 6-month intermission. The first treatment block consisted of 9 sessions and the second block of 10 sessions. B.'s speech, language, and cognitive problems required an approach that would not rely on comprehension of complex instructions, and considerable monitoring of speech production. Thus, most treatment techniques developed for adults with developmental stuttering could not be used with this client. Based on observation, it was decided to use a paced speech approach, with visual and tactile feedback from a six-square pacing board (▶ Fig. 17.4), complemented with low-level cognitive restructuring.

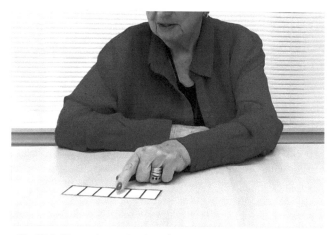

Fig. 17.4 Client using pacing board.

The first treatment block focused on learning to use the pacing board and regain confidence when speaking to other people. Each session started with spontaneous conversation without the pacing board to establish a baseline fluency measure. Then the pacing board was introduced. The client was encouraged to tap on a square on the pacing board with her finger, for each syllable that she produced. During the training phase, the use of the pacing board was modeled by the speech therapist. Then B. was encouraged to repeat what the speech-language pathologist was saying, using unison speech with the clinician while tapping along. The same sentence was repeated a couple of times, and the therapist gradually provided less guidance. First, the therapist stopped tapping along on the pacing board, then fully stopped tapping along, and finally stopped the unison speech.

Once the pacing led to consistent fluency during sentence repetition, this technique was applied during spontaneous conversation. B. regularly needed reminders and modeling to continue using the pacing technique. During this activity, her fluency markedly improved (▶ Fig. 17.5 and ▶ Video 17.3). Next, the names of family members were gradually introduced into the conversation and practiced. This step was added as B.'s fluency during conversation was often interrupted by word-finding pauses when trying to say family member's names.

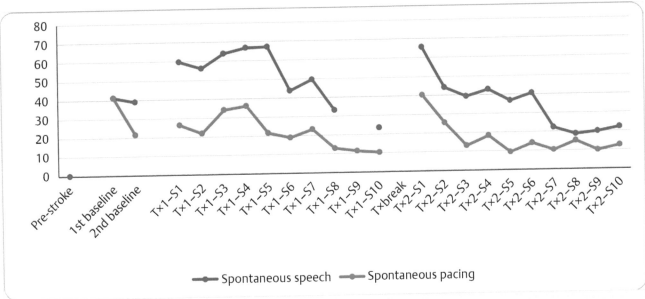

Fig. 17.5 Overview of the number of stuttering disfluencies per 100 syllables during spontaneous conversation and paced speech across sessions.

During the sessions, strategies to increase B.'s confidence and decrease her anxiety when talking to others were discussed. B. reported always feeling rushed and under pressure to speak quickly. She indicated that she would feel more comfortable if people knew that she needed more time. Therefore, the following text was printed on the back of the pacing board: "My name is B. I had a stroke. Please give me time to talk. Thank you for your patience." B. was taught to show this to new conversation partners before starting a conversation, and she was reminded that it was okay to take her time whenever she started to rush her speech. Later in the treatment sessions, B's frustration about getting stuck was addressed and strategies—relaxation through deep breathing, self-imposed time-out, and easy onset—to address this were implemented using modeling.

At the end of the first treatment block, B. had made significant gains in fluency. This was reflected in a reduction in disfluencies from 41 to 24% SS during spontaneous (non-paced) conversation, a decline in stuttering severity from moderate to mild on the SSI-4, and a decrease in secondary behaviors. In addition, she had markedly more confidence when speaking. Treatment was then paused for 6 months due to significant events occurring in B.'s life. When treatment restarted, she reported not to have worked on her speech during the break. Her disfluencies during spontaneous conversation had returned to pretreatment levels (66% SS, moderate severity). B. also reported to be socially isolated and did not want to participate in any activities organized at the retirement village. Using a shared goal-setting approach, the end goal of the second treatment block was increased participation in activities in her community.

After quickly regaining the ability to use paced speech, B.'s treatment sessions focused on skill transfer and generalization. To encourage this, a family member and a close friend underwent conversation partner training during the last five sessions, and B. practiced using her techniques with them. The conversation partner training consisted of instructed demonstration of pacing and self-monitoring strategies so conversation partners could remind B. to use these strategies. During transfer sessions, B.'s speech improved from baseline (22% SS, mild

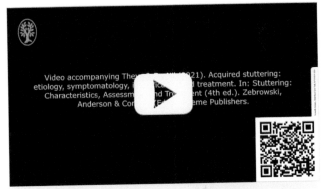

Video 17.3 This video provides supporting information for the case study in the chapter. The selected video clip shows B. while using the paced speech approach toward the end of the first treatment block. It shows the increase in fluency while using this technique.

severity; ▶ Fig. 17.5), but did not reach the same fluency levels as during the conversations with the speech therapist alone. More importantly, increasing B.'s awareness about the importance of participating in community activities, and working on her confidence levels when speaking, led to a steady increase in activity participation. Over the course of the second treatment block, B. started to attend gatherings and outings organized in her retirement village as well as weekly gym classes. As the treatment sessions progressed, B. said she was more confident and willing to engage with others.

17.7 Concluding Remarks

This chapter provides a review of the various forms of acquired stuttering that may be seen in clinical practice, especially by clinicians working in a hospital or rehabilitation environment. Acquired neurogenic stuttering is a speech fluency disorder that affects individuals who most often, but not exclusively, have experienced a stroke, TBI, or neurodegenerative disease.

In addition, acquired stuttering can be functional in nature as well as factitious or malingered. Although acquired stuttering is seen mainly in adults, it can also occur in younger individuals.

We have described principles of assessment and options for intervention. Regardless of the nature of the acquired stuttering, assessment and intervention approaches will need to be highly individualized based on the characteristics of the fluency problem, as well as any other communication or health conditions. As clinicians become more aware of the potential presence of acquired stuttering in the clients they serve, and the impact this may have on their clients' personal and professional life, they will be more likely to recognize and diagnose the disorder, and researchers will be able to provide a more accurate picture of its incidence and prevalence. This, in turn, should lead to a more thorough understanding of the nature of the disorder and ultimately to investigations of effective intervention approaches that not only target speech disfluencies but also focus on communicative competence, participation, and quality of life.

Acknowledgments

The preparation of this chapter was supported in part by a grant from the Natural Sciences and Engineering Research Council of Canada (awarded to LDN) and the Royal Society of New Zealand Marsden Fund (awarded to CT).

References

[1] Chang SE, Garnett EO, Etchell A, Chow HM. Functional and neuroanatomical bases of developmental stuttering: current insights. Neuroscientist. 2019; 25 (6):566–582

[2] Stone J, Carson A, Hallett M. Explanation as treatment for functional neurologic disorders. Handb Clin Neurol. 2016; 139:543–553

[3] Bass C, Wade DT. Malingering and factitious disorder. Pract Neurol. 2019; 19 (2):96–105

[4] Seery CH. Differential diagnosis of stuttering for forensic purposes. Am J Speech Lang Pathol. 2005; 14(4):284–297

[5] Theys C, van Wieringen A, De Nil LF. A clinician survey of speech and non-speech characteristics of neurogenic stuttering. J Fluency Disord. 2008; 33 (1):1–23

[6] De Nil LF, Theys C, Jokel R. Stroke-related acquired neurogenic stuttering. In: Coppens PP, J., ed. Aphasia Rehabilitation: Clinical Challenges. Burlington, MA: Jones & Bartlett Learning; 2018

[7] Lundgren K, Helm-Estabrooks N, Klein R. Stuttering following acquired brain damage: a review of the literature. J Neurolinguist. 2010; 23(5):447–454

[8] Koller WC. Dysfluency (stuttering) in extrapyramidal disease. Arch Neurol. 1983; 40(3):175–177

[9] Hertrich I, Ackermann H. Acoustic analysis of speech prosody in Huntington's and Parkinson's disease: a preliminary report. Clin Linguist Phon. 1993; 7(4): 285–297

[10] Lebrun Y, Leleux C, Retif J. Neurogenic stuttering. Acta Neurochir (Wien). 1987; 85(3–4):103–109

[11] Lebrun Y, Rétif J, Kaiser G. Acquired stuttering as a forerunner of motor-neuron disease. J Fluency Disord. 1983; 8(2):161–167

[12] Decker BM, Guitar B, Solomon A. Corpus callosum demyelination associated with acquired stuttering. BMJ Case Rep. 2018; 2018:bcr-2017-223486

[13] Dinoto A, Busan P, Formaggio E, et al. Stuttering-like hesitation in speech during acute/post-acute phase of immune-mediated encephalitis. J Fluency Disord. 2018; 58:70–76

[14] Sudo D, Doutake Y, Yokota H, Watanabe E. Recovery of brain abscess-induced stuttering after neurosurgical intervention. BMJ Case Rep. 2018; 2018:bcr-2017-223259

[15] Kaplan PW, Stagg R. Frontal lobe nonconvulsive status epilepticus: a case of epileptic stuttering, aphemia, and aphasia: not a sign of psychogenic nonepileptic seizures. Epilepsy Behav. 2011; 21(2):191–195

[16] Picillo M, Vincos GB, Sammartino F, Lozano AM, Fasano A. Exploring risk factors for stuttering development in Parkinson disease after deep brain stimulation. Parkinsonism Relat Disord. 2017; 38:85–89

[17] Burghaus L, Hilker R, Thiel A, et al. Deep brain stimulation of the subthalamic nucleus reversibly deteriorates stuttering in advanced Parkinson's disease. J Neural Transm (Vienna). 2006; 113(5):625–631

[18] Thiriez C, Roubeau B, Ouerchefani N, Gurruchaga J-M, Palfi S, Fénelon G. Improvement in developmental stuttering following deep brain stimulation for Parkinson's disease. Parkinsonism Relat Disord. 2013; 19(3):383–384

[19] Brady JP. Drug-induced stuttering: a review of the literature. J Clin Psychopharmacol. 1998; 18(1):50–54

[20] Van Borsel J. Acquired stuttering: a note on terminology. J Neurolinguist. 2014; 27(1):41–49

[21] Theys C, van Wieringen A, Sunaert S, Thijs V, De Nil LF. A one year prospective study of neurogenic stuttering following stroke: incidence and co-occurring disorders. J Commun Disord. 2011; 44(6):678–687

[22] Rachamallu V, Haq A, Song MM, Aligeti M. Clozapine-induced microseizures, orofacial dyskinesia, and speech dysfluency in an adolescent with treatment resistant early onset schizophrenia on concurrent lithium therapy. Case Rep Psychiatry. 2017; 2017:7359095

[23] Helm-Estabrooks N. Stuttering associated with acquired neurological disorders. In: Curlee RF, ed. Stuttering and Related Disorders of Fluency. 2nd ed. New York, NY: Thieme Medical Publishers; 1999:255–268

[24] Quinn PT, Andrews G. Neurological stuttering-a clinical entity? J Neurol Neurosurg Psychiatry. 1977; 40(7):699–700

[25] Wong PP, Dornan J, Schentag CT, Ip R, Keating M. Statistical profile of traumatic brain injury: a Canadian rehabilitation population. Brain Inj. 1993; 7(4):283–294

[26] Ludlow CL, Rosenberg J, Salazar A, Grafman J, Smutok M. Site of penetrating brain lesions causing chronic acquired stuttering. Ann Neurol. 1987; 22(1): 60–66

[27] Jokel R, De Nil L, Sharpe K. Speech disfluencies in adults with neurogenic stuttering associated with stroke and traumatic brain injury. J Med Speech-Lang Pathol. 2007; 15(3):243–262

[28] Tani T, Sakai Y. Analysis of five cases with neurogenic stuttering following brain injury in the basal ganglia. J Fluency Disord. 2011; 36(1):1–16

[29] Van Borsel J, Van Coster R, Van Lierde K. Repetitions in final position in a nine-year-old boy with focal brain damage. J Fluency Disord. 1996; 21(2):137–146

[30] Aram DM, Meyers SC, Ekelman BL. Fluency of conversational speech in children with unilateral brain lesions. Brain Lang. 1990; 38(1):105–121

[31] Saeedi MJ, Esfandiary E, Almasi Dooghaee M. Childhood neurogenic stuttering due to bilateral congenital abnormality in globus pallidus: A case report and review of the literature. Iran J Child Neurol. 2016; 10(4):75–79

[32] Chang S-E, Synnestvedt A, Ostuni J, Ludlow CL. Similarities in speech and white matter characteristics in idiopathic developmental stuttering and adult-onset stuttering. J Neurolinguist. 2010; 23(5):455–469

[33] Van Borsel J, van der Made S, Santens P. Thalamic stuttering: a distinct clinical entity? Brain Lang. 2003; 85(2):185–189

[34] Theys C, De Nil L, Thijs V, van Wieringen A, Sunaert S. A crucial role for the cortico-striato-cortical loop in the pathogenesis of stroke-related neurogenic stuttering. Hum Brain Mapp. 2013; 34(9):2103–2112

[35] Kalia LV, Lang AE. Parkinson's disease. Lancet. 2015; 386(9996):896–912

[36] Hartelius L. Incidence of developmental speech dysfluencies in individuals with Parkinson's disease. Folia Phoniatr Logop. 2014; 66(3):132–137

[37] Whitfield JA, Delong C, Goberman AM, Blomgren M. Fluency adaptation in speakers with Parkinson disease: a motor learning perspective. Int J Speech Lang Pathol. 2018; 20(7):699–707

[38] Levenson J, Sharpe M. The classification of conversion disorder (functional neurologic symptom disorder) in ICD and DSM. Handb Clin Neurol. 2016; 139:189–192

[39] Baumgartner J, Duffy JR. Psychogenic stuttering in adults with and without neurologic disease. J Med Speech-Lang Pathol. 1997; 5:75–96

[40] Espay AJ, Aybek S, Carson A, et al. Current concepts in diagnosis and treatment of functional neurological disorders. JAMA Neurol. 2018; 75(9): 1132–1141

[41] American Psychiatric Association. Diagnostic and Statistical Manual of Mental Disorders (DSM-5). Washington, DC: American Psychiatric Association Publishing; 2013

[42] Edwards MJ, Stone J, Lang AE. From psychogenic movement disorder to functional movement disorder: it's time to change the name. Mov Disord. 2014; 29(7):849–852

[43] Roth CR, Aronson AE, Davis LJ, Jr. Clinical studies in psychogenic stuttering of adult onset. J Speech Hear Disord. 1989; 54(4):634–646

[44] Carson A, Hallett M, Stone J. Assessment of patients with functional neurologic disorders. Handb Clin Neurol. 2016; 139:169–188

[45] Baizabal-Carvallo JF, Jankovic J. Speech and voice disorders in patients with psychogenic movement disorders. J Neurol. 2015; 262(11):2420–2424

[46] Van Borsel J, Taillieu C. Neurogenic stuttering versus developmental stuttering: an observer judgement study. J Commun Disord. 2001; 34(5):385–395

[47] Penttilä N, Korpijaakko-Huuhka A-M, Kent RD. Disfluency clusters in speakers with and without neurogenic stuttering following traumatic brain injury. J Fluency Disord. 2019; 59:33–51

[48] Canter GJ. Observations on neurogenic stuttering: a contribution to differential diagnosis. Br J Disord Commun. 1971; 6(2):139–143

[49] Max L, Kadri M, Mitsuya T, Balasubramanian V. Similar within-utterance loci of dysfluency in acquired neurogenic and persistent developmental stuttering. Brain Lang. 2019; 189:1–9

[50] Nowack WJ, Stone RE. Acquired stuttering and bilateral cerebral disease. J Fluency Disord. 1987; 12(2):141–146

[51] Juste FS, Sassi FC, Costa JB, de Andrade CRF. Frequency of speech disruptions in Parkinson's disease and developmental stuttering: a comparison among speech tasks. PLoS One. 2018; 13(6):e0199054

[52] Krishnan G, Tiwari S. Differential diagnosis in developmental and acquired neurogenic stuttering: do fluency-enhancing conditions dissociate the two? J Neurolinguist. 2013; 26(2):252–257

[53] Theys C, Van Wieringen A, Tuyls L, De Nil L. Acquired stuttering in a 16-year-old boy. J Neurolinguist. 2009; 22(5):427–435

[54] Attanasio JS. A case of late-onset or acquired stuttering in adult life. J Fluency Disord. 1987; 12(4):287–290

[55] Chung DS, Wettroth C, Hallett M, Maurer CW. Functional speech and voice disorders: case series and literature review. Mov Disord Clin Pract (Hoboken). 2018; 5(3):312–316

[56] Mahr G, Leith W. Psychogenic stuttering of adult onset. J Speech Hear Res. 1992; 35(2):283–286

[57] Mattingly EO. Dysfluency in a service member with comorbid diagnoses: a case study. Mil Med. 2015; 180(1):e157–e159

[58] Ward D. Sudden onset stuttering in an adult: neurogenic and psychogenic perspectives. J Neurolinguist. 2010; 23(5):511–517

[59] Folstein MF, Folstein SE, Messer MA, White T. Mini-Mental State Examination: MMSE-2. Lutz, FL: Psychological Assessment Resources; 2010

[60] Nasreddine ZS, Phillips NA, Bédirian V, et al. The Montreal Cognitive Assessment, MoCA: a brief screening tool for mild cognitive impairment. J Am Geriatr Soc. 2005; 53(4):695–699

[61] Goodglass H, Kaplan E, Barresi B. BDAE-3: Boston Diagnostic Aphasia Examination, Third edition. Philadelphia, PA: Lippincott Williams & Wilkins; 2001

[62] Swinburn K, Porter G, Howard D. Comprehensive Aphasia Test. New York, NY: Psychology Press; 2004

[63] Kaplan E, Goodglass H, Weintraub S. Boston Naming Test. Austin, TX: Pro-Ed; 2001

[64] Enderby PM, Palmer R. Frenchay Dysarthria Assessment: Examiner's manual. Austin, TX: Pro-ed; 2008

[65] Dabul B. ABA-2: Apraxia Battery for Adults. Austin, TX: Pro-Ed; 2000

[66] Lowit A, Kent RD. Management of dysarthria. In: Papathanasiou I, Coppens P, eds. Aphasia and Related Neurogenic Communication Disorders. Vol. 2. Burlington, MA: Jones and Bartlett; 2016:527–56

[67] Miller N, Wambaugh J. Acquired apraxia of speech. In: Papathanasiou I, Coppens P, eds. Aphasia and Related Neurogenic Communication Disorders. Vol. 2. Burlington, MA: Jones and Bartlett; 2016:431–57

[68] Yaruss JS, Quesal RW. Overall Assessment of the Speaker's Experience of Stuttering (OASES): documenting multiple outcomes in stuttering treatment. J Fluency Disord. 2006; 31(2):90–115

[69] Andrews G, Cutler J. Stuttering therapy: the relation between changes in symptom level and attitudes. J Speech Hear Disord. 1974; 39(3):312–319

[70] Vanryckeghem M, Brutten GJ. Behaviour Assessment Battery for Adults Who Stutter. San Diego, CA: Plural Publishing Inc.; 2018

[71] Baylor C, Yorkston K, Eadie T, Kim J, Chung H, Amtmann D. The Communicative Participation Item Bank (CPIB): item bank calibration and development of a disorder-generic short form. J Speech Lang Hear Res. 2013; 56(4):1190–1208

[72] Roth CR, Cornis-Pop M, Beach WA. Examination of validity in spoken language evaluations: adult onset stuttering following mild traumatic brain injury. NeuroRehabilitation. 2015; 36(4):415–426

[73] Duffy JR. Motor Speech Disorders. Substrates, Differential Diagnosis, and Management. 4th ed. Amsterdam: Elsevier; 2020

[74] Schnellbacher S, O'Mara H. Identifying and Managing Malingering and Factitious Disorder in the Military. Curr Psychiatry Rep. 2016; 18(11):105

[75] Norman RS, Jaramillo CA, Eapen BC, Amuan ME, Pugh MJ. Acquired stuttering in veterans of the wars in Iraq and Afghanistan: the role of traumatic brain injury, post-traumatic stress disorder, and medications. Mil Med. 2018; 183(11–12):e526–e534

[76] Market KE, Montague JC, Jr, Buffalo M, Drummond SS. Acquired stuttering: Descriptive data and treatment outcome. J Fluency Disord. 1990; 15(1):21–33

[77] Stewart T, Rowley D. Acquired stammering in Great Britain. Eur J Disord Commun. 1996; 31(1):1–9

[78] Marshall RC, Neuburger SI. Effects of delayed auditory feedback on acquired stuttering following head injury. J Fluency Disord. 1987; 12(5):355–365

[79] Balasubramanian V, Cronin KL, Max L. Dysfluency levels during repeated readings, choral readings, and readings with altered auditory feedback in two cases of acquired neurogenic stuttering. J Neurolinguist. 2010; 23(5):488–500

[80] McClean MD, McLean A, Jr. Case report of stuttering acquired in association with phenytoin use for post-head-injury seizures. J Fluency Disord. 1985; 10(4):241–255

[81] Tykalová T, Rusz J, Čmejla R, et al. Effect of dopaminergic medication on speech dysfluency in Parkinson's disease: a longitudinal study. J Neural Transm (Vienna). 2015; 122(8):1135–1142

[82] Ahlberg E, Laakso K, Hartelius L. Perceived changes in communication as an effect of STN surgery in Parkinson's disease: a qualitative interview study. Parkinsons Dis. 2011; 2011:540158

[83] Hopp JL, LaFrance WC, Jr. Cognitive behavioral therapy for psychogenic neurological disorders. Neurologist. 2012; 18(6):364–372

[84] Eastwood S, Bisson JI. Management of factitious disorders: a systematic review. Psychother Psychosom. 2008; 77(4):209–218

[85] Bass C, Halligan P. Factitious disorders and malingering: challenges for clinical assessment and management. Lancet. 2014; 383(9926):1422–1432

[86] Riley GD. SSI-4: Stuttering Severity Instrument. 4th ed. Austin, TX: Pro-Ed; 2009

[87] Friederici AD, Gierhan SM. The language network. Curr Opin Neurobiol. 2013; 23(2):250–254

Further Readings

Acquired Stuttering

Duffy JR. Motor Speech Disorders. Substrates, Differential Diagnosis, and Management. 4th ed. Edinburgh: Elsevier; 2020

Norman RS, Jaramillo CA, Eapen BC, Amuan ME, Pugh MJ. Acquired stuttering in veterans of the wars in Iraq and Afghanistan: the role of TBI, post-traumatic stress disorder, and medications. Mil Med. 2018; 183(11–12): 526–e534

Van Borsel J. Acquired stuttering: a note on terminology. J Neurolinguist. 2014; 27(1):41–49

Ward D. Sudden onset stuttering in an adult: neurogenic and psychogenic perspectives. J Neurolinguist. 2010; 23(5):511–517

Acquired Neurogenic Stuttering

Brady JP. Drug-induced stuttering: a review of the literature. J Clin Psychopharmacol. 1998; 18(1):50–54

Canter GJ. Observations on neurogenic stuttering: a contribution to differential diagnosis. Br J Disord Commun. 1971; 6(2):139–143

De Nil LF, Rochon E, Jokel R. Adult-onset neurogenic stuttering. In: McNeil MR, ed. Clinical Management of Sensorimotor Speech Disorders. New York, NY: Thieme; 2008

De Nil LF, Theys C, Jokel R. Stroke-related acquired neurogenic stuttering. In: Coppens P, Patterson J, eds. Aphasia Rehabilitation: Clinical Challenges. Burlington, MA: Jones & Bartlett Learning; 2018

Helm-Estabrooks N. Stuttering associated with acquired neurological disorders. In: Curlee RF, ed. Stuttering and Related Disorders of Fluency. 2nd ed. New York, NY: Thieme Medical Publishers; 1999

Juste FS, Sassi FC, Costa JB, de Andrade CRF. Frequency of speech disruptions in Parkinson's disease and developmental stuttering: a comparison among speech tasks. PLoS One. 2018; 13(6):e0199054

Lundgren K, Helm-Estabrooks N, Klein R. Stuttering following acquired brain damage: a review of the literature. J Neurolinguist. 2010; 23(5):447–454

Ludlow CL, Rosenberg J, Salazar A, Grafman J, Smutok M. Site of penetrating brain lesions causing chronic acquired stuttering. Ann Neurol. 1987; 22(1):60–66

Theys C, De Nil L, Thijs V, van Wieringen A, Sunaert S. A crucial role for the cortico-striato-cortical loop in the pathogenesis of stroke-related neurogenic stuttering. Hum Brain Mapp. 2013; 34(9):2103–2112

Theys C, van Wieringen A, Sunaert S, Thijs V, De Nil LF. A one year prospective study of neurogenic stuttering following stroke: incidence and co-occurring disorders. J Commun Disord. 2011; 44(6):678–687

Van Borsel J, Taillieu C. Neurogenic stuttering versus developmental stuttering: an observer judgement study. J Commun Disord. 2001; 34(5):385–395

Whitfield JA, Delong C, Goberman AM, Blomgren M. Fluency adaptation in speakers with Parkinson disease: a motor learning perspective. Int J Speech Lang Pathol. 2018; 20(7):699–707

Acquired Functional Stuttering

Baumgartner J, Duffy JR. Psychogenic stuttering in adults with and without neurologic disease. J Med Speech-Lang Pathol. 1997; 5(2):75–95

Chang S-E, Synnestvedt A, Ostuni J, Ludlow CL. Similarities in speech and white matter characteristics in idiopathic developmental stuttering and adult-onset stuttering. J Neurolinguist. 2010; 23(5):455–469

Duffy J. Functional speech disorders: clinical manifestations, diagnosis, and management. In: Hallett M, Stone J, Carson A, eds. Handbook of Clinical Neurology. Amsterdam: Elsevier; 2016

Edwards MJ, Stone J, Lang AE. From psychogenic movement disorder to functional movement disorder: it's time to change the name. Mov Disord. 2014; 29(7):849–852

Jokel R, Wolf U. When a duck is not a duck: non-organic bases for aphasia and dementia. Aphasiology. 2017; 31(1):100–121

Mahr G, Leith W. Psychogenic stuttering of adult onset. J Speech Hear Res. 1992; 35 (2):283–286

Factitious Stuttering/Malingering

Bolat N, Yalçin Ö. Factitious disorder presenting with stuttering in two adolescents: the importance of psychoeducation. Noro Psikiyatri Arsivi. 2017; 54(1):87–89

Seery CH. Differential diagnosis of stuttering for forensic purposes. Am J Speech Lang Pathol. 2005; 14(4):284–297

Index

Note: Page numbers set **bold** or *italic* indicate headings or figures, respectively.